# INFECTIOUS AGENTS AND HOST REACTIONS

*Edited by*

## STUART MUDD, M. A., M. D.

Professor Emeritus of Microbiology,
The University of Pennsylvania School of Medicine;
Past President, The International Association of
Microbiological Societies; Chief, Microbiologic Research
Program, Veterans Administration Hospital, Philadelphia

1970   W. B. SAUNDERS COMPANY

*Philadelphia · London · Toronto*

W. B. Saunders Company:   West Washington Square
Philadelphia, Pa. 19105

12 Dyott Street
London W.C.1

1835 Yonge Street
Toronto 7, Ontario

Infectious Agents and Host Reactions

THE UNIVERSITY OF LIVER⌐

# Contributors

SIR CHRISTOPHER HOWARD ANDREWES, M.D. (London and Lund), LL.D. (Aberdeen), F.R.C.P. (Lond.), F.R.S.
> Formerly Deputy Director, National Institute for Medical Research, Mill Hill, London. Honorary Consultant to Common Cold Research Unit, Salisbury, England

ABRAM S. BENENSON, M.D.
> Professor of Preventive Medicine (Epidemiology) and Professor of Microbiology, Jefferson Medical College, Philadelphia, Pennsylvania. Formerly Director, Pakistan-SEATO Cholera Research Laboratory, Dacca, East Pakistan

ROBERT VINCENT BLANDEN, M.D.S.
> Visiting Investigator, Trudeau Institute, Inc., Saranac Lake, New York

SIR F. MACFARLANE BURNET, M.D., Ph.D.
> Emeritus Professor of Experimental Medicine, University of Melbourne, Melbourne, Australia

GILBERT DALLDORF, M.D.
> Formerly Director, Division of Laboratories and Research, New York State Department of Health. Member Emeritus, Sloan-Kettering Institute, New York, New York

ALLAN W. DOWNIE, M.D., D.Sc., F.R.S.
> Visiting Professor, Pediatric Department, Medical Center, University of Colorado, Denver, Colorado

WILBUR G. DOWNS, M.D.
> Associate Director, Rockefeller Foundation. Professor of Epidemiology, Yale University School of Medicine; Director, Yale Arbovirus Research Unit, New Haven, Connecticut

MONROE D. EATON, M.D.
> Professor of Bacteriology and Immunology, Harvard Medical School, Boston, Massachusetts

BERNICE E. EDDY, Ph.D.
> Chief, Section on Experimental Virology, Division of Biologics Standards, National Institutes of Health, Bethesda, Maryland

JOANNE FINSTAD, M.S.
  Research Fellow, United States Public Health Service, University of Minnesota, Minneapolis, Minnesota

RICHARD A. GATTI, M.D.
  Special Fellow, United States Public Health Service, University of Minnesota, Minneapolis, Minnesota

HAROLD S. GINSBERG, M.D.
  Professor of Microbiology and Chairman, Department of Microbiology, School of Medicine, University of Pennsylvania, Philadelphia, Pennsylvania

ROBERT A. GOOD, M.D., Ph.D.
  American Legion Memorial Heart Research Professor of Pediatrics and Microbiology, University of Minnesota, Minneapolis, Minnesota

MAURICE HILLEMAN, Ph.D., D.Sc.
  Division of Virus and Cell Biology Research, Merck Institute for Therapeutic Research, West Point, Pennsylvania

GEORGE A. HOTTLE, Ph.D.
  Lecturer in Public Health, School of Public Health, University of California, Berkeley. Assistant Director, Naval Biological Laboratory

ANN G. KUTTNER, M.D. †
  Associate Professor of Pediatrics, Emeritus, New York University Medical Center, New York, New York

REBECCA C. LANCEFIELD, Ph.D.
  Professor Emeritus, Microbiology, The Rockefeller University, New York, New York

GEORGE B. MACKANESS, M.B., D.Phil.
  Director, Trudeau Institute, Inc., Saranac Lake, New York

COLIN M. MACLEOD, M.D.
  Vice President for Medical Affairs, The Commonwealth Fund, New York, New York

NORMAN B. McCULLOUGH, Ph.D., M.D.
  Professor of Microbiology and Public Health and Professor of Medicine, Michigan State University, East Lansing, Michigan

GARDNER MIDDLEBROOK, M.D.
  Professor of International Medicine, University of Maryland School of Medicine, Baltimore, Maryland

COUNCILMAN MORGAN, M.D.
  Department of Microbiology, Columbia University College of Physicians and Surgeons, New York, New York

STUART MUDD, M.A., M.D.
  Professor Emeritus of Microbiology, School of Medicine, University of Pennsylvania. Chief, Microbiologic Research Program, Veterans Administration Hospital, Philadelphia, Pennsylvania

† Deceased

ARYEH LEO OLITZKI, M.D.
>    Professor Emeritus, Hebrew University-Hadassah Medical School, Jerusalem, Israel

JOHN R. PAUL, M.D. Sc.D.
>    Professor (Emeritus) of Preventive Medicine and Epidemiology, Yale University School of Medicine; Associate Physician, Yale-New Haven Medical Center, New Haven, Connecticut

MARGARET PITTMAN, Ph.D.
>    Research Microbiologist (Medical), Chief of Laboratory of Bacterial Products, Division of Biologics Standards, National Institutes of Health, Bethesda, Maryland

JOSEPH STOKES, Jr., M.D., D.Sc.
>    Emeritus Professor of Pediatrics, School of Medicine, University of Pennsylvania, Henry Phipps Institute, Philadelphia, Pennsylvania

THOMAS B. TURNER, M.D., Sc.D. (Hon.)
>    Professor of Microbiology, The Johns Hopkins University School of Medicine; Physician, Outpatient Department, The Johns Hopkins Hospital, Baltimore, Maryland

NEYLAN ANTHONY VEDROS, Ph.D.
>    Associate Professor of Medical Microbiology and Immunology, School of Public Health, University of California, Berkeley. Director, Naval Biological Laboratory

W. BARRY WOOD, Jr., M.D.
>    Professor of Microbiology, The Johns Hopkins University School of Medicine, Baltimore, Maryland

# Preface

Investigation of infectious agents and host reactions during the past half century has undergone a rapid evolution, with emergence and growth of numerous and flourishing subspecies of research interest and teaching emphasis. Some observers of the changing scene have expressed concern lest intense preoccupation with specialized aspects, however essential for advancing frontiers through research, should limit the knowledge and insight of our young scientists and medical practitioners into diseases as holistic phenomena. It is with such a concern that the Editor of this volume has appealed to colleagues whose professional lifework has been investigation of infectious diseases in depth. The response of these colleagues has been magnificent, as a close study of the chapters of this volume will make clear.

My hope for this book is that it may help to bring into focus the ecology of parasitic disease in its great breadth and depth: that one may imagine with Sir Macfarlane Burnet and Robert Good the origin of adaptive immunity in the surveillance of inimical somatic mutations; that one may perceive as an integrated whole the mechanisms of immunity through activated cells of the lymphocytic system and through circulating antibodies, mechanisms subtle and complex, yet exquisitely coordinated in the total defense of the macroorganism; that one may follow the diverse adaptations of microparasites toward coexistence in the ecosystem of the host, from those of free-living bacteria to those of the viruses which can subvert and exploit the synthetic machinery of host cells.

This hope must be tempered with realism, however. For it would, indeed, be naïve to suppose that one book could deal adequately with all aspects of parasite-host interaction. The present volume, for instance, gives inadequate attention to genetic factors of either parasite or host in relation to resistance to disease.

Another significant modulating influence on resistance to which little attention has been directed in the present volume is the homeostatic influence of the endocrine system on the reticuloendothelial apparatus, which is of such critical importance in resistance. A long series of studies of modulation of reticuloendothelial function by endocrine action has been published by Professor T. Nicol and his collaborators at the University of London (Nicol, T., et al., J. Endocr. 1964, *30*:277–291; 1965, *33*:365–383; 1966, *34*:163–178, 377–386).

Nicol, Vernon-Roberts, and Quantock have written (Nicol, T., B. Vernon-Roberts, and D. C. Quantock. 1966. Effect of orchidectomy and ovariectomy on survival against lethal infections in mice. Nature *211*:1091–1092): "The present results provide additional evidence in support of our earlier postulate that oestrogen is the principal natural stimulant of bodily defence in both the male and female, and further that oestrogen treatment would seem to be of clinical value in the treatment of acute bacterial infections." Broad though present horizons are in relation to the ecology of disease, obviously the horizons open to future exploration are far broader.

Editing this volume has, indeed, been a learning experience. Certainly the most striking lesson to me has been to appreciate that resistance to infectious disease is a far more inclusive complex of interrelated factors than ordinarily realized. Explicitly I, and obviously many others of my generation of teachers and investigators, have tended to think of resistance as *essentially* a function either of circulating antibodies or of activated reticuloendothelial cells. Examples of the former are pneumococcal pneumonia, in which the "crisis" occurred, at least in preantibiotic days, when measurable anticapsular antibodies appeared in the circulation, or measles, in which the clinical disease can be ameliorated or aborted by injection of gamma globulin. The prime example of essentially cellular immunity has been tuberculosis (although less orthodox views about tuberculosis are expressed in Chapter 10 by Dr. Gardner Middlebrook). A modern integration of mechanisms of host resistance is of course presented in the opening chapters of this volume.

Consideration of the chapter by two eminent investigators of streptococcal infection, Drs. Ann G. Kuttner and Rebecca C. Lancefield, is illuminating. In their chapter, "Unsolved Problems of the Nonsuppurative Complications of Group A Streptococcal Infections," two clinical diseases are dealt with: rheumatic fever and acute glomerulonephritis. With respect to the pathogenesis of acute glomerulonephritis the following pertinent facts are brought out.

Outbreaks of acute glomerulonephritis in many parts of the world have been found to be due to specific nephritogenic serotypes of Group A streptococci. These nephritogenic strains fall into five serotypes of the known 55 serotypes of Group A streptococci. Antibodies of the specific nephritogenic type have been found "bound to electron-dense deposits in the glomerular tissue of nephritic patients, but no binding was noted in the glomerular tissues obtained from normal individuals or from patients with other types of renal disease." The reaction with the glomerular basement membrane "is accompanied by marked decrease in serum complement and an accumulation of polymorphonuclear leukocytes which conjointly may be responsible for the disease and is considered to be the cause of the renal lesion." The attack of acute glomerulonephritis is preceded from 7 to 21 days by infection of pharynx or skin by a nephritogenic strain of Group A streptococcus, but, in contrast to rheumatic fever, prior sensitization of the patient is not required. There is complete recovery.

These facts, in the minds of the authors (and the Editor), clearly lead to the conclusion that acute glomerulonephritis is caused by reactions of an antigen on the glomerular basement membrane with specific antibody, followed by accumulation of complement and polymorphonuclear leukocytes and damage to the membrane.

In contrast to glomerulonephritis, the following pertinent facts are presented with reference to rheumatic fever.

Rheumatic fever may be brought on by successive attacks of pharyngitis by any of the known 55 serotypes of Group A streptococci. Prior sensitization of the individual is essential. Serum complement is normal. Prophylaxis is mandatory to prevent recurrent attacks. Attempts to immunize either human subjects or rabbits with various nonliving products of Group A streptococci have not produced rheumatic fever. However, the authors were unwilling to commit themselves to any explicit hypothesis regarding the pathogenesis of rheumatic fever.

I venture to carry this discussion a step further. Kaplan and associates and Zabriskie, Freimer, and Seegal have demonstrated cross reactive antigens between Group A streptococcal cells and human heart tissue. Chase and Rapaport (Chase, R. M., and F. T. Rapaport. 1965. The bacterial induction of homograft sensitivity. I. Effects of sensitization with Group A streptococci. J. Exper. Med. *122*:721–732) have sensitized guinea pigs to Group A streptococci of various serotypes and shown that such sensitized animals reject skin homografts in a manner which is indistinguishable from that which results from sensitization with homologous tissues. Sensitization with streptococci of Lancefield groups B, C, D, E, G, H, L, and O or pneumococcus types II, III, and XIV was ineffective in inducing such graft rejection (Rapaport, F. T., and R. M. Chase. 1965. The bacterial induction of homograft sensitivity. II. Effects of sensitization with staphylococci and other microorganisms. J. Exper. Med. *122*: 733–744).

Taking all these observations together, I venture to propose the hypothesis that rheumatic fever is mediated by a phenomenon essentially resembling graft rejection. The prior attacks of streptococcus pharyngitis sensitize the subject to one or more antigens of the streptococcus which cross react with heart tissue, and the precipitating streptococcal pharyngitis induces both immune reaction to the streptococcus and a reaction of rejection against heart tissue, which has an antigenic determinant in common with streptococci of Group A (cf. Rapaport, F. T. 1967. Heterologous cross-reactions in mammalian transplantation, and discussion following. *In:* Trentin, J. (Ed.): Cross-Reacting Antigens and Neoantigens. Williams & Wilkins Co., Baltimore).

Viewed in this way, the nonsuppurative complications of streptococcal infection would seem to fall essentially into two categories: (1) classic antigen-antibody-complement reactions in acute glomerulonephritis, and (2) reactions of rejection essentially cell-mediated (see Chapter 2) in rheumatic fever.

Circulating antibodies are enormously useful in the diagnosis of infection by viruses. Moreover the efficacy of immunization procedures against viruses is often evaluated in terms of antibody titers (Chapter 5). However, viruses are obligate intracellular parasites. What of delayed hypersensitivity, and the ability of cells of the lymphoid-macrophage system to inactivate intracellular disease agents? Practical measures in immunizing against viral infections got off to quite a dramatic start with reference to hypersensitivity:

"It is remarkable that variolous matter, when the system is disposed to reject it, should excite inflammation on the part to which it is applied more speedily than when it produces the Small Pox. Indeed it becomes almost a criterion by which we can determine whether the infection will be received or not. It seems as if a change, which endures through life, had been produced in the action, or disposition to action, in the vessels of the skin; and it is remarkable too, that whether this change has been effected by the Small Pox, or the Cow Pox, that the disposition to sudden cuticular inflammation is the same on the application of variolous matter." (Jenner, E. 1798. An Inquiry into the Causes and Effects of the Variolae Vaccinae. London, p. 13.)

Is something of vital importance being underemphasized in modern virological lore? Dr. Allan Downie in Chapter 21 indicates that the pox viruses of animals and smallpox virus in man multiply during the incubation period in the reticuloendothelial cells of lymph glands, spleen, liver, and bone marrow. In the opening chapters of this book it is emphasized that the efficacy of the reticuloendothelial defense can be significantly augmented by first inducing a state of delayed hypersensitivity and then activating with homologous antigen. The macrophages thus activated are nonspecifically effective in the destruction of intracellular disease agents. Can this nonspecific mechanism be exploited against viruses which have a multiplication period in the reticuloendothelial system?

We have obtained a positive answer in one trial system. Mice rendered hypersensitive to tuberculosis by H37Ra and further stimulated by O. T. injections are being shown to be significantly more resistant to vaccinia virus than control mice. (Mudd, S., P. Zappasodi, and J. H. Taubler. 1969. Bact. Proc. M16.)

As Editor I express my profound appreciation and gratitude to the authors who have contributed so richly to this volume, and I think it is not too much to believe that a generation of teachers, investigators, and students will share this gratitude for these records of experience and insight into the interaction of parasite and host.

STUART MUDD, M.D.

# Contents

# INFECTIONS BY GRAM-POSITIVE PATHOGENS

# INFECTIONS BY GRAM-NEGATIVE PATHOGENS

## INFECTIONS BY VIRUSES

# Chapter 1

# THE NEWER IMMUNOLOGY: AN EVOLUTIONARY APPROACH

SIR MACFARLANE BURNET

*School of Microbiology, University of Melbourne, Melbourne, Australia*

## THE CHANGING ACCENT IN IMMUNOLOGY

My first published investigation was on the H and O agglutinins present in the serum of typhoid fever patients (Burnet, 1924) and ever since then I have been deeply interested in immunology. Immunological memory fascinated me from the beginning and I remember in 1923 covering sheets of paper in an attempt to apply Semon's mnemic theroy of memory to immune phenomena. So I can claim to have had an open and enquiring mind on the subject as well as a ringside seat from which to watch the development of immunology over 45 years. Changes in outlook have been as deep seated as in any other field of medical science over the wonderful years since 1920.

In retrospect there have been striking changes during that period in the topics which on the one hand guided the practical applications of immunology to medicine and, on the other, held the center of the stage for scholarly investigation. At the practical level, immunization against diphtheria dominated the picture from 1922 to 1930, with serum treatment of pneumonia probably coming next in importance in that decade. In the 1930's the use of serological methods to elucidate the epidemiology of yellow fever and the development of a live virus vaccine probably held most attention. Other virus infections, notably influenza, also became susceptible to immunological study in the late 30's and 40's and the concept of immunological drift as a factor emerged. In 1940, Landsteiner and Wiener discovered the Rh antigen and the rapid elucidation of hemolytic disease of the newborn followed. Blood transfusion became a standard type of treatment and a vast collection of immunological anomalies and catastrophes became known. With the development of tissue culture techniques a whole new world of possibilities in preventing viral disease arose in the early 1950's with the Salk vaccine against poliomyelitis and tissue culture titration of poliomyelitis antibody as the first fruits. Since 1960 the growing edge of practical application has turned to renal transplantation and the immunosuppressive drugs, and on the other side of the same coin, as it were, to the study and chemotherapeutic treatment of autoimmune disease.

Laboratory investigations have gone in parallel with the practical topics but have had many other interests, some of which at one time or another tended to dominate activity. One may mention the great increase in the study of transplantation that followed the discovery of experimental immunological tolerance by Medawar's group in 1953 (Billingham, Brent, and Medawar, 1953). Similarly, the thymus suddenly became the center of immunological interest with Miller's work on neonatal thymectomy in 1961.

One can almost sum up the situation in half a dozen sentences. Immunology was born from the demand for protection against infectious disease. Effectively what was needed has been provided. Today, immunology is concerned essentially with the way the normal body maintains its structural and biochemical integrity, how that integrity can be broken down by autoimmune disease and the various forms of malignancy, and how methods to counter these calamities may be devised. At a more active level the challenge of organ transplantation has now been accepted. Here the problem is how to circumvent the normal processes of immune homeostasis and compel the body to accept an alien tissue.

My objective in this essay is to attempt to present to readers interested in the way immunology has developed over the last 30 or 40 years, a tentative picture of the place of immunology in relation to living function in general, in other words, to express the nature and development of adaptive immunity in evolutionary terms. I believe that in the last few years it has become possible for the first time to approach such a discussion with the feeling that there are at least *some* facts on which it can be based. There is also the progressive acceptance as a theoretical basis of the genetic origin of immune pattern in antibody. Throughout this chapter I am adopting the approach which emerged as the predominant one at the Cold Spring Harbor Symposium on Antibodies in June, 1967. It was expressed both in my opening remarks and in Jerne's final summary at that meeting. I still prefer to think of that approach as clonal selection theory but others would prefer it to be called simply the modern genetic approach to antibody pattern. A full account of my own elaboration of the approach can be found in *Cellular Immunology* (Burnet, 1969).

## THE PHYLOGENETIC APPROACH

### LIMITATIONS OF ADAPTIVE IMMUNITY TO VERTEBRATES

The most important finding of comparative immunology is that adaptive immunity is confined to the vertebrates. No invertebrate produces antibody and when tested by a suitable technique any invertebrate will accept tissue from another individual of the same species as readily as autologous tissue.

Invertebrates must exist in the same world as vertebrates, amidst a myriad of pathogenic and potentially pathogenic microorganisms. In general they survive like vertebrates without overt evidence of infection.

It seems logical, then, to look at the evolutionary origin of the apparatus of immunity as being initiated by some other need than protection against infection by microorganisms. Judging, as we must, by the reactions of modern forms, the appearance of immune apparatus came early in vertebrate history. Of the two existent groups of agnathous vertebrates, hagfishes and lampreys, the first show no evidence of any antibody production. The lamprey has produced agglutinins to *Brucella* and rejected homografts. In crude form it shows, according to Good and Papermaster (1964), all the essentials that go with adaptive immunity—immunoglobulin, circulating lymphocytes, and a thymus-like structure in the pharyngeal region. All cartilaginous and bony fishes conform much more closely to the standard vertebrate pattern. Elasmobranchs have immunoglobulins of 19S and 7S types although these are antigenically similar and probably correspond essentially to mammalian IgM (Marchalonis and Edelman, 1965). Lymphocytes are readily recognizable and there is a thymus. Antibody production is poor by mammalian standards in all cold-blooded animals but homograft rejection is very well marked in those bony fishes in which it has been tested. There is a hint here, to be developed in later pages, that the capacity to produce antibody is a later development arising from a basic mechanism that is expressed experimentally in the phenomena of homograft rejection, and is mediated wholly by cells.

Immunoglobulin production has been well established in the fishes and there is already some evidence of a progressive complexity and effectiveness of the antibody mechanism as we come up to the higher mammals. When laboratory methods of determining amino acid sequences in antibody chains have developed a little further, they should provide almost a precise picture of the evolution of the immunoglobulins. In principle the plasma proteins of all the forms from hagfish to man are available for study. A full series of mammalian K and L light chains and their evolutionary precursors could provide data of unique evolutionary interest. It is already evident that the type L light chains of mice have an amino acid structure quite strikingly similar to that of L light chains of man (Kabat, 1967).

It is very clear that the evolution of the adaptive immune system—the thymus, lymphocyte, immunoglobulin, antibody, plasma cell system—did not mean the disappearance of the invertebrate system of defense against microorganisms. Polymorphs and macrophages are still vital for mammalian defense and those subtle and complex functions of blood and blood vessels that deal with hemorrhage and minimize infection after superficial trauma are at the same time essential and virtually unrelated to adaptive immunity.

The art of the theoretical immunologist—if we can use such a phrase —is to unravel the evolutionary story of how and why adaptive immunity appeared and to interpret the progressive mutual coordination and interaction of the primitive and the new systems. It is a program of pure biological research which might cause eyebrows to be lifted today. But if we allow ourselves a little unfashionable optimism it may yet prove to be a typical major topic for academic study in the affluent years ahead when scholarly work need no longer be judged by its apparent relevance to human needs.

### THE ORIGINS OF ADAPTIVE IMMUNITY

In the absence of a great corpus of scholarly work on comparative immunology we are reduced to speculation, and what logic is possible, in dealing with the sparse experimental material we have. If, when primitive vertebrates began to develop to the stage represented by the modern lamprey, there was no new need for defense against microbial infection, we have to look for some other basic function that the immune mechanism was "invented" by nature to fulfill.

The first answer to that question was suggested by Thomas in 1959. In the laboratory, immunological research is concerned with models of natural infection by microorganisms, and with a great variety of manipulation which has no direct bearing on any aspect of mammalian life that could have had evolutionary significance—such things as the injection of alien blood and of artificial antigens and adjuvants, and transplantation of tissues or organs from other races or species. In looking for immunologically significant phenomena which might have an evolutionary relevance, Thomas seized on two, the relation of fetus to mother in placental mammals and the very widespread vertebrate character of susceptibility to spontaneous malignant disease.

Placental reproduction evolved late in vertebrate history long after the appearance of immunoglobulins and the rest. Adaptive immunity clearly did not evolve as an answer to the problems of placentation and we are left with the possibility that malignant disease or its equivalent was in some way concerned. Strictly speaking we should be seeking evidence for such a hypothesis in lampreys and sharks rather than in laboratory mammals but we know vastly more about mice than about dogfish. Both mice and goldfish reject a transplant of foreign skin or scales and show accelerated rejection on a retest with tissue from the same donor. Such homograft immunity has two necessary aspects. On the one hand, each individual of a species has its characteristic pattern of histocompatibility antigens which is in general distinct from that of any other individual. When two individuals are derived from the same zygote, as in human identical twins, the antigens will be the same, but in any other natural circumstances the chances of all antigens being the same is vanishingly small. Animals artificially bred as pure line strains are of immense importance as laboratory tools but they are outside the order of nature. The second complementary aspect is that each individual can recognize at least one antigen in any other individual as foreign and produce specifically patterned immunocytes or antibodies against it. Since transplantation of normal tissues is something unknown in vertebrate evolution we have to seek some logic for this two-sided capacity to assert individuality. In a slight elaboration of Thomas's point of view I have looked for the source of the evolutionary initiative in changes that were bound to develop in the genetic situation of somatic cells when animals became larger, lived longer, and developed more elaborate and labile mechanisms for differentiation

(Burnet, 1962). Under such circumstances, somatic mutation in the broad sense introduces both new dangers and the potentiality of dealing with these dangers.

Somatic mutation, used in a broad sense to include both point mutation and any other chromosomal anomalies that are inheritable and randomly occurring, must be frequent in any large long-lived animal species. By far the most likely explanation of most malignant conditions in man is that they arise by a process of sequential somatic mutation (see Burnet, 1957b). For the present it is reasonable to take malignant disease as the natural danger which adaptive immunity evolved to counteract. There were two basic requirements needed to minimize the biological significance of malignant disease. The first was a lability, in the germ cell line, of the genes concerned with the detailed structures of the lipoprotein surface of somatic cells —the molecular structures which we now speak of as histocompatibility antigens. A high degree of neutral polymorphism in the genetic sense could so develop. The second requirement was that the capacity of the wandering mesenchymal cells to recognize gross foreignness be sharpened so that mutant cells within the body could be recognized and effectively dealt with. One can dramatize the situation by saying that without these two characteristics all superficially located malignant disease would be contagious, particularly to the young.

On this view the initial capacity to arise would be an ability of wandering cells, lymphocyte progenitors, to react with any surface component of another cell that could be recognized as foreign. The beginning of adaptive immunity, on this view, was initially an adaptation of cell surface to recognize anomaly in another cell surface. This may be a general statement of considerable importance for the understanding of a number of immunological fields. It is underlined by recent work in which it has been shown that if cells as disparate as HeLa cells and mouse lymphocytes can be induced by Sendai virus to abrogate surface activity and become heterokaryons, the nuclei flourish in the composite cytoplasm and may even fuse to form a hybrid nucleus (Harris, 1966). Cellular incompatibility is wholly a surface matter.

## HOMOGRAFT REJECTION AND DELAYED HYPERSENSITIVITY

Most immunologists are willing to recognize the close similarities or analogies of homograft immunity and delayed hypersensitivity. Both are associated with cells and there is little or no evidence that antibody plays a significant part in either.

If ideas of cell to cell contact can provide an evolutionary basis for adaptive immunity they are obviously relevant to the phenomena of delayed hypersensitivity. I have developed this approach extensively in another context (Burnet, 1969) and believe that it can cover in an interesting fashion the phenomena as observed by conventional techniques in man and the common laboratory animals.

In any systematic consideration of delayed hypersensitivity or homograft immunity—or for that matter any other immunological process—we are necessarily concerned with two aspects.

1. The process by which contact with sensitizing antigen leads to the hypersensitive state, i.e., how a population of sensitive immunocytes is built up.

2. The process by which in the sensitive or immune animal active immunocytes reach the site of challenge and induce the observable inflammatory changes or tissue rejection.

## Induction of the Hypersensitive State

Delayed hypersensitivity in the broad sense is specially characteristic of tuberculosis and some other chronic infections, the response to certain protein-reactive simple chemicals, and homograft immunity. In all these instances it is reasonable to consider the likelihood that *the antigenic determinant involved is brought to the draining lymph node incorporated in the surface of a mobile cell.* We should first point out that it is a general rule that to produce delayed hypersensitivity the antigen must be present in the tissues, whereas tolerance or desensitization is much more easily achieved by the intravenous route. Concentrating, then, on antigen applied peripherally, we can pay chief attention to the draining lymph node.

The active agent in tuberculin is a small molecular weight protein or polypeptide ($\pm$ 5000 m.w.), and the agent of experimental allergic encephalomyelitis is a considerably smaller one; picryl, dinitrofluorobenzene, and similar skin-sensitizing chemicals are small molecules. The histocompatibility antigens are intrinsic parts of the lipoprotein structures of the cell surface and the differences are rather probably related to changes in small molecular groupings. The working hypothesis I want to examine is that to induce delayed hypersensitivity and equivalent immunological states the antigenic determinant must be incorporated into the surface lipoprotein of a mobile cell. Cells so modified pass in the lymph stream to the draining node and there lodge in the paracortical region (Oort and Turk, 1965), which is identical with the thymus-dependent area of Parrott et al. (1966). Here they will find opportunity for the antigenic determinants they carry to react with any lymphocytes (immunocytes) bearing receptors (or bound antibody) of appropriate immune specificity. The result is to stimulate the immunocytes to activity so that after conversion to the pyroninophil blast form descendant clones of sensitized lymphocytes are produced. It is likely that antigen-carrying cells are also stimulated by such contact, and there is indirect evidence to be mentioned later that in one way or another some or all of the antigen on one cell can pass to the surface of other mobile cells.

I think it will be obvious how such an hypothesis arises naturally from the picture we have been developing of the first stages of the evolution of adaptive immunity. What is needed is a way by which a mobile cell surface can "recognize" abnormality in the surface of another cell. It is axiomatic that in the healthy organisms contact of a mobile cell with a fixed cell must not induce a damaging reaction. When animals became large enough and lived long enough for somatic mutation (again in the broad sense) to become a significant occurrence, two things began to happen:

1. Histocompatibility antigens of mutant form appeared in a small proportion of tissue cells, and

2. The genes coding for a globulin component of the surface of the mobile cells ancestral to immunocytes became subject to somatic mutation or equivalent process which could significantly modify the globulin structure. As a result the possibility arose that some of these cells could react *differently* with mutant molecules when they encountered them. This is the sort of material which evolution through mutation and selection, the "great constructors" of Konrad Lorenz, can mold until it becomes a functional system of adaptive immunity.

Our hypothesis would envisage delayed hypersensitivity as arising by a relatively limited elaboration from the primitive form of intercellular contact I have described. The essential development was an expansion and specialization of the capacity of the mobile cells to produce a diversity of globulin patterns. This allowed much more specific powers of recognition (by complementary steric union) for anomalous patterns on the surface of other cells. In addition, a mutually stimulating and damaging effect of specific contact must have evolved.

I have discussed the character of delayed hypersensitivity in relation to this hypothesis quite extensively in the book already referred to (Burnet, 1969) and here it is only necessary to present a summary account of the main arguments. The physical character of the haptens and antigens which most readily provoke delayed hypersensitivity has already been mentioned. Evidence from sensitization reactions produced by specific chemicals points to an important role of the draining lymph nodes in which there is a rapid accumulation of pyroninophilic blast cells in the paracortical area a few days after the sensitizing application. According to Turk (1967) this reaction is characteristic also of homograft reactions and is quite different from the response to a typical immunizing nonsensitizing antigen like pneumococcal polysaccharide. Parrott et al. (1966) have found that the same area of the lymph node is characteristically depleted after neonatal thymectomy and they refer to it as the thymus-dependent area. The plasmablasts can be shown by appropriate labelling to develop not into plasma cells but into lymphocytes and in the case of homograft reactions it can be shown that cells newly formed in regional lymph nodes do in fact infiltrate the homograft (Gowans et al., 1963).

## Hypothesis of the Immunogen in the Cell Surface

An interpretation of these findings could take the following form. In the paracortical areas most lymphocytes and other cells brought in by afferent lymph paths lodge temporarily. Here there are also many lymphocytes from the adjacent lymph follicles and indirectly from the circulating blood. Having regard to the high intrinsic mobility of the small lymphocyte, the paracortical region is a common mixing ground for all mobile cells in the lymph node. On the surfaces of these cells there will be a wide variety of lipoprotein-associated chemical configurations including the standard histocompatibility patterns typical of the individual. All those lymphocytes which have undergone differentiation to immunocytes will also carry immune pattern receptors which can be thought of as firmly held IgM antibody molecules synthesized according to the restricted genetic capacity of the clone.

These are all "normal" cells. In addition there are lymphocytes which as a result of somatic mutation carry a variant histocompatibility pattern and any cells with surface abnormalities resulting from attachment to or damage by foreign substances entering naturally or as a result of experimental manipulations including tissue grafting. It is in line with general biological experience of cell surfaces to assume a high metabolic activity of the surface layer and reversible liberation and readsorption of many of the surface components. There is good reason to believe that all immunocytes release from their surface immunoglobulin of one specific type in amount ranging from below the detectable level to the profuse activity of the plasma cell (van Furth, 1964). There is very little evidence that lymphocytes adsorb antibody produced by other cells. It will be helpful, perhaps necessary, to assume that there is significant ability for histocompatibility and equivalent patterns to pass from the surface of one cell to another, perhaps mainly as a result of actual contact but not excluding liberation into and reabsorption from body fluids.

Direct evidence for this is almost nonexistent but there is a good deal of indirect. If one makes the credible assumption that crude "RNA-" made by phenol extraction may also contain significant amounts of histocompatibility antigens from the surface of the extracted cells and that these can be taken up by mobile (or fixed?) cells of an animal injected with the extract, a simple explanation of some otherwise exotic phenomena becomes available. Jones and Lafferty (1965), for instance, studying normal lymphocytic transfer (NLT) reactions between individual sheep, showed that RNA extracts of lymphocytes from sheep A would produce a reaction similar to NLT in sheep B but not in the donor (A) of the "RNA." Mannick and Egdahl (1962) produced rather similar results in rabbits by exposing lymphocytes to "RNA" in vitro before injection.

Transfer of foreign pattern adsorbed to cells has not, as far as I am aware, been studied directly but, as I have discussed elsewhere, seems to be the only possible way of interpreting Lawrence's transfer factor experiments (Lawrence, 1955, 1960). It is difficult, too, to conceive how a protein-reactive sensitizing chemical painted on the skin reaches the draining lymph node unless the effective antigen can be transferred to mobile cells. With modern radioisotope techniques it should be very easy to establish the existence and extent of this transfer process. For the present we can adopt the hypothesis that delayed hypersensitivity of classic form is possible only when the antigen can be actively adsorbed to lymphocyte surface in a reversible reaction with a low dissociation coefficient, so that a slow but progressive transfer of antigen to the surface of other lymphocytes is the rule.

## The Situation in the Draining Lymph Node

After this interpolation we can look again at the situation which develops in the paracortical area of the draining lymph node after painting
the skin with oxosalone (Oort and Turk, 1965). Cells heavily loaded with
the antigen-complex reach the area and other lymphocytes will receive it by
transfer. Some will move to other lymphoid accumulations. If there are
any progenitor immunocytes with appropriate pattern in the body, contact
between an antigen-carrying cell and an immunocyte will take place. The
specific union generates a signal, presumably by liberation of pharmocologi-
cally active agents which induce conversion of both cells to pyroninophil
blasts from which descendant cells, lymphocytes, arise. This will result in
a rapid increase of the number of specific immunocytes but will have only a
minor effect in dispersing antigen. The overall result will be (1) proliferation of specific immunocytes in the form of specifically sensitized lymphocytes
and their dispersion throughout the lymphoid accumulations and circulating
cells in the body; (2) proliferation of cells carrying specific antigen, which
will result in an increase in the number of lymphocytes and a nonspecific
increase in immunoglobulins—there is a suggestion that IgA-type immunocytes may be preferentially involved in guinea pigs (Rothman and Lidén,
1965), perhaps in both specific and nonspecific stimulation; and (3) activation of adjacent immunocytes not carrying antigen or specific immune pattern
to a similar low level of proliferation and antibody production.

## The Response of the Sensitized Animal to Challenge

To turn now from the problems of the genesis of a population of sensitized lymphocytes to the effector side, what is the mechanism by which
such delayed hypersensitivity reactions as an intradermal Mantoux test,
a cutaneous reaction to a simple chemical in a sensitive individual, or the
accelerated rejection of a homograft, are mediated? In attempting to answer
this I shall draw largely on two recent reviews by Uhr (1966) and Humphrey
(1967). Both agree that the response results from a damaging interaction
of antigen with specifically sensitized lymphocyte and the activation, with
superficial damage, of adjacent mobile cells, lymphocytes, and monocytes
from pharmacological agents liberated by the antigen-sensitive cell interaction.
There is much to be said for the claim by Willoughby et al. (1964) that
their lymph node permeability factor (LNPF) may be the responsible mediator. This is extractable from lymph nodes and from the cellular exudate
of typical hypersensitivity reactions in guinea pigs. LNPF appears to be a
protein, it is antigenic, and antibody produced in rabbits against guinea pig
LNPF can sharply diminish the response of a sensitized animal.

There is probably near unanimity among immunologists in regard to
this broad interpretation of the delayed hypersensitivity response in the
challenged animal but there is an infinite amount of detail to be fitted into
a definitive picture of the reaction. Only a few of these aspects can be touched

on here and again the approach will be general rather than particular. For manifestation of the challenge response the antigenic determinant (AD) must be associated with an appropriate carrier. In experiments using synthetic hapten-carrier combinations, Schlossman and Levine (1967) showed that DNP combined with polylysine with six or fewer lysine residues was not capable of effective challenge. When the polylysine component was of seven or more units a full reaction was produced in sensitized guinea pigs. There is a similar limitation of immunogenicity in guinea pigs which holds for capacity to produce either Arthus-type or delayed hypersensitivity. Arthus-type *responses,* however, can be elicited with the hapten combined with smaller numbers of lysine residues.

When hapten-carrier combinations are under study it is regularly found that the "combining site" associated with DH is larger, involving both hapten and carrier, than that concerned in antibody which may have specificity solely concerned with the hapten.

In tissue transplantation reactions it is general and probably legitimate to regard the cells concerned with both homograft rejection and graft-versus-host (GVH) reactions as sensitized lymphocytes which along with nonspecific activated lymphocytes are damaged by contact with the histocompatibility antigens of the graft in the homograft rejection situation and liberate pharmacological agents which are directly responsible for the damage to target cells. In the GVH reaction a similar process is initiated by specific immunocytes from the donor but in the early stages also involves some of the associated nonspecific donor lymphocytes and a little later, host cells reaching the focus from the circulation.

Desensitization resulting from appropriately administered extra antigen (usually given intravenously or by mouth) is a complex process. In part it results from lethal damage to specific immunocytes scattered so diffusely through the body that no local signs are evident but in many cases it probably depends on the development of circulating antibody which by combining with antigen can reduce its effective concentration below that necessary to give a demonstrable DH reaction.

To summarize this discussion of the phenomena of delayed hypersensitivity and homograft immunity: Both represent relatively primitive cellular responses involving immunocytes with receptors capable of reaction with a relatively large antigenic determinant and probably because of this making a relatively high-affinity union. To stimulate progenitor immunocytes to proliferation the antigenic determinant must be presented on the surface of a mobile cell in the paracortical region of lymph nodes. The essence of the DH reaction to challenge is damaging response of a sensitive immunocyte to antigen contact with involvement of relatively large numbers of adjacent cells.

### LAWRENCE'S TRANSFER FACTOR

If leukocytes are obtained from a person showing a very active tuberculin response and injected subcutaneously in a tuberculin-negative recipient, the latter within 18 or 24 hours shows a generalized tuberculin reactivity. The "transfer factor" responsible is not dependent on viable leukocytes and is present in the clear supernatant from an extract of frozen and thawed leukocytes. So far it has been impossible to isolate and characterize the factor (Lawrence, 1959).

This phenomenon is one of the most baffling in the whole corpus of experimental immunology. It is demonstrable with leukocytes from persons showing DH reactions to coccidioidin, streptococcal M antigen, and dinitrofluorobenzene and with accelerated rejection of skin from a specific donor. It has never been successfully demonstrated in any animal species and there is no accepted interpretation of the phenomenon.

As will be apparent from the approach I have adopted, an interpretation seems to be implicit in the hypothesis of specific antigen, incorporated reversibly in the surface of mobile cells. The whole picture is that of an exquisitely sensitive *active* response to antigen of optimal quality rather than a passive distribution of antibody or something equivalent which can react with antigen. The prolonged persistence of the transferred reactivity—up to a year in some cases—speaks strongly for this. The suggestion, then, is that a high degree of hypersensitivity in the donor means that in this individual, large numbers of mobile cells carry small amounts of reversibly held specific antigen. The function of this antigen is to stimulate appropriate immunocytes to proliferate and maintain an adequate level of sensitive lymphocytes in the body. By hypothesis the antigen is passed on to other lymphocytes after lysis of the carrying cell. In the classic transfer experiment the antigen in its optimally immunogenic form is transferred to circulating lymphocytes and monocytes, perhaps to polymorphonuclears. This is followed by a rapid stimulation to activity of any available immunocytes with the appropriate specificity and their proliferation.

One is almost driven to the conclusion that there must be a substantial number of preexistent immunocytes of the correct specificity in the human recipients even if they have no sign of a positive tuberculin test. One suggestion as to why this transfer of tuberculin sensitivity fails in all laboratory mammals may be simply that adult human beings with negative tuberculin reactions have not in fact wholly escaped infection and possess a considerable number of potentially reactive clones.

## IMMUNOLOGICAL SURVEILLANCE

If the system of adaptive immunity arose because of the demand for some means of maintaining the integrity of the body against the potential danger of mutant somatic cells, one must expect this function still to be evident in the higher mammals. The topic of immune reactions against malignant cells and tissues has been widely discussed in recent years and the concept of immunological surveillance has gradually emerged. I believe that I was the first to use the term in 1960 when I suggested that it was a function of the immune system "to maintain a surveillance over the orthodoxy of (the body's) chemical structure and to stamp out heresy before it could spread" (Burnet, 1961). The concept was reviewed in some detail more recently (Burnet, 1964, 1967). It was concluded that there was evidence from many sources to indicate that there was in fact a process by which the incidence of tumors was kept far below what would be the case in its absence. An interesting addition to the evidence for which I am indebted to Dr. D. A. Long is his recognition that in man, monkeys, and guinea pigs, the three types in which delayed hypersensitivity reactions are readily manifested, spontaneous cancer is very much rarer than in mice, rats, and rabbits, which are able to synthesize ascorbic acid (a relevant association in Long's opinion) and show much less well defined delayed hypersensitivity.

# THE EVOLUTION OF ANTIBODY PRODUCTION

## THE MODERN GENETIC APPROACH TO ANTIBODY PRODUCTION

Any discussion of antibody production from the evolutionary angle must take for granted the modern approach which I like to call clonal selection theory. Others with some justification suggest that things have moved so fast and far in immunology in the last decade that it is illegitimate to claim that a modern theoretical approach could still be basically the same as what was suggested in 1957 (Burnet, 1957a).

In my view the essence of the modern approach is as follows:

1. The specific immune pattern of antibody is determined by genetic information in the genome of the synthesizing cell as it is for any other enzyme or protein.

2. The diversity of patterns within the competence of an individual arise by genetic processes taking place during the postzygotic period: the nature of these processes and their genetic background are matters for current discussion.

3. There is a very wide but not infinite range of immune patterns that can be produced by an individual but once a cell has become a recognizable immunocyte it produces only one pattern and only one type of immunoglobulin.

4. All descendants of an immunocyte produce or can potentially produce the same pattern: phenotypic restriction persists throughout the clone.

5. The only function of the antigenic determinant is by reversible union with a cell receptor of the same specificity as an antibody combining site, to act as a specific stimulant to cell function, the most characteristic type of cell behavior so induced being proliferation to form a plasma cell clone actively synthesizing antibody.

My impression after the Symposium on Antibodies at Cold Spring Harbor in June, 1967, was that there would have been virtually unanimous agreement on that summary. Perhaps the most impressive new finding presented was Eisen's work with a myeloma protein which behaved as if it was (and therefore *was*) an anti-DNP antibody.

### Antibody in Lower Vertebrates

In discussing the specificity of delayed hypersensitivity I assumed mainly for ease of exposition that the receptors involved could be thought of as IgM antibody molecules incorporated in the cell surface. This is as likely to be true as any alternative but all that it is strictly permissible to say is that something structurally and therefore genetically equivalent to antibody combining site is serving as a receptor.

Whatever the detail, it is very much in line with the process of evolution to say that "when nature grasped the idea" that diversity of pattern in a globulin could serve a useful function the way was open for progressive elaboration of the idea. Until we know a great deal more than we do now of the structure and special functions of IgM, IgG, and IgA and of the physical nature of the antibody combining site, which seems to be common to antibodies irrespective of their immunoglobulin type, it will be impossible to trace any evolutionary sequence in detail. The fact that the single *antigenic* type of immunoglobulin in elasmobranchs seems to be equivalent to IgM though present in both 17S and 7S, pentamer and monomer form, justifies our choice of IgM as the most primitive form and therefore likely to be related to the receptor for DH reactivity. No firm decision has been made as to whether the transition from IgM to IgG, which is characteristic of the response to most types of primary immunization, results from individual cells initially IgM producers, switching to IgG production or from a new series of IgG clones being brought into action as the peak activity of IgM clones is falling. I can see no evolutionarily valid reason why both should not be correct.

The most striking feature of antibody production from the genetic point of view is the strict phenotypic restriction, beautifully demonstrated in the homogeneity of myeloma proteins, by which only one immunoglobulin is produced under normal and near normal circumstances. I have wondered not very seriously whether the knobs on the "clock face" nucleus of a mature plasma cell represent the number of chromosomes subject to a Lyon type of restriction including autosomes as well as the X chromosome, and representing a physical concomitant of strict phenotypic restriction.

Speaking again with far too little in the way of hard facts, it seems that at the level of cartilaginous and bony fishes, homograft immunity, as shown, e.g., by Hildemann and Owen's (1956) work with goldfish, is specific and effective, but in all cold-blooded vertebrates the antibody response is relatively meager and greatly enhanced when the temperature is raised. On the other hand, the mammal par excellence for production of highly specific antibody is the rabbit. Here, delayed hypersensitivity is inconspicuous. There are many antigens that produce typical delayed hypersensitivity in a guinea pig but little antibody, yet are good antibody producers in the rabbit.

### The Induction of Antibody in Mammals

One of the important discoveries in immunology of the last 5 years is the recognition by Ada, Nossal, and their collaborators of the function of the dendritic phagocytic cells of lymph follicles, whether in lymph nodes, Peyer's patches and similar collections, or spleen (Ada et al., 1964; Nossal et al., 1964; Ada et al., 1967). I have adopted and generalized their interpretation that soluble antigens draining into a lymph node are taken up in part by standard macrophages particularly in the medullary and paracortical regions and in part by the dendritic phagocytic cells (DPC) supported on the reticulin fibers of the lymph follicles. Here the antigen, possibly after some form of pretreatment, is held on the surface of the DPC, in contrast to the way it is engulfed and digested in the phagolysosomes of the standard macrophages. In the opinion of Nossal's group the antigen held on the dendritic extensions of the DPC is directly concerned in the standard process of antibody production. With regard to the high mobility of lymphocytes and the known active turnover of lymphocytes entering and leaving the lymph node, one can picture the lymph follicles in life as a continually mixing and changing mass of moving lymphocytes, "a bag of worms," in which each cell has repeated opportunities of making contact with antigenic determinants held superficially on the processes of DPC's. Here, when specific union of antigenic determinant and receptor is made, the lymphocyte is activated to blast form and, if it lodges in an appropriate niche, proliferation to an antibody-producing plasma cell clone will follow.

As in every field of immunology, that simple statement requires qualification in various directions. In all probability appropriate lodgment of antigen on the DPC requires that there be at least a minute amount of circulating antibody. Immunofluorescent studies indicate the presence of mixed immunoglobulins in germinal centers which are distributed in a reticular fashion suggesting association with the dendritic processes of these cells. It is known that the presence of antibody is inhibitory to IgM production but much less so to IgG production and it may well be that the process we are discussing is mostly concerned with the stimulation of committed immunocytes to produce IgG antibody. There are too many resemblances between IgM and IgG production, however, to make it conceivable that completely different modes of induction exist and the best current opinion is to ascribe the stimulation of progenitor (uncommitted) immunocytes to IgM production, to the same process.

The role of the DPC can obviously be regarded from the evolutionary angle as a specialized development of the process which has been postulated for the induction of delayed hypersensitivity. It represents a logical progression from the first primitive capacity of a cell surface to recognize anomaly in the surface of another cell on which we have based the whole evolution of adaptive immunity. If presentation of antigen on DPC surface is the standard stimulus for antibody production it does not necessarily follow that all other types of contact between antigenic determinant and the corresponding combining site of antibody or cell receptor are inert. Nothing in cellular interactions is ever 100 per cent; there is always a soft edge, a margin for error. Contact of antigenic determinant with a corresponding immune receptor may have many different results, from acute destruction of the immunocyte to the classic differentiation to an antibody-producing clone of plasma cells that we have taken as the norm. There are numerous indications to tell us something of the likelihood of immunocyte destruction and of whether cells sensitized to give delayed hypersensitivity, plasmacytes, or lymphocytic memory cells will be produced, under this or that mode of presentation of the antigen. Experience suggests, however, that even with theoretically perfect experimental techniques the observed result of administering a well defined pure antigen would have to be expressed as the respective *probabilities* that effects a, b, c, and so on would be observed.

### The Function of Antibody

It is not as easy as it was 20 years ago to define the primary function of antibody. After all there are many invertebrates, large and small, that seem to be perfectly able to resist casual infection by microorganisms without antibody. It was a real shock to immunologists to observe that children with congenital agammaglobulinemia showed a normal course of measles and subsequent immunity against reinfection. And it is self-evident that when antibody would seem to be most helpful—as in an adult first exposed to virulent yellow fever—it is absent.

In a sense this is sophistry. Agammaglobulinemic children always died of bacterial infection in the days before antibiotics. Calves receiving no maternal antibody in colostrum suffer severely from bowel infections, and antitoxin is often curative in diphtheria. Nevertheless there is much to be said beyond the facile statement that the function of antibody is to cure first infections and prevent subsequent reinfection by the same organism.

1. Protection of the newborn. Perhaps the best established function of antibody is its capacity to transfer an improved chance of survival to the newborn. Confining ourselves to mammals, we find that there is no evidence of any transfer of *specific* immunological competence except in the form of antibody. When transferred across the placenta, as in man, it is in the form of IgG; when provided wholly in colostrum, as in sheep and cattle, IgA antibodies are concerned.

A good example of the influence of maternal antibody against a ubiquitous parasite, the virus of herpes simplex, is to be found in the investigation by Anderson and Hamilton (1949), on the natural history of herpes infection in an orphanage. Virtually 100 per cent of children under 6 months showed measurable virus-inactivating antibody of maternal origin. By 9 months it was usually below a detectable level, yet infection, whether symptomatic with stomatitis or subclinical and recognized only by a rise in antibody titer, took place essentially over the period 12 to 20 months. Environmental factors, including the shift from infant cribs to the toddlers' ward, undoubtedly played a part but maternal antibody was almost certainly responsible for the delay in primary infection.

It seems highly probable that the classic immunity of the native-born to yellow fever was equally based on low-grade infection at a time of falling maternal antibody levels plus the general finding that the mortality of young children from an infection encountered for the first time is lower than is seen in adolescents and young adults.

A recent observation of considerable interest is the finding of Kerman et al. (1967) that newborn mice from mothers immunologically paralyzed with pneumococcal SSS (Felton's phenomenon) differed significantly from normal infant mice. When the two groups of baby mice were injected with graded doses of SSS it was found that the minimal doses needed to produce immunity and to establish immune paralysis were both an order of 10 smaller in the offspring of paralyzed mothers than in normal animals. The basis of the difference is almost certainly the absence in the offspring of paralyzed mice of any trace of antibody to assist either removal of antigen from circulation or its establishment on DPC surfaces.

2. The immunosuppressive function of antibody.   Another function of antibody which has only recently been clearly recognized and which has both theoretical and practical importance is its *immunosuppressive* effect. There is now an extensive literature on the way in which antibody, especially IgG, can prevent response to a standard dose of the corresponding antigen (Möller, 1964; Möller and Wigzell, 1965; Finkelstein and Uhr, 1964; Rowley and Fitch, 1965; Wigzell, 1966). The most striking effect, and possibly the only significant one, is the capacity of preformed antibody, either 7S or, less effectively, 19S, to stop the recruitment of progenitor immunocytes to the ranks of antibody producers. The effect can be seen either as a reduction in the number of plaque-forming cells producing IgM or in the observed production of new antibody. Wigzell's (1966) work with 7S (IgG) plaque-forming cells showed that the effect of antibody in reducing their number had a lag of 48 to 72 hours. The hint is that these 7S PFC are the product of an earlier process which is the one directly inhibited by antibody. It seems that inhibition by antibody in high enough concentration functions by combination of the antibody with antigen in such a fashion that it can no longer stimulate progenitor immunocytes.

There may well be a real biological function behind these experimental findings. This may be to help ensure that any relatively prolonged infection shall not result in a complete crowding out of immunocyte populations that are unable to react with antigens of the microorganism concerned. When young rats are given closely spaced injections of sheep red cells for some weeks there is very little further production of antibody after the initial response, and according to Rowley and Fitch (1966) this is mainly due to the homeostatic action of antibody in preventing the recruitment of uncommitted cells.

## PRACTICAL ASPECTS OF THE NEW IMMUNOLOGY

The theme of this book is the way in which microbiological and immunological science over the last 30 or 40 years has brought us to our present level of practical control and theoretical understanding of the processes at work in infectious disease of man. It is undoubtedly true that present fashions in immunological research have moved rather far from the old concentration on infectious disease. I suspect that if there had been no antibiotics we should know more than we do about the processes of natural cure in bacterial disease. There seems, in fact, curiously little to say on this subject that was not said 30 years ago.

I shall conclude this paper, therefore, by making a modest attempt to indicate some of the practical applications which are relevant to or based on the newer concepts in immunology. For obvious reasons I shall make no attempt to discuss aspects of immunology concerned with topics remote from infectious disease. Autoimmune disease and the immunological problems of tissue or organ transplantation and blood transfusion are immensely important but they belong to a different universe of medicine and will not be considered. Even at the theoretical level it may have been noted that I have made no significant reference to two topics that have concerned me closely, the function of the thymus and immune tolerance.

## Prevention of Rh Disease

It has something of an air of paradox to use antibody to prevent antigens from stimulating antibody production. Yet though there has only recently been much experimental work on the topic it has been known for many years that if a mother has a relatively high titer of diphtheria antitoxin, toxoid given to her newborn infant will not immunize (Osborne et al., 1952).

The first practical use of this phenomenon is the method initiated by Finn et al. (1961) of preventing hemolytic disease of the newborn by the administration of anti-D serum to Rh− mothers who have just been delivered of an Rh+ infant. This is based on the well established finding that fetal cells are frequently injected in small amount into the mother's circulation during labor. In the presence of anti-D these D/d cells are rapidly removed and fail to sensitize the mother. This is a new development and it is too early to say that it has been proved effective in preventing "Rh disease." Reports to date are, however, uniformly favorable and the method has all the indications of becoming one of the great lifesaving discoveries of our time.

There have been suggestions that what is required to ensure lack of immune response against a homograft in man is that the recipient be immunized, preferably by the intravenous route, with purified histocompatibility antigens of the donor. The presence of circulating antibody, equivalent to the enhancement effect in experimental cancer research, is expected to inhibit the response of immunocytes against the cell-bound antigen of the transplanted tissue.

## The Optimal Time for Immunization

If one were trying to develop from first principles what was the best age for immunization against an endemic infection, the following points would need consideration:

1. The mother is by hypothesis immune; antibody will be passively transferred to the infant and will become ineffective some time before the

end of the first year. The actual time will depend mainly on the height of the concentration reached in the infant's blood if, as is reasonable, one assumes the half-life of maternal globulin is approximately the same in all infants.

2. There is evidence that viral, bacterial, and combined viral-bacterial infections tend to cause the highest mortality at young adult age in completely unprotected individuals. With some infections, such as poliomyelitis, most cases in very young children are subclinical.

3. Excessive reactions to antigens present in immunizing preparations are rare before adolescence.

4. Unless there is occasional restimulation by the immunizing antigen, either natural or artificial, the capacity to produce antibody will gradually disappear.

The solution logically derived from these points is to give the course of immunization when the maternal antibody is too low to interfere with immunogenicity but still exists in sufficient amount to provide an opsonizing effect. The optimal time would therefore be between 3 and 9 months of age; this is a thoroughly orthodox conclusion. When the subjects are likely to escape casual infection during childhood it is desirable to reinforce immunity with a booster injection at some appropriate age. Once again it appears that very little that is new and useful in the practice of immunization has emerged in 20 years.

## CONCLUSION

Around 1890 it seemed clear that everything important was known in physics and that research was henceforth to be a matter of refining the quantitative aspects and garnering unconsidered trifles. I can believe at times that the present position in regard to the understanding and control of infectious disease of man is basically similar. Environmental hygiene and quarantine were well understood at the turn of the century, the principles of immunization were known by 1930, and the significant antibiotics were in full use by 1950. Since poliomyelitis vaccine was proved effective in 1954 not much of fundamental importance has happened.

My own generation, active in investigation from immediately after the first world war to 1960, showed what a magnificent contribution laboratory research could make to preventive and curative medicine. That phase is over and the next generation must have a different approach. We combined the scholarly and the practical; in the future the approaches will move apart.

Already the scholarly approach to the biomedical sciences has moved into fields as irrelevant to human affairs as the families of fundamental particles that occupy the physicists. The intellectual attraction of microbiology and immunology today is at the level of molecular biology and biochemical genetics. Especially when combined with an evolutionary approach—as I have attempted in this chapter—the modern approach has an immense fascination for the scholar. The greatest modern work in biology has included the elucidation of the genetic code, the geometric structure of viruses, the amino acid sequences of the immunoglobulins, and the complete structural chemistry of several of the smaller proteins. It is a magnificent continuing achievement and it has no bearing whatever on human needs.

At the other end of the scale are the immensely more difficult and urgent problems at the human level. We have still to eliminate from the world many infections that could be eliminated, to feed adequately those who need food, and to tackle all the evil things that are either intrinsic to our species, based on genetic anomaly, or forced on us by cultural pressures: war, poverty, racial discrimination, delinquency, and crime. Especially important to us who have been concerned with the control of infectious disease are overpopulation and long-term genetic deterioration. Human biology in the broadest sense is the science of the future, and the electronic computer is the tool that came when it was most needed to provide human intellects with the means of tackling the human problems.

I hope the world will allow our successors to go on exploring the ways and the history of life in scholarly fashion—above all to expose the full picture of the evolution of immunity that I have tried to sketch. But it is even more urgent that an increasing proportion of men with first-rate capacity move away from the laboratories to the direct and practical but still scholarly applications of biological science to men and their problems.

# *References*

Ada, G. L. , Nossal, G. J. V., and Pye, J. (1964). Antigens in immunity. III. Distribution of iodinated antigens following injection into rats *via* the hind footpads. Aust. J. Exp. Biol. Med. Sci. *42:*295–310.

Ada, G. L., Parish, C. R., and Lang, P. G. (1967). The cellular localization and immunogenicity of antigen and antigen fragments. *In:* Cold Spring Harbor Sympos. Quant. Biol. Vol. 32.

Anderson, S. G., and Hamilton, J. (1949). The epidemiology of primary herpes simplex infection. Med. J. Aust. *i:*308–311.

Billingham, R. E., Brent, L., and Medawar, P. B. (1953). 'Actively acquired tolerance' of foreign cells. Nature *172:*603–606.

Burnet, F. M. (1924). Preliminary note on a new method of serological investigation in cases of suspected typhoid fever. Med. J. Aust. *i:*205–208.

Burnet, F. M. (1957a). A modification of Jerne's theory of antibody production using the concept of clonal selection. Aust. J. Sci. *20:*67–69.

Burnet, F. M. (1957b). Cancer—a biological approach. II. The significance of somatic mutation. Brit. Med. J. *i:*779–786.

Burnet, F. M. (1961). Immunological recognition of self (Nobel Lecture, Dec. 12, 1960). Science *133:*307–311.

Burnet, F. M. (1962). Symposium on specificity of cell differentiation and interaction. Summary. J. Cell Comp. Physiol. *60:*Supp. I, pp. 201–206.

Burnet, F. M. (1964). Immunological factors in carcinogenesis. Brit. Med. Bull. *20:*154–158.

Burnet, F. M. (1967). Immunological aspects of malignant disease. Lancet, *i:*1171–1174.

Burnet, F. M. (1969). Cellular Immunology. Cambridge and Melbourne University Presses.

Finkelstein, M. S., and Uhr, J. W. (1964). Specific inhibition of antibody formation by passively administered 19S and 7S antibody. Science *146:*67–69.

Finn, R., Clarke, C. A., Donohoe, W. T. A., McConnell, R. B., Sheppard, P. M., Lehane, D., and Kulke, W. (1961). Experimental studies on the prevention of Rh haemolytic disease. Brit. Med. J. *i:*1486–1490.

Good, R. A., and Papermaster, B. W. (1964). Ontogeny and phylogeny of adaptive immunity. Advances Immun. 4:1–115.

Gowans, J. L., McGregor, D. D., and Cowen, D. M. (1963). The role of small lymphocytes in the rejection of homografts of skin. In: Ciba Foundation Study Group No. 16. Churchill, London, p. 20–29.

Harris, H. (1966). Hybrid cells from mouse and man: a study in genetic regulation. Proc. Roy. Soc. B 166:358–368.

Hildemann, W. H., and Owen, R. D. (1956). Histocompatibility genetics of scale transplantation. Transplant. Bull. 3:132–134.

Humphrey, J. H. (1967). Cell-mediated immunity—general perspectives. Brit. Med. Bull. 23: 93–97.

Jones, M. A. S., and Lafferty, K. J. (1965). The inflammatory reaction induced in sheep by homologous lymphocytes and an RNA fraction extracted from homologous lymphocytes. In: Twelfth Congress Internat. Soc. Blood Transfusion, Sydney, Abstracts, p. 45.

Kabat, E. A. (1967). The paucity of species-specific amino acid residues in the variable regions of human and mouse Bence-Jones proteins and its evolutionary and genetic implications. Proc. Nat. Acad. Sci. 57:1345–1349.

Kerman, R., Segre, D., and Myers, W. L. (1967). Altered response to pneumococcal polysaccharide in off-spring of immunologically paralyzed mice. Science, 156:1514–1515.

Landsteiner, K., and Wiener, A. S. (1940). An agglutinable factor in human blood recognized by immune sera for Rhesus blood. Proc. Soc. Exp. Biol. Med. 43:223.

Lawrence, H. S. (1955). The transfer in humans of delayed skin sensitivity to streptococcal M substance and to tuberculin with disrupted leucocytes. J. Clin. Invest. 34:219–230.

Lawrence, H. S. (Ed.) (1959). The transfer of hypersensitivity of the delayed type in man. In: Cellular and Humoral Aspects of the Hypersensitive State. Hoeber, New York, pp. 279–318.

Lawrence, H. S. (1960). Some biological and immunological properties of transfer factor. In: Wolstenholme, G. E. W., and O'Connor, M. (Eds.): Cellular Aspects of Immunity. Ciba Foundation Symposium. Churchill, London, pp. 243–279.

Mannick, J. A., and Egdahl, A. R. (1962). Ribonucleic acid in "transformation" of lymphoid cells. Science 137:976–977.

Marchalonis, J., and Edelman, G. M. (1965). Phylogenetic origins of antibody structure. I. Multichain structure of immunoglobulins in the smooth dogfish (Mustelus canis). J. Exp. Med. 122:601–618.

Möller, G. (1964). Antibody induced depression of the immune response: a study of the mechanism in various immunological systems. Transplantation, 2:405–415.

Möller, G., and Wigzell, H. (1965). Antibody synthesis at the cellular level: antibody-induced suppression of 19S and 7S antibody response. J. Exp. Med. 121:969–989.

Nossal, G. J. V., Ada, G. L., and Austin, C. M. (1964). Antigens in immunity. IV. Cellular localization of $^{125}$I- and $^{131}$I-labelled flagella in lymph nodes. Aust. J. Exp. Biol. Med. Sci. 42:311–330.

Oort, J., and Turk, J. L. (1965). A histological and autoradiographic study of lymph nodes during the development of contact sensitivity in the guinea-pig. Brit. J. Exp. Path. 46: 147–154.

Osborne, J. J., Dancis, J., and Julia, J. F. (1952). Studies of the immunology of the newborn infant. 1. Age and antibody production. Pediatrics 9:736–744.

Parrott, D. M. V., de Sousa, M. A. B., and East, J. (1966). Thymus-dependent areas in the lymphoid areas of neonatally thymectomized mice. J. Exp. Med. 123:191–204, Pl. 39.

Rothman, U., and Lidén, S. (1965). Isolation of a lymphoid-cell protein with relation to delayed hypersensitivity. Nature 208:389–390.

Rowley, D. A., and Fitch, F. W. (1965). The mechanism of tolerance produced in rats to sheep erythrocytes. II. The plaque-forming cell and antibody response to multiple injections of antigen begun at birth. J. Exp. Med. 121:683–695.

Rowley, D. A., and Fitch, F. W. (1966). Clonal selection and inhibition of the primary response by antibody. In: Cinader, B. (Ed.): Regulation of the Antibody Response. Thomas, Springfield, Illinois.

Schlossman, S. F., and Levine, H. (1967). Immunochemical studies on delayed and Arthus-type hypersensitivity reactions. I. The relationship between antigenic determinant size and antibody combining site size. J. Immun. 98:211–219.

Thomas, L. (1959). Discussion. In: Lawrence, H. S. (Ed.): Cellular and Humoral Aspects of the Hypersensitive State. Symposia of the Section of Microbiology. The New York Academy of Medicine No. 9. Cassell, London, p. 529.

Turk, J. L. (1967). Cytology of the induction of hypersensitivity. Brit. Med. Bull. 23:3–8.

Uhr, J. W. (1966). Delayed hypersensitivity. Physiol. Rev. *46:*359–419.

van Furth, R. (1964). The formation of immunoglobulins by human tissues in vitro. Thesis, Leiden.

Wigzell, H. (1966). Antibody synthesis at the cellular level: antibody-induced suppression of 7S antibody synthesis. J. Exp. Med. *124:*953–969.

Willoughby, D. A., Spector, W. G., and Boughton, B. (1964). A lymph-node permeability factor in the tuberculin reaction. J. Path. Bact. *87:*353–363.

# Chapter 2

# CELLULAR IMMUNITY*

G. B. MACKANESS and R. V. BLANDEN

*The Trudeau Institute Medical Research*
*Laboratories, Saranac Lake, New York*

## I. INTRODUCTION

More often than not the term "cellular immunity" will be found written within quotation marks, as if to signify ambiguity or doubt in the mind of the author. There is reason enough for this, for the concept is vague, the underlying immunological processes are ill-defined, and the term has been used with two entirely different connotations. Students of infectious disease use it to describe a form of acquired anti-microbial resistance in which the host's mononuclear phagocytes show increased destructive capacity for ingested organisms. This form of "cellular immunity" can be transferred with cells, but not with serum;[151, 2, 144, 115] it is evoked by way of a specific immunological reaction, but is non-specific in its anti-microbial effects.[108] Once it has been established, it can combat infections caused by unrelated organisms.[108, 109, 88, 54]

The term has been used in a different sense by those wishing to explain the rejection of solid tissue grafts, organ-specific auto-immune reactions, or the phenomenon of delayed-type hypersensitivity. These immunological reactions do not conform to classical immunology in that no antibody has been found which will passively immunise normal recipients. When, therefore, it became evident that immunity of this type could be conferred adoptively with living cells, "cellular immunity" acquired a second meaning.

It is obvious that the microbiologist has been preoccupied with the end-effect of an immune response, namely, with the change in host macrophages upon which anti-microbial resistance finally depends. The tissue immunologist, being uncertain of the way in which immunity against tissue components is ultimately expressed, implied no more in his use of the term than the apparent requirement for living cells in the adoptive transfer of immunological

---

* Reprinted from Progr. Allergy, vol. 11, pp. 89–140 (Karger, Basel/New York 1967)

reactivity. More recently, however, it has become increasingly clear that cells may be needed in anti-tissue immunity, not merely for the synthesis of recognition factors (antibody), but also for active transport of antibody into the target area and even for the execution of the immunological attack.

There is, then, a fundamental difference of meaning between the anti-microbial and anti-tissue forms of cellular immunity. Nonetheless, the two are linked in the minds of many immunologists because immunity in each case is accompanied by the phenomenon of delayed-type hypersensitivity.[108, 112, 103] Indeed, many writers appear to use the terms "cellular immunity" and "delayed-sensitivity" as if they were synonymous.

It is the purpose of this review to examine certain problems concerning the nature of acquired cellular resistance to infectious agents, its relationship to the mechanisms involved in the immunological destruction of tissues and organs, and the underlying significance of delayed-type hypersensitivity in each of these forms of immunity.

## II. THE BASIC PROBLEM

It might seem, at first, that the elimination of microbial parasites and the focal or diffuse destruction of indigenous or foreign tissues are so dissimilar that any comparison would be highly artificial. In both cases, however, the problem resolves itself into the question of how the body achieves the death of viable structures by immunological means.

Acquired cellular resistance to microbial parasites has been seriously invoked as the essential mechanism of immunity only in those infectious diseases in which the parasite is normally capable of surviving in host phagocytes, and in which anti-bacterial antibody cannot be shown to exert any significant degree of protection.[109] Here the essential problem for the host is to achieve the augmentation of phagocyte function necessary to ensure the ultimate death of ingested organisms. In the destruction of living tissues the problem seems somewhat different. The immunological dissolution of organised tissues is not obviously an intra-phagocytic event, though the case may well be different with dissociated cellular transplants.[16, 129] For the most part, the processes of phagocytosis and intracellular digestion are not conspicuously involved in the expression of intolerance towards target tissues. Nevertheless, the macrophage (which is finally responsible for the death of facultative intracellular parasites) also figures in almost every description that has been given of the cellular elements which congregate in tissues that are the subject of immunological attack.[112, 178, 179, 139] The possibility exists, therefore, that the final destruction of healthy tissue and the inactivation of facultative intracellular parasites may devolve upon the same cell type. It is perhaps too soon to attempt a real comparison between these two immunological situations; but the exercise may be worthwhile if it does no more than clarify the issues involved in the use of the term "cellular immunity."

# III. THE ANTI-MICROBIAL FORM OF CELLULAR IMMUNITY

## A. Nature of Acquired Cellular Resistance

It is well known that Metchnikoff would countenance nothing but a cellular mechanism to explain the phenomena of acquired anti-microbial immunity. He felt that acquired resistance to infectious agents resulted from "the perfecting of the phagocytic and digestive powers of the leucocytes."[114] A modified form of Metchnikoff's concept persists to this day. Since the evidence for the existence of a cellular form of anti-microbial resistance has been well and extensively reviewed in recent years[105, 161] it will not be discussed here in detail. However, some published observations have not completely excluded the possibility that anti-bacterial antibody, firmly bound to the cell surface, may confer "immunity" on macrophages without the necessity for an enhancement of their intrinsic microbicidal ability.[92, 169] For this reason certain more recent findings deserve comment.

Evidence has been obtained from studies conducted both *in vivo* and *in vitro* that the killing of ingested bacteria proceeds at a much faster rate and in a higher proportion of macrophages obtained from infected animals than it does in cells from normal animals. For example, the inactivation of *Salm. typhimurium* in the cells of actively infected mice commences almost immediately after ingestion and proceeds rapidly until virtually every intracellular organism has been killed, a process that takes about 15 minutes. In cells from normal mice, inactivation of this organism does not even commence for 9 to 12 min after ingestion, and seldom accounts for the death of more than 50 to 60% of phagocytosed bacteria.[21] Although we do not know the exact reasons for the difference between the cells of normal and infected animals, we do know that it is not due to specific anti-bacterial antibody. This is indicated by the fact that cells from animals infected with *Listeria monocytogenes* or *Salm. typhimurium* are equally microbicidal for *Salm. typhimurium* despite the absence of demonstrable anti-Salmonella antibody either in the serum or adsorbed to the cells of the Listeria-infected mice.[21] This exemplifies one of the most notable features of acquired cellular resistance. The augmented activity of cells, once established, is not specifically directed against the infectious agent which induced it.[21, 54, 62, 108, 109] This helps greatly our understanding of the cross-resistance which develops between taxonomically[83, 84] and antigenically[88] unrelated organisms. The list of organisms which cause cross-protection is quite extensive. Examples which are supported by quantitative data include the observations that mice, at certain stages of infection with *Br. abortus*[108, 109] or *Salm. typhimurium*,[21] can eliminate *L. monocytogenes* from their tissues with great rapidity; they can do it more rapidly, in fact, than mice which are convalescing from infection with *L. monocytogenes* itself.[107] In addition, the isolated macrophages of Listeria-infected mice can inactivate *Salm. typhimurium in vitro*,[21] while those from Brucella-infected animals are extremely active against *Listeria monocytogenes*.[108]

These facts alone strongly suggest that macrophages of the actively-infected host undergo intrinsic changes in functional ability. Furthermore, copious evidence of such changes has accumulated since the 19th century, when Delezenne showed that cells taken from the peritoneal cavities of dogs injected with gelatin possess an increased capacity to digest this substance.[114] Until recently, however, there had been no unequivocal evidence that the immune macrophage can inactivate organisms with added efficiency.

The mononuclear phagocytes of infected animals differ in many ways from their normal counter-parts. The morphological, metabolic and functional changes found in the macrophages of tuberculous animals have been discussed by Lurie;[105] similar changes in the cells of animals infected with other intracellular parasites have been described by Suter and Ramseier.[161] One of the most notable is the observed increase in their content of acid hydrolases. This increase in enzyme content is attended by an increased content of lysosomes,[39, 122] and an ability to discharge them more rapidly into the phagocytic vacuoles which form around ingested organisms.[127] But the significance of these differences is not clear, for we know virtually nothing of the way in which organisms are killed within mononuclear phagocytes. However, the recent findings of Cohn and Benson[37, 38] may lead us to a better understanding. These workers have found that the pinocytotic activity of mouse macrophages increases in proportion to the concentration of foreign serum used in the culture medium. Different sera vary in their stimulatory effect, calf serum being among the most active. After 24 h in the presence of 50% new-born calf serum the pinocytotic activity was approximately 20 times greater than that produced by the same serum at a concentration of 1%. After 48 hours' exposure to the higher concentration, mouse macrophages showed an enormous increase in their content of various acid hydrolases. The changes are reversible,[38] suggesting that they are merely an expression of altered physiological activity.

Similar changes in the enzyme content of cells occurs *in vivo* when calf serum is introduced into the peritoneal cavity of a normal mouse.[36] Most significantly, the cells obtained 48 h after an intraperitoneal injection of 0.5 ml of foetal calf serum were found to possess microbicidal properties for *Salm. typhimurium* comparable with those found in the immune cells of actively infected mice.[20] It is inferred that the microbicidal ability of cells can be enhanced by non-immunological processes and that the physiological state of macrophages is markedly influenced by factors in their environment.

The foregoing discussion has focussed attention upon the fact that enhancement of the microbicidal ability of macrophages is accompanied by a coincident increase in the synthesis of lysosomal enzymes. A similar relationship between enzyme content and microbicidal activity has been demonstrated in macrophages stimulated with endotoxin.[8] Similar anatomical and chemical changes occur when lymphocytes from tuberculin-sensitive humans are exposed to tuberculin *in vitro*. Prior to mitosis the cell undergoes a morphological transformation involving, among other things, the development of cytoplasmic granules containing acid phosphatase.[85] Phytohaemagglutinin produces a similar effect on the lymphocytes of normal individuals.[86] More will be said of the significance of these observations in a later section. They are mentioned now merely to emphasise that antigenic stimulation of cells can produce changes in their physiological activity similar to those produced by infection.

It is of interest that macrophages from rabbits given intravenous injections of Triton WR 1339 can destroy ingested tubercle bacilli *in vitro*,[106] a fact which may explain the increased resistance to tuberculosis found in Triton-treated animals.[44] Since Triton WR 1339 has been shown to accumulate in the lysosomes of the Kupffer cells of treated rats,[182] it is probable that it would also be present in high concentration in the phagocytic vacuoles formed around tubercle bacilli ingested by rabbit macrophages. In this situation it would be favourably placed to comply with the suggestion of Hart and Rees,[81] that the anti-tuberculous properties of Triton may depend upon its ability to make the hydrophobic surface of the tubercle bacillus accessible to the innate antibacterial mechanisms of the cell. Fulton[70] has also reported evidence for enhanced resistance of Triton-treated hamsters to infection with *Leishmania donovani*, a protozoan intracellular parasite. This indicates that the effect of Triton is not specific for the tubercle bacillus. However, similar treatment of mice did not increase their resistance to *Listeria monocytogenes*.[20] This failure would seem to be due to the parasite and not to the host species, because Cornforth *et al.*[44] used mice in their original demonstration of the anti-tuberculous effect of Triton. These facts support the idea that Triton may merely supplement the normal anti-bacterial mechanisms of macrophages without causing any intrinsic change in cell function of the sort produced by endotoxin[8] or high concentrations of foreign serum.[36, 20]

It should not be inferred from the foregoing discussion that inactivation of organisms within macrophages is a simple process of enzymic degradation. All that can be said at present is that parallel changes have been observed in the enzymic and microbicidal potential of macrophages under a variety of conditions.

## B. The Immunological Basis of Acquired Cellular Resistance

The factors responsible for the changes which occur in the structure and function of macrophages during an infectious disease are not precisely known. There seems little doubt, however, that an immunological process is involved.[108]

There is always a delay before increased anti-microbial properties can be detected in the cells of animals infected for the first time with organisms known to induce this type of acquired resistance. This delay occurs regardless of the number of organisms injected. Resistant macrophages persist in the tissues for as long as the animal remains infected, but they rapidly disappear once the tissues have become sterile again. Resistance reappears more quickly during re-infection with the same organism, but develops at the normal rate if the re-infecting organism is unrelated to the one used to induce resistance in the first instance.[108] It can be said, therefore, that the recall of cellular resistance is immunologically specific.

Mice which have fully recovered from a listeria infection show this accelerated response to re-infection during the first 12 weeks of convalescence.

During this period, however, the time taken for resistance to be re-established increases progressively. By 12 weeks the animals have reverted to normal and are no longer hypersensitive to listeria antigens. In this and other respects immunity to *L. monocytogenes* resembles the second-set response to homografts of skin. The accelerated rejection of a second graft also diminishes with time,[157] and is antigenically specific.[112]

It is inferred from these and similar observations that infected animals respond immunologically during the initial stages of the infection and remain, for a time, hyper-reactive to antigens specific for the infecting organism. The immunological nature of the hyper-reactive state has not been clearly defined, but circumstantial evidence suggests that the delayed type of hypersensitivity which can be elicited in the immune animal is mediated by the same mechanism. Since delayed-type hypersensitivity is a recurrent theme in what is to follow, it should be understood that we refer to a form of immunological reactivity with the following features:

(1) A maximum local response 18 to 24 h after the injection of specific antigen,

(2) persistence of the response beyond this time,

(3) a mononuclear cell infiltrate at the reaction site,

(4) a dependence upon living cells for its passive transfer to normal recipients.

Hypersensitivity of this type occurs in mice infected with *L. monocytogenes*,[107] *Br. abortus*,[108, 96] and a variety of Salmonella species.[40, 137] In all of these infections a significant time relationship is found between the onset of hypersensitivity and the development of host resistance. Delayed-type hypersensitivity also occurs in every other infectious disease in which this type of anti-microbial resistance has been sought and found, e.g. tuberculosis[105, 161] and tularaemia.[165, 166] In none of these diseases has clear evidence been adduced for the passive transfer of resistance with serum. In some of them, however, resistance has been successfully transferred with cells.[151, 2, 144, 115] These facts are compatible with a mechanism similar to that involved in the mediation of delayed-type hypersensitivity. So also is the fact that immunisation with killed vaccines of *L. monocytogenes*[110, 1] or *Br. abortus*[110, 32] fails to induce delayed-type hypersensitivity and has little if any immediate effect on the level of host resistance.

It should be clearly understood that the foregoing observations, though tending to implicate a particular form of hypersensitivity, do not preclude the possibility that other types may also be involved. It is entirely possible, for instance, that an Arthus-type reaction at the infective focus could produce environmental conditions leading to a change in the physiological state of macrophages similar to that produced by a high concentration of foreign serum.[37] Inflammation, however, is not a necessary condition for the development of acquired cellular resistance. Following intravenous infection with *L. monocytogenes*[107] or *Br. abortus*,[108] the cells of the peritoneal cavity become profoundly altered in the absence of any local infection or evidence of an inflammatory reaction. Whatever the nature of the stimulus which produces the change in cells, its effects are felt in areas remote from the sites of active infection.

## C. The Role of Antigen in Acquired Cellular Resistance

Although it is clear that acquired cellular resistance to infectious agents requires the prior sensitisation of the host, hypersensitivity alone does not produce anti-microbial resistance. This occurs only in the presence of sustained antigenic stimulation. Three typical intracellular infections will be used to illustrate this point. After intravenous injection, *L. monocytogenes* produces an acute infectious disease. The bacterial population multiplies rapidly in the liver and spleen for a period of three days. Delayed-type hypersensitivity is first detected on the 4th day.[107] This coincides with the appearance of resistant macrophages in the peritoneal cavity, and the onset of bacterial inactivation in the tissues. Thereafter, the organisms are rapidly eliminated, and within a short time resistant cells disappear from the tissues. Hypersensitivity, however, persists for many weeks.[1] *Br. abortus* grows much more slowly in the spleen and liver, but delayed-type hypersensitivity appears by the 4th day of infection. However, the bacterial population continues to increase for a further 8 days. Thereafter, resistant macrophages appear in the peritoneal cavity. Similar changes are presumed to occur in the phagocytic cells of the spleen and liver, for at this time the viable count in these organs begins to decrease. When the bacterial population has been reduced to small proportions, host resistance and the proportion of resistant macrophages decrease, but the level of hypersensitivity continues to rise.[108]

Attenuated strains of *Myco. tuberculosis* also multiply slowly *in vivo*.[133] The rate of development of tuberculin sensitivity, however, is not clearly known. It was already firmly established when tests were first performed by Boyden[24] on the 11th day of a BCG infection in guinea pigs. There is reason to think, however, that it may develop much earlier than this. In animals injected with Freund's *complete* adjuvant, Shaw *et al.*[152] found that tuberculin sensitivity was clearly evident 4 days after immunisation. Although tuberculin sensitivity probably develops very early in BCG-infected mice, significant numbers of highly resistant cells may never appear in the peritoneal cavity.[110] A BCG infection differs from the other two in one important respect: The number of infecting organisms always remains relatively small.[133]

All of the foregoing observations are consistent with the view that delayed-type hypersensitivity develops on or about the 4th day of immunisation, but that host-resistance and cell changes do not develop until the bacterial population has reached critical dimensions. This suggests that one factor in determining the level of host resistance is the intensity of the antigenic stimulation it is receiving. Many observations support this view. For example, the injection of a large number of BCG into BCG-sensitised mice causes a prompt and marked increase in the level of host resistance to challenge with *L. monocytogenes*. No such effect is seen when the same dose of BCG is injected into unsensitised animals.[108, 109] It is consistent with this observation that host resistance in BCG-vaccinated animals does not develop until the virulent organisms of the challenge infection have had time to multiply.[104] The re-injection of *Br. abortus* into mice with a latent brucella infection causes a sudden drop in the number of residual organisms persisting in the tissues. Even dead organisms, though incapable of influencing resistance in normal animals, have a similar effect on organisms surviving in the tissues of minimally infected mice. They are so effective, in fact, that a latent infection may be abolished by this manoeuvre.[110]

The level of host resistance in Salmonella-infected mice appears to be controlled in a similar way. Mice which have been actively infected with a standard dose of *Salm. typhimurium* commonly show a wide variation in the numbers of organisms present in the tissues at any one time. When a group of such mice were challenged with *L. monocytogenes*, an inverse relationship was found between the numbers of *Salm. typhimurium* and *L. monocytogenes* present in the liver and spleen 4 and 28 h later. The larger the number of Salmonella present, the more rapid was the inactivation of *L. monocytogenes*.[21] A similar phenomenon was observed in mice infected with *Salm. montevideo*. Since this organism persists in the tissues at a level which varies according to the infecting dose, it is possible to produce experimental infections in which the numbers of organisms in the tissues can be varied over a wide range. When animals were injected with different infecting doses of *Salm. montevideo* and were subsequently challenged with virulent *Salm. enteritidis*, it was found that resistance to the challenge infection varied inversely with the size of the resident population of *Salm. montevideo*.[41] In both of the foregoing experiments the organisms used to challenge were antigenically unrelated to the immunising organism, so that the variation in the level of host resistance could not have been due to differences in antibody titer, nor to stimulation of sensitised cells by the antigens of the challenging organism. The observed differences must be attributed, therefore, to inequalities in the intensity of the stimulus provided by microbial populations of differing size. This adds further emphasis to the importance of antigenic stimulation as a factor in determining the level of host resistance.

### D. The Mechanism of Macrophage Stimulation

The scant attention that has been given to this aspect of acquired cellular resistance is regrettable. Much of the evidence relating to the stimulation of cells of the reticulo-endothelial system by microbial antigens concerns the effects of bacterial endotoxin. Unfortunately, the validity of using this evidence in the present context is questionable, since we are not yet entirely certain that all of the biological effects of endotoxin have an immunological basis. It is true, however, that germ-free animals[93] and specific pathogen-free mice[93, 149] are highly resistant to the effects of endotoxin, but acquire the sensitivity of conventional animals after exposure to the full gamut of their microbial flora.[93] It seems likely, then, that some effects of endotoxin are due to immunological sensitisation. If we can assume with Stetson[158] that the mechanism involved is basically a delayed type of hypersensitivity, it is possible to discuss the host's response to endotoxin as an illustration of the effect of microbial antigens on sensitised tissues. Since this subject has engaged the attention of many workers for many years, what follows is an eclectic's view of a highly complex subject.

The effect of most bacterial endotoxins on the cells of the reticuloendothelial system can range from a mild stimulation of physiological activity[184] to one of frank destruction.[64] The end effect depends, among other things, upon the dose of endotoxin and the sensitivity of the subject.

A subcutaneous injection of 0.1 $LD_{50}$ of endotoxin severely damages the free macrophages in the peritoneal cavity of normal mice.[64] Within a few hours free macrophages may disappear completely and remain absent from the peritoneal fluid for 48 h or more. It is presumed that phagocytic cells elsewhere in the tissues are similarly affected, thus accounting both for the faulty blood clearance of particulate material and the increased susceptibility to infection that is found soon after treatment with endotoxin. The cytolytic effect of endotoxin is less significant, however, than its stimulatory effects. Small doses of endotoxin produce an increase in metabolic activity,[192] an increased rate of DNA synthesis,[64] a rise in acid phosphatase content[8] and a general increase in phagocytic and microbicidal activity.[8]

These effects of endotoxin on mononuclear phagocytes are significant in relation to the problem of acquired cellular resistance, for similar changes occur when microbial antigens other than endotoxin are injected into specifically sensitised animals. The macrophages of tuberculous animals, which are the subject of constant antigenic stimulation, show a similar augmentation of their metabolic and functional activities,[105] and an increase in their content of acid hydrolases.[145] In regard to the latter, it is interesting to note from the studies of Saito and Suter[145] that the enzyme content of mouse macrophages begins to increase on the 8th day of a BCG injection. By 10 to 14 days the peritoneal macrophages and the blood plasma show a twofold or greater increase in their content of acid phosphatase, protease and β-glucuronidase. The content of acid phosphatase and lipase in the alveolar phagocytes of animals repeatedly injected with BCG is also increased to a similar extent.[39] The injection of tuberculin or endotoxin causes a further, and highly significant, increase in the level of certain acid hydrolases in the serum of BCG-infected animals.[145] This presumably reflects the hyperplasia and increased enzyme content of phagocytic cells in the tissues of the infected animals. It also draws attention to the sensitivity of these cells to the lytic effects of endotoxin.

As was mentioned in a previous section, the treatment of lymphocytes with an antigen to which they are specifically sensitised leads to a build-up in lysosomal acid phosphatase prior to mitosis.[85, 86] The mitotic rate of macrophages in animals infected with BCG does not appear to have been studied; but the macrophages of animals infected with L. monocytogenes and Br. abortus show a progressive increase in mitotic activity during the course of infection.[96] Furthermore, the injection of specific antigens in the form of living organisms or culture filtrates leads to a further sudden increase in mitotic activity.[96, 109] It is not intended to argue a causal relationship between a rising enzyme content and cell division.[3] Nevertheless a progressive increase in enzyme levels and mitotic rates occurs in cells stimulated with antigen in vitro. This seems to be analogous to similar changes which occur in the macrophages of sensitised animals under the influence of antigenic stimulation in vivo, changes which are attended by an increase in their microbicidal ability.

The relationship of the foregoing phenomena to the state of delayed-type hypersensitivity is suggested by the observation[65] that a subcutaneous injection of bovine serum albumin into mice sensitised by immunisation with Freund's *complete* adjuvant, produces a similar mitotic response in peritoneal macrophages. This response does not occur in mice immunised with soluble antigen,[110] a procedure which does not normally lead to the production of delayed-type hypersensitivity (Section III, B).

### E. TRANSFER OF RESISTANCE BETWEEN CELLS

The passive transfer of a form of cellular resistance has been reported by two groups of workers. Fong and his collaborators[62, 60, 63, 61, 59] have found that the ability of both rabbit and mouse macrophages to resist the necrotising effect of virulent tubercle bacilli *in vitro* could be transferred to the cells of a normal animal by the injection of living immune cells or ribosomes from these cells,[60, 61] and by ribosomal RNA itself.[60] Trypsin treatment of immune macrophages rendered them as susceptible as normal cells to the necrotising effect of tubercle bacilli, yet their resistance could be restored with anti-mycobacterial, anti-brucella or anti-salmonella serum, suggesting that a nonspecific surface protein may be responsible.[63, 161] There was no interspecies barrier between the mouse, the rabbit and the guinea pig in that the two former could be used as donors of immune cells, or cell extracts, for transferring resistance to the cells of recipient guinea pigs, mice or rabbits.[61] However, one of the puzzling features of these experiments was the anomalous behaviour of guinea pig macrophages. Though demonstrated to acquire anti-tuberculous resistance during a BCG infection, these cells were unable to confer their resistance upon the cells of rabbits, mice, or even other guinea pigs. Yet guinea pig macrophages which had acquired their resistance passively from immune mouse or rabbit cells, *were* capable of transferring resistance.[61] Inconsistencies of this sort require further explanation.

Another difficulty concerns the specificity of the mechanisms involved in Fong's experimental model. The macrophages and sub-cellular fractions obtained from rabbits immunised with BCG were found to confer on normal rabbit macrophages, resistance to both virulent tubercle bacilli and virulent brucellae. However, brucella-immune cells, although themselves resistant to both organisms were unable to confer this ability on other cells.[62] The latter differed from BCG-immune cells in an additional way. Whereas virulent tubercle bacilli were said to undergo attenuation within BCG-immune cells, no such effect was seen with cells obtained from brucella-infected animals.[59]

The durable nature of the "transfer factor" in BCG-immune cells or ribosomal fractions thereof, was demonstrated by its serial passage through rabbits. Its effect persisted in normal recipients for a period of 6 months. However, resistance transferred with RNA from immune cells was not so enduring. Though fully effective in the first recipient, resistance conferred in this way could not be passed on to other cells.[62]

The resistance of immune macrophages to the cytotoxic effects of intra-cellular tubercle bacilli or brucellae, described above, has not been demonstrated to depend upon any increase in the microbicidal ability of cells which have been rendered resistant passively; nor have their altered properties *in vitro* been examined for an effect on host resistance *in vivo*. In the circumstances it is difficult to see how they relate to an immune mechanism based on a change in the physiological activity of macrophages and dependent upon antigenic stimulation of specifically sensitised tissues.

A transfer factor similar to that described by Fong and his collaborators (also RNA in nature) has been reported by a group of Japanese workers.[118, 143, 148] In these studies *Salm. enteritidis* was used as the test organism. It was found that resistance to damage by intracellular *Salm. enteritidis* could be conferred on mouse macrophages by ribonuclease-sensitive extracts obtained from immune cells. It is possible that this example of cell resistance can be explained by the induction of antibody synthesis. This is suggested by the finding of Gelzer and Suter[71] that anti-somatic antibody to *Salm. typhimurium* will protect mouse macrophages from the cytotoxic effects of this organism. However, the results of Fong and his co-workers are difficult to interpret in this way because of the haphazard nature of the cross-resistance and transferability that seems to exist between the bacterial and animal species so far employed.

# IV. DELAYED-TYPE HYPERSENSITIVITY

The next question of importance concerns the nature of the immune response that forms the basis of the anti-microbial form of acquired cellular immunity. Reasons have already been given for believing that the state of delayed-type hypersensitivity may be an essential part of the immune mechanism. This provides yet another reason for wishing to know more about the nature of delayed-type hypersensitivity.

Whenever serum fails to effect the passive transfer of a particular immunological reaction, its mediation is usually ascribed to cells. However, the mere fact that reactivity can be transferred with living lymphoid cells leaves unanswered the question of whether or not antibody is involved.[159] Nor does it establish that the transferred cells themselves actually participate in the immunological reaction. Great ingenuity has been exercised in efforts to decide whether they do or not. It seems that a good case has been made for the active participation of transferred lymphoid cells in the tuberculin reaction.[123, 57] But in other instances, the evidence to date rejects the notion that the transferred cells themselves are the vectors by which the immune state is distributed systemically throughout the passively sensitised recipient. This has been concluded from experiments with labelled cells from sensitised donors. Experiments of this sort have failed to show a preferential accumulation of transferred cells in skin grafts[124, 125] or a reaction site in subjects which have been adoptively immunised against haptenic sensitising agents.[125] Despite this disappointment, the conviction remains that the ability to react is in some way associated with cells.

We have seen in connection with acquired cellular resistance to microbial parasites a need for specific antibody. Its role is to confer on the free and fixed cells of the reticulo-endothelial system the sensitivity to microbial antigens which is necessary for the induction of cell changes. Two classes of antibody molecule qualify for this role by virtue of their affinity for the surface of mononuclear cells. The first is the so-called cytophilic antibody of Boyden and Sorkin.[29, 30, 26] Although this antibody has not yet been characterised, it is said to constitute no more than 1 per cent of the free antibody of serum. The other possible mediator is $\gamma$M-immunoglobulin; this molecular species of antibody also qualifies by virtue of its ability to become attached to the surface of mononuclear phagocytes. It is pertinent, therefore, to examine these two classes of antibody more closely for a possible role in the mediation of delayed-type hypersensitivity.

Boyden[28] has demonstrated in guinea pigs the production of a cytophilic antibody to red cell antigens. It could be detected on macrophages or in the serum of immunised animals only when Freund's *complete* adjuvant had been used for immunisation. It was never found in animals which did not respond to homologous red cell antigens with hypersensitivity reactions of delayed type. The antibody was detected by virtue of its ability to cause the adherence of homologous red cells to the macrophages of immunised subjects or of normal subjects after treatment with immune serum. Tests conducted on immune cells in the presence of normal serum were negative, suggesting that cytophilic antibody combines reversibly with cells and can exchange with free antibody present in the serum.

The co-existence of cytophilic antibody and the state of delayed-type hypersensitivity is of great theoretical interest. So, too, is another important finding: neither of these responses occurred when mycobacteria were omitted from the immunising mixture. In their absence, high titers of haemagglutinating antibody and Arthus-type hypersensitivity developed. In Boyden's experimental model the hypersensitivity to red cell antigens was exclusively of delayed-type during the early stages of sensitisation. At this time, no haemagglutinating antibody could be detected in the serum.[28] When it did appear, an Arthus component was added and the hypersensitivity displayed the features of a compound reaction involving immediate and delayed reactions. The same theme will constantly recur: When some or all of the antibody is bound to cell surfaces, a delayed component is found in the sensitivity reaction.

This concept of delayed-type hypersensitivity is consistent with all its known features. If we assume that cells bearing antibody of appropriate specificity are free to circulate, it follows that eventually some will pass in the vicinity of the corresponding antigen in a skin test site, a homograft or any other immunological target. In effect, the immunological reagent (bound to cells) arrives at the reaction site one quantum at a time. If antibody were delivered in this manner the tempo of local events would be much slower than in immediate-type reactions in which excess antibody is available to combine with antigen as rapidly as diffusion rates permit.

The cytophilic antibody described above seems to differ in one respect from another antibody-like substance with similar potential as a mediator of delayed-type hypersensitivity. It has been suspected for some time that mononuclear cells from animals showing delayed-type hypersensitivity to microbial antigens show specific sensitivity when exposed to them *in vitro*.[56, 177] This subject has created much interest of late through the studies of David and his collaborators.[47, 48, 49, 50] These authors, in reviewing previous work, point out that tests conducted on isolated mononuclear phagocytes *in vitro* have often revealed an effect of antigen that could be correlated with the state of delayed-hypersensitivity in the cell donor. But the low sensitivity and apparent lack of specificity have detracted from the significance of earlier observations. Adapting the method of George and Vaughan,[72] David and co-workers have devised a much more sensitive test. In essence, it measures the inhibitory influence of antigen on the centrifugal migration of aggregated macrophages from hypersensitive subjects. There is reason to think that the test is a subtle measure of the agglutinating effect of antigen on specifically sensitised macrophages. This is suggested by the finding that re-aggregation of cells occurs when antigen is introduced *after* the macrophages have become separated from each other by migration.[47] (An entirely analogous phenomenon occurs when listeria antigens are introduced into dispersed monolayers of macrophages from specifically sensitised mice.[110]) Trypsinisation of sensitive cells destroys their ability to respond in this test.[50] However, continued incubation restores their reactivity, indicating that antibody at the cell surface is replenished, but its source is still unknown. Sensitivity to antigen can be passively conferred on normal macrophages by the admixture of a very small percentage of cells from a sensitised donor.[49] This implies that the majority of cells in any population acquire their reactivity by passive means, perhaps from cells engaged in active synthesis of antibody. This form of reactivity, like that described by Boyden, is specific, and present only in animals appropriately immunised for the production of delayed-type hypersensitivity. The reaction appears to differ from that described by Boyden in that serum will not passively confer reactivity upon normal cells. This difference should not be over-emphasised, for Boyden's test is conducted at 4°C and in the absence of serum. It is possible that antibody adsorbed at this temperature by cells maintained in the absence of serum would not be degraded or exchanged during the period of test. In the method used by David and co-workers, passively adsorbed antibody could be destroyed at 37°C, or be exchanged for antibody of different specificity under the experimental conditions used.

These two experimental systems provide an important link between the state of delayed-type hypersensitivity and the development of acquired cellular resistance by animals stimulated with microbial antigens to which they are sensitised. Their importance rests upon the unequivocal fact that the presence of *circulating* antibody of the same specificity does not automatically confer reactivity upon host macrophages. This occurs only under special conditions of immunisation. And as we have seen, acquired cellular resistance does not develop when animals are immunised with dead vaccines that do not produce delayed-type hypersensitivity. Further discussion of the significance of cell-bound antibody in relation to acquired cellular resistance will be deferred until the nature of this antibody has been considered in more detail (Section V, B).

# V. THE ANTI-TISSUE FORM OF CELLULAR IMMUNITY

The similarities between transplantation immunity and tuberculin-type hypersensitivity have received frequent comment and critical appraisal.[112, 103, 159, 5] There are three points of comparison: (1) Both types of immunity depend for their induction upon special conditions of immunisation; (2) sensitivity reactions to microbial and histocompatibility antigens are similar in all their features; (3) in most instances, there is a requirement for living cells in the adoptive transfer of the reactive state from immune donor to normal recipient. Although this sharing of common characteristics is not sufficient in itself to establish the identity of these two forms of immunity, it does provide a basis for further discussion of important problems relating to the anti-microbial and anti-tissue forms of cellular immunity.

## A. THE INDUCTION OF ANTI-TISSUE IMMUNITY

It should be recalled at the outset that the induction of acquired cellular resistance to infectious agents, and of delayed-type hypersensitivity to the corresponding microbial antigens, usually requires the use of living vaccines or a method of immunisation that makes use of special adjuvant mixtures. It is highly significant that similar conditions of immunisation apply to the induction of anti-tissue immunity. The first indication of this stems from the recognition that a marked difference exists in the nature of the immune response obtained by immunisation with living and dead tissue. Early studies showed that grafts of living tissue provoked an immune response leading to accelerated graft rejection and the appearance of delayed-type hypersensitivity to specific transplantation antigens.[112] Dead tissues, on the other hand, produced an abundance of haemagglutinating antibodies of the same specificity, but no evidence of transplantation immunity.[17, 155] More recent studies with transplantable tumours have shown that the immune response to lyophilised tissue is, in fact, biphasic.[34] The first phase is associated with evidence of heightened resistance; the second with a more permanent state of graft enhancement. The significance of the biphasic character of the immune response to transplantation antigens will be considered later in relation to the two established phases of antibody production.

The second indication that anti-tissue immunity requires special conditions of immunisation emerged from efforts to produce experimental autoimmune disease. It was recognised historically that soluble antigens seldom give rise to an unequivocal form of delayed-type hypersensitivity. When incorporated in Freund's *complete* adjuvant, however, protein antigens were known to produce the classical features of delayed-type hypersensitivity.[136] It is not important that hypersensitivity produced in this way is usually accompanied by Arthus reactivity as well.[28] What is significant is that the immune response becomes changed in character when the antigen is presented in a special way. The fundamental significance of this has been clearly demonstrated by experiments designed to establish the optimal conditions necessary for the induction of experimental auto-immune disease. The incorporation of thyroid or brain tissue in Freund's *complete* adjuvant leads to the production of delayed-type hypersensitivity to thyroglobulin[139] or the basic protein antigen of myelin sheath;[152] and, *pari passu*, to the development of experimental thyroiditis or experimental allergic encephalomyelitis (EAE). The study of these two experimental diseases has been particularly rewarding.

Close enquiry into the immunising conditions necessary for the induction of EAE has revealed a counter influence between the immune responses provoked by the same antigen administered in two forms. Brain extracts injected in Freund's *complete* adjuvant, or its equivalent,[153] leads to demyelinating disease. The omission of mycobacteria from the adjuvant mixture not only fails to induce the disease, but actively protects against its subsequent production by a procedure that would otherwise be effective.[4] This is only one of many instances of immunological interference. It is presumed in this case that the primary response to antigen and *incomplete* adjuvant was not merely lacking in some essential quality necessary for the production of lesions, but was actively antagonistic to the effector mechanism responsible for demyelination. An explanation of the protective effect of prior immunisation with *incomplete* adjuvant seems to have been supplied by the work of Paterson and his collaborators.[131, 132] These workers have shown that serum from animals immunised with *incomplete* adjuvant will passively protect normal recipients against the induction of EAE. The protective serum has been shown to contain a $\gamma_2$-globulin that fixes complement in the presence of brain extracts. In an earlier study[164] an inverse relationship had been found between the titer of this antibody in the serum and the incidence of demyelinating lesions in the central nervous system of dogs. In addition, two strains of rats were found which differed in their susceptibility to the induction of EAE.[132] This difference between strains was related to their relative capacities to produce the protective antibody. Moreover the disease could not be induced for a second time in rats which had developed complement-fixing anti-brain antibody in their serum at the time of recovery. These observations point to the existence of a species of antibody molecule which can actively interfere with the process of demyelination.

The immunological induction of experimental allergic thyroiditis appears to be basically similar. Here, too, lesions seldom arise unless Freund's *complete* adjuvant is used for immunisation.[139] Even the use of alum precipitated antigen does not suffice for the induction of thyroiditis.

Having said that the induction of an immunological attack upon intact tissues requires conditions of immunisation similar to those required for the induction of acquired cellular resistance to microbial parasites, it is necessary to consider the peculiarities of the immune response that are attributable to the addition of mycobacteria to Freund-type adjuvants.

## B. The Mediation of Anti-Tissue Reactions

The tissue reaction resulting from the use of Freund's *complete* adjuvant has been described in detail.[68, 7, 150] The most significant feature is the intense stimulation of mononuclear phagocytes that is produced by the addition of mycobacteria to the immunising emulsion, resulting in the formation of epi-thelioid-cell granulomas at the injection site and in remote tissues. This type of tissue reaction is common to most devices that have been used for the induction of delayed-type hypersensitivity.[52, 150, 136]

Although it is commonly accepted that antibody titers tend to be higher following immunisation with Freund's *complete* adjuvant than they are when mycobacteria or other microbial extracts are omitted from the adjuvant mix-ture, the difference in titer is often not conspicuous.[28] There are, however, marked differences of another sort. *Complete* adjuvant tends to promote the production of $7S\gamma_2$-immunoglobulins of slow electrophoretic mobility. Im-munisation without adjuvant, on the other hand, results predominantly in the production of a fast moving $7S$ $\gamma_1$-immunoglobulin.[14] Since there are marked differences in the biological properties of these two classes of anti-body,[22] the predominance of one or the other may explain some of the observed differences in the type of immunological reactivity that results from these two methods of immunisation. But there is no known relationship between either of these two classes of 7S antibody and the state of delayed-type hy-persensitivity; nor is there any established tendency for either of them to be adsorbed to cell surfaces. For these reasons it seems necessary to look for some other difference to explain the induction of delayed-type hypersensitivity with adjuvants containing mycobacteria or other microbial products.[153]

Immunisation with Freund's *complete* adjuvant has been shown to pro-mote a greater and more sustained production of 19S γ-M-immunoglobulin.[150] In searching for the mediator of delayed-type hypersensitivity reactions and the immunological processes that they control, a role for macroglobulin anti-bodies deserves very close scrutiny.[159] A relationship in time and an affinity for cell surfaces are the main reasons for directing attention to 19S antibody as a likely mediator of this form of immunological reactivity.

There is no need to emphasise that γM-immunoglobulin is produced exclusively during the initial stages of the immune response to most antigens. Its production appears to continue so long as antigenic stimulation persists.[171, 163] Some antigens produce predominantly this type of antibody[12, 102] but others do not produce it at all.[128] The kinetics of γM- and γG-antibody production vary from one antigen to another and are affected by its physical form and the route of inoculation. In general, however, the initiation of γM-immuno-globulin synthesis is very rapid.[170, 162, 163] Cells actively producing this antibody have been detected within 8 to 15 h of the administration of antigen,[102, 121, 187] while its presence in the serum has been detected within 2 to 3 days. These facts are important in relation to the rate of appearance of delayed-type hypersensitivity.

Uhr, Salvin and Pappenheimer[173] showed that small amounts of diphtheria toxoid or of ovalbumin complexed with homologous antibody, are capable of inducing delayed-type hypersensitivity in guinea pigs. Skin sensitivity could be detected by the 4th day, and sometimes persisted for 6 weeks or more in the absence of detectable antibody. This state of hypersensitivity could be adoptively transferred with lymph node cells. Salvin[146] studied the rate of development of delayed-type hypersensitivity in relation to serum antibody titers following the injection of varying, but small, amounts of protein antigen in Freund's *incomplete* adjuvant. There was a latent period of 2 to 4 days before delayed-type sensitivity could be elicited. Skin sensitivity remained exclusively of delayed-type for a varying period. The duration of this phase of the immune response varied inversely with the dose of antigen. An extremely small dose produced a relatively protracted state of pure delayed-type hypersensitivity. Progressively larger doses produced an immune response that gave way with increasing rapidity to an Arthus-type of hypersensitivity. These findings are extremely interesting in relation to the kinetics of $\gamma$M-globulin production.

The use of sensitive methods of assay have revealed that $\gamma$M-globulin alone is produced when the dose of antigen is sufficiently small.[170] If the antigenic stimulus is sustained at a low level, production of this class of antibody may continue indefinitly, but if larger doses are used synthesis usually switches to the production of $\gamma$G-immunoglobulins. The observations of Salvin on the sequential changes in skin reactivity can be readily explained if delayed-type hypersensitivity and Arthus sensitivity are mediated respectively by $\gamma$M- and $\gamma$G-immunoglobulins.

There is a further argument in support of this view. Salvin and Smith[147] have shown that the development of Arthus sensitivity can be suppressed by doses of X-irradiation which do not influence the development of delayed-type hypersensitivity to diphtheria toxoid. This is significant in view of the finding of Svehag and Mandel[163] that 19S antibody production is resistant to doses of X-irradiation sufficient to suppress the production of 7S antibody.

It would be convenient at this stage to consider several studies in which a relationship has been established between the rate of development of delayed-type hypersensitivity and the appearance of the anti-microbial or anti-tissue forms of cellular immunity.

During primary infection of mice with *L. monocytogenes* the parasite multiplies progressively in the tissues for the first three days. By the 4th day the host develops classical delayed-type hypersensitivity to listeria antigens, and a high percentage of its macrophages become resistant to infection *in vitro*. At this time the parasite ceases to multiply. The type of antibody responsible for host resistance has not been identified for want of an appropriate test; however, neither agglutinins nor precipitating antibodies can be detected in the serum at this or later stages of infection.[107] In analogy with what is known of the immune response to most antigens, it is a reasonable assumption that the onset of delayed sensitivity and of acquired cellular resistance occurs at a time when the immune response is in the phase of 19S antibody production.

Essentially the same conclusion can be reached from recent studies showing a correlation between delayed-type hypersensitivity to a basic protein component of myelin and the development of experimental allergic encephalomyelitis.[152] Immunisation was performed with purified encephalitogenic agent incorporated in Freund's *complete* adjuvant. Delayed-type hypersensitivity to this antigen (and to tuberculo-protein as well) first appeared on the 4th day following immunisation; it increased in intensity until the 10th or 12th day. A strong correlation was found between the intensity of the hypersensitivity on day 10 and the incidence and severity of the demyelinating lesions which subsequently developed. Animals which failed to develop skin sensitivity uniformly failed to develop EAE. Those with mild reactions failed to develop clinical signs, but showed microscopic evidence of demyelination. Parallel studies[4] revealed that induction of EAE and delayed-type hypersensitivity were both suppressed when animals were pre-treated by the injection of the encephalitogenic protein in *incomplete* adjuvant.

This raises questions regarding the nature of the inhibitory effect of prior immunisation with antigen presented in a non-sensitising form. As mentioned previously, Paterson and co-workers[132] have demonstrated a protective effect of serum containing complement-fixing anti-brain antibodies. The precise identity of the antibody responsible for inhibiting the immunological attack is not known, though Alvord *et al.*[4] have presented evidence that it is specific for the encephalitogenic protein. The expressed view[130] that it is a 19S antibody is not convincing, since the evidence depends mainly upon sensitivity to 2-mercaptoethanol which can interfere with complement fixation by 7S antibody.[185] Moreover, the protective antisera were not specific for the encephalitogenic agent; they must be presumed to have contained antibodies to other brain antigens as well.

The presence of circulating antibody to tuberculo-protein has been shown to suppress the development of a delayed skin reaction to this antigen. Boyden[24] found that prior immunisation with a purified protein derivative of tuberculin prevented the development of tuberculin sensitivity in guinea pigs infected with BCG; the pre-immunised animals developed, instead, an Arthus-type of hypersensitivity. The same phenomenon has been demonstrated by Crowle and Hu[45] who found that passive transfer of humoral antibody, or prior immunisation with soluble antigen, effectively prevented the induction of delayed-type hypersensitivity to ovalbumin or bovine serum albumin when animals were subsequently immunised with water-in-oil emulsions. Here, as in Salvin's experiments, the presence of precipitating antibody, actively or passively acquired, produced Arthus-type hypersensitivity and suppressed the development of delayed-type hypersensitivity.

There are two ways in which circulating antibody could interfere with the development of delayed-type hypersensitivity mediated by $\gamma$M-immunoglobulin. One is by direct combination with the eliciting dose of antigen thereby preventing its subsequent interaction with antibody attached to cells. Direct evidence that interference can occur in this way is to be discussed later. Another, and potentially more significant mechanism depends upon the inhibitory effect of 7S antibody on the synthesis of 19S antibody. The passive administration of 7S antibody to phage $\phi$X174, when given 3 days after immunisation, was shown by Finkelstein and Uhr[58] to depress the 19S and abolish the 7S antibody response in guinea pigs. Möller and Wigzell,[121] investigating this phenomenon at the cellular level, found that 7S antibody to sheep red cells, if given prior to immunisation, completely prevents the appearance of plaque-forming cells in the spleen. Since the plaquing technique of Jerne appears to detect only cells producing 19S antibody, it was concluded that 7S antibody interferes in some way with the induction of cells capable of synthesising 19S antibody. If 19S antibody is the mediator of delayed-type hypersensitivity, as the time of its appearance suggests, the effect of prior immunisation or of passive serum transfer on the development of delayed-type hypersensitivity is plausibly explained by the suppressive effect of 7S antibody on the synthesis of 19S antibody.

## C. CELLULAR TRANSPORTATION OF ANTIBODY

There is no doubt that antibody, in one form or another, enters into the mechanism of anti-tissue immunity. The arguments for the direct involvement of antibody in graft rejection have been well stated by Stetson,[159] but there are many serious impediments to acceptance of the simple proposition that cytotoxic antibody, in conjunction with complement, is sufficient in itself to explain all the phenomena of anti-tissue immunity. It is true that dissociated cellular grafts which are completely sensitive to the cytolytic effects of iso-antibody *in vitro* are effectively prevented from establishing themselves in recipients protected passively with immune serum.[95] But what is true of dissociated cells cannot be unreservedly applied to solid vascularised grafts, or to the immunological destruction of intact organs *in situ*. Excellent reasons exist for thinking that antibody and complement, regardless of their cytolytic potential, do not gain ready access by diffusion to the constituent cells of solid tissues.[159, 5] Solid tissues are nonetheless vulnerable to immunological destruction. Delayed-type hypersensitivity, experimental auto-allergic disease and transplantation immunity can all be adoptively transferred between compatible donors with modest numbers of living lymphoid cells. This must surely signify that the antibodies which mediate these reactions are functionally available in the recipient of immune cells to a degree which cannot be reproduced by the passive transfer of immune serum. It is the business of immunologists to explain the reason for this.

The fact that reactive cells implanted in the skin can impart local sensitivity at the site of implantation[113] indicates that the transferred cells themselves can mediate a delayed-type hypersensitivity reaction *in situ*. But their ability to confer cutaneous hypersensitivity after intravenous injection[35, 13] demands something more. The transferred cells must enter the reaction site themselves, as has been claimed[123] and denied[167] in the case of tuberculin sensitivity, or they must synthesise a recognition factor which reaches the reaction site by some other means. That something is actively synthesised after cell transfer is suggested by the finding of Bloom *et al.*[23] who showed that the transfer of hypersensitivity with active cells was prevented by their prior treatment with mitomycin C. However, the crucial question is not so much concerned with antibody synthesis as with its mode of transport to the site of an eliciting dose of antigen in the skin, a graft of foreign tissue or a target tissue in auto-immune disease.

It is improbable that the effective antibody formed after adoptive immunisation is free in the serum. If it were, it should also exist in the serum of a sensitive donor at a far greater concentration than is achieved in the serum of cell recipients. Yet the serum of sensitive donors is usually inert in the passive transfer of these forms of immunological reactivity. The only alternative is to suppose that the antibody is transported in or on the formed elements of the blood.

We believe that it is important to distinguish between antibody that is transported by cells which are actively engaged in the synthesis of antibody, and cells which have acquired reactive antibody by passive adsorption. There is ample evidence that cells do serve as "active" or "passive" vectors of antibody.

(1) CELLS AS "PASSIVE" VECTORS. Reasons have been given for believing that the delayed reactions which can be elicited for varying intervals after immunisation with small antigenic stimuli are mediated by γM-immunoglobulins. To sustain this argument it would be necessary to establish that 19S antibody can attach itself to a convenient cell population. Although the evidence for this is not extensive there is no doubt that γM-immunoglobulin is particularly prone to adhere to cell surfaces, and to the surface of monocytes and macrophages in particular. The most direct demonstration of the passive adsorption of 19S antibody by macrophages is contained in the studies of Turner, Jenkin and Rowley.[169] These workers showed in mice that the antibodies synthesised during the first two weeks of infection with an attenuated strain of *Salm. typhimurium* were exclusively γM-immunoglobulins. During this period large amounts of 19S antibody could be eluted from the peritoneal cells of the infected mice.[142] The adsorbed antibody was shown, by density gradient centrifugation and sensitivity to 2-mercaptoethanol, to be a 19S immunoglobulin. Treatment of macrophages with trypsin destroyed their opsonic activity for *Salm. typhimurium*, but this could be restored by re-suspending the cells in immune serum containing 19S antibody. Late in the infection, when 7S antibody alone was present in the serum, there was no indication of antibody activity associated with macrophages.

The observations of Friedman[69] in relation to 19S and 7S anti-ø X antibody are also relevant. Normal rabbit lymph node cells were treated with immune serum containing either 19S or 7S antibodies. After 5 washings at 4°C antibody activity could be eluted at 37°C from cells treated with 19S antibody, but not from those treated with 7S antibody.

The decay rates of passively transferred antibody show differences in the catabolic destruction of 19S and 7S antibody.[55] What is more significant, however, is the biphasic nature of the decay curve of passively transferred 19S antibody.[162] The first phase of its disappearance after passive transfer is short lived, but very steep. The rapid initial fall in 19S antibody titer cannot be accounted for by simple equilibration with extracellular fluid since 7S antibody, though smaller in molecular weight, disappears much more slowly during equilibration. A more likely explanation is that during this period the specific macroglobulin antibody exchanges with a larger pool of cell-associated macroglobulins of different specificity. Presumably the process occurs on cell surfaces exposed to the circulation. This would include most of the elements of the reticulo-endothelial system.

Many other observations indicate that antibody is carried on the surface of macrophages. It has already been noted that trypsin destroys the capacity of macrophages to respond to antigen in the macrophage immobilisation test described by David *et al.*[50] Additional indications of specific reactivity in macrophages include the following observations: The mononuclear phagocytes of tuberculin-sensitive animals disappear from the free fluid of the peritoneal cavity (by adherence to serosal surfaces) when tuberculin is injected subcutaneously into sensitised guinea pigs.[126] A similar reaction occurs when animals have been sensitised to protein antigens; but it occurs only when the animal has been immunised with Freund's *complete* adjuvant and shows delayed-type hypersensitivity. Lymphocytes do not participate in the peritoneal response to antigen.[126] A proteolytic enzyme is released into the medium when pure cultures of macrophages from immunised animals are exposed to specific antigen *in vitro*.[82] A cell-fixed antibody has been detected in the blood of tuberculin-sensitive human subjects. The antibody, which is haemagglutinating, correlates quantitatively with the level of cutaneous hypersensitivity.[67] Pure cultures of macrophages from mice which have been immunised with bovine serum albumin (BSA) showed an increased rate of DNA synthesis when exposed to BSA *in vitro*.[141] The macrophages of immunised mice have been shown to adhere specifically to target cells in monolayer cultures, to lyse them and be themselves destroyed in the process[79] (Section VI. B. 2).

Mention has been made of only a few of the many observations which show that mononuclear phagocytes can acquire specific immunological reactivity. Some of these observations leave no doubt that their reactivity is passively acquired. Indeed there is no acceptable evidence that cells of the monocyte-macrophage series are capable of antibody synthesis.

(2) CELLS AS "ACTIVE" VECTORS. Gowans and McGregor[77] have reviewed the evidence which establishes that immunologically committed cells are present in peripheral blood. These are cells which have been primed for the synthesis of specific immunoglobulin. The unequivocal identification of such cells in the systemic circulation calls for positive demonstration of their ability to synthesise antibody molecules. This has been done by Hulliger and Sorkin[90] and by Hirschhorn *et al*.[85] both of whom have presented convincing evidence of the synthesis of antibody by peripheral blood leucocytes *in vitro*. The cells were obtained from hyper-immunised animals and included a variety of mature and immature plasmacytes. There is other evidence, however, of circulating cells which are certainly not plasma cells, but which contain $\gamma$G- and $\gamma$M-globulins in concentrations high enough to be demonstrated by immunofluorescence. These cells have been described by Van Furth.[175] They present the morphological features of lymphocytes. In addition, cells with the ultrastructural characteristics of antibody-forming cells (plasmacytes) have been found in thoracic duct lymph[194] and peripheral blood.[33] These, too, were found after hyper-immunisation, and are of less significance than those which circulate after more moderate degrees of antigenic stimulation. That such cells exist in the peripheral blood is suggested by the functional capacity of peripheral leucocytes from immunised donors to effect, months later, the accelerated rejection of grafts in normal recipients.[18, 19]

There is a further possible indicator of committed cells in the peripheral circulation. When antigen is introduced into cultures of peripheral leucocytes obtained from specifically immunised human subjects a proportion of the cells undergo transformation and division. However, mitosis *in vitro* can be induced in many ways[94] and is not absolute evidence that reacting cells are immunologically committed.

The evidence leaves no doubt that cells which are active in the synthesis of antibody, or capable of this response when re-stimulated with specific antigen, appear in the peripheral blood under appropriate conditions of immunisation. These cells provide a second potential vector for the transportation of antibody. The ontogenetic identity of these cells is of particular interest. If those with the morphology of plasma cells are excluded on the grounds that they are perhaps a product of intensive immunisation, we are left with the distinct impression that most of the antibody forming cells in the peripheral blood are lymphocytes.[175] They correspond, in fact, to the description given by Rauch and Raffel[138] of the cells in regional lymph nodes that stain specifically for anti-encephalitogenic antibody after immunisation with this antigen. Morphologically, they resemble the progeny of the pyroninophilic cells that arise during graft-versus-host reactions[78] or the response to haptenic sensitising agents.[168]

### D. FUNCTIONAL SIGNIFICANCE OF THE CELLULAR TRANSPORTATION OF ANTIBODY

Virtually all studies reporting the successful transfer of homograft immunity by humoral antibody have been performed with serum obtained at an early stage of graft rejection. For this, and other reasons, Stetson[159] and Kaliss[95] have emphasised the fact that antibody produced early in the immune response to transplantation antigens may be of critical importance. This is further emphasised by the well established fact that antibody produced by hyper-immunisation is rather consistent in its graft-enhancing effect.[95] The point is well demonstrated in the studies of Chantler and Batchelor[34] who found that immunisation of mice with a lyophilised ascites tumour produced an effect which varied according to the interval of time between immunisation and challenge. Grafts implanted 8 days after pre-treatment were destroyed at an accelerated rate; those implanted at 16–19 days showed enhancement. At intervening times a variable response was found. This is yet another example of an antagonistic effect between the antibodies produced during early and late phases of the immune response.

If it is conceded that antibody produced early in the immune response tends to become attached to cells, many of the enigmatic features of transplantation immunity are resolved. It would explain, for instance, why serum transfer of anti-tissue immunity is so difficult to achieve, even with serum obtained quite early in the immune response. For every mobile cell which is capable of adsorbing transferred antibody, the tissues must contain many more that are completely sessile. It is difficult to imagine how sessile cells could make any contribution to an immunological event enacted elsewhere in the body.

In connexion with the role of cellular vectors in immunological processes an important fact has recently emerged. Cell labelling with tritiated thymidine has revealed that the mononuclear cells which enter a mild inflammatory reaction,[73] a skin window,[176] a demyelinating lesion in EAE,[180] a tolerated graft during its rejection by competent cells from an isogeneic donor,[78] or delayed sensitivity reactions in the skin,[98, 99] are almost exclusively young cells derived by recent mitotic division. Unfortunately we know little concerning the identity of these cells. A high proportion of them are undoubtedly monocytes;[73, 176] some are probably not.[180] It is extremely likely that the cells which infiltrate reaction sites are formed outside the vasculature and migrate into the circulation not long before they are called upon to participate in the events occurring at a reactive focus. This may mean that only those cells which have recently gained access to the circulation are available for an immunological commission. All those which have been circulating for longer periods may already be otherwise committed, perhaps in a variety of directions, by passive adsorption of antibody molecules of differing specificity. Among them may be antibodies produced for the purpose of recognising self components. Boyden has proposed a mechanism of this sort for the removal of effete cells,[25] and to explain some aspects of the inflammatory response to traumatic injury.[27]

How the newly circulating cell acquires its immunological direction is a moot point. It could do so by adsorbing free antibody from the serum. This would be likely to occur if antibody with the physical properties of $\gamma$M-immunoglobulin were freely available in the plasma. In some circumstances, however, the only available source of a specific antibody might be from circulating cells which are actively engaged in its synthesis, but incapable of secreting it into the plasma. The cells which we have dubbed "active vectors" would qualify in this regard. Transfer of reactivity to "passive vectors" would then depend on random contacts between cells in circulation.

The observations of Prendergast[135] and of McCluskey et al.[111] are particularly relevant to the foregoing problem which deals essentially with the mechanism responsible for encouraging the accumulation of immunologically reactive cells in a target area. The former author showed by autoradiographic means that mononuclear cells *originating in the lymph node draining a first-set skin graft* entered two other grafts applied at the same time. One graft was from the same donor, the other from a donor of different genotype. Labelled cells were preferentially selected from the blood; but their entry into the test grafts was not dictated by information obtained in the stimulated node from which the cells took origin. This conclusion was necessary in view of the finding that labelled cells entered *in equal numbers* into grafts from both donors. There is no doubt that the cells which entered these grafts were not a random sample of the circulating cell population. They differed from the vast majority of peripheral leucocytes in one important respect—they had only recently entered the blood from a particular lymph node. It seems highly probable that whatever influences young cells to enter grafts ahead of other circulating cells is either inherent in *all* young cells or a property acquired by them after they enter the circulation. The latter is the more satisfying explanation. In the circulation they would be equally exposed to antibody, or "active vectors," specific for either graft. Analogous observations were made in the experiments of McCluskey et al.[111] who studied the cells which entered delayed skin reactions to two unrelated antigens. The implications are quite clear: if cells enter reaction sites for immunological reasons, most of them have been influenced to do so by passive means.

The foregoing discussion is significant in relation to experiments performed by Najarian and Feldman.[124] These authors showed that spleen and lymph node cells taken at the height of the immune response to a first set homograft of skin can produce an accelerated rejection of homologous grafts when segregated in a diffusion chamber and implanted in the peritoneal cavity of normal recipient mice. The mouse is unique among laboratory animals in having a large population of resident mononuclear phagocytes free in its peritoneal cavity.[116] They are capable of intense mitotic activity[109, 96, 65] and hence of sustaining their numbers despite their constant migration from the peritoneal cavity. Antibody synthesised by immunologically committed cells within a diffusion chamber would encounter this mobile cell population as it diffused into the peritoneal fluid. Unlike the majority of cells that would be encountered by the $\gamma$M-immunoglobulin contained in an intravenous infusion of immune serum, most of the cells in the peritoneal cavity might be expected to be unsaturated with antibody and freely mobile. For these two reasons they would seem to be better placed to function as passive vectors of an immune reaction than would the fixed cells of the reticulo-endothelial system, no matter how heavily charged with specific antibody.

The strategic advantages provided by amoeboid cells for the deployment of antibody needs little emphasis.[183, 5] There is a possibility, however, that the availability of specifically reactive vector cells may sometimes impose a limit upon the efficiency of graft rejection. This is one possible explanation for the findings of Ballantyne and Stetson[10] and of Converse *et al.*[42] Despite the demonstration that there was no impairment of the immune response of rats to massive grafts of skin, large grafts were found to survive long after the death of small "third party" grafts. Since the requirement for vector cells would vary with the size of the immunological target, large grafts would be expected to persist until sufficient vector cells became available.

### E. THE PHENOMENON OF DESENSITISATION

There is one other important indication that certain immune reactions are mediated by cellular vectors. It is well recognised that tuberculous subjects sometimes become anergic in the terminal stages of the disease. The phenomenon can be reproduced experimentally. The systemic injection of antigen, given at the same time or prior to the intradermal injection of a skin test dose, will specifically and completely prevent development of a reaction in the skin, and leave the subject non-reactive for several days.[108, 1, 152] Uhr and Pappenheimer[172] have shown that this suppressive effect of antigen is dose-dependent. It is difficult to explain the phenomenon in terms of the neutralisation of humoral antibody. An explanation based on the destruction or deviation of cellular vectors is easier to visualise, and is supported by direct experimental evidence. It has been mentioned that the injection of tuberculin or other protein antigen to which guinea pigs have been rendered sensitive, causes immobilisation[126] or even death[109] of detached mononuclear cells in the peritoneal cavity. The immobilisation of sensitised cells exposed to specific antigen *in vitro*[46] is an equivalent response. Presumably the systemic injection of antigen affects sensitised cells everywhere, and denies them temporarily or permanently the opportunity of participating in a reaction at the skin test site. The depression, by anti-leucocyte serum, of delayed reactions to tubercu-lin[91, 181] or haptenic sensitising agents[181, 188] is an even more compelling argu-ment that reactivity depends upon circulating cells.

The practical importance of the deviation of cellular vectors is illustrated by its effect on graft survival[191] and the production of experimental allergic encephalomyelitis.[152] A single injection of 0.5 mg of the encephalitogenic protein, given before the onset of symptoms and at a time corresponding to the peak level of skin sensitivity to the antigen, completely suppressed skin sensitivity and delayed the onset of EAE. Daily injections abolished both skin sensitivity and the development of lesions. The relationship is very striking. It implies that the demyelinating mechanism can be temporarily or permanently interrupted by interference with the transportation of the im-munological reactant.

It is interesting that in the foregoing experiments of Shaw et al.[152] the onset of demyelination was accompanied by a partial loss of skin sensitivity. A similar loss of sensitivity occurs in brucella-infected mice.[108, 96] It is observed during the period when organisms are being inactivated most rapidly in the spleen and liver. Release of excess antigen is the most obvious explanation for these examples of spontaneous desensitisation; its effects could be quite important. In the case of EAE it would provide a stimulus for the synthesis of competing antibodies—those which interfere with the demyelinating mech-anism. This may be the reason why the experimental disease is sometimes self-limiting.[132] In infectious disease, on the other hand, the release of antigen provides the antigenic stimulus to sensitised macrophages upon which the level of host resistance depends.[108]

# VI. EFFECTOR MECHANISMS

## A. ANTI-MICROBIAL IMMUNITY

There is no dispute concerning the effector cells responsible for acquired cellular resistance to microbial agents. The activated mononuclear phagocytes seem almost exclusively involved in the final expression of immunity against a variety of intracellular parasites. However, the augmentation of their mi-crobicidal powers is only one aspect of their added potential to serve the host's defenses. Their ability to converge on the parasite, and their tendency to proliferate[107, 96] under the influence of antigen, are two others. The former is referred to[105] as "accelerated tubercle formation" in the case of myco-bacterial infections. The same phenomenon is evident whenever the infectious agent causes delayed-type hypersensitivity. It is particularly well seen in listeriosis[107] and brucellosis.[31] This tendency for cells to congregate in relation to the infective agent is no more than a multi-focal expression of delayed-type hypersensitivity. The fact that the cells involved are almost exclusively mono-nuclear phagocytes is indication that in the anti-microbial form of cellular immunity this cell type greatly outnumbers all others (lymphocytes) which might be equipped to participate by virtue of their antibody content. This is an important point to consider in relation to the following discussion of effector mechanisms in anti-tissue immunity.

There is one other respect in which recent *in vitro* studies have a bearing on the response of cells *in vivo*. The immobilisation of sensitised macrophages that occurs in the presence of specific antigen[47] appears to contribute to the cohesiveness of cells that go to make the mononuclear cell lesions which form at infective foci. The phenomenon is very conspicuous in monolayers of mouse macrophages obtained from animals infected with *L. monocytogenes*. Unlike normal cells those from an immune host do not remain discrete when soluble listeria antigens are introduced into the medium. Instead they congregate in a number of tight-packed aggregates just as they do *in vivo*.[110] This is presumably due to the cross-linking effect of antigen molecules on cells that are sensitised at the surface by adsorbed antibody.

## B. Anti-Tissue Immunity

The effector mechanisms in anti-tissue immunity are more obscure, but there is much about them that is reminiscent of those which operate in the anti-microbial form of cellular immunity. Most observers agree that tissue damage is contingent upon infiltration of the target by blood-borne cells,[179, 178, 77, 139] but the identity of these cells is still in doubt. We have postulated two categories of cells, "active" and "passive" vectors, equipped to detect a foreign antigen. The former seem to answer to the definition of lymphocytes,[77] and the latter to be cells of the monocyte-macrophage class. Unfortunately the inter-relations between these two categories of cells are quite unknown. For the moment it would seem wisest to regard them as ontogenetically unrelated. Both are represented in the cellular infiltrate that forms within an immunological target. What are their respective functions?

Recent studies have done much to clarify this issue. Histological and ultrastructural observations suggest that the dissolution of cellular elements in homografts,[178, 186] tumour grafts,[5] or in organs under immunological attack[180, 139, 134] is spatially related to the immigrant cells. The morphological evidence suggests, in fact, that one process of cell damage depends on "contactual" interaction between the target and effector cells. It is interesting, therefore, that lymphocytes and macrophages have both been demonstrated to be capable of inflicting lethal damage upon specific target cells in tissue culture. The evidence for this will now be discussed.

(1) Lymphocytes as effector cells. The lymphocyte, as a cytocidal agent, seems somewhat less efficient than the macrophage.[79] However, the recent quantitative studies of Wilson[190] give new perspective to the problem. His experiments, which measured the destructive effect of immune lymphoid cells on target kidney cells *in vitro*, have revealed a log-linear relationship between the numbers of target cells destroyed and the numbers of lymphocytes present in the system. The data show that lymphocyte populations vary in their content of functionally competent cells. Lymph nodes draining a skin graft site are relatively rich in active cells, and reach a peak on the 6th or 7th day. Active lymphocytes were not detected in the thoracic duct lymph until the 9th day and never approached in numerical efficiency the cells

obtained from regional nodes. Since the dose-response relationship was exponential, Wilson suggests that the inactivation process has the characteristics of a "single-hit" phenomenon, implying that one *activated* lymphocyte is capable of destroying one target cell. It follows that the numerical differences observed in the efficiency of cells obtained from different sources is due to variation in their content of *activated* cells. This suggests again the possibility that only those lymphocytes which have been actively engaged in antibody synthesis are functionally competent to damage target cells, and cannot acquire this property by passive means.

In the elegant studies of Rauch and Raffel[138] the proportion of *specifically fluorescent lymphocytes* in the regional nodes and spleens of animals immunised with encephalitogenic antigen ranged between 5 and 10% of all cells. These figures for the percentage of cells containing specific immunoglobulin are in surprisingly good agreement with the computed percentage of cells with cytocidal properties found by Wilson[190] in the regional nodes of rats immunised with homologous skin. This, too, suggests the likelihood that the cytocidal lymphocytes are those which contain demonstrable antibody.

The capacity of immune lymphocytes to inflict damage on specific target cells *in vitro* has now been reported from many laboratories.[119, 76, 140, 97, 189, 174] Most observers concur in the view that a high multiplicity of lymphocytes to target cells is necessary to achieve high mortality rates; that the reaction is specific; and that complement is not required. It appears, moreover, that the introduction of specific immune serum into the system does not enable the lymphocytes of un-immunised subjects to damage cellular targets. However, if the cells can be made to adhere with heterologous anti-leucocyte serum[120] or with phytohaemagglutinin[120, 87] target cell damage is said to occur. A role for antibody in promoting cellular contact is clearly indicated,[120] even though circulating antibody does not suffice for this purpose. Of this matter, more will be said later.

(2) MONOCYTES AND MACROPHAGES AS EFFECTOR CELLS. It has been indicated that only some of the cells in any given population of immune lymphocytes are equipped as effector cells to act *directly* on target cells. The position may be quite different in the case of mononuclear phagocytes. These cells have been shown by Granger and Weiser[79] to be capable of mediating the cytolytic destruction of specific target cells *in vitro*. In these studies experiments were performed with monolayers composed either of target cells or immune macrophages. The addition of macrophages or target cells to restricted areas of appropriate monolayers caused specific adhesion between the two cell populations, a process which took no more than 4 min. Cell death, affecting both macrophages and target cells, occurred within 12 to 24 h. It resulted in complete cell lysis and the production of discrete plaques. Cultures which were washed after cell adhesion had occurred still yielded zones of complete lysis within the target area. Although the experiments of Granger and Weiser were not meant to be quantitative, they leave no doubt that virtually every immune macrophage was capable of exerting a cytocidal effect. The reaction was entirely specific and highly discriminative. This was shown with monolayers containing a mixture of target cells of differing antigenicity. In mixed cells populations only partial lysis occurred in the areas exposed

to mono-specific immune macrophages; the antigenically appropriate cells were destroyed, but the others survived. Normal macrophages were inert in the presence of normal or hyper-immune serum.

The destruction of target cells by immune macrophages occurs without obvious evidence of phagocytosis;[79] though this phenomenon has also been described.[129] There is, however, a requirement for very intimate contact between cells. Immune macrophages[79] or lymphocytes[190] do no damage to target cells located on the opposite side of a diffusion membrane. This has led to a suggestion,[120] which is supported by ultrastructural findings,[134] that cell death is due to the fusion of plasma membranes and an exchange of cytoplasmic contents.

The studies with immune macrophages emphasise an important point. It is almost inconceivable that virtually every macrophage in an immune population could acquire its reactivity towards a given antigenic target except by passive means. It is significant that the macrophages used in the experiments of Granger and Weiser[79] were obtained 10 days after immunisation; that is to say, at an early stage of the immune response. At this time γM-immunoglobulins are usually still in production and can be eluted from the surface of macrophages.[142] So far no tests have been made to determine whether serum obtained at this, or even earlier, stages of the immune response contains antibody which can sensitise normal macrophages. The immune serum used by Granger and Weiser[79] was obtained from hyper-immunised donors. It was ineffective when tested with normal macrophages, and actually tended to inhibit the cytocidal effect of immune macrophages. It is by no means certain that early immune serum would prove to be any more effective for passive sensitisation of macrophages. Its ability to do so would depend upon the availability of antibodies with an affinity for cell surfaces. These may not always appear in the serum in significant concentrations because of their rapid removal by a large (and expanding) population of cells capable of adsorbing them at the source. This, indeed, may be one of the major reasons why serum transfer experiments have seldom met with success. Other reasons have already been given (Section V). There is little doubt, however, that effective antibodies do appear in the serum under suitable conditions of immunisation.[159, 160, 156] It would be worthwhile, therefore, to examine serum taken at intervals during the immune response for the presence of antibody capable of conferring on normal macrophages the cytocidal properties found in macrophages obtained from actively immunised donors.

Important differences between antibodies produced early and late in the immune response to histocompatibility antigens have already received frequent comment in this review. A further illustration of the functional differences between antibodies of similar specificity is provided by the inhibitory effect of hyper-immune serum on the cytocidal properties of immune lymphocytes in tissue culture.[119, 190] Workers who have used this experimental approach have obtained their immune lymphocytes within 6 to 10 days of the commencement of immunisation. Möller[119] found that lymphocytes from the regional node reached peak activity within 10 days. It was the cytocidal activity of cells obtained at this time which was suppressed completely by hyper-immune serum obtained from donors repeatedly injected with living homologous tumour cells. Needless to say it was proposed by Möller that this is one obvious mechanism of graft enhancement. A similar view has been expressed by Gorer[74] and by Batchelor and Silverman[11] who have given thoughtful consideration to the counter-influence of humoral and sessile antibody in the mechanism of graft rejection.

Experimental results obtained *in vitro* are always more compelling when supported by evidence that the same phenomenon occurs *in vivo*. Such evidence exists to corroborate the evidence that macrophages are lethal for target cells in tissue culture. A direct interaction between immune macrophages and tumour target cells was demonstrated in the peritoneal cavity of mice.[9] Death of both cell populations occurred much as it does *in vitro*;[79] the phenomenon has been described as "allergic death" by Gorer and Boyce.[75] More recently, Bennett[15] has reported the complete suppression of tumour growth by purified macrophage suspensions containing fewer than 0.5% residual lymphocytes. The immune macrophages and tumour cells were mixed together prior to injection into the skin of non-immune recipients.

It is obviously more difficult to demonstrate that lymphocytes are also capable of a direct attack on target cells *in vivo*. The problem is complicated by the small percentage of competent lymphocytes even in the most active populations available; and by the developmental cycle that the lymphocyte embarks upon under the influence of antigenic stimulation,[77] making its movements difficult to trace. The best evidence that lymphocytes participate at all in the destructive attack on tissue targets is their presence in the lesions. However, the most detailed study of this problem is that of Wiener *et al.*[186] who have expressed the view that the cells most intimately involved are unidentifiable. They were described, for this reason, as "graft rejection cells," and were depicted as having an ultrastructural morphology midway between that of macrophages and lymphocytes.

As mentioned earlier (Section V. D), studies with tritiated thymidine have shown that most of the participating cells are very young. Moreover, they continue to proliferate within the reaction site.[180, 99, 98] This may account for their nondescript morphology. During strong antigenic stimulation of hypersensitive mice large numbers of unclassifiable cells appear in the peritoneal cavity to the accompaniment of an intense mitotic response.[109] Many of these cells are basophilic (pyroninophilic). They were originally thought to arise from lymphocytes. If placed in tissue culture, however, they differentiate into typical macrophages.[110] At one stage in this process of maturation they resemble intermediate lymphocytes (Figs. 3 and 4 of ref. 7). It now seems likely that the unidentifiable cells which appeared to arise by the transformation of lymphocytes were actually young macrophages derived by a quick succession of cell divisions. The same may be true of many of the cells observed in immunological reaction sites *in vivo*. Indeed, Waksman[180] has described a similar maturation of cells resembling lymphocytes in the lesions of EAE. If this interpretation is correct it means that a majority of the cells which infiltrate an immunological reaction site are of monocyte-macrophage type. This view makes it simpler to explain why most of the cells which enter lesions are young; and why cells labelled in the lymph node in which the primary immune response occurs are no more likely to arrive in the skin graft which provided the initial stimulus than in another, unrelated graft.[135]

## VII. GRAFT-VERSUS-HOST REACTIONS

A discussion dealing with the behaviour of mononuclear phagocytes during the reactive phase of an immunological response would be incomplete without reference to the graft-*versus*-host reaction. There are several unexplained features of the assault which lymphoid grafts can make on hosts which cannot retaliate. One is the nature of the splenomegaly which is so characteristic of graft-*versus*-host reactions.[154] To the surprise of most observers this is due mainly to the proliferation of host cells. Davies and Doak[51] and Gorer and Boyse[75] interpreted it as a histiocytic response on the part of the host; but Howard, Michie and Simonsen[89] were puzzled by the pyroninophilic nature of so many of the cells involved. Cells of this type have come to be associated in the minds of immunologists with the inductive phase of the immune response. Since host cells have no immunological reason to respond to histocompatibility antigens present in the graft, there must be some other explanation for proliferation of host cells.

It is likely that the mechanisms employed by graft cells in their immunological attack upon the host are similar to those which operate in host against graft reactions. They would involve, at least in the early stages, the synthesis of antibodies of a type which would mediate delayed-type hypersensitivity against host antigens. It has been argued that such antibodies have a special affinity for the mononuclear phagocytes of the reticulo-endothelial system. We know of no reason why antibody molecules produced by the lymphoid graft should not become associated with host macrophages as readily as they would with equivalent cells of graft origin (if macrophages were represented in the lymphoid implant). This would mean that, during graft-*versus*-host reactions, the host's own phagocytic cells become vicariously sensitised to the histocompatibility antigens of the host. In these circumstances there would be two reasons for expecting host cell proliferation. Firstly, it has been suggested that antibody acting on target cells may sometimes serve to stimulate mitosis rather than cytolysis.[74] Lymphocytes, for instance, have been observed to mitose under the influence of anti-leucocyte serum.[80] Since macrophages are more resistant to the cytolytic effects of antibody than other cells of the lympho-reticular tissues,[15] it is likely that host histiocytes would survive and multiply under the stimulus of an antibody directed against their constituent antigens. Less resistant cells, such as lymphocytes, would be more likely to succumb (lymphoid atrophy is, in fact, a feature of the graft-versus-host reaction). The second, and potentially more important, reason for host cell proliferation is the mitogenic effect of specific antigen on the macrophages of animals with delayed-type hypersensitivity. Although there is no direct evidence that antigen causes mitosis in *passively* sensitised macrophages, it certainly does have this effect on lympho-reticular tissues[53] and especially on the macrophages[109, 65, 96] of *actively* sensitised subjects. It is reasonable to assume, therefore, that host macrophages, sensitised by antibodies elaborated by the graft, would proliferate under the influence of the host's own antigens. In addition they may even play the major part in the destructive processes involved in the immunological attack on the host, for they could serve as the "passive" vectors of what is really a disseminated delayed-type hypersensitivity reaction. This is essentially the way in which Gorer and Boyse[75] described the tissue reactions observed in graft-*versus*-host reactions. Since cellular proliferation is a recognised feature of the delayed-type hypersensitivity reaction,[179] many of the histological features of graft-*versus*-host reactions are plausibly explained in this way.

There remains the problem of pyroninophilia in cells of host origin. In the preceding section it was explained that rapidly proliferating macrophages take on the basophilia and nuclear features of blast cells. In this undifferentiated state they are unclassifiable. There is, then, no reason to suppose that the pyroninophilic cells are not a part of the histiocytic response. An indirect indication of the histiocytic nature of the cellular hyperplasia in graft-versus-host reactions is the heightened resistance to infection that has been reported by Cooper and Howard.[43] It is also an excellent illustration of the non-specific nature of the anti-microbial mechanisms responsible for acquired cellular resistance to infectious disease.

## SUMMARY

A difference in meaning between two uses of the term "cellular immunity" requires that distinction be drawn between its anti-microbial and anti-tissue forms. It is proposed, however, that there is a basic similarity between the two forms in that each is mediated by cell-associated antibodies. Delayed-type hypersensitivity, which is invariably associated with cellular immunity, is also most plausibly explained in terms of an antibody which is normally transported by cellular vectors. It is suggested that these vectors may be "active" or "passive." The former appear to be cells of lymphocyte type containing antibody which they themselves have synthesised; the latter are cells of the monocyte-macrophage type which have acquired their immunological reactivity by passive adsorption of specific antibody. Experimental evidence is cited to justify a distinction between these two classes of vector cells. Both types are potentially capable of functioning also as "effector" cells in the anti-tissue form of cellular immunity, for each has been shown capable of inflicting damage on target cells. Numerically, however, the monocyte (or macrophage) appears to predominate. In the anti-microbial form of cellular immunity, on the other hand, "effector" cells are exclusively of the monocyte-macrophage type because phagocytosis is an essential step in the process of bacterial inactivation. Passive sensitisation of mononuclear phagocytes equips them with the reactivity needed to ensure the accumulation of cells at an infective focus or in a target tissue. However, it does not impart the increased microbicidal ability that is characteristic of acquired cellular resistance against infectious agents. This requires, in addition, that host phagocytes be stimulated to increased physiological activity. The action of antigen on sensitised macrophages appears to provide this stimulus. This view is supported by experimental evidence which shows that the functional and metabolic changes characteristic of anti-microbial immunity occur only during sustained antigenic stimulation.

Evidence is cited to support a suggestion that γM-immunoglobulins have biological properties in keeping with a role as the mediators of both types of cellular immunity. The kinetics of synthesis of this class of immunoglobulins correspond with the rate of development of delayed-type hypersensitivity. Their propensity to become cell-associated is also consistent with a role in cellular immunity.

Considerable emphasis has been placed on the competition which exists between antibodies with different biological properties. γG-immunoglobulins are known to interfere with cellular mechanisms of immunity by sequestering antigen. It is suggested that they may also interfere because of their known ability to suppress γM-immunoglobulin production.

# *References*

1. Ackerman, V. P.: Delayed-type hypersensitivity and acquired resistance in listeriosis. Ph.D. Thesis, Australian National University (1964).
2. Allen, W. P.: Immunity against tularemia: passive protection of mice by transfer of immune tissues. J. exp. Med. *115*:411 (1962).
3. Allison, A. C., and Mallucci, L.: Lysosomes in dividing cells, with special reference to lymphocytes. Lancet, Lond. *i*:1371 (1964).
4. Alvord, E. C., Shaw, C., Hruby, S., and Kies, M. W.: Encephalitogen-induced inhibition of experimental allergic encephalomyelitis: prevention, suppression and therapy. Ann. N.Y. Acad. Sci. *122*:333 (1965).
5. Amos, D. B.: The use of simplified systems as an aid to the interpretation of mechanisms of graft rejection. Progr. Allergy *6*:468 (1962).
6. Asherson, G. L., and Stone, S. H.: Selective and specific inhibition of 24 hour skin reactions in the guinea pig. I. Immune deviation: description of the phenomenon and the effect of splenectomy. Immunology *9*:205 (1965).
7. Askonas, B. A., and White, R. G.: Sites of antibody production in the guinea pig. The relation between *in vitro* synthesis of anti-ovalbumin and γ-globulin and distribution of antibody-containing plasma cells. Brit. J. exp. Path. *37*:61 (1956).
8. Auzins, I., and Rowley, D.: On the question of specificity of cellular immunity. Austr. J. exp. Biol. med. Sci. *40*:283 (1962).
9. Baker, P., Weiser, R. S., Julita, J., Evans, C. A., and Blandau, R. J.: Mechanisms of tumor homograft rejection: The behavior of sarcoma I ascites tumor in the A/JAX and the C57BL/6K mouse. Ann. N.Y. Acad. Sci. *101*:46 (1963).
10. Ballantyne, D. L., and Stetson, C. A.: Serologic reactions to skin homografts of various sizes in the rat. Ann. N.Y. Acad. Sci. *102*:7 (1964).
11. Batchelor, J. R., and Silverman, M. S.: Further studies on interactions between sessile and humoral antibodies in homograft reactions, *in* Ciba Found. Symposium on Transplantation, p. 216 (Churchill, London 1962).
12. Bauer, D. C., and Stavitsky, A. B.: On the different molecular forms of antibody synthesized by rabbits during the early response to a single injection of protein and cellular antigens. Proc. Nat. Acad. Sci. *47*:1667 (1961).
13. Bauer, J. A., and Stone, S. H.: Isologous and homologous lymphoid transplants. I. The transfer of tuberculin hypersensitivity in inbred guinea pigs. J. Immunol. *86*:177 (1961).
14. Benacerraf, B., Ovary, Z., Bloch, K. J., and Franklin, E. C.: Properties of guinea pig 7S antibodies. I. Electrophoretic separation of two types of guinea pig 7S antibodies. J. exp. Med. *117*:937 (1963).
15. Bennett, B.: Specific suppression of tumor growth by isolated peritoneal macrophages. Fed. Proc. (Abst.) *24*:305 (1965).
16. Bennett, B., Old, L. J., and Boyse, E. A.: Opsonisation of cells by isoantibody *in vitro*. Nature, Lond. *198*:10 (1962).

17. Billingham, R. E., Brent, L., and Medawar, P. B.: 'Enhancement' in normal homografts, with a note on its possible mechanism. Transpl. Bull. *3*:84 (1965).

18. Billingham, R. E., Silvers, W. K., and Wilson, D. B.: Adoptive transfer of transplantation immunity by means of blood-borne cells. Lancet, Lond. *i*:512 (1962).

19. Billingham, R. E., Silvers, W. K., and Wilson, D. B.: Further studies on adoptive transfer of sensitivity to skin homografts. J. exp. Med. *118*:397 (1963).

20. Blanden, R. V.: Unpublished observation (1965).

21. Blanden, R. V., Mackaness, G. B., and Collins, F. M.: Mechanisms of acquired resistance in mouse typhoid. J. exp. Med. *124*:585 (1966).

22. Bloch, K. J.: Heterogeneity in biologic function of antibodies: implications for immunologic tumor enhancement. Fed. Proc. *24*:1030 (1965).

23. Bloom, B. R., Hamilton, L. D., and Chase, M. W.: Effects of mitomycin C on the cellular transfer of delayed-type hypersensitivity in the guinea pig. Nature, Lond. *201*:689 (1964).

24. Boyden, S. V.: The effect of previous injections of tuberculo-protein on the development of tuberculin sensitivity following B.C.G. vaccination in guinea pigs. Brit. J. exp. Path. *38*:611 (1957).

25. Boyden, S.: Cellular recognition of foreign matter. Internat. Rev. exp. Path. *2*:31 (1963).

26. Boyden, S. V.: Cytophilic antibody. *In* Cell-bound antibodies. p. 7 (Wistar Institute Press, Philadelphia 1963).

27. Boyden, S.: Autoimmunity and inflammation. Nature, Lond. *201*:200 (1964).

28. Boyden, S. V.: Cytophilic antibody in guinea pigs with delayed-type hypersensitivity. Immunology *7*:474 (1964).

29. Boyden, S. V., and Sorkin, E.: The adsorption of antibody and antigen by spleen cells *in vitro*. Immunology *3*:272 (1960).

30. Boyden, S. V., and Sorkin, E.: The adsorption of antibody and antigen by spleen cells *in vitro*. Some further experiments. Immunology *4*:244 (1961).

31. Braude, A.: Studies in the pathology and pathogenesis of experimental brucellosis. J. infect. Dis. *89*:76 (1951).

32. Braun, W., Kessel, R. W. I., and Pomales-Lebron, A.: Failure of vaccination with killed brucellae to modify monocyte-bacterium interactions. Proc. Soc. exp. Biol. N.Y. *109*:875 (1962).

33. Braunsteiner, H., and Pakesch, F.: Electron microscopic studies on the problem of blood plasma cells. Wien. Z. inn. Med. *41*:58 (1960).

34. Chantler, S. M., and Batchelor, J. R.: Changes in the host response following treatment with lyophilized tissue. Transplantation *2*:75 (1964).

35. Chase, M. W.: Models for hypersensitivity studies. *In* Cellular and humoral aspects of the hypersensitive states. p. 251 (Hoeber-Harper, New York 1959).

36. Cohn, Z. A.: Personal communication. (1965).

37. Cohn, Z. A., and Benson, B.: The *in vitro* differentiation of mononuclear phagocytes. II. The influence of serum on granule formation, hydrolase production and phagocytosis. J. exp. Med. *121*:835 (1965).

38. Cohn, Z. A., and Benson, B.: The *in vitro* differentiation of mononuclear phagocytes. III. The reversibility of granule and hydrolytic enzyme formation and the turnover of granule constituents. J. exp. Med. *122*:455 (1965).

39. Cohn, Z. A., Hirsch, J. G., and Wiener, E.: The cytoplasmic granules of phagocytic cells and the degradation of bacteria. *In* Ciba Found. Symposium on Lysosomes, p. 126 (Churchill, London 1963).

40. Collins, F. M., and Mackaness, G. B.: Unpublished observations (1965).

41. Collins, F. M., Mackaness, G. B., and Blanden, R. V.: Infection-immunity as the basis of resistance to Salmonella infections. J. exp. Med. *124*:601 (1966).

42. Converse, J. M., Siegel, W. H., and Ballantyne, D. L.: Studies in antigenic overloading with massive skin homografts in rats. Plastic reconstruct. Surg. *31*:9 (1963).

43. Cooper, G. W., and Howard, J. G.: An effect of the graft-versus-host reaction on resistance to experimental bacteraemia. Brit. J. exp. Path. *42*:558 (1961).

44. Cornforth, J. W., Hart, P. D., Rees, R. J. W., and Stock, J. A.: Antituberculous effect of certain surface-active polyoxyethylene ethers in mice. Nature, Lond. *168*:150 (1951).

45. Crowle, A. J., and Hu, C. C.: Interference by pre-immunisation of mice with induction of delayed hypersensitivity. Fed. Proc. (abst.) *24*:183 (1965).

46. David, J. R., Al-Askari, S., Lawrence, H. S., and Thomas, L.: *In vitro* studies on delayed hypersensitivity and homograft immunity. Ann. N.Y. Acad. Sci. *120*:393 (1964).

47. David, J. R., Al-Askari, S., Lawrence, H. S., and Thomas, L.: Delayed hypersensitivity

*in vitro.* I. The specificity of inhibition of cell migration by antigens. J. Immunol. *93:* 264 (1964).

48. David, J. R., Al-Askari, S., Lawrence, H. S., and Thomas, L.: *In vitro* studies on delayed hypersensitivity and homograft immunity. Ann. N.Y. Acad. Sci. *120:*393 (1964).

49. David, J. R., Lawrence, H. S., and Thomas, L.: Delayed hypersensitivity *in vitro.* II. Effect of sensitive cells on normal cells in the presence of antigen. J. Immunol. *93:*274 (1964).

50. David, J. R., Lawrence, H. S., and Thomas, L.: The *in vitro* desensitization of sensitive cells by trypsin. J. exp. Med. *120:*1189 (1964).

51. Davies, A. J. S., and Doak, S. M. A.: Fate of homologous adult spleen cells injected into newborn mice. Nature, Lond. *187:*610 (1960).

52. Dienes, L.: The specific immunity response and the healing of infectious diseases: Significance of active immunity and the connections between the immunity response and the anatomical lesions. Arch. Path. *21:*357 (1936).

53. Dutton, R. W., and Pearce, J. D.: An antigen-dependent stimulation of synthesis of deoxyribonucleic acid in spleen cells from immunised rabbits. Nature, Lond. *194:*93 (1962).

54. Elberg, S. S., Schneider, P., and Fong, J.: Cross immunity between *Brucella melitensis* and *Mycobacterium tuberculosis:* Intracellular behavior of *Brucella melitensis* in monocytes from vaccinated animals. J. exp. Med. *106:*545 (1957).

55. Fahey, J. L., and Sell, S.: The immunoglobulins of mice. V. The metabolic (catabolic) properties of five immunoglobulin classes. J. exp. Med. *122:*41 (1965).

56. Favour, C. B.: Cell injury in allergic inflammation. Int. Arch. Allergy *10:*193 (1957).

57. Feldman, J. D., and Najarian, J. S.: Dynamics and quantitative analysis of passively transferred tuberculin hypersensitivity. J. Immunol. *91:*306 (1963).

58. Finkelstein, M. S., and Uhr, J. W.: Specific inhibition of antibody formation by passively administered 19S and 7S antibody. Science *146:*67 (1964).

59. Fong, J., Chen, D., and Elberg, S. S.: Studies on tubercle bacillus-histiocyte relationship. IV. Effects of passage in normal and immune systems upon virulent bacilli. J. exp. Med. *114:*75 (1961).

60. Fong, J., Chen, D., and Elberg, S. S.: Studies of tubercle bacillus-histiocyte relationship. VI. Induction of cellular resistance by ribosomes and ribosomal RNA. J. exp. Med. *118:*371 (1963).

61. Fong, J., Chen, D., and Vickery, H. M.: Studies of tubercle bacillus-histiocyte relationship. VII. Homologous and heterologous transfer of cellular resistance. J. exp. Med. *118:* 727 (1963).

62. Fong, J., Chen, D., and Elberg, S. S.: Studies of tubercle bacillus-histiocyte relationship. VIII. Comparative study of cellular resistance induced by brucella and mycobacteria. J. exp. Med. *120:*885 (1964).

63. Fong, J., Schneider, P., and Elberg, S. S.: Studies on tubercle bacillus-monocyte relationship. II. Induction of monocyte degeneration by bacteria and culture filtrate. Specificity of serum and monocyte effects on resistance to degeneration. J. exp. Med. *105:*25 (1957).

64. Forbes, I. J.: Induction of mitosis in macrophages by endotoxin. J. Immunol. *94:*37 (1965).

65. Forbes, I. J., and Mackaness, G. B.: Mitosis in macrophages. Lancet *ii:*1203 (1963).

66. Fox, M.: Cytological estimation of the proportion of proliferating donor cells during graft-versus-host disease in $F_1$ hybrid mice injected with parental spleen cells. Nature, Lond. *195:*1024 (1962).

67. Freedman, S. O., Turcotte, R., Fish, A. J., and Sehon, A. H.: The *in vitro* detection of 'cell-fixed' haemagglutinating antibody to tuberculin purified protein derivative (PPD) in humans. J. Immunol. *90:*52 (1963).

68. Freund, J.: The mode of action of immunologic adjuvants. Adv. Tuberc. Res. *7:*130 (1956).

69. Friedman, R.: Quoted by Uhr, J. W. *in* Cell-bound antibodies, p. 16 (Wistar Institute Press, Philadelphia 1963).

70. Fulton, J. D.: Treatment of *Leishmania donovani* infections with surface-active agents. Nature, Lond. *187:*1129 (1960).

71. Gelzer, J., and Suter, E.: The effect of antibody on intracellular parasitism of *Salmonella typhimurium* in mononuclear phagocytes *in vitro.* Prolonged survival of infected monocytes in presence of antibody. J. exp. Med. *110:*715 (1959).

72. George, M., and Vaughan, J. H.: *In vitro* cell migration as a model for delayed sensitivity. Proc. Soc. exp. Biol. N.Y. *111:*514 (1962).

73. Goldman, A. S., and Walker, B. E.: The origin of cells in the infiltrates found at the sites of foreign protein injection. Lab. Invest. *11:*808 (1962).

74. Gorer, P. A.: Interactions between sessile and humoral antibodies in homograft reactions. *In* Cellular Aspects of Immunity, p. 330 (Churchill, London 1959).

75. Gorer, P. A., and Boyse, E. A.: Pathological changes in $F_1$ hybrid mice following trans-

plantation of spleen cells from donors of the parental strains. Immunology *2:*182 (1959).

76. Govaerts, A.: Cellular antibodies in kidney homotransplantation. J. Immunol. *85:*516 (1960).

77. Gowans, J. L., and McGregor, D. D.: The immunological activities of lymphocytes. Progr. Allergy *9:*1 (1965).

78. Gowans, J. L., McGregor, D. D., Cowen, D. M., and Ford, C. E.: Initiation of immune responses by small lymphocytes. Nature, Lond. *196:*651 (1962).

79. Granger, G. A., and Weiser, R. S.: Homograft target cells: specific destruction *in vitro* by contact interaction with immune macrophages. Science *145:*1427 (1964).

80. Gräsbeck, R., Nordman, C. T., and De la Chappelle, A.: The leucocyte-mitogenic effect of serum from rabbits immunized with human leucocytes. Acta med. Scand. *175:* Suppl. *412:*39 (1964).

81. Hart, P. D., and Rees, R. J. W.: Influence of certain surface-active agents on the host-parasite relationship in experimental tuberculosis. *In* Ciba Found. Symposium on Experimental Tuberculosis, p. 299 (Churchill, London 1955).

82. Hayashi, H., Tokuda, A., and Ukeda, K.: Biochemical study of cellular antigen-antibody reaction in tissue culture. I. Activation and release of a protease. J. exp. Med. *112:*237 (1960).

83. Henderson, D. W.: Bacterial interference. Bact. Rev. *24:*167 (1960).

84. Henderson, D. W.: Mixed populations *in vivo* and *in vitro*. Symp. Soc. gen. Microbiol. *14:*241 (1964).

85. Hirschhorn, K., Bach, F., Kolodney, R. L., Firschein, I. L., and Hasheim, N.: Immune response and mitosis of human peripheral blood lymphocytes *in vitro*. Science *142:* 1185 (1963).

86. Hirschhorn, R., Kaplan, J. M., Goldberg, A. F., Hirschhorn, K., and Weissmann, G.: Acid phosphatase-rich granules in human lymphocytes induced by phytohemagglutinin. Science *147:*55 (1965).

87. Holm, G., Perlmann, P., and Werner, B.: Phytohemagglutinin-induced cytotoxic action of normal lymphoid cells on cells in tissue culture. Nature, Lond. *203:*841 (1964).

88. Howard, J. G.: Resistance to infection with *Salmonella paratyphi* C in mice parasitized with a relatively avirulent strain of *Salmonella typhimurium*. Nature, Lond. *191:*87 (1961).

89. Howard, J. G., Michie, D., and Simonsen, M.: Splenomegaly as a host response in graft-versus-host disease. Brit. J. exp. Path. *42:*478 (1961).

90. Hulliger, L., and Sorkin, E.: Synthesis of antibodies by blood leucocytes of the rabbit. Nature, Lond. *198:*299 (1963).

91. Inderbitzin, T.: The relationship of lymphocytes, delayed cutaneous allergic reactions and histamine. Int. Arch. Allergy *8:*150 (1956).

92. Jenkin, C. R., and Rowley, D.: Basis for immunity to typhoid in mice and the question of 'cellular immunity.' Bact. Rev. *27:*391 (1963).

93. Jensen, S. B., Mergenhagen, S. E., Fitzgerald, R. J., and Jordan, H. V.: Susceptibility of conventional and germ-free mice to lethal effects of endotoxin. Proc. Soc. exp. Biol. N.Y. *113:*710 (1963).

94. Johnson, G. J., and Russell, P. S.: Reaction of human lymphocytes in culture to components of the medium. Nature, Lond. *208:*343 (1965).

95. Kaliss, N.: Immunological enhancement and inhibition of tumour growth: relationship to various immunological mechanisms. Fed. Proc. *24:*1024 (1965).

96. Khoo, K. K., and Mackaness, G. B.: Macrophage proliferation in relation to acquired cellular resistance. Austr. J. exp. Biol. med. Sci. *42:*707 (1964).

97. Koprowski, H., and Fernandes, M. V.: Autosensitisation reaction *in vitro*. Contactual agglutination of sensitised lymph node cells in brain tissue culture accompanied by destruction of glial elements. J. exp. Med. *116:*467 (1962).

98. Kosunen, T. U., and Dvorak, H. F.: The transfer reaction in the rabbit. II. A radioautographic study. Lab. Invest. *12:*628 (1963).

99. Kosunen, T. U., Waksman, B. H., Flax, M. H., and Tihen, W. S.: Radioautographic study of cellular mechanisms in delayed hypersensitivity. I. Delayed reactions to tuberculin and purified proteins in the rat and guinea pig. Immunology *6:*276 (1963).

100. Kretschmer, R. R., and Perez-Tamayo, R.: The role of humoral antibodies in rejection of skin homografts in rabbits. II. Passive transfer of transplantation immunity by sensitised lymph node cells within diffusion chambers. J. exp. Med. *116:*879 (1962).

101. Kurashige, S., Orawa, N., Kawakami, M., and Mitsuhashi, S.: Cell-bound antibody of mouse

mononuclear phagocytes in experimental salmonellosis. Proc. 19th Kanto Branch Meeting, Japan Bacteriol. Assoc. p. 19–20 (1964).

102. Landy, M., Sanderson, R. P., and Jackson, A. L.: Humoral and cellular aspects of the immune response to the somatic antigen of *Salmonella enteritidis*. J. exp. Med. *122:* 483 (1965).

103. Lawrence, H. S.: Similarities between homograft rejection and tuberculin-type allergy. Ann. N.Y. Acad. Sci. *64:*826 (1957).

104. Lévy, F. M., Conge, G. A., Pasquier, J. F., Mauso, H., Dubos, R. J., and Schaedler, R. W.: The effect of BCG vaccination on the fate of virulent tubercle bacilli in mice. Am. Rev. Respir. Dis. *84:*28 (1961).

105. Lurie, M. B.: Resistance to tuberculosis: experimental studies in native and acquired defensive mechanisms (Harvard University Press, Cambridge, 1964).

106. Mackaness, G. B.: Artificial cellular immunity against tubercle bacilli. An effect of polyoxyethylene ethers (Triton). Amer. Rev. Tuberc. *69:*690 (1954).

107. Mackaness, G. B.: Cellular resistance to infection. J. exp. Med. *116:*381 (1962).

108. Mackaness, G. B.: The immunological basis of acquired cellular resistance. J. exp. Med. *120:*105 (1964).

109. Mackaness, G. B.: The behaviour of microbial parasites in relation to phagocytic cells *in vitro* and *in vivo*. *In* Symposium Soc. gen. Microbiol. *14:*213 (1964).

110. Mackaness, G. B.: Unpublished observations (1965).

111. McCluskey, R. T.: Benacerraf, B., and McCluskey, J. W.: Studies on the specificity of the cellular infiltrate in delayed hypersensitivity reactions. J. Immunol. *90:*466 (1963).

112. Medawar, P. B.: The immunology of transplantation. Harvey Lecture *52:*44 (1956).

113. Metaxas, M. N., and Metaxas-Buehler, M.: Studies on the cellular transfer of tuberculin reactivity in the guinea pig. J. Immunol. *75:*333 (1955).

114. Metchnikoff, E.: Immunity in infective diseases. (University Press, Cambridge 1905).

115. Miki, K., and Mackaness, G. B.: The passive transfer of acquired resistance to *Listeria monocytogenes*. J. exp. Med. *120:*93 (1964).

116. Mims, C. A.: The peritoneal macrophages of mice. Brit. J. exp. Path. *45:*37 (1964).

117. Mitsuhashi, S.: Cell-bound antibody in mouse mononuclear phagocytes. Allergy *13:*198 (1964).

118. Mitsuhashi, S., and Saito, K.: *In vitro* transfer of cellular immunity of mouse phagocytes in experimental Salmonellosis. J. Bact. *84:*592 (1962).

119. Möller, E.: Antagonistic effects of humoral isoantibody on the *in vitro* cytotoxicity of immune lymphoid cells. J. exp. Med. *122:*11 (1965).

120. Möller, E.: Contact induced cytotoxicity by lymphoid cells containing foreign isoantigens. Science *147:*873 (1965).

121. Möller, G., and Wigzell, H.: Antibody synthesis at the cellular level: Antibody-induced suppression of 19S and 7S antibody response. J. exp. Med. *121:*969 (1965).

122. Myrvik, Q. N., Leake, E. S., and Oshima, S.: A study of macrophages and epithelioid-like cells from granulomatous (BCG-induced lungs) of rabbits. J. Immunol. *89:*745 (1962).

123. Najarian, J. S., and Feldman, J. D.: Passive transfer of tuberculin sensitivity by tritiated thymidine-labeled lymphoid cells. J. exp. Med. *114:*779 (1961).

124. Najarian, J. S., and Feldman, J. D.: Passive transfer of transplantation immunity. I. Tritiated lymphoid cells. II. Lymphoid cells in millipore chambers. J. exp. Med. *115:*1083 (1962).

125. Najarian, J. S., and Feldman, J. D.: Observations on the passive transfer of transplantation immunity and delayed hypersensitivity with lymphoid cells in millipore chambers. Transplantation *1:*495 (1963).

126. Nelson, D. S., and Boyden, S. V.: The loss of macrophages from peritoneal exudates following the injection of antigen into guinea pigs with delayed-type hypersensitivity. Immunology *6:*264 (1963).

127. North R. J., and Mackaness, G. B.: Electron microscopical observations on the peritoneal macrophages of normal mice and mice immunised with *Listeria monocytogenes*. II. Structure of macrophages from immune mice and early cytoplasmic response to the presence of ingested bacteria. Brit. J. exp. Path. *44:*608 (1963).

128. Nossal, G. J. V., Ada, G. L., and Austin, C. M.: Antigens in immunity. II. Immunological properties of flagella, polymerized flagellin and flagellin in the primary response. Austr. J. exp. Biol. med. Sci. *42:*283 (1964).

129. Old, L. J., Boyse, E. A., Bennett, B., and Lilly, F.: Peritoneal cells as an immune population in transplantation studies. *In* Cell-bound antibodies, p. 89 (Wistar Institute Press, Philadelphia 1963).

130. Paterson, P. Y., Coia, E. M., and Jacobs, A. F.: Complement-fixing antibrain antibodies and allergic encephalomyelitis. I. Characterisation of the antibodies. Ann. N.Y. Acad. Sci. 122:256 (1965).

131. Paterson, P. Y., and Harwin, S. M.: Suppression of allergic encephalomyelitis in rats by means of antibrain serum. J. exp. Med. 117:755 (1963).

132. Paterson, P. Y., Jacobs, A. F., and Coia, E. M.: Complement-fixing antibrain antibodies and allergic encephalomyelitis. II. Further studies concerning their protective role. Ann. N.Y. Acad. Sci. 124:292 (1965).

133. Pierce, C. H., Dubos, R. J., and Schaefer, W. B.: Differential characteristics in vitro and in vivo of several substrains of BCG. III. Multiplication and survival in vivo. Amer. Rev. Tuberc. and Pul. Dis. 74:683 (1956).

134. Porter, K. A.: Morphological aspects of renal homograft rejection. Brit. med. Bull. 21:171 (1965).

135. Prendergast, R. A.: Cellular specificity in the homograft reaction. J. exp. Med. 119:377 (1964).

136. Raffel, S.: Delayed hypersensitivities. Progr. Allergy 4:173 (1954).

137. Raffel, S.: Immunity. 2nd ed. (Appleton-Century-Crofts, New York 1963), p. 333.

138. Rauch, H. C., and Raffel, S.: Antigen uptake by specifically reactive cells in experimental allergic encephalomyelitis. Ann. N.Y. Acad. Sci. 122:297 (1965).

139. Rose, N. R., Kite, J. H., Doebbler, T. K., Spier, R., Shelton, F. R., and Witebsky, E.: Studies on experimental thyroiditis. Ann. N.Y. Acad. Sci. 124:201 (1965).

140. Rosenau, W., and Moon, H. D.: Lysis of homologous cells by sensitised lymphocytes in tissue culture. J. nat. Cancer Inst. 27:471 (1961).

141. Rowley, D. and Leuchtenberg, C.: Antigen-stimulated desoxyribonucleic-acid synthesis in vitro by sensitised mouse macrophages. Lancet, Lond. ii:734 (1964).

142. Rowley, D., Turner, K. J., and Jenkin, C. R.: The basis for immunity in mouse typhoid. 3. Cell-bound antibody. Austr. J. exp. Biol. med. Sci. 42:237 (1964).

143. Saito, K., and Mitsuhashi, S.: Experimental Salmonellosis. VI. In vitro transfer of cellular immunity of mouse mononuclear phagocytes. J. Bact. 90:629 (1965)

144. Saito, K., Nakano, M.; Akiyama, T., and Ushiba, D.: Passive transfer of immunity to typhoid by macrophages. J. Bact. 84:800 (1962).

145. Saito, K., and Suter, E.: Lysosomal acid hydrolases in mice infected with BCG. J. exp. Med. 121:727 (1965).

146. Salvin, S. B.: Occurrence of delayed hypersensitivity during the development of Arthus type hypersensitivity. J. exp. Med. 107:109 (1958).

147. Salvin, S. B., and Smith, R. F.: Delayed hypersensitivity in the development of circulating antibody. The effect of X-irradiation. J. exp. Med. 109:325 (1959).

148. Sato, L., Kato, E., and Mitsuhashi, S.: In vitro transfer of cellular immunity by ribosomal fraction of mouse mononuclear phagocytes. Proc. 19th Kanto Branch Meeting, Japan bact. Assoc. p. 20 (1964).

149. Schaedler, R. W., and Dubos, R. J.: The susceptibility of mice to bacterial endotoxins. J. exp. Med. 113:559 (1961).

150. Schoenberg, M. D., Stavitsky, A. B., Moore, R. D., and Freeman, M. J.: Cellular sites of synthesis of rabbit immunoglobulins during primary response to diphtheria toxoid-Freund's adjuvant. J. exp. Med. 121:577 (1965).

151. Sever, J. L.: Passive transfer of resistance to tuberculosis through use of monocytes. Proc. Soc. exp. Biol. and Med. 103:326 (1960).

152. Shaw, C., Alvord, E. D., Kaku, J., and Kies, M. W.: Correlation of experimental allergic encephalomyelitis with delayed-type skin hypersensitivity to specific homologous encephalitogen. Ann. N.Y. Acad. Sci. 122:318 (1965).

153. Shaw, C., Alvord, E. C., Fahlberg, W. J., and Kies, M. W.: Substitutes for the mycobacteria in Freund's adjuvants in the production of experimental 'allergic' encephalomyelitis in the guinea pig. J. Immunol. 92:28 (1964).

154. Simonsen, M.: Graft versus host reactions. Their natural history, and applicability as tools of research. Progr. Allergy 6:349 (1962).

155. Snell, G. D.: The immunogenetics of tumor transplantation. Cancer Res. 12:543 (1952).

156. Steinmuller, D.: Passive transfer of immunity to skin homografts in rats. Ann. N.Y. Acad. Sci. 99:629 (1962).

157. Stetson, C. A.: The role of antibody in the rejection of homografts. In Mechanisms of Hypersensitivity. p. 569 (Churchill, London 1958).

158. Stetson, C. A.: Endotoxins and bacterial allergy. In Cellular and humoral aspects of the hypersensitive states. p. 442 (Hoeber-Harper, New York 1959).

159. Stetson, C. A.: The role of humoral antibody in the homograft reaction. Adv. Immunol. *3*:97 (1963).

160. Stetson, C. A., and Demopopoulos, R.: Reactions between skin homografts and specific immune sera. Ann. N.Y. Acad. Sci. *73*:687 (1958).

161. Suter, E., and Ramseier, H.: Cellular reactions in infection. Adv. Immunol. *4*:117 (1964).

162. Svehag, S., and Mandel, B.: The formation and properties of poliovirus-neutralizing antibody. I. 19S and 7S antibody formation: differences in kinetics and antigen dose requirement for induction. J. exp. Med. *119*:1 (1964).

163. Svehag, S., and Mandel, B.: The formation and properties of poliovirus-neutralizing antibody. II. 19S and 7S antibody formation: differences in antigen dose requirement for sustained synthesis, analysis, and sensitivity to X-irradiation. J. exp. Med. *119*:21 (1964).

164. Thomas, L., Paterson, P. Y., and Smithwick, B.: Acute disseminated encephalomyelitis following immunization with homologous brain extracts. I. Studies on the role of circulating antibody in the production of the condition in dogs. J. exp. Med. *92*:133 (1950).

165. Thorpe, B. D., and Marcus, S.: Phagocytosis and intracellular fate of *Pasteurella tularensis*. I. *In vitro* studies with rabbit peritoneal mononuclear phagocytes. J. Immunol. *92*:657 (1964).

166. Thorpe, B. D., and Marcus, S.: Phagocytosis and intracellular fate of *Pasteurella tularensis*. II. *In vitro* studies with rabbit alveolar and guinea pig alveolar and peritoneal mononuclear phagocytes. J. Immunol. *93*:558 (1965).

167. Turk, J. L.: The passive transfer of delayed hypersensitivity in guinea pigs by the transfusion of isotopically-labelled lymphoid cells. Immunology *5*:478 (1962).

168. Turk, J. L., and Stone, S. H.: Implications of the cellular changes in lymph nodes during the development and inhibition of delayed-type hypersensitivity. *In* Cell-bound antibodies, p. 51 (Wistar Institute Press, Philadelphia 1963).

169. Turner, K. J., Jenkin, C. R., and Rowley, D.: The basis for immunity to mouse typhoid. 2. Antibody formation during the carrier state. Austr. J. exp. Biol. med. Sci. *42*:229 (1964).

170. Uhr, J. W.: The heterogeneity of the immune response. Science *145*:457 (1964).

171. Uhr, J. W., and Finkelstein, M. S.: Antibody formation. IV. Formation of rapidly and slowly sedimenting antibody and immunological memory to bacteriophage øX 174. J. exp. Med. *117*:457 (1963).

172. Uhr, J. W., and Pappenheimer, A. M.: Delayed hypersensitivity. III. Specific desensitization of guinea pigs sensitized to protein antigens. J. exp. Med. *108*:891 (1958).

173. Uhr, J. W., Salvin, S. B., and Pappenheimer, A. M.: Delayed hypersensitivity. II. Induction of hypersensitivity in guinea pigs by means of antigen-antibody complexes. J. exp. Med. *105*:11 (1957).

174. Vainio, T., Koskimies, O., Perlmann, P., Perlmann, H., and Klein, G.: *In vitro* cytotoxic effect of lymphoid cells from mice immunized with allogeneic tissue. Nature, Lond. *204*:453 (1964).

175. Van Furth, R.: Quoted by Gowans, J. L., and McGregor, D. D.: The immunological activities of lymphocytes. Progr. Allergy *9*:1 (1965).

176. Volkman, A., and Gowans, J. L.: The production of macrophages in the rat. Brit. J. exp. Path. *46*:50 (1965).

177. Waksman, B. H.: The toxic effects of the antigen-antibody reaction on the cells of hypersensitive reactors. *In* Cellular and humoral aspects of the hypersensitive states. p. 123 (Hoeber-Harper, New York 1959).

178. Waksman, B. H.: A comparative histopathological study of delayed hypersensitive reactions. *In* Ciba Found. Symposium on Cellular aspects of immunity. p. 280 (Churchill, London 1960).

179. Waksman, B. H.: The local reaction of cellular hypersensitivity. Ann. N.Y. Acad. Sci. *116*:1045 (1964).

180. Waksman, B. H.: Animal investigation in autosensitisation: nervous system. Ann. N.Y. Acad. Sci. *124*:299 (1965).

181. Waksman, B. H., Arbouys, S., and Arnason, B. G.: The use of specific 'lymphocyte' antisera to inhibit hypersensitive reactions of the 'delayed' type. J. exp. Med. *114*:997 (1961).

182. Wattiaux, R., Wibo, M., and Baudhuin, P.: Influence of the injection of Triton WR-1339 on the properties of rat-liver lysosomes. *In* Ciba Found. Symposium on Lysosomes, p. 176 (Churchill, London 1963).

183. Weiser, R. S.: *In* Cell-bound antibodies, p. 71 (Wistar Institute Press, Philadelphia 1963).

184. Whitby, J. L., Michael, J. G., Woods, M. W., and Landy, M.: Symposium on bacterial

endotoxins. II. Possible mechanisms whereby endotoxins evoke increased nonspecific resistance to infection. Bact. Rev. *25:*437 (1961).

185. Wiedermann, G., Miescher, P. A., and Franklin, E. C.: Effect of mercaptoethanol on complement binding ability of human 7S gamma globulin. Proc. Soc. exp. Biol. N.Y. *113:* 609 (1963).

186. Wiener, J., Spiro, D., and Russell, P. S.: An electron microscopic study of the homograft reaction. Amer. J. Path. *44:*319 (1964).

187. Wigzell, H., Möller, G., and Andersson, B.: Studies at the cellular level of the 19S immune response. Acta Path. Microbiol. Scandinav. *66:*530–540 (1966).

188. Wilhelm, R. E., Fischer, J. P., and Cooke, R. A.: Experimental depletion of mononuclear cells for the purpose of investigating reactions of the allergic contact type. J. Allergy *29:*493 (1958).

189. Wilson, D. B.: The reaction of immunologically activated lymphoid cells against homologous target tissue cells *in vitro*. J. cell. compl. Physiol. *62:*273 (1963).

190. Wilson, D. B. Quantitative studies on the behaviour of sensitised lymphocytes *in vitro*. I. Relationship of the degree of destruction of homologous target cells to the number of lymphocytes and to the time of contact in culture and consideration of the effects of isoimmune serum. J. exp. Med. *122:*143 (1965).

191. Woodruff, M. F. A., and Anderson, N. F.: The effect of lymphocyte depletion and administration of antilymphocytic serum on the survival of skin homografts in rats. Ann. N.Y. Acad. Sci. *120:*119 (1964).

192. Woods, M. W., Landy, M., Whitby, J. L., and Burk, D.: Symposium on bacterial endotoxins. III. Metabolic effects of endotoxins on mammalian cells. Bact. Rev. *25:*447 (1961).

193. Zeiss, I. M., and Fox, M.: Donor and host contribution to splenomegaly in homologous mouse chimeras. Nature, Lond. *197:*673 (1963).

194. Zucker-Franklin, D.: The ultrastructure of cells in human thoracic duct lymph. J. Ultrastruct. Res. *9:*325 (1963).

# Chapter 3

# THE MECHANISM OF MACROPHAGE ACTIVATION

G. B. MACKANESS

*The Trudeau Institute Medical Research*
*Laboratories, Saranac Lake, New York*

Previously I have given reasons for thinking that insight into the mechanisms involved in antituberculous immunity might come more easily through the study of other intracellular infections than by studying tuberculosis itself. Now I would like to present the results of some experiments which have been performed in the intervening years in efforts to explore the nature of the antibacterial immunity developed against the tubercle bacillus.

In its resting state, the mononuclear phagocyte is a mobile cell of relatively simple structure; but it is capable of responding to a variety of stimuli which provoke it into a state of intense physiological activity. This is accompanied by changes in function and morphology which have been referred to as "differentiation." But since the process is reversible, it seems more appropriate to speak of the phenomenon as "macrophage activation." Cohn[1] has shown, in elegant studies, that activation of macrophages occurs *in vitro*, and studies in many other laboratories have shown that a similar process also occurs *in vivo*. It has become clear, in fact, that this potential for functional hypertrophy of macrophages is exploited by the host in its defense against a variety of infectious diseases, and that one mechanism of macrophage activation is under immunological control. Moreover, the phenomenon does not appear to be restricted to defense against infectious disease; for it seems that activated macrophages appear in other important immunological processes such as the graft-versus-host reaction and transplantation immunity.

It has long been known from the studies of Lurie[4] that the macrophages of tuberculous animals possess properties which distinguish them from those of normal animals. It is only recently, however, that we have learned of the magnitude of the change which can develop in their functional capacity, and of the importance of activated macrophages in acquired immunity. The subject will be discussed under several broad headings, beginning with a description of the features which distinguish an activated macrophage from its normal counterpart.

# THE CHARACTERISTICS OF ACTIVATED MACROPHAGES

Macrophages taken from animals at certain stages of infection with any of a variety of facultative intracellular parasites are found to differ from normal cells in morphology, behavior *in vitro*, phagocytic activity, metabolic activity, content of hydrolytic enzymes, microbicidal ability, and cytopeptic activity. Figure 1 shows a comparison between macrophages obtained from the peritoneal cavities of normal (A) and BCG-infected mice (B). They are phase-contrast micrographs taken, at the same magnification, 12 hours after the cells had been isolated in culture at 37°C. A difference in size, tendency to spread, and content of cytoplasmic organelles is clearly apparent. The activated cells were obtained 12 days after the intravenous injection of $5 \times 10^7$ viable BCG. The most distinguishing features of the activated macrophages from the infected animal are their content of mitochondria (filamentous phase-dense bodies), lysosomes (spherical phase-dense granules), and pinocytic activity. The latter is revealed by the numbers of phase-lucent vesicles which can be seen in living cultures to arise in the periphery of the cell and migrate toward the center where they fuse to form larger vesicles. From the studies of Cohn and his collaborators[1] we know that pinocytic vesicles acquire hydrolytic enzymes and become consolidated into the dense granules which are often a conspicuous feature of the activated macrophage.

The foregoing differences in morphology can also be seen in the electron micrographs of Figure 2, which also show that the activated cell (B) has an enlarged Golgi complex. It usually contains more free ribosomes and a more elaborate endoplasmic reticulum than is seen in the unstimulated cell (A).

The second distinguishing feature of the activated macrophage is the extreme rapidity with which it spreads on glass surfaces when first isolated from the peritoneal cavity. This is illustrated in Figure 3 which shows that macrophages from a BCG-infected animal (B) were fully and circumferentially spread after only 15 minutes of incubation, whereas those of normal mice (A) were not completely spread after 3 hours and had assumed an elongated rather than a rounded form.

North[2] has made interesting studies in recent years which show that the spreading of a macrophage is an expression of its capacity to perform mechanical work, and that the degree to which a cell spreads is related to its phagocytic capacity. It is not surprising, therefore, that the activated macrophage displays a markedly increased phagocytic ability which appears to be due to an intrinsic property of the cell. Thus, the activated macrophages produced during a *Listeria* infection can ingest *Salmonella typhimurium* in the absence of specific antibody, whereas those of normal mice cannot.[3]

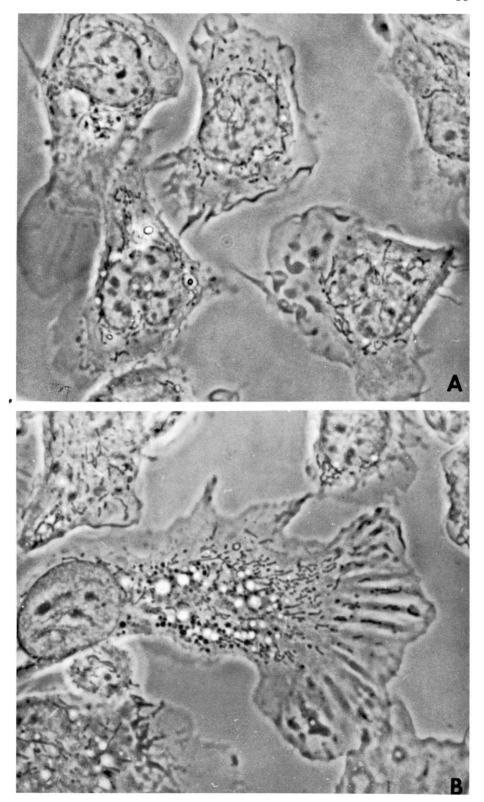

*Figure 1.*  For explanation see text.

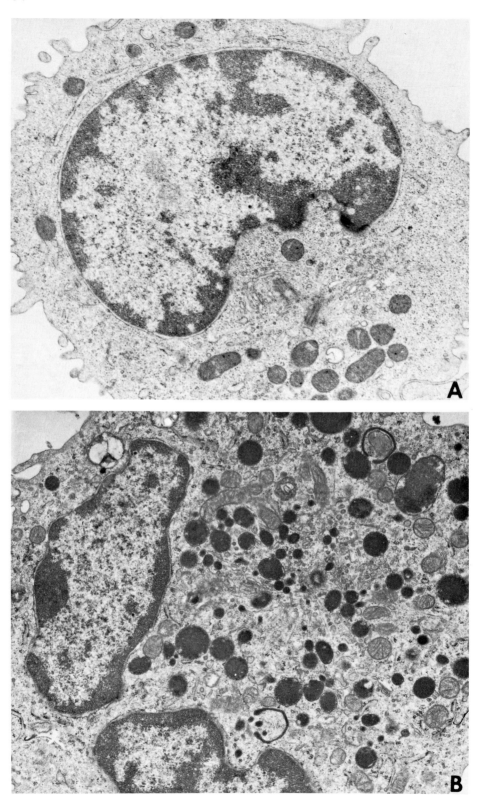

*Figure 2.*   For explanation see text.

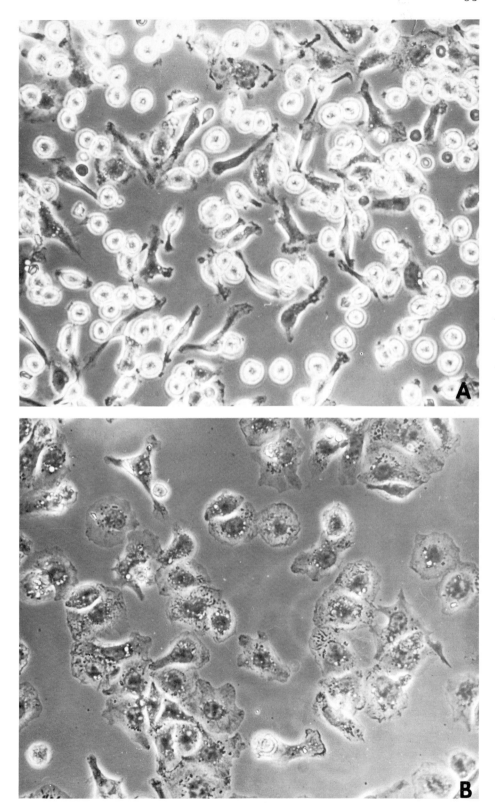

*Figure 3.* For explanation see text.

The metabolic activity of fully activated macrophages has never been the subject of detailed study. It is known, however, that a variety of enzymic activities are increased in cells obtained from actively infected animals.[4] But the observations have usually been performed on cells taken at a late stage of infection, and have shown only slight differences from normal. As we shall see, highly activated macrophages exist for only a limited period during the course of most infectious diseases. We know very little about the metabolism of macrophages at this time of heightened activity.

The increased pinocytic activity and content of hydrolytic enzymes[1] suggest that the synthetic activity of the activated macrophage is high. Both of these functions require an abundant and continuous supply of metabolic energy. Moreover, the greatly enhanced capacity of the cell to spread and to ingest particulate material suggests that the activated cell possesses a fund of energy which is immediately available to it. The studies of North[2] suggest that this energy may exist in the form of free adenosine triphosphate (ATP), which has a marked stimulating effect on spreading and phagocytosis. The energy metabolism of activated macrophages deserves further detailed investigation.

From the viewpoint of infectious disease, the most important attribute of the activated macrophage is its enhanced microbicidal activity. This property can be demonstrated convincingly only by using special techniques, because the rapid phagocytosis of which activated cells are capable can be misinterpreted as enhanced microbicidal activity. In order to measure intracellular killing it is necessary to distinguish between phagocytic and postphagocytic events. When this is done, the activated macrophage is found to kill a variety of microorganisms more rapidly and more completely than normal. Macrophages obtained at certain stages of *Listeria* or *Brucella* infections are uniformly microbicidal for *Listeria monocytogenes* when studied by a plaquing technique which measures the proportion of ingested bacteria which are irreversibly inactivated.[5, 6] This method, however, does not measure the *rate* of bacterial inactivation. If Maaløe's technique, in which intracellular and extracellular bacteria are counted independently, is used to study the intracellular fate of *S. typhimurium* in the peritoneal cavity, it is found that the rate of intracellular bacterial inactivation is slower and less complete in normal cells than in the activated macrophages found in *Listeria, Salmonella*, or BCG-infected mice. This is illustrated in Figure 4.[3] Intracellular death of *S. typhimurium* does not

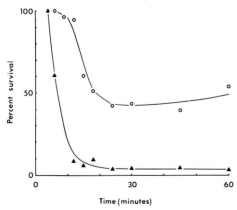

*Figure 4.* Curves showing rates of intracellular death of *S. typhimurium* in normal ( o —— o) and activated (▲ —— ▲) macrophages. In both cases the organisms were opsonized with specific antiserum.

begin for 9 minutes after ingestion by normal cells and only about 50 per cent are finally inactivated. In the activated macrophages, on the other hand, killing begins even before the first reading can be obtained 2.5 minutes after first contact between cells and organisms. From this time on bacterial inactivation proceeds rapidly until 98 per cent of all ingested organisms are killed, a process which takes about 15 minutes.

In addition to the increased rate of bacterial inactivation there are indications that the rate of bacterial degradation is also greater in the activated macrophage. The difference, however, is not spectacular in comparison with the difference in the rate of killing.[12]

## TIME-COURSE OF MACROPHAGE ACTIVATION

All of the foregoing observations, and many others, show that the macrophages of actively infected animals can become much more active physiologically. It must not be inferred, however, that marked changes are always found, or that macrophages become activated uniformly throughout the reticuloendothelial system. The cells of infected animals change more or less gradually to reach a peak of activity and then return toward normal. The tempo of events depends upon the infecting organism and the size of the infecting dose. Cell changes develop rapidly in acute intracellular infections such as listeriosis, and more slowly in chronic infections such as brucellosis or tuberculosis. However, if the infecting dose is very large, even the tubercle bacillus can bring about rapid and dramatic changes in host macrophages.

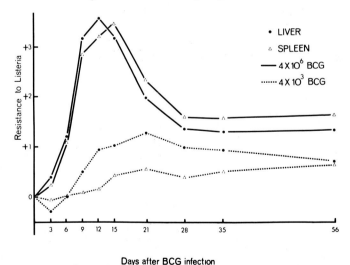

Days after BCG infection

*Figure 5.* Curves depicting the progressive changes in the index of resistance to *L. monocytogenes* in the livers and spleens of mice during primary infection with BCG administered at two dose levels. Each point represents the mean difference (Log$_{10}$) between the increase or decrease in viable count of *L. monocytogenes* found in the organs of control and BCG-infected animals 24 hours after intravenous challenge. Data from Blanden, Lefford, and Mackaness.[7]

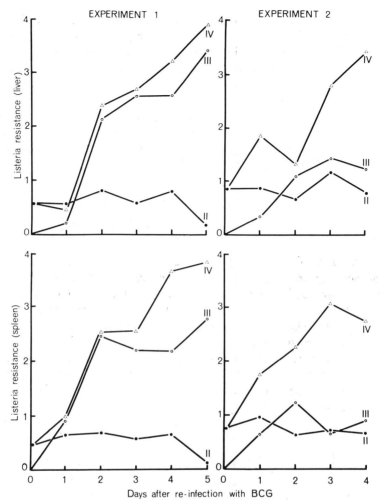

*Figure 6. Disregard Experiment 1. Experiment 2:* Curves showing progressive changes in the index of resistance to *L. monocytogenes* in liver and spleen (See Fig. 5 for description) during primary and secondary BCG infection in mice. The mice were immunized with $1 \times 10^4$ BCG 23 days prior to day 0 (II); $1 \times 10^7$ BCG on day 0 (III); or $1 \times 10^4$ BCG 23 days prior to day 0 and re-infected with $1 \times 10^7$ BCG on day 0 (IV). Data from Blanden, Lefford, and Mackaness.[7]

The host response to a mycobacterial infection can be illustrated by experiments in which *L. monocytogenes* and *S. typhimurium* were used to measure the effects of living BCG on host resistance and macrophage activity.[7] Different doses of BCG were compared with respect to the effects produced on the macrophages of the spleen and liver, and on those in the peritoneal cavity of the mouse. With small infecting doses ($10^3$ to $10^6$) the cells of the peritoneal cavity remained morphologically and functionally normal, but in those in the spleen an increased level of activity developed after 10 to 20 days. During this interval the macrophages of the spleen were morphologically similar to those illustrated in Figure 1. Coinciding with this period of altered cell morphology, the ability of the spleen and the liver to inactivate an inoculum of *L. mono-*

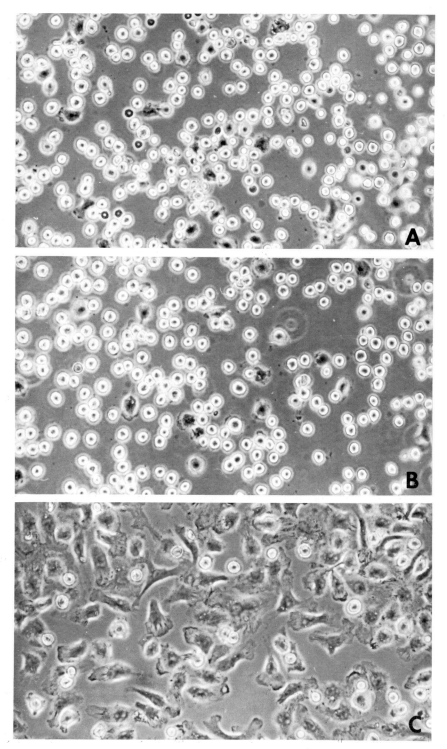

*Figure 7.* For explanation see text.

*cytogenes* was greatly increased. This is illustrated in Figure 5 which shows the progressive changes in the behavior of an intravenous inoculum of *L. monocytogenes* in the organs of normal and BCG-infected mice. The plot shows the differences ($\log_{10}$) in the viable counts found in spleens and livers 24 hours after challenge. It is apparent that in mice injected with $4 \times 10^6$ living BCG a high level of resistance to *Listeria* developed in the interval 9 to 15 days after infection; those receiving $4 \times 10^3$ BCG were much less resistant.

When larger doses of BCG ($10^7$ to $10^8$) were injected into mice, morphological and functional changes *did* develop in the macrophages of the peritoneal cavity. These changes appeared at the time when peak resistance to *Listeria* was reached in the spleen and liver. The cells illustrated in Figure 1 were taken on the twelfth day after the intravenous injection of $5 \times 10^7$ viable BCG. At this time the peritoneal macrophages were also found to be highly microbidical for *S. typhimurium.*

The foregoing observations indicated that the free macrophages of the peritoneal cavity of the mouse become activated only during a very heavy infection with BCG. However, much smaller numbers were found to produce effects in peritoneal cells of previously vaccinated mice. Animals injected intravenously with a small, sensitizing dose of BCG ($1 \times 10^4$) were found to be highly sensitive to tuberculin when tested 23 days later. Half of them and half of an equal number of normal mice were then given an intravenous injection of BCG ($1 \times 10^7$). The other two halves of each group were used as normal and hypersensitive controls. Each day after the second injection of BCG ten mice from each of the four groups received an intravenous injection of *L. monocytogenes* to measure host resistance in spleen and liver. It was found that the index of resistance to this organism rose much more rapidly in the hypersensitive mice (Fig. 6, Experiment 2). Moreover, the macrophages in the peritoneal cavity of the reinfected mice became morphologically and functionally hyperactive within 24 hours of the second injection of BCG (Fig. 7C), and became even more active over the next 3 days. By contrast, the cells of normal mice remained uninfluenced by this dose of BCG (Fig. 7B). The effects seen in the peritoneal cavities of the hypersensitive mice were due entirely to the second injection of BCG because the cells of the hypersensitive controls remained normal throughout the period of observation (Fig. 7A). The cells illustrated in Figure 7 had been incubated for 15 minutes. Only the cells of reinfected mice showed spreading and increased microbicidal activity for *S. typhimurium.*[7]

## THE IMMUNOLOGICAL BASIS OF MACROPHAGE ACTIVATION

There are many reasons for thinking that the sharp increase in host resistance and the rapid changes observed in the macrophages of reinfected mice are somehow related to the phenomenon of delayed-type hypersensitivity. The first indication of this came from studying the rate at which hypersensitivity and resistance develop in *Listeria*-infected mice. The onset of delayed hypersensitivity to *Listeria* culture filtrate coincides with the appearance of activated macrophages in the peritoneal cavity.[5] A similar time relationship exists between the development of tuberculin sensitivity and the appearance of increased resistance to *L. monocytogenes* in the spleens and livers of BCG-infected mice.[7]

A second indication that delayed-type hypersensitivity might be involved in the production of activated macrophages was the finding that resistance to intracellular parasites arises only when the method used for immunization also produces this type of immunological reactivity. Living organisms provoke both delayed-type hypersensitivity and increased resistance to infection. Dead organisms, on the other hand, are relatively or absolutely inert as immunizing agents unless they are administered in Freund-type adjuvant which alters the type of immune response and directs it toward the production of delayed hypersensitivity.

The difference in host response to living and dead organisms is well illustrated in mice injected with BCG. Figure 8 shows a difference in the effect of living and dead BCG on resistance to challenge with *L. monocytogenes*. The living organism ($7 \times 10^7$), when injected intravenously, produced a rapid and marked increase in resistance to *Listeria*. The same number of partially heat-inactivated BCG (56°C. for 30 minutes) had no such effect. Figure 8 also shows that in animals given the same number of living BCG while under treatment with isoniazid resistance began to develop, but was rapidly lost. The initial effect observed in isoniazid-treated mice may have been due to the lag in the bactericidal action of this drug. Whatever the reason, it is clear that

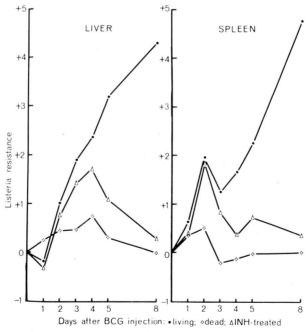

*Figure 8.* Curves showing progressive changes in the index of resistance to *L. monocytogenes* in the livers and spleens of mice given $7 \times 10^7$ viable BCG on day 0 (●); of mice given the same dose of living BCG but treated with isoniazid throughout the experiment (△); and mice given the same number of heat-inactivated BCG (◇). Data from Blanden, Lefford, and Mackaness.[7]

living organisms are much more effective in producing the type of immune response which leads to increased host resistance. The inertness of killed organisms cannot be due to destruction of heat-labile antigens or to any deficiency in the dose of antigens delivered by nonmultiplying organisms. This is deduced from the fact that dead organisms cause an increase in resistance if they are administered in a Freund-type adjuvant (unpublished observations).

There is one more apparently conclusive indication that acquired cellular resistance is dependent upon the phenomenon of delayed-type hypersensitivity. Figure 9 records the results of an experiment which illustrates some important features of the immunology of acquired cellular resistance.[11] The passive transfer of serum from actively infected donors is incapable of transferring resistance against *L. monocytogenes* (Fig. 9B). However, living lymphoid cells prepared from the spleens of the same donors did confer a high level of resistance upon the spleens and livers of normal recipients (Fig. 9A). Frenkel[8] has also shown that living lymphoid cells from immunized donors can protect mice against infection with *Besnoitia jellisoni*. In the *Listeria* experiments dissociated spleen cells were filtered through cotton wool to remove all preformed macrophages. The resulting suspension of "lymphoid" cells made normal

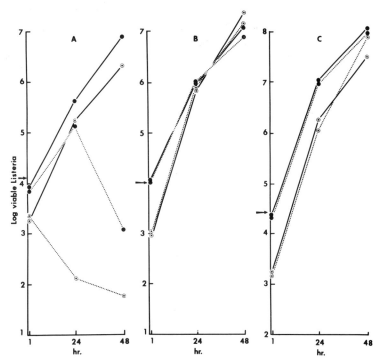

*Figure 9.* Curves showing growth or inactivation of *L. monocytogenes* in the liver ( ● ) and spleens ( ⊙ ) of mice challenged intravenously.

A, Mice treated with $10^8$ spleen cells from normal (———) or immune (·······) donors. Immune cells taken on day 8 of a primary *Listeria* infection.

B, Mice treated with 1.0 ml. of serum from the normal (———) or immune (·······) donors.

C, Mice given normal (———) or immune (·······) spleen cells ($10^8$) which had been disrupted by ultrasound. Data from Mackaness.[11]

recipients hypersensitive to *Listeria* culture filtrate, and protected them against intravenous challenge when given intravenously in a dose equivalent to the cell content of a single spleen (Fig. 9A). The resistance that developed in the recipients was dependent upon the numbers of cells injected (Fig. 10) and the stage of the infection at which they were harvested (Fig. 11). The cells were active only in a living condition (Fig. 10C) and lost most of their activity when preincubated with mitomycin C.

The passive protection afforded by living lymphoid cells suggests that acquired resistance to *Listeria*, which is known to be due to activation of host macrophages,[5] depends upon a cell-mediated form of immunological reactivity. This suggests more strongly and more directly than other evidence already cited that acquired cellular resistance is somehow dependent upon delayed-type hypersensitivity. This view gains further support from studies on the specificity of the immunity which can be transferred with living lymphoid cells.

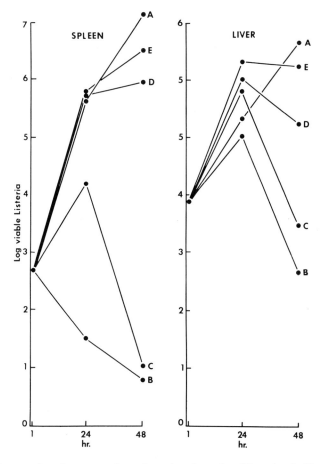

*Figure 10.* Curves showing growth or inactivation of a *Listeria* challenge in livers and spleens of mice injected intravenously with normal spleen cells (*A*) in a dose of $2 \times 10^8$, or immune spleen cells from *Listeria*-infected donors in doses of $2 \times 10^8$ (*B*), $4 \times 10^7$ (*C*), $8 \times 10^6$ (*D*) and $2 \times 10^6$ (*E*). The high 24 hour counts in liver may have been due to transfer of *L. monocytogenes* with the immune spleen cells which were obtained while the donors were still actively infected. Data from Mackaness.[11]

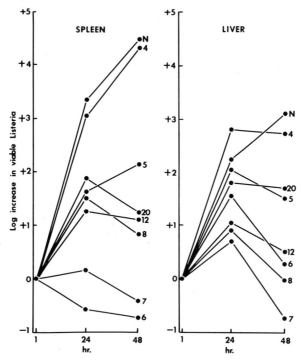

*Figure 11.* Curves showing the growth or inactivation of a *Listeria* challenge in spleens and livers of mice receiving spleen cells in a dose of $10^8$ from normal donors (N) or from immune donors at different stages of an immunizing *Listeria* infection. The curves are numbered according to the day of the infection upon which the cells were harvested. Maximum protection was afforded by cells obtained on the sixth to the eighth day of a *Listeria* infection. Data from Mackaness.[11]

The resistance which can be transferred with immune lymphoid cells appears to be specific for the infecting agent used to immunize the donor. In this respect, the immunity conferred adoptively is completely different from that which exists in the donor, because this is known to be nonspecific.[6] When spleen cells from BCG-immunized animals were transferred to normal recipients they conferred tuberculin sensitivity upon the recipients, but did not protect them against a *Listeria* challenge. Figure 12 shows this and two other significant facts: (1) the BCG-immunized cell donors were in fact nonspecifically resistant to *L. monocytogenes* (Fig. 12E); (2) the recipients of BCG-sensitized cells (Fig. 12B) developed a measurable degree of resistance to *Listeria* when injected with a dose of BCG which had no effect upon mice receiving cells from normal mice (Fig. 12D). Apparently the macrophages in the spleens of animals which have been passively sensitized with lymphoid cells from BCG-sensitive donors become altered only in the presence of the organism (BCG) to which the donor had been rendered sensitive.

Although this finding indicates that macrophage activation takes place during a delayed-type hypersensitivity reaction, the exact mechanism is still obscure. It is tempting to speculate that a stimulating substance is released by the sensitive lymphoid cell when exposed to specific antigen. However, attempts

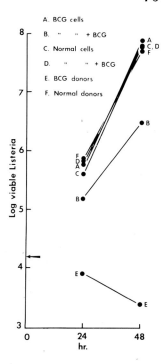

*Figure 12.* The curves illustrate the behavior of a population of *L. monocytogenes* in the spleens of mice which had received $10^8$ normal (*C* and *D*) or BCG-immunized spleen cells (*A* and *B*); and in the spleens of the normal (*F*) or immune (*E*) donors. Half of the recipients of normal (*D*) and immune (*B*) cells were also injected with a small dose of BCG at the same time. The curves show that the immune donors were *Listeria* resistant (*E*). However, the recipients of cells from these donors were no more resistant than normal animals (*F*) or the recipients of normal cells (*C*); but the injection of BCG produced a statistically significant increase in resistance only in the recipients of BCG-sensitized lymphoid cells (*B*). This dose of BCG had no effect on the resistance of recipients given normal cells (*D*).

to demonstrate a stimulating substance analogous to the macrophage migration inhibition factor of David[9] and Bloom and Bennett[10] have been unsuccessful.

# References

1. Cohn, Z. A., and Benson, B. (1965). The *in vitro* differentiation of mononuclear phagocytes. II. The influence of serum on granule formation, hydrolase production and pinocytosis. J. Exp. Med., *121*:835–848.
2. North, R. J. (1968). The uptake of particulate antigens. J. Retic. Soc. *5*:203–229.
3. Blanden, R. V., Mackaness, G. B., and Collins, F. M. (1966). Mechanisms of acquired resistance in mouse typhoid. J. Exp. Med. *124*:585–600.
4. Lurie, M. B. (1964). Resistance to Tuberculosis. Harvard University Press, Cambridge, Massachusetts.
5. Mackaness, G. B. (1962). Cellular resistance to infection. J. Exp. Med. *116*:381–406.
6. Mackaness, G. B. (1964). The immunological basis of acquired cellular resistance. J. Exp. Med. *120*:105–120.
7. Blanden, R. V., Lefford, M. J., and Mackaness, G. B. (1969). The host response to Calmette-Guérin bacillus infection in mice. J. Exp. Med. *129*:1079–1106.
8. Frenkel, J. F.: (1967). Adoptive immunity to intracellular infection. J. Immun. *98*:1309–1319.
9. David, J. R. (1966). Delayed hypersensitivity *in vitro*: its mediation by cell-free substances formed by lymphoid cell-antigen interaction. Proc. Nat. Acad. Sci. *56*:72–77.
10. Bloom, B. R., and Bennett, B. (1966). Mechanism of a reaction *in vitro* associated with delayed-type hypersensitivity. Science *153*:80–82.
11. Mackaness, G. B. (1969). The influence of immunologically committed lymphoid cells on macrophage activity *in vivo*. J. Exp. Med. *129*:973–992.
12. Blanden, R. V. (1968). Modification of macrophage function. J. Retic. Soc. *5*:179–202.
13. Wigzell, H., Möller, G., and Andersson, B. (1966). Studies at the cellular level of the 19S immune response. Acta. Path. Microbiol. Scand. *66*:530–540.

# Chapter 4

# BULWARKS OF THE BODILY DEFENSE*

ROBERT A. GOOD, JOANNE FINSTAD, and RICHARD A. GATTI

*Pediatric Research Laboratories and Departments of Microbiology and Pediatrics, Variety Club Heart Hospital, University of Minnesota, Minneapolis, Minnesota*

As one might expect of a major contributor to survival, immunity has proved to be a most complicated process, the understanding of which is only beginning to emerge. To understand fully immune participation in the bodily defense one must consider cellular and molecular bases of immune reactions, the interrelations of the various cellular systems involved in immunity, and the biologic systems by which these interactions can be amplified to achieve an effective defense. The mammalian host survives in a sea of bacteria, viruses, and fungi, many of which possess the capacity to invade and utilize bodily cells and fluids for their own nutrition and replication. The products of the micro-organismal metabolism are often toxic to Eutherian hosts, the placental mammals. Defense against invasion by encapsulated extracellular pyogenic bacterial pathogens, facultative intracellular pyogenic bacteria, fungi, and viruses, as well as against invasion by neoplastic cells, represents a major role for the immune reactions and their biologic amplification systems. Included in the latter must be the complement system, the inflammatory response, amplification of the cell-mediated immune response, microphagic and macrophagic phagocytic cells, and mechanisms for intracellular destruction of the invaders.

Using evidence gathered in recent years from the study of patients with hereditary immune deficiencies, immunologic deficiencies associated with malignancies of the lymphoreticular apparatus, and experimentally produced immune deficiencies, we hope to delineate some of the major bulwarks of bodily

* Aided by The National Foundation–March of Dimes, U.S. Public Health Service (AI-08677, HE-06314, and AI-00798), American Heart Association, and the Minnesota Chapter of the Arthritis Foundation.

defense and in the process suggest constellations of infection that may assist the practicing physician in recognizing new syndromes of infectious disease. We further hope in this chapter to provoke a new approach to the classification of Eutherian pathogens and, subsequently, to their treatment.

# DIFFERENTIATION OF TWO LYMPHOID SYSTEMS

Several lines of inquiry provide compelling evidence that the major roles in immunologic defense are to be divided into two separate systems of lymphoid cells, each of which employs different amplification systems to achieve its full potential in the bodily defense.[66] Figure 1 summarizes our current view relating anatomic structure to physiologic function of the lymphoid system in terms of the developmental relationships. It seems clear that the hematopoietic tissues, e.g., yolk sac, fetal liver, and bone marrow, contain a multipotent progenitor cell. Depending upon its preceding complex history, this cell can respond to inducing influences of different microchemical environments and thereby differentiate along a variety of lines representing the definitive hematologic components. For example, these cells can differentiate to erythrocytes, granulocytes, megakaryocytes, eosinophils, or basophils depending upon the microchemical environment in which the progenitor cell finds itself during the developmental process. Another direction of differentiation is to a lymphoid stem cell, which may develop in the yolk sac, fetal liver, or marrow. This lymphoid stem cell, a pivotal point in the development of the lymphoid system, can be further

THYMUS SYSTEM DEVELOPMENT

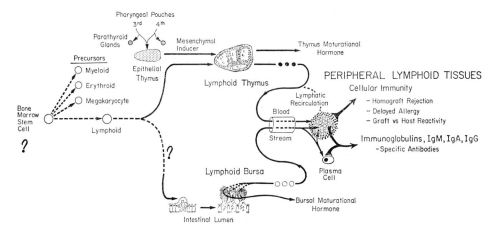

BURSAL SYSTEM DEVELOPMENT

*Figure 1.* Schematic diagram illustrating development of dual-component immunologic system. (From Hoyer, J. R., et al. 1968. Lymphopenic forms of congenital immunologic deficiency diseases. Medicine *47*:201–226.)

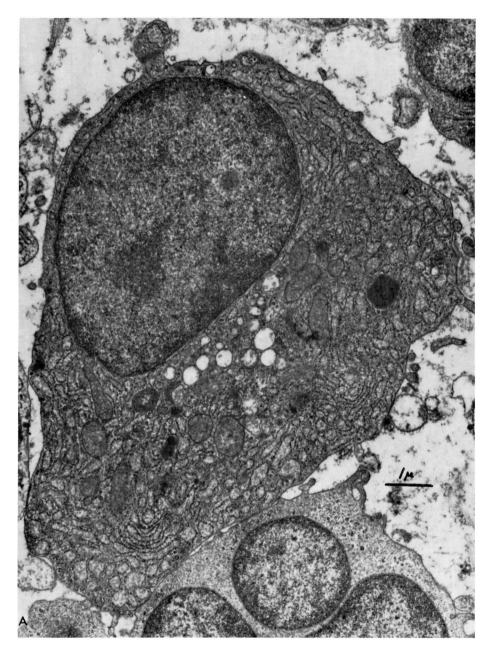

*Figure 2.* *A,* Electromicrograph of normal plasma cell showing eccentrically placed nucleus, well developed endoplasmic reticulum, and prominent Golgi apparatus (18,000×). *B,* Electromicrograph of normal small lymphocyte showing scant cytoplasm with absence of endoplasmic reticulum (16,000×). (Courtesy of C.C. Clawson.)

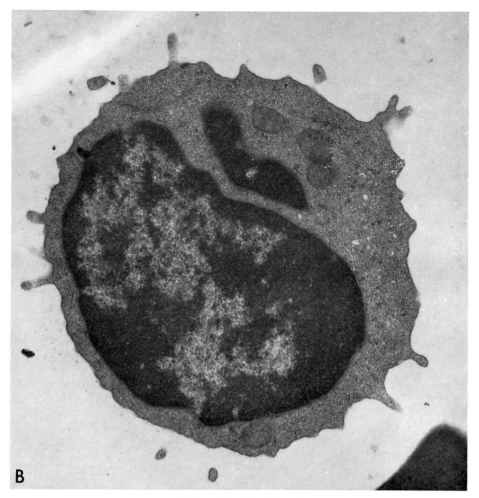

B

*Figure 2.* Continued.

differentiated into either of two separate populations of lymphoid cells, depending upon the nature of a second differentiative environment. One of these populations, differentiated under thymic influence, probably actually within the microchemical environment of the thymus, represents a system of small, long-lived lymphocytes that percolate through the lymphoid tissues and circulate and recirculate through peripheral lymphoid tissues and in lymph and blood. This system of cells, in its fully differentiated form, has a strong propensity to reside in specialized areas or zones in the peripheral lymphoid organs, e.g., in lymph nodes and spleen and along the gastrointestinal tract. It represents a readily mobile system that acts as a veritable "flying squadron" of cells capable of subserving the functions of cell-mediated immunity.

This lymphocytic system is to be sharply separated from a second system of lymphoid cells which in fully differentiated form represents a more sessile population of cells responsible for production of circulating antibodies. This population of cells, too, tends to be located within rather specialized areas of the peripheral lymphoid organs. In fully differentiated form these cells

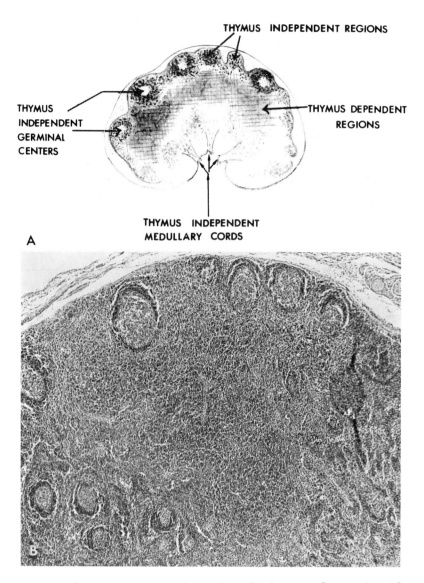

*Figure 3.   A*, Schematic diagram of lymph node showing thymus-dependent and thymus-independent regions. *B*, Normal human lymph node showing thymus-dependent and thymus-independent regions.

represent veritable factories for production and secretion of the immunoglobulin molecules and the antibodies they represent. The site or sites in man where differentiation to the antibody-secreting, immunoglobulin-producing cells occurs is not known, but in birds it appears to be confined to a peculiar lymphoepithelial organ located at the posterior end of the gastrointestinal tract, the bursa of Fabricius. The cells representing this line of differentiation possess an admirable machinery for protein synthesis and secretion and to the morphologist have the appearance of plasma cells (Fig. 2). It seems to us no longer germane to argue whether it is lymphocytes or plasma cells that synthesize antibodies—they both do, but when they are capable of executing this function they represent the end result of a specific line of differentiation which separates them distinctly from the line of differentiation of the population of long-lived small lymphocytes responsible for the cell-mediated immune responses.

## THYMUS-DEPENDENT AND THYMUS-INDEPENDENT AREAS OF PERIPHERAL LYMPHOID ORGANS

The population of small lymphocytes developing under thymic influence tends to reside in regions in the peripheral lymphoid organs and tissues that are rather specialized and that are separate (although overlapping of territories surely exists) from the regions in the lymph nodes and spleen that house the cells which produce antibodies. Figure 3 shows a typical regional lymph node illustrating the thymus-dependent and thymus-independent regions of the lymph node. Such organization within the lymph nodes holds for mice,[127] rabbits,[156] and guinea pigs,[162] and man[65, 75] and thus represents an organization widespread in nature. In lymph nodes, the thymus-dependent regions are located in the deep cortical or paracortical zones whereas the far external cortical regions, the juxtamedullary areas, and the medullary cords represent thymus-independent regions of the nodes. It is regularly within the thymus-independent areas that germinal centers appear, and germinal centers represent thymus-independent structures.

The populations of lymphoid cells in the peripheral lymphoid organs can be induced to proliferative expansion by antigenic stimulation. If one chooses antigens appropriately one can expand the dual lymphoid populations separately.[75, 126, 163] For example, after intradermal injection of pneumococcal polysaccharide into the guinea pig or rabbit, which will bring about only antibody production, the lymphoid cells in the thymus-independent regions proliferate and plasma cells develop in the medullary cords. By contrast, stimulation of the regional node at the base of the ear by topical application of 2,4-dinitrochlorobenzene (DNCB) or intradermal injection of DNP-bovine gamma globulin brings about proliferation of cells in the deep cortical region of the node without producing proliferative response in the far cortical regions or in medullary cords, and plasma cell formation is minimal or does not occur at all. In other words, appropriate antigenic stimulation which brings about either cell-mediated immunity or antibody formation, but not both, will stimulate independent proliferation and further differentiation of either the thymus-dependent or thymus-independent system of cells. However, most antigenic stimuli provoke both cell-mediated immunities and antibody production, leading to expansion of both populations of lymphoid cells.

## EFFECT OF NEONATAL THYMECTOMY

In 1960 and 1961, we in Minneapolis[4, 64, 108] and at approximately the same time Miller in England[118] independently discovered that removal of the thymus in rabbits or rodents in the immediate neonatal period will interfere with development of immunologic capacity. In mice, considerable strain differences have been observed in this influence and the cleanest models have been obtained in both mice and rabbits when sublethal, total-body irradiation is given in the neonatal period to the thymectomized animals.[111, 112, 120] Although some confusion was introduced by the fact that the discovery of thymic influence was made with respect to antibody production,[4] it soon became apparent that the major influence of thymic extirpation was on ability to develop and execute the cell-mediated immune responses.[64, 108] Mice thymectomized as neonates or, better, thymectomized and irradiated as neonates, develop as profound immunologic cripples. Such animals cannot develop delayed allergy or reject homografts of skin. The lymphoid cells from their blood, thoracic duct, lymph nodes, or spleen will not initiate a graft-versus-host reaction[38] and they cannot resist infections with certain bacteria, fungi, and viruses.[139] By contrast, such animals have normal amounts of each of the known immunoglobulins and can make antibodies as well as can normal animals when stimulated with appropriate antigens, e.g., Brucella, Salmonella H, or flagellin.

Neonatally thymectomized mice and rabbits, however, are defective in producing antibodies to sheep red blood cells (SRBC) as well as to certain soluble protein antigens, but it has become clear that even with these thymus-dependent antibody responses the actual production of antibody is achieved by thymus-independent lymphoid cells and plasma cells.[39, 119, 122] Mosser et al.,[120] Lemmel et al.[102, 111] in Minneapolis, and Sinclair and Elliott[145] have presented evidence that the thymus-dependent lymphoid cells exert only a helping role in this regard, and most likely this does not imply the existence of antigen-sensitive cells which exchange information with antigen-insensitive cells of the thymus-independent system.[62] In mice thymectomized at birth and in addition given near-lethal x-irradiation, the antibody production to SRBC is minimal, but small amounts of antibody are always produced. If such mice are given larger numbers of SRBC or are repeatedly stimulated with SRBC, antibody responses will occur and will achieve titers approximately equal to those of mice that have undergone sham operations and that possess an intact thymus-dependent system of cells. Neonatally thymectomized and irradiated mice respond with antibody synthesis as do normal mice or those that have had sham operations to antigenic stimulation with Brucella or Salmonella H antigens.

Figure 4 shows the lymph node of an 8 week old neonatally thymectomized mouse.

## THYMUS-INDEPENDENT LYMPHOID SYSTEM

Plasma cell production, germinal center development, and lymphocyte concentrations in the far cortical regions are normal in mice from which the thymus has been removed (either in the neonatal period or in adulthood) that have also been subjected to near-lethal, total-body irradiation. Such animals are very prone to infections with fungi, viruses, and pyogenic pathogens of otherwise low-grade virulence. When they become infected they can often achieve marked elevations of immunoglobulin levels and seem very likely to develop autoimmune phenomena and amyloidosis.[155, 157]

The apparently paradoxical relationships derived from study of immunoglobulin levels, immune responses, lymphoid tissue reactions, and development of amyloidosis in neonatally thymectomized rodents led us to a desire to clarify these relationships in model systems where control of development of immuno-globulins, antibody production, and plasma cells could be achieved separately from the cell-mediated immunities in neonatally thymectomized rodents. Incentives for our investigations of the chickens were derived primarily from the studies of Glick and his associates.[58] Glick et al. had discovered that extirpation of the bursa of Fabricius early in life prevents development of normal ability to produce circulating antibodies against bacterial antigens. His experiments were elegantly confirmed by Wolfe and his collaborators with a variety of antigens[8, 121] and by Warner and Szenberg[167, 168] in Australia. The latter group, comparing hormonally bursectomized birds and hormonally and surgically thymectomized birds, had concluded that in chickens the bursa functions primarily to influence the development of antibody-synthesizing capacity while the thymus functions primarily in the development of homograft rejection capacity.

These early results were confusing[59] because the apparently cell-mediated delayed allergy had been grouped with antibody production under bursal influence and graft-versus-host reactions did not seem to be under either bursal or thymic influence.[167, 168] Already in 1962, Waksman and his associates in Boston[7, 91, 166] were arguing that for the rat all antibody synthesis and all forms of cellular immunities were to be dissociated and that all cellular immunities were under thymic influence. In an extensive series of experiments summarized in detail elsewhere,[66, 70, 74, 131] Cooper et al.[33-35] and Perey et al.[128] showed clearly that in chickens antibody and immunoglobulin synthesis develop under control of the bursa of Fabricius whereas cell-mediated immunities, including ability to develop and express delayed allergy, solid tissue homograft rejection, and ability to initiate graft-versus-host reactions, are dependent upon

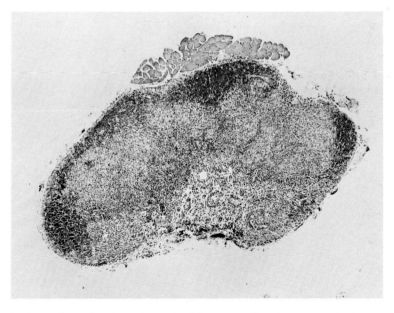

*Figure 4.* Lymph node of an 8 week old neonatally thymectomized mouse illustrating depletion of lymphoid elements in thymus-dependent regions.

the thymus. The thymus-dependent system of lymphoid cells in the chicken includes small lymphocytes in circulating blood and concentrations of small lymphocytes in the classic white pulp of the spleen and in the tiny little lymph nodes of these animals. By contrast, the bursal-dependent system of lymphocytes and plasma cells includes the germinal center type follicles of spleen, lymph nodes, and gut-associated lymphoid tissue and the plasma cells in all locations of the body.

Chickens exposed to near-lethal irradiation at hatching often grow up agammaglobulinemic, lacking both IgG and IgM immunoglobulins, and are unable to form antibodies even after repeated antigenic stimulation. On the other hand, such chickens do possess circulating lymphocytes which will initiate graft-versus-host reactions after intravenous injection into chick embryos, and they can develop and exhibit normal delayed allergic skin reactions and homograft rejections. Indeed, they can achieve homograft rejection reactions to the degree of white graft rejection.[128] By contrast, chickens irradiated and thymectomized in the newly hatched period develop with normal concentrations of both IgG and IgM immunoglobulin, make antibodies to numerous antigens only slightly less vigorously than do intact chicks, and possess normal numbers of plasma cells and germinal centers in their spleen and lymph nodes. Such chickens, however, cannot develop delayed allergy, reject skin homografts, or launch a graft-versus-host reaction. In both neonatally thymectomized rodents and irradiated thymectomized chickens the lymphoid cells show deficient responses in vitro to phytohemagglutinin (PHA), to antigens with which the host has previously been stimulated, and to allogeneic cells.[116] Chickens that have been irradiated and bursectomized at hatching possess circulating lymphocytes that respond normally to PHA, allogeneic cells, or antigens.[115] Thus, in both groups of experimental animals the proliferative responses of peripheral blood lymphocytes to antigenic stimulation sort out with the cell-mediated, thymus-dependent immune responses and are to be separated from the humoral immune responses. Figure 5 illustrates the respective cellular deficits in chickens that have been irradiated and either bursectomized or thymectomized at hatching.

During the course of these investigations, we observed that a few chickens subjected only to bursal extirpation just after hatching became dysgammaglobulinemic (Fig. 6). Such animals possessed normal or increased concentrations of IgM immunoglobulins, but lacked entirely the IgG immunoglobulin band. Similar findings had been mentioned earlier in an abstract by Ortega and Der.[124] It was at this time that the experimental embryologist, Van Alten, came to our laboratory and in collaborative study with Cooper and Cain carried out an important series of experiments employing bursectomy in ovo.[20, 28, 165]

To be absolutely certain that the development of capacity for immunoglobulin and antibody synthesis was dependent upon the bursa of Fabricius, it was desirable to avoid the unknown and unanalyzable influences of x-irradiation or of the hormones 19-nortestosterone and testosterone propionate. In short, the Minnesota workers were able to demonstrate that complete in ovo removal of the bursa of Fabricius prior to the seventeenth day of embryonation often produced animals with both 19S IgM and 7S IgG hypo-

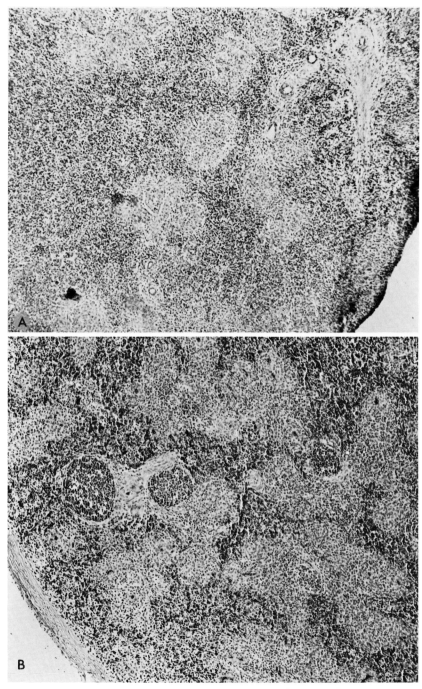

*Figure 5.* *A,* Spleen of bursectomized, irradiated chicken showing absence of lymphoid follicles. *B,* Spleen of thymectomized, irradiated chicken showing depletion of lymphoid elements in thymus-dependent areas. Note presence of lymphoid follicles, which are absent in *A.* (From Cooper, M. D., et al. 1966. The functions of the thymus system and the bursa system in the chicken. J. Exp. Med. *123:* 75–102.)

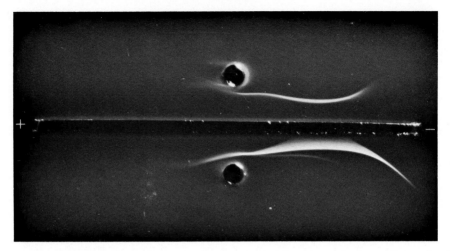

*Figure 6.* Immunoelectrophoretic patterns contrasting serum from 6 week old dysgammaglobulinemic chicken which was bursectomized at hatching (top) with serum of normal chicken (bottom). Note absence of 7S immunoglobulin in dysgammaglobulinemic chicken. Goat antiserum to chicken gamma globulin in center trough. ( From Cooper, M. D., et al. 1966. The functions of the thymus system and the bursa system in the chicken. J. Exp. Med. *123:*75–102).

gammaglobulinemia or agammaglobulinemia. These animals also lacked both plasma cells and germinal centers. If the bursectomy was completed after the seventeenth day but before the nineteenth or twentieth day of embryonation the chicks were frequently dysgammaglobulinemic, lacking 7S IgG immunoglobulins and possessing apparently normal amounts of IgM immunoglobulin. Such chickens, when they could be studied 6 to 9 weeks after hatching, possessed normal or near-normal numbers of plasma cells, made IgM antibodies normally, and showed both primary and secondary memory responses restricted to IgM type antibody; however, they lacked IgG and IgG antibodies, and germinal center development was extremely deficient.[36, 63]

## THE GERMINAL CENTER

These provocative findings relate in still another way to the enigma of the germinal center. The germinal centers have been related to memory phenomena in immune responses by studies of Thorbecke et al.[160] and to 7S IgG synthesis by observations obtained in the course of our phylogenetic analysis.[136] In the latter studies, we have found that the development of capacity for germinal center formation was not present in phylogenetic forms immediately preceding the avians but may have appeared earlier in forms ancestral to modern lungfishes[47] and amphibians.[153] The latter two groups are the most primitive vertebrates with the ability to synthesize immunoglobulins having both 19S and 7S types of heavy chains.[106, 107] In the sharks, paddlefish, Amia calva, and marine teleosts 19S and 7S immunoglobulins and antibodies are to be found, but these immunoglobulins appear to possess a common heavy chain and thus do not represent antecedents of the two separate IgM and IgG immunoglobulins.[23, 47, 106, 137, 153] Such animals have not been found to possess a germinal center type organization. By contrast, the lymphoid tissues of both amphibians and lungfishes seem to possess structures strikingly similar to the germinal centers found in mammalian lymphoid tissues.

Consequent to this series of investigations, we have viewed germinal centers as specialized sites in which apparently wasteful proliferation of lymphoid cells may occur in the presence of a mechanism for concentrating both antigen and antigen-sensitive cells. This apparently wasteful proliferation, similar to that which occurs in the thymus and probably in cortical areas of bursal follicles, may be necessary to achieve dilution of some kind of derepressor and permit the lymphoid cells to arrive at a point in differentiation where a switch from IgM to IgG immunoglobulin synthesis can occur.[27]

From this perspective, it has been of interest to study germinal centers in clinical and experimental analysis. We have shown that germinal centers of man and rabbit contain antigen together with IgM or IgG antibodies and complement. These accumulations of immunoglobulin are capable of fixation of additional complement and thus of acting as antigen-antibody complexes.[50, 51] The latter are not contained within cells, but the immunoglobulin-antigen-complement complexes can be readily eluted, apparently from the surfaces of the dendritic reticulum cells.

Thus, we visualize the bursa and its equivalent in mammals as providing a differentiative influence that makes possible development of antigen-sensitive cells. These cells, without further differentiation, are capable of producing, upon contact with antigen, specific 19S antibodies. Either by providing greater numbers of antigen-sensitive cells which can be further differentiated by antigen contact in the peripheral lymphoid tissues or by providing a different level of differentiation of antigen-sensitive cell as a consequence of longer residence in the bursa of Fabricius, this organ is essential for development of lymphoid cells that produce 7S immunoglobulin.

In further experiments, Cain et al.[19] have been able to show that bursectomy carried out even after hatching selectively prevents production of certain kinds of antibodies and responses to certain specific antigens but will not influence responses that develop earlier. Among the late-developing immune responses that can be inhibited by late extirpation of the chicken bursa is formation of antibody of the anaphylactic type. Analysis of the questions raised by these experiments obviously will require much additional study, but the experiments indicate clearly that the final chapter in the story of the sequential influences of the bursa of Fabricius in development of the several types of immunoglobulin-producing cells has not yet been written.

## The Mammalian Bursal Equivalent

Of course, in analyzing the major bulwarks of bodily defense for the Eutherian, we must be careful not to misinterpret or overemphasize these important studies in chickens. The lessons learned from the study of chickens, which present a definitive site of differentiation of the immunoglobulin-producing cells, have made it abundantly clear that the design of experimental models in mammals will be a crucial factor in obtaining equally penetrating results and avoiding misinterpretation of data suggesting a bursal equivalent in the mammal.

Studies with mice and rabbits, irradiated and thymectomized in the neonatal period, and of these same animals irradiated and thymectomized at more advanced ages indicate clearly that for mammals an equally sharp contrast between thymus-dependent and thymus-independent components of lymphoid tissue exists.[111, 112, 120] Consequently, it has become a major challenge to determine the location in mammals of the differentiative influence that provides the focus for development of immunoglobulin- and antibody-producing cells. Recent studies indicate that certain reptiles[142] possess a bursa of Fabricius, and a precursor of the bursa may be present in the lungfish and coelacanth.[47] Although efforts to define the bursal equivalent in mammals have proceeded now for several years, full definition is not yet at hand except for the rabbit. In the rabbit, there is considerable morphological evidence, as well as evidence from study of the bursa's proliferative characteristics, immunohistochemical analyses, and analyses from extirpative studies performed during development and in conjunction with heavy-dose, total-body irradiation, that suggests that the bursal equivalent site, as a major component of the critical site, resides in certain gut-epithelium-associated lymphoid tissue (GALT).[5, 6, 31, 32, 129, 130, 154] By inference, then, the lymphoid tissue of appendix, Peyer's patches, and intestinal tonsils or sacculus rotundus could very possibly represent the bursal equivalent of other mammals and man.

Like the chickens subjected *in ovo* to bursectomy, rabbits subjected in early life to complete extirpation of the GALT, or to irradiation plus extirpation, are very prone to infection and thus are most difficult to raise.[130] Perhaps the most meaningful experiments that lend support to inference of GALT as the bursal equivalent site are the rabbit experiments carried out by Cooper et al.[31, 32] and Perey et al.[129,130] These investigators showed that complete extirpation of the appendix, Peyer's patches, and sacculus rotundus in the immediate neonatal period interferes with normal development of immunoglobulin levels and results in a striking depression in the ability to synthesize antibody. Perey et al.,[129] in a most crucial series of experiments, analyzed recovery of ability to mount a primary response to Brucella antigen following supralethal irradiation. After irradiation with 1250 R, the rabbits were salvaged by administration of hematopoietic cells from the liver of fetal rabbits of 19 and 20 days' embryonation. Groups of animals were subjected to either complete thymectomy or appendectomy, removal of sacculus rotundus (S), appendix (A), and every Peyer's patch (PP), or a sham operation including removal of pieces of intestine plus spleen and lymph nodes. One month after recovery from the surgery, these rabbits were given injections of Brucella antigen, immediately exposed to supralethal irradiation, and 24 hours later given intravenous injections of liver cells from rabbit fetuses of 19 or 20 days' embryonation (at this point in embryonic development rabbits have not yet developed the capacity to synthesize immunoglobulins or antibody to the antigen used). The experimental observations were clear cut. Only those animals previously subjected to SAPP extirpation failed to develop the ability to exercise a primary response to Brucella antigen. All other groups, including a control group of nonirradiated animals subjected to the SAPP extirpation, responded well to the antigen. The appendectomized rabbits developed their responsiveness somewhat slowly but reached levels of agglutinin production within the range of the controls that had had the sham operation. Thus, in these experiments the GALT seemed to play a crucial role in development of capacity for antibody response in the rabbit.

Whether in other mammals and man this function is concentrated in the GALT is not known at present. Silverstein, however, has presented rather compelling evidence from extirpation of the gut during embryonation in sheep which indicates that in this mammal no area along the gastrointestinal tract plays a determinant role in development of the antibody-forming cells.[143]

To us, it is not crucial that differentiation of the thymus-independent cells be attributable to GALT in all mammals at all stages of embryonic development. A quick glance, for example, in both phylogenetic and ontogenetic perspective reveals that several distinct sites have provided the differentiative influence for red blood cell development. Yolk sac and fetal liver and marrow are the successive sites for this differentiative influence in ontogenetic development, and anterior kidney, gonad, and spleen play the same critical role in red blood cell differentiation during phylogenetic development prior to the time when bone marrow becomes the focus of this activity. Only quite late in phylogeny does the differentiative influence move to bone marrow. The important point from these analyses is that the differentiative influence for development of antigen-responsive lymphoid cells and for immunoglobulin synthesis can be separated from the influence for development of cells subserving cell-mediated immunity. Studies to date indicate that this important dichotomy exists in all mammals and man as well as in the birds.

## PRIMARY IMMUNE DEFICIENCY DISEASES OF MAN

The genetically determined primary immune deficiency diseases of man have so far provided the single most important experience for development of our views concerning the separate bulwarks of the bodily defense. They also serve as the prime support for the two-component immunologic model described here.[141] Summarized in Figure 7 is our analysis of the levels of block in immunologic development thus far defined in the primary immunologic deficiencies of man. It will be seen from the figure that patients have been described whose immunologic deficiency may be attributed to a block at the basic progenitor cell. In such patients not only lymphocytes and plasma cells fail to develop but also granulocytes and red blood cells. This condition has thus far been extremely rare and the patients have survived only a few days; consequently, they have not been sufficiently studied. The extreme nature of this lack of cells that serve as bulwarks against infection is implicit, however, in the rapid demise of these infants even when maintained in the most protected environment.

Two genetic variants that reflect a block at the lymphoid stem cell stage (blocks 2 and 3 in our theoretical scheme) are now well known. In one of these groups the genetic fault is transmitted as an autosomal recessive characteristic. Both lymphocyte lines fail to develop normally and plasma cells and

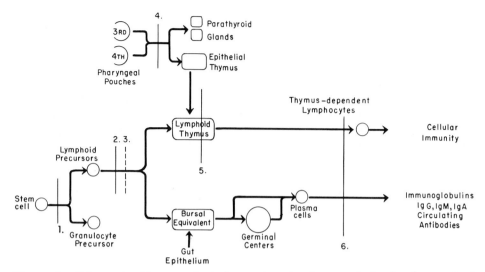

*Figure 7.* Schematic diagram depicting points in immunologic development at which blocks might occur leading to various immunologic disorders. (From Hoyer, J. R., et al. 1968. Lymphopenic forms of congenital immunologic deficiency: Clinical and pathologic patterns. *In* R. A. Good and D. Bergsma (eds.). Immunologic Deficiency Diseases in Man. Birth Defects Original Article Series, vol. 4. National Foundation Press, New York.)

small lymphocytes are virtually absent from peripheral blood, marrow, and peripheral lymphoid systems. The thymus is epithelial and represents an apparent early embryonic arrest in development of this organ. This condition has been called the Swiss type agammaglobulinemia because Swiss investigators published the initial description and analysis;[82, 161] it has also been called lymphopenic agammaglobulinemia syndrome. The patients are inordinately susceptible to infections with all manner of bacteria, fungi, pneumocystis, and viruses and rarely survive beyond 1 year of age. They cannot produce antibodies normally, cannot reject homografts of skin, and cannot develop delayed allergic responses to chemicals like 2,4-dinitrofluorobenzene (DNFB) 2,4-dinitrochlorobenzene (DNCB), tuberculin, or antigens of other organisms that infect them.[82, 88, 89] Their circulating lymphocyte counts are regularly very low, there are almost no small lymphocytes, and the peripheral blood leukocytes will not respond by blast transformation or proliferation to PHA, allogeneic cells, or antigens with which prior stimulation has been attempted. These patients often die of overwhelming vaccinia infection as a consequence of prophylactic efforts to provide immunity by live virus vaccine.[49] Since both systems of immunologic lymphoid cells are lacking in the patients, development of the lymphoid system must be arrested sometime before the establishment of the cellular dichotomy. Figure 8 shows the lymphoid tissues of a typical case of Swiss type agammaglobulinemia. One of the common causes of death in these patients is graft-versus-host disease initiated by transfusions of fresh blood or lymphoid cells from donors who differ from the patients by antigens determined at the HLA histocompatibility locus.[86]

Similar to these patients but somewhat more variable in the extremeness

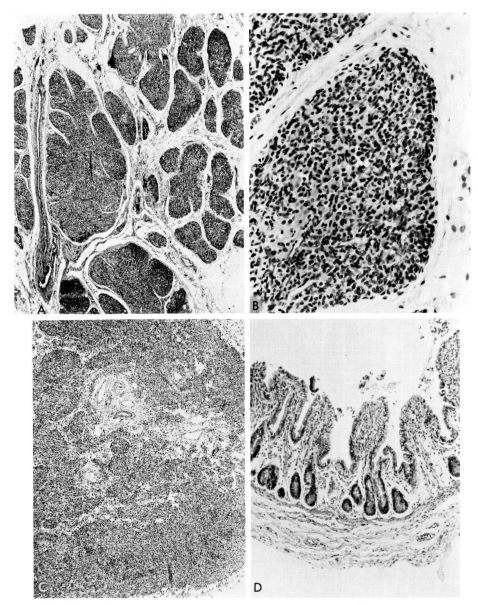

*Figure 8.* *A,* Thymus of patient with Swiss type lymphopenic agammaglobuline-mia (under low power), showing vestigial small lobules and small blood vessels. Note lack of differentiation into cortex and medulla and absence of Hassall's cor-puscles. *B,* Thymus of patient with Swiss type lymphopenic agammaglobulinemia (under high power), showing lack of differentiation into cortex and medulla, marked depletion of lymphoid elements, and lack of Hassall's corpuscles. *C,* Lymph node of patient with Swiss type lymphopenic agammaglobulinemia, showing marked depletion of lymphocytes in thymus-dependent areas and absence of ger-minal centers in cortical (thymus-independent) regions. Such nodes also lack plasma cells. *D,* Appendix from patient with Swiss type lymphopenic agamma-globulinemia, showing absence of lymphoid follicles and lymphocytes in lamina propria. Plasma cells also were lacking.

of the lymphoid tissue deficit are patients suffering from dual-system immunologic deficiency inherited as either a sex-limited or sex-linked recessive trait.[56] These patients have similar deficiencies of their lymphoid and plasma cell systems in both central and peripheral lymphoid organs, their circulating lymphocyte counts are regularly low, and the numbers of small lymphocytes in the blood are clearly deficient. The thymus is very small and poorly developed in patients with sex-linked immunologic deficiency syndrome, but it has usually descended into the mediastinum; in patients with the autosomal recessive form of lymphopenic agammaglobulinemia, the thymus is usually found high in the neck and is less completely developed. In several cases studied in Minneapolis, smears of the marrow from patients with sex-linked lymphopenic immunologic deficiency revealed normal numbers of cells that looked like small lymphocytes. Still, the peripheral blood and all lymphatic tissues showed profound deficiencies of the small lymphoid elements, although perhaps morphologically less complete than are seen in the autosomal recessive disease. Like the patients with Swiss type agammaglobulinemia, patients with sex-linked lymphopenic immunologic deficiency cannot survive and death is attributable to infection with a variety of pathogens including many different kinds of bacteria, viruses, fungi, and Pneumocystis. Some of these patients may produce small amounts of one or another of the immunoglobulins and their condition is then sometimes referred to as lymphopenic dysgammaglobulinemia —a term that we have shunned.[141] These patients, too, are extremely vulnerable to the induction of graft-versus-host reactions from blood transfusions or from injections of hematopoietic or lymphoid cells that have been given in attempts to correct their immunologic deficiencies.

Because of the combined immunologic deficiency underlying the inability of such children to survive, we reasoned that both the autosomal recessive Swiss type and the sex-linked form must involve an abnormal lymphoid stem cell (see Fig. 7). Initial efforts to exploit this analysis led to catastrophe, although sometimes there was a dramatic correction of the immunologic deficit before demise. The developing donor lymphoid system, once established to immunologic vigor, launched a graft-versus-host reaction that was fatal to the host.[87] At this juncture, our previous experiences with manipulation of transplantation barriers in experimental animals were of great value. We had been working for some years with manipulation of the so-called weak transplantation barrier.[73] In our studies, as well as in those of several other investigators, fatal graft-versus-host reactions could not be launched in mice unless the recipient differed from the donor by antigens genetically controlled by the $H_2$ major histocompatibility locus. [144, 152, 164, 172]

Recently, we[54, 61] and subsequently others[40] have restored complete immunologic competence of both thymus-dependent and thymus-independent systems of lymphoid cells in several patients with lymphopenic immunologic deficiency. This restoration has been associated with a decrease in susceptibility to infection, elimination of apparent ongoing graft-versus-host reaction produced by the mother's lymphocytes, establishment of plasma cells in marrow and lamina propria of the gut, development of ability to produce all types of immunoglobulins, development of ability to respond with all the different forms of cell-mediated immunity, and development of a population of small lymphocytes in circulating blood which are able to respond to PHA, to antigen to which the host has been previously sensitized, and to allogeneic cells *in vitro*. When this can be analyzed, all responding cells in the blood are found to be of the donor karyotype.[71, 114] Thus, providing a functional stem cell source has permitted us to reconstruct the defects in immunologic responsiveness and bodily defense in patients with lymphopenic agammaglobulinemia. This is a dramatic clinical achievement indeed, and one that provides strong support for the experimental analysis of two-component immunologic system which made it possible for us to focus the immunologic deficiency at the level of the lymphoid stem cell.

A third type of immunologic deficiency is the so-called DiGeorge syndrome.[43, 44, 103] Infants suffering from this disease fail to develop epithelial anlagen derived from the third and fourth pharyngeal pouches. These anlagen, after full differentiation, develop into thymus, parathyroids, and probably those clear cells of the thyroid responsible for calcitonin production. Infants with DiGeorge syndrome are generally brought to the pediatrician with hypoparathyroidism expressed as neonatal tetany. Thus, it is possible to recognize them, to analyze their immunology deficiencies early, and to treat their deficiencies. Unfortunately, critical immunologic studies have not yet been performed on patients with DiGeorge syndrome in the neonatal period. At a few months of age the children have been found to have normal or elevated immunoglobulin levels, normal antibody responses to a variety of antigens, normal plasma cell development, and normal primary lymphoid follicle and germinal center development in far cortical regions of the nodes.[98] Their lymph nodes show dramatically the same deficiencies present in the nodes of mice or rabbits that have been thymectomized and irradiated in the neonatal period. Although they have normal immunoglobulin levels and normal antibody responses, children with DiGeorge syndrome do not reject allografts of skin, do not develop delayed allergy to DNFB, and do not possess lymphocytes that can respond normally *in vitro* to stimulation with PHA, allogeneic cells, or antigens to which the patients have previously been sensitized. Further, these patients without a thymus and thymus-dependent system cannot cope normally with many kinds of infection. They have proved to be vulnerable to progressive infections with fungi, e.g., Candida. They cannot control infection with atypical acid-fast organisms of low-grade virulence and they often succumb to generalized infections with low-grade pyogenic pathogens, vaccinia virus, the virus of cytomegalic inclusion disease, or the measles virus. The granulocytes of patients with both lymphopenic immunologic deficiency and the DiGeorge syndrome when exposed to opsonized bacteria will phagocytize and kill the ingested organisms normally.

As was the case with children who suffer from the combined-system immunologic deficiency, it was the study of experimental models that led us to postulate that the deficiency of patients with DiGeorge syndrome might be cured if an appropriate thymic transplant could be achieved.[60] Following directly this line of reasoning, Cleveland in Florida transplanted a thymus from a human fetus to a patient with DiGeorge syndrome. The operation resulted in prompt establishment of immunologic function and progressive development of a circulating population of small lymphocytes and a lymphocyte population that reconstituted the thymus-dependent, deep cortical regions of the lymph node.[25] This child with DiGeorge syndrome has now been immunologically normal for approximately 2 years,[24] even though the developing immunologic responsiveness attributable to the host cells resulted in complete rejection of the thymic transplant. These findings have subsequently been confirmed in almost every detail by a successful transplant of fetal thymus in the patient described by August et al.[9]

Studies with mice can perhaps help us anticipate the future of these patients. When reconstitution of neonatally thymectomized mice is accomplished by transplant of thymus from a syngeneic donor, the thymus transplant is permanently successful and immunologic reconstitution is attributable to host cells.[151] Similarly, reconstitution of neonatally thymectomized mice with a thymus transplant from a donor differing from the recipient at a non-$H_2$ (minor) histocompatibility locus is long-lasting and the thymus persists in an apparently tolerant recipient.[150] If, however, a neonatally thymectomized mouse is given a thymus from a donor differing from the recipient by strong histocompatibility antigens, controlled by the $H_2$ locus, the host is at first reconstituted immunologically by donor cells, but then cells of the recipient become progressively more abundant until the thymus, essential to the reconstitution, is recognized as being foreign and is completely rejected. The mice maintain the immunologic restoration for approximately 150 days and then it begins to wane; the selective immunologic deficiency of the thymus-dependent system is reestablished usually by 170 to 200 days after restoration of this function.[150] Thus we would predict that if the process in man continues to be similar to that in the mouse and chicken, those patients with DiGeorge syndrome in whom reconstitution has been accomplished by fetal thymus transplants obtained from HLA-incompatible donors should eventually reject their thymus transplants, after immunologic vigor has been restored, and ultimately become immunologically defective again. Figure 9 illustrates the reconstitution of the lymph node, particularly the thymus-dependent regions, associated with correction of the immunologic defect by thymic transplant in a child with the DiGeorge syndrome.

Another primary immunologic deficiency of major importance in considering the bulwarks of bodily defense is the agammaglobulinemia first described by Bruton.[17, 72, 77] One form of this disease is sex-linked, is of very infrequent occurrence, and is associated with defects of immunologic function that are strikingly selective for the humoral immunities. These patients produce immunoglobulins very poorly or not at all and lack both plasma cells and germinal centers in their lymphoid tissues. Further, they cannot be induced to produce plasma cells or antibodies even after repeated antigenic stimulation. By contrast, their circulating lymphocytes are normal in number and morphology. They have normal or near-normal capacity to develop all of the cell-mediated immunities. They can reject homografts of skin, and can develop delayed allergy to antigens such as diphtheria toxoid, mumps, poison ivy, and 2,4-dinitrofluorobenzene. The lymphocyte populations in the thymus-dependent regions of the peripheral lymph nodes are normal (Fig. 10). Study of the thymus from several of these children has revealed no differences in size or morphologic structure from the thymus of normal children of the same age.

The clinical course in these patients reveals no hazard from blood trans-

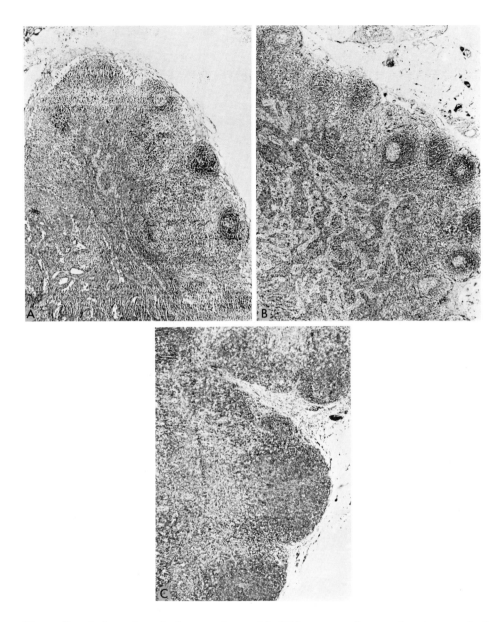

*Figure 9.* A, Lymph node from patient with DiGeorge syndrome, showing marked depletion of lymphoid elements in deep cortical, thymus-dependent regions as compared with intact cortical thymus-independent regions where germinal follicles can be clearly seen. Plasma cells are present in abundance in medullary cords and around periphery of germinal centers. B, Lymph node of same patient 1 month after reconstitution with fetal thymus transplant. Note increased cell density in thymus-dependent regions. C, Lymph node of same patient 6 months after transplantation. Note progressive filling-in of thymus-dependent regions by small lymphocytes.

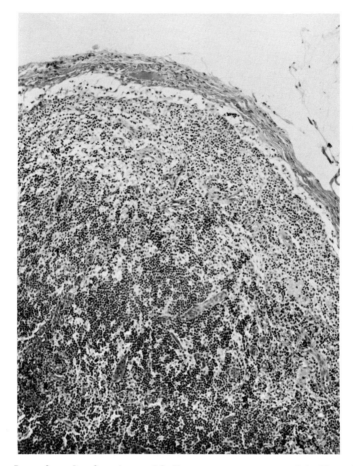

*Figure 10.*   Lymph node of patient with Bruton type agammaglobulinemia showing intact thymus-dependent region filled with lymphocytes as compared with depleted thymus-independent cortical areas where germinal centers are absent. Plasma cells also are lacking in such nodes.

fusions. The patterns of infection that plague these children are dramatically different from those that prove fatal to children with DiGeorge syndrome or either form of lymphopenic immunologic deficiency syndrome. First of all, children with Bruton type agammaglobulinemia are rarely sick during the first 6 months of their life since they are protected by antibodies derived from their mothers. By contrast, patients with lymphopenic agammaglobulinemia start with infections during the early weeks. Secondly, the infections that develop in Bruton patients who have not been treated by injections of gamma globulin are predominantly those attributable to the high-grade, encapsulated, pyogenic pathogens. Pneumococci are the most frequent offenders; Haemophilus influenzae, Streptococcus, meningococcus sp., and Pseudomonas aeruginosa also produce frequent infections.[13, 57, 72] On the other hand, BCG vaccination,[100] histoplasmosis, Candida and Brucella infections, and infections with many viruses evoke a normal response in these patients.[72] They can be immunized by vaccination with vaccinia virus. The reactions to vaccination develop as do those of normal persons into typical primary immune reactions.[57, 72] Upon subsequent exposure to vaccinia virus an accelerated immune reaction will occur and upon still greater exposure an immediate reaction often is encountered.[49] These immune reactions may develop in complete absence of demonstrable antibody titers for the virus. These patients can develop immunity to both chickenpox and measles; they develop the typical exanthema, and yet antibody responses to these agents may not be demonstrable.

In contrast to their extreme susceptibility to pneumonia, septicemia, meningitis, skin infections, conjunctivitis, and sinopulmonary infections with the encapsulated pyogenic pathogens, patients with Bruton type agammaglobulinemia have little clinical trouble with recurrent viral or fungal infections or infections with Enterobacteriaceae, Klebsiella, or Serratia marcescens. They do, however, seem to be unusually susceptible both to infection with hepatitis virus and its progressive destructive effects[125] and occasionally to Pneumocystis carinii.[52] In our own experience, we have observed both fulminating progressive viral hepatitis and rapidly progressive chronic active hepatitis infections in children with Bruton type agammaglobulinemia.[125] For reasons as yet unclear, defense against virus hepatitis, unlike defense against certain other viruses, requires an intact system of antibody-producing cells. It is not so difficult to understand how defense against encapsulated pyogenic pathogens might require ability to form opsonins and a vigorous antibody response that could utilize the complement system for amplification of phagocytosis and even direct destruction of these organisms. By contrast, a major bulwark against fungus infections and infections by low-grade pyogenic pathogens, particularly the facultative intracellular pyogenic pathogens, is provided by cell-mediated immune responses which utilize the amplification mechanism of the extraordinarily activated or "angry" macrophages[15, 104, 105] nonspecifically stimulated by a process set in motion by the thymus-dependent lymphocytes. How the patients with virtual absence of gamma globulins, who are unable to produce circulating antibodies, defend themselves so effectively against many viruses is far from clear, but from the study of the infections to which patients with Bruton type agammaglobulinemia are most prone, together with study of patients with other immunologic deficiencies, it is quite clear that a major bulwark of the bodily defenses against most viruses resides in the functions of the thymus-dependent lymphoid system and in the biologic amplification system or systems that cell-mediated immunity can muster. Nonetheless, these patients also teach us that immunity to and recovery from some virus and Pneumocystis infections cannot be primarily attributed either to interferon or to cell-mediated responses. Much additional work needs to be done to meet the important challenge placed before us by this experiment of nature in clinical immunobiology.

An example of the new definition of defense mechanisms that have been derived from clinical studies of immunologically deficient patients is represented by the children with the sex-linked recessive Wiskott-Aldrich syndrome. From the studies of Cooper et al.,[29] confirmed and extended by Blaese et al.,[14] it is now clear that these children suffer from a primary immunologic deficiency disease based upon failure to handle and respond normally to polysaccharide antigens. Rather paradoxically, there also develops in such patients a progressive deficiency of cell-mediated immunities that is apparently secondary to their difficulty in handling the polysaccharide antigens. These children also are born with profound deficiency of production of blood platelets. At present, the fact that they cannot survive seems to be due both to their extreme susceptibility to infections with a wide variety of bacteria, viruses, and fungi and to an extraordinary susceptibility to lymphoid malignancy.[30, 158] Definition of the precise nature of the immunologic deficiency underlying their susceptibility to infection and malignancy requires more study, but it is already very clear that when defined it will surely represent a major component of one of the bulwarks of defense against a constellation of microorganisms of broad scope. To fully interpret the meaning of this experiment of nature also requires careful delineation of the pathogens responsible for the many infections they experience. An inborn error of metabolism linking together platelet production, preparation of polysaccharide antigens, susceptibility to infection with a wide range of microorganisms, and progressive deficiency of cell-mediated immunities would certainly teach us much about thrombopoiesis, defense against infection, and cellular immunity. Preliminary results of studies by Baldini suggest that this inborn error may involve an inadequate energy source in these cell lines, possibly a hexokinase deficiency.[12] Therapeutically, Bach et al.[10] have recently achieved a long-lasting bone marrow transplant from a matched sibling which seems to have corrected, at least in part, some of the defects of a child with the Wiskott-Aldrich syndrome.

Until Thieffry,[159] surveying immunologic parameters, discovered the association of ataxia-telangiectasia and absence of IgA in serum, the repeated sinopulmonary infections in patients with ataxia-telangiectasia were considered to be a function of the inadequate respiratory exchange consequent to the progressive neuromuscular disease in these patients. However, it is now clear that approximately 60 per cent of patients with ataxia-telangiectasia[132–134, 171] lack IgA in the circulation, in their saliva, and in both nasopharyngeal and gastrointestinal secretions. In addition, extensive immunologic investigations have revealed that patients with ataxia-telangiectasia form antibodies poorly against certain relatively weak antigens and have a rather feeble ability to reject homografts of skin.[132, 134] Until very recently, the progressive sinopulmonary infections in these patients seemed most readily explained by their inability to form IgA in normal amounts. Indeed, a good correlation was established between the IgA deficiency and the susceptibility to frequent sinopulmonary infections in these patients.[147]

However, the recent discovery that certain patients having sinopulmonary disease and often bronchiectasis possess normal amounts of IgA, but lack IgE, whereas patients with genetically determined complete absence of IgA do not have recurrent or progressive sinopulmonary infection when they possess normal amounts of IgE, has made us focus on the possibility that it is IgE rather than or along with IgA that acts as a major bulwark protecting the upper and lower respiratory apparatus from repeated or continuous low-grade viral and bacterial infections.[18] These observations led us to restudy the patients with ataxia-telangiectasia, and found that all the patients with this syndrome who also have recurrent sinopulmonary infection lack demonstrable amounts of IgE in their skin. Indeed, lack of IgE in these patients correlated better with the progressive and recurrent sinopulmonary infections than did the absence of IgA.[3] In the meantime, Heremans and his associates obtained evidence implicating IgA as a bulwark of defense of the gastrointestinal tract.[37, 80] At present writing, the best interpretation seems to be that IgE, in addition to providing the basis for most allergic reactions,[90, 92] has as its major protective function in the body economy the defense of the respiratory tract. The details of the process by which IgE carries out this role are obscure but certainly the field represents a fruitful area for concentrated study. On the other hand, IgA seems particularly to participate in defense of the glands of external secretion and the bowel. That IgA does not function significantly in defense of the respiratory apparatus, of course, cannot be concluded, but its role in defense in this arena does not seem so dominant as it did only a few months ago.[146] Although many relationships remain to be worked out, interpretation of the natural experiments at this stage of our knowledge seems to indicate that the late-developing immunoglobulins IgA and IgE, which either do not utilize the complement amplification system at all or use it less efficiently than do immunoglobulins IgM and IgG, which develop earlier in ontogeny, play major roles in defending the respiratory and gastrointestinal surfaces of the body against virus and bacterial pathogens.

## SECONDARY IMMUNOLOGIC DEFICIENCIES

The secondary immunologic deficiencies accompanying the several malignancies of the lymphoreticular system provide additional support for interpretations concerning the major defense mechanisms against infections. Only a few of the best-studied examples will be considered here. Patients with Hodgkin's disease have long been known to express peculiar vulnerability to tuberculosis, to fungal infections, and perhaps to infections with certain viruses.[140] These patients likewise show a selective defect of immunologic functions which becomes worse with progression and dissemination of the malignant disease.[1, 16, 21, 95, 96, 101] Infrequent expression of delayed allergic reactions to antigens that revealed a high frequency of positive reactions in members of the general population as well as several populations of sick controls was the first demonstration of deficient cell-mediated immunity in this disease.[140] Patients with Hodgkin's disease fail to develop delayed allergy to protein antigens and chemical irritants that produce active cell-mediated immunity in normal persons and other hospitalized controls. In addition, they often fail to reject allografts of skin with the vigor shown by normal persons and in some instances a skin allograft may persist on a patient with Hodgkin's disease as though it were an autograft.[95, 96] The immunologic deficiency of the patient with Hodgkin's disease is peculiar in that transfer of cellular immunity to the patient with Hodgkin's disease using intact cells from highly sensitive donors regularly fails, in contradistinction to regular transferability of this form of allergy to nonsensitive, but immunologically normal persons. On the other hand, untreated patients with Hodgkin's disease usually have at least normal levels of each of the known immunoglobulins. Although minimal deficiencies of primary antibody response in Hodgkin's disease patients have been described, most untreated patients with this disease produce antibodies well to many antigens. Further, they possess plasma cells and achieve plasma cell proliferation and germinal center formation after antigenic stimulation as do immunologically normal persons. Even though the thymus is quite normal in most patients with Hodgkin's disease, it must be concluded that their immunologic deficiency represents a perturbation of function of the thymus-dependent lymphoid system.[41,42] Since the malignancy of Hodgkin's disease clearly does not involve the lymphoid cells directly, but rather represents malignant transformation of the reticulum cells in the lymphoreticular apparatus, it seems most likely that the progressive deficiency selective for the thymus-dependent lymphoid system represents an indirect influence perhaps of the agent responsible for this malignant adaptation.

In rather striking opposition to the set of immunologic deficiencies observed in patients suffering from Hodgkin's disease are those encountered in patients with multiple myeloma. In this malignant disorder, involving the thymus-independent plasma cell line of differentiation, one sees great perturbation of immunoglobulin synthesis and humoral immune functions. In this disorder monoclonal spikes of one or another of the immunoglobulins are the rule. But what are the deficits to be recorded in these patients? Regardless of the cells and the type of immunoglobulins present in excess, deficiencies of antibody production and synthesis of each of the normal immunoglobulin classes is the rule.[41, 42, 109] By contrast, cell-mediated immunities, e.g., delayed allergy and allograft immunity, often show normal vigor.[173] In contradistinction to the kinds of infections experienced by patients with Hodgkin's disease, patients with myeloma, like the children with Bruton type agammaglobulinemia, suffer from recurrent episodes of pneumococcal pneumonia, septicemia, and meningitis.[173] As with the hypogammaglobulinemic adults and agammaglobulinemic children, their deficit of humoral immune responses predisposes them to life-threatening infections primarily with the encapsulated, extracellular, pyogenic pathogens.

Patients with chronic lymphatic leukemia, too, experience profound and often progressive secondary immunologic deficiencies.[41, 42] Like the children with lymphopenic agammaglobulinemia, adults with chronic lymphatic leukemia have dual-system immunologic deficiencies[26] even early in the course of their hematologic disease. They do not develop delayed allergy well. They show deficient responses of lymphocytes *in vitro* to PHA, to allogeneic cells, and to antigens to which prior stimulation has been given. Immunoglobulin levels are often low and antibody production deficient (reviewed by Dent et al.[41, 42]). These patients are inordinately susceptible to virus, fungus, Pneumocystis, and facultative intracellular bacterial pathogens. At the same time, however, they show inordinate vulnerability to the encapsulated extracellular pyogenic pathogens as well.

Surprisingly, children with acute lymphatic leukemia usually have normal immunoglobulin levels and they usually can form circulating antibodies quite well. They are able to reject allografts of skin with vigor and to develop and express cell-mediated immunities as do normal persons.[99, 117] Of course, following prolonged antileukemic and immunosuppressive treatment they may develop iatrogenic hypogammaglobulinemia and immunologic deficiency.[48] Looking again at the deficiencies that accompany their disease, one notes that the cellular defects primarily associated with their malignant transformation include deficiency of red blood cells, platelets, and granulocytes. We do not at this time know the nature of the so-called lymphoblastic cells that accumulate in their blood, marrow, and lymphoreticular tissues. It seems a prudent guess that these lymphoblasts do not represent stem cells that have deviated from a normal differentiation pattern that includes lymphocytes and plasma cells. More likely, the malignant cell in this disease is a deviation of a stem cell of another line. Perhaps the malignant perturbation in this disease deviates stem cells that are destined to become red blood cells, granulocytes, and platelets.[41, 42]

We would conclude from study of the secondary immunologic deficiencies of man and from the infections characteristically associated with each of these diseases that the specific immunologic inadequacies and the constellations of infection that develop in patients with malignancies of the lymphoreticular apparatus provide firm support for the view that certain subcomponents of the immune response are especially concerned with defense of the body against a particular set of microorganisms. A corollary to this view is that one can begin to derive a classification of microorganisms in terms of the specific form of bodily defense which the mammalian organism has evolved to cope with potential invasion and injury by specific groups of pathogens. Since analyses of both microorganisms and constellations of infection are only beginning, the ultimate usefulness of this approach as compared, for example, to Gram staining cannot yet be appreciated. Its basis in fundamental ecological interrelationships makes this an attractive basis for classification.

## BIOLOGICAL AMPLIFICATION SYSTEMS

The cell-mediated immunities do not utilize in any demonstrable way the complement system. This complex system of interacting proteins, polypeptides,

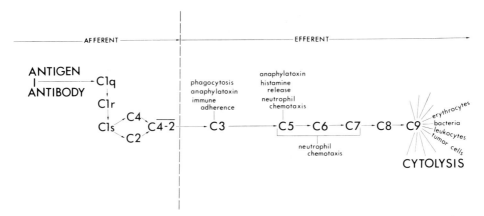

*Figure 11.* Schematic representation of complement system showing sequence from antibody recognition by C'1q to activation of the efferent limb by C'$\overline{4\text{-}2}$ complex. Once activated, the separate components serve to amplify the host's humoral response, ultimately leading to cell wall destruction and cytolysis.

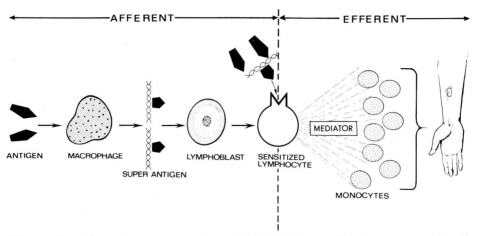

*Figure 12.* Schematic representation of biological amplification system of cell-mediated immune response. Macrophage ingests and processes antigen, and produces a "super antigen" capable of sensitizing lymphocytes which then initiate chemotactic mediator(s). Monocytes are summoned into an area by such mediator (s). (Modified after Chilgren, R. A., et al. 1969. The cellular immune defect in chronic mucocutaneous candidiasis. Lancet *1:*1286–1288).

and enzymes represents an extraordinary biologic amplification mechanism for those humoral immune responses that are based on production of IgM and IgG immunoglobulins. Discussion of the complement system has been extensively reviewed elsewhere[55] and will not be considered further in this chapter (Fig. 11).

Antibodies do not execute biologic effects except by combination and activation of other biologic systems. Consequently, the means by which destruction of microorganisms is achieved as a consequence of cell-mediated immunity are of great interest to clinicians. In recent years, a whole galaxy of cellular products has been described which are involved in cellular or humoral responses. These factors may be produced by, or called into play by, lymphocytes reacting with specific antigen in cell-mediated immune responses (Fig. 12). Whether there are many such factors, e.g., the migration inhibition factor (MIF), cytotoxic factor (CIF), macrophage stimulation factor (MSF), chemotactic factor (CF), or a recruitment factor such as transfer factor (TF) or *in vitro* transfer factor (ITF), or whether these observations reflect a number of different biologic assays for one or several mediators, will be determined by future comparative biochemistry studies and comparative bioassays. Perhaps from these studies will come further understanding of other mechanisms of bodily defense afforded by cell-mediated immune reactions.

The details of the intimate relationship of lymphocytes to histiocytic cells and macrophages in inflammation also will require further intensive analysis. There can be no doubt, however, from the recent studies of Mackaness and his associates that activation of macrophages represents one means by which cell-mediated immunities can alter the capacity of the body to rid itself of micro-organisms.[15, 104, 105] These investigations show that specific cellular immunity associated with delayed allergy can bring into play extraordinary amplification mechanisms in the bodily defense by activating histiocytic cells or macro-phages to increased vigor in destroying a number of different facultative intra-cellular bacterial pathogens. The changes induced in the macrophage popula-tion that bring about increased capacity for killing Listeria monocytogenes, BCG organisms, and other facultative intracellular bacterial pathogens include: (1) increase in size and mobility of the phagocytic cells, (2) increase in numbers and size of the cytoplasmic organelles, e.g., lysosomal particles, and (3) increase in phagocytic activity. These changes of the macrophage occur only after stimulation by lymphoid cells which have themselves been aroused by contact with a specific antigen to which cell-mediated immunity has been induced. This nonspecific change in an effector cell population represents another extraordinary biologic amplification system which, like the complement system, can be brought to bear by specific immunologic reaction. In this in-stance, however, it is cellular immunity rather than IgG- or IgM-dependent humoral immunity which activates the nonspecific host response to achieve the increased destruction of the microorganisms.

It seems likely that this mechanism stands as a major bulwark not only against the facultative intracellular bacterial pathogens, but also against fungi. Could this also be the means by which cellular immunity defends against certain viruses? It can be said almost without argument that virus-neutralizing antibodies represent one major element of defense against both recurrent and continuing virus infection. It also seems almost axiomatic that interferon[113] represents an important nonspecific bulwark of defense that can be brought to bear on facilitating recovery from virus infection. While accepting the biologic importance of these mechanisms, it is most provocative that defense against many virus infections, as seen through the clinical experiments of nature, involves cell-mediated immunity in a most fundamental and essential way. Progressive vaccinia, overwhelming Hecht's pneumonia as a reflection of rubeola infection, fatal varicella infection, progressive inclusion body virus disease, and perhaps a host of other infections like generalized fungal infections, BCG infections, and progressive destructive infection by other facultative intra-cellular pyogenic pathogens seem to relate more to cell-mediated immune deficiencies than to ability to produce circulating antibodies and immuno-globulins. The *modus operandi* of the bodily defense and of the amplification resources used in the cellular defenses against viruses has not yet been clarified. The role of "angry" macrophages and other means of cellular destruc-tion that might be brought to bear on host cells containing virus or against viruses directly needs much further analysis. It seems certain that clinical experience will play a crucial role in achieving this understanding.

Studies of the genetic perturbations of the biologic amplification systems and the significance of these disturbances as a basis for increased susceptibility to infection is only beginning to be recognized. In these experiences, as in study of specific immunologic deficiency, evidence of specialization within the systems for major roles of defense against particular sets of pathogens has already been forthcoming. An inherited abnormality of granule morphology and doubtless of lysozymal function, as yet poorly defined, appears to underlie the increased susceptibility to infection observed in the Chediak-Higashi syn-drome.[22, 81, 169, 170] Similarly, abnormalities in capacity of polymorphonuclear leukocytes and monocytes to kill phagocytized fungi or bacteria normally underlie the lethality of fatal or chronic granulomatous disease of childhood.[76] A correctable deficiency of a stabilizer or inhibitor of the activation of the third component of the complement system has been implicated in a syndrome featured by recurrent pulmonary and other infections.[2] Many more clinical diseases will be found to be associated with defective chemotaxis, phagocytosis, bactericidal action, lysosomal function, and biochemical machinery associated with intracellular destruction of microorganisms. It might be useful here to take but a single example of an inherited defect in bodily defense and show how it may unify an otherwise apparently diverse group of microorganisms and, at the same time, reveal a major line of bodily defense.

### Leukocyte Bactericidal Function

Chronic granulomatous disease of childhood is an inherited disease that may be transmitted as either an autosomal recessive, sex-limited, or sex-linked disorder.[76] The majority of active cases occur in male children and the clinical features of the disease are recurrent, often life-threatening granulomatous or septic infections with low-grade pyogenic bacteria. Organisms that usually cause the infections in these children are staphylococci, Klebsiella sp., Aerobacter aerogenes, Serratia marcescens, Candida, and Aspergillus. Because these include highly mutable organisms that are highly pathogenic for these children, the disease, especially in males, is often lethal during early or mid childhood. An organism resistant to all antibiotics is ultimately encountered and it causes a fatal pulmonary or more disseminated infection. The specific functional defect in these children is inability to kill, at normal rate, organisms ingested by the phagocytic granular and monocytic leukocytes.[85, 138] This functional deficit, most likely a consequence of a single, as yet undefined, enzyme defect, is associated with metabolic abnormalities of phagocytizing leukocytes.[11, 84] The leukocytes ingest bacteria at a normal or even excessive rate. In addition to their defective killing of the organisms, leukocytes from patients with fatal granulomatous disease fail to exhibit the usual increase in respiration, hexose monophosphate pathway activity, and hydrogen peroxide production that occurs in leukocytes of normal persons during phagocytosis. The latter reaction is thought to be bactericidal.[97] Although the evidence has been disputed, it has been demonstrated that the granular leukocytes of children with fatal granulomatous disease do not show normal rates of degranulation following phagocytosis.

We have discovered in these patients a perturbation of a basic mechanism of the bodily defense which stands against a restricted population of potential microbial pathogens all of which are catalase producers. These patients have no unusual problem in resisting streptococcal, pneumococcal, and Haemophilus influenzae organisms and the incidence of tuberculosis or viral infection is not unusually high in them. Instead, life to them is an unending succession of episodes of skin, lung, liver, bone, lymphatic, or visceral granulomatous and septic disease caused by this strange family of low-grade pathogens. The leukocytes of these children ingest and kill opsonized streptococci and pneumococci normally.[93] In addition their serum can opsonize staphylococci and Enterobacteriaceae normally for killing by leukocytes of normal persons. All the components of complement are present and function normally according to present methods of assay.

The infections these children experience are caused by the same organisms against which their phagocytic cells fail to function *in vitro*. In this experiment of nature, we see revealed in bold relief a major bulwark of the bodily defense that groups together what might otherwise appear to be a heterogeneous group of microorganisms. The unifying characteristic of these organisms is that they all produce catalase. Since hydrogen peroxide production by the leukocytes is thought to be bactericidal, it has been suggested that the antagonistic effects of a catalase-producing microorganism on cells already deficient in hydrogen peroxide production may be responsible for the inordinate susceptibility of these patients to infection. This metabolic characteristic of the organisms that reflects the Achilles heel of these children may be the clue to this important bulwark of the bodily defense. (See Table 1.)

## IMMUNOLOGIC SURVEILLANCE AGAINST MALIGNANCY

Although extensive discussion of the mountain of evidence that has accumulated indicating both the reality and importance of immunologic surveillance against cancer is possible, only a brief summary of clinical evidence of the nature of this bulwark against internal invasion will be given here. The

TABLE 1. *Constellations of Infection*: Three groups of microorganisms arranged according to primary mechanism of host defense against each pathogen. These constellations of infection have been assembled mainly from clinical experience with patients suffering from immunologic deficiency diseases and chronic granulomatous disease of childhood.

| PATHOGENS | PRIMARY BODILY DEFENSE MECHANISM |
| --- | --- |
| Pneumococcus<br>Haemophilus influenzae<br>Streptococcus<br>Meningococcus sp.<br>Pseudomonas aeruginosa<br>Hepatitis virus<br>Pneumocystis carinii | Humoral immune responses |
| Rubeola<br>Varicella<br>Vaccinia<br>Cytomegalic inclusion body virus<br>Mycobacterium tuberculosis<br>Candida albicans<br>Histoplasmosis | Cellular immune responses |
| Staphylococcus<br>Klebsiella sp.<br>Aerobacter aerogenes<br>Serratia marcescens<br>Candida albicans<br>Aspergillus<br>Nocardia | Leukocyte bactericidal function |

incidence of cancer in patients with each of the different kinds of primary immunologic deficiency is far in excess of that in members of the general population. In those with Bruton type agammaglobulinemia only "lymphatic leukemia" develops.[126] This complicating disorder has occurred five times to our knowledge among approximately 30 such patients. These children lack only humoral immunities. Carcinomas, epitheliomas, solid tissue sarcomas, and Hodgkin's disease have not yet been found in them. On two occasions there was massive thymus involvement with the leukemia and apparently the disease either began in the thymus or involved the thymus-dependent lymphoid system in major ways. In this regard, it is of interest that Gorer long ago presented evidence in experimental animals that circulating antibodies can represent a major form of immunity against leukemias which for solid tumors may not be so important.[78] The inordinate susceptibility to leukemia of children with a genetically determined lack of antibody-producing capacity further serves to argue that the humoral immune mechanism may represent a major bulwark against occurrence of malignancy involving dispersed hematopoietic or lymphoid cells.

Patients with late-occurring immunologic deficiency, Wiskott-Aldrich syndrome, and ataxia-telangiectasia syndrome by contrast have broadly based immunologic deficiencies, each differing in basic mechanism from the other. In each of these genetically-determined diseases malignancy has occurred in a variety of forms. The malignancies occurring in patients with the late-occurring immunologic deficiency, whose deficiency involves both cellular and humoral systems, have included gastric and colonic carcinomas, epitheliomas, reticulum cell sarcomas, lymphomas, and leukemias. Indeed, nearly the whole range of those malignancies that occur with greatest frequency in man have turned up in such patients. Similarly, patients with ataxia have had malignancies of a wide range of types including lymphosarcomas, reticulum cell sarcomas, Hodgkin's disease, and carcinomas. In the Wiskott-Aldrich syndrome, in which the inherited deficit seems to involve the afferent limb of the immune response, the malignancies appear to be quite uniformly reticulum cell sarcomas and lymphomas. The incidence of successful malignant adaptation in these three groups of patients has exceeded 10 per cent and may reach even higher levels as reporting becomes more complete. At any rate, the incidence of cancer in these patients is far greater than can be explained by chance alone. Malignancy has also occurred in lymphopenic agammaglobulinemia and recently a patient with the rare DiGeorge syndrome has been found to have a lymphoreticular malignancy. Thus, in all forms of primary immune deficiency of man, malignancy occurs with inordinate frequency; this finding is commensurate with the view that the immunologic system stands as a major bulwark against malignant adaptation.

Recent studies of patients receiving immunosuppressive therapy to prolong or prevent allograft rejection have indicated that they have a susceptibility to transplantation of cancer as well as to the development of primary malignancies.[67, 68] During the past several years more than 17 primary malignancies have been encountered among patients under effective immunosuppression, often including antilymphocyte serum. This incidence of cancer far exceeds that expected for persons of the same age in the general population. The kinds of primary malignancies observed under these conditions include the full gamut of malignancies that are frequent in man, e.g., lymphomas, reticulum cell sarcomas, leukemias, anaplastic carcinomas, epitheliomas, and Hodgkin's disease.[110, 149] This experiment of nature in a test situation again provides substantial evidence that an intact immune system stands as a major bulwark of defense against cancer.

In clinical medicine further support for this view derives from evidence of the flagging of immunologic vigor that occurs with aging.[45, 46, 53, 149] This loss of immunologic vigor is reciprocal to the increasing incidence of cancer with aging in both man and animals. Further, once a malignancy has developed in a person, the chances of a second primary cancer developing are very great. This finding is consistent with observations that indicate that cell-mediated immunities may become progressively deficient with the extension of malignancy in man.[101, 148] Further, evidence has recently been accumulated by the Hellstroms in Seattle which argues strongly that the lymphoid cells of patients with neuroblastoma exhibit an immunity to the tumor tissue which is somehow neutralized by an antibody or antibody-like substance circulating in the serum of these patients.[79]

From studies in experimental cancer biology, the immunologic bulwark against the internal invasion represented by cancer has gained abundant support and it has even appeared reasonable to postulate an essential relationship between malignancy, the lymphoid system, and immunity.[53, 68, 61] Basically, the reflection of this bulwark argues that for cancer to succeed, immunologic surveillance must fail. The failure of immunologic surveillance may be generalized or local and may represent a highly specific deficiency or a more broadly based one.

It seems eminently clear that major bulwarks of the bodily defense stand as well against neoplastic invasion from within as they do against microbial invasion from without. The dissection and resolution of the specific details of the nature of the bulwarks against specific forms of internal invasion and the extension of analysis of the defenses against external invasion by microorganisms will surely continue to depend heavily on those extraordinary experiments of nature represented by genetic faults that reveal specific deficits and their biologic implications so clearly.

# *References*

1. Aisenberg, A.C. 1962. Studies on delayed hypersensitivity in Hodgkin's disease. J. Clin. Invest. *41:*1964–1970.
2. Alper, A., N. Abramson, R. B. Johnston, C. E. McCall, J. H. Jandl and F. S. Rosen. 1968. Increased susceptibility to infection associated with a defect of complement metabolism. J. Clin. Invest. *47:*1a.
3. Ammann, A. J., W. A. Cain, R. Hong and R. A. Good. Immunoglobulin E deficiency in ataxia-telangiectasia. New Eng. J. Med. In press.
4. Archer, O. K., and J. C. Pierce. 1961. Role of the thymus in development of the immune response. Fed. Proc. *20:*26.
5. Archer, O. K., D. E. R. Sutherland and R. A. Good. 1963. Appendix of the rabbit: A homologue of the bursa in the chicken? Nature *200:*337–339.
6. Archer, O. K., D. E. R. Sutherland and R. A. Good. 1964. The developmental biology of

lymphoid tissue in the rabbit. Consideration of the role of thymus and appendix. Lab. Invest. *13*:259–271.

7. Arnason, B. J., B. D. Jankovic, B. H. Waksman and C. Wennersten. 1962. Role of the thymus in immune reactions in rats. II. Suppressive effect of thymectomy at birth on reactions of delayed (cellular) hypersensitivity and the circulating small lymphocyte. J. Exp. Med. *116*:177–186.

8. Aspinal, R. L., R. K. Meyer, M. A. Graetzer and H. R. Wolfe. 1964. Effect of thymectomy and bursectomy on the survival of skin homografts in chickens. J. Immunol. *90*:872–877.

9. August, C. S., F. S. Rosen, R. M. Filler, C. A. Janeway, B. Markowski and H. E. M. Kay. 1968. Implantation of a foetal thymus restoring immunological competence in a patient with thymic aplasia (DiGeorge's syndrome). Lancet *2*:1210–1211.

10. Bach, F. H., R. J. Albertini, P. Joo, J. L. Anderson and M. M. Bortin. 1968. Bone marrow transplantation in a patient with Wiskott-Aldrich syndrome. Lancet *2*:1364–1366.

11. Baehner, R. L. and D. G. Nathan. 1967. Leukocyte oxidase: defective activity in chronic granulomatous disease. Science *155*:835–836.

12. Baldini, M. G. 1969. Platelet defect in Wiskott-Aldrich syndrome. New Eng. J. Med. *281*:107.

13. Barandum, S., H. Cottier, A. Hassig and G. Riva. 1959. Das Antikörper-Mangelsyndrom. Benno Schwabe & Co., Basel and Stuttgart.

14. Blaese, R. M., W. Strober, R. S. Brown, and T. A. Waldmann. 1968. The Wiskott-Aldrich syndrome. A disorder with a possible defect in antigen processing or recognition. Lancet *1*:1056–1060.

15. Blanden, R. V., M. J. Lefford and G. B. Mackaness. 1969. The host response to Calmette-Guérin bacillus infection in mice. J. Exp. Med. *129*:1079–1107.

16. Brown, R. S., H. A. Haynes, H. T. Foley, H. A. Godwin, G. W. Berard and P. P. Carbone. 1967. Hodgkin's disease: Immunologic clinical and histologic features in 50 untreated patients. Ann. Int. Med. *67*:291–302.

17. Bruton, O. C. 1952. Agammaglobulinemia. Pediat. *9*:722–728.

18. Cain, W. A., A. J. Ammann, R. Hong, K. Ishizaka and R. A. Good. 1969. IgE deficiency associated with chronic sinopulmonary infection. (Abstract.) J. Clin. Invest. *48*:12a.

19. Cain, W. A., M. D. Cooper and R. A. Good. 1969. Relationship between ability to synthesize immunoglobulins and antibodies against different antigens in bursectomized chicks. (Abstract.) Feb. Proc. *28*:432.

20. Cain, W. A., M. D. Cooper, P. J. Van Alten and R. A. Good. 1969. Development and function of the immunoglobulin-producing system. II. Role of the bursa in the development of humoral immunological competence. J. Immunol. *102*:671–678.

21. Chase, M. W. 1966. Delayed-type hypersensitivity and the immunology of Hodgkin's disease, with a parallel examination of sarcoidosis. Cancer Res. *26*:1097–1120.

22. Chediak, M. 1952. Nouvelle anomalie leucocytaire de caractère constitutionnel et familial. Rev. Hémat. *7*:362–367.

23. Clem, L. W. and P. A. Small. 1967. Phylogeny of immunoglobulin structure and function. I. Immunoglobulins of the lemon shark. J. Exp. Med. *125*:893–920.

24. Cleveland, W. W., B. Fogel, W. T. Brown and H. E. M. Kay. 1968. Foetal thymic transplant in a case of DiGeorge's syndrome. Lancet *2*:1211–1214.

25. Cleveland, W. W., B. J. Fogel and H. E. M. Kay. 1968. Implant of fetal thymus in an infant with the 3rd and 4th pharyngeal pouch syndrome. (Abstract.) J. Clin. Invest. *47*:20a.

26. Cone, L. and J. W. Uhr. 1964. Immunological deficiency disorders associated with chronic lymphocytic leukemia and multiple myeloma. J. Clin. Invest. *43*:2241–2248.

27. Cooper, M. D. Effects of environmental factors on the ontogenetic sequence of immunoglobulin synthesis. To be submitted.

28. Cooper, M. D., W. A. Cain, P. J. Van Alten and R. A. Good. 1969. Development and function of the immunoglobulin producing system. I. Effect of bursectomy at different stages of development on germinal centers, plasma cells, immunoglobulins and antibody production. Int. Arch. Allerg. *35*:242–252.

29. Cooper, M. D., H. P. Chase, J. T. Lowman, W. Krivit and R. A. Good. 1968. Wiskott-Aldrich syndrome: An immunologic deficiency disease involving the afferent limb of immunity. Am. J. Med. *44*:499–513.

30. Cooper, M. D., H. P. Chase, J. T. Lowman, W. Krivit and R. A. Good. 1968. Immunologic defects in patients with Wiskott-Aldrich syndrome. *In* R. A. Good and D. Bergsma (eds.). Immunologic Deficiency Diseases in Man. Birth Defects Original Article Series, vol. 4. National Foundation Press, New York, p. 378–387.

31. Cooper, M. D., D. Y. Perey, A. E. Gabrielsen, D. E. R. Sutherland, M. F. McKneally and R. A. Good. 1968. Production of an antibody deficiency syndrome in rabbits by neonatal removal of organized intestinal lymphoid tissues. Int. Arch. Allerg. *33*:65–88.

32. Cooper, M. D., D. Y. Perey, M. F. McKneally, A. E. Gabrielsen, D. E. R. Sutherland and R. A. Good. 1966. A mammalian equivalent of the avian bursa of Fabricius. Lancet 1: 1388–1391.

33. Cooper, M. D., R. D. A. Peterson and R. A. Good. 1965. Delineation of the thymic and bursal lymphoid system in the chicken. Nature 205:143–146.

34. Cooper, M. D., R. D. A. Peterson, M. A. South and R. A. Good. 1966. The functions of the thymus system and the bursa system in the chicken. J. Exp. Med. 123:75–102.

35. Cooper, M. D., M. M. Schwartz and R. A. Good. 1966. Restoration of gamma globulin production in agammaglobulinemic chickens. Science 151:471–473.

36. Cooper, M. D. and E. M. Weller. 1969. Developmental suppression of germinal centers and IgG production by prednisolone and 6-mercaptopurine. In L. Fiore-Donati and M. G. Hanna (eds.). Lymphatic Tissue and Germinal Centers in Immune Response. Adv. in Exp. Med. and Biol., Vol. 5. Plenum Press, New York, pp. 277–284.

37. Crabbé, P. A. and J. F. Heremans. 1966. Lack of gamma A-immunoglobulin in serum of patients with steatorrhea. Gut 7:119–127.

38. Dalmasso, A. P., C. Martinez and R. A. Good. 1964. Studies of immunological characteristics of lymphoid cells from thymectomized mice. In R. A. Good and A. E. Gabrielsen (eds.). The Thymus in Immunobiology. Hoeber-Harper, New York, pp. 478–489.

39. Davies, A. J. S., E. Leuchars, V. Wallis, R. Marchant and E. V. Elliot. 1967. The failure of thymus-derived cells to produce antibody. Transplantation 5:222–231.

40. De Koning, J., L. J. Dooren, D. W. van Bekkum, J. J. van Rood, K. A. Dicke and J. Radl. 1969. Transplantation of bone marrow cells and foetal thymus in an infant with lymphopenic immunological deficiency. Lancet 1:1223–1227.

41. Dent, P. B., A. E. Gabrielsen, M. D. Cooper, R. D. A. Peterson and R. A. Good. 1969. The secondary immunologic deficiency diseases associated with lympho-proliferative disorders. In P. A. Miescher and H. J. Muller-Eberhard (eds.). Textbook of Immunopathology. Grune & Stratton, New York, pp. 385–405.

42. Dent, P. B., R. D. A. Peterson and R. A. Good. 1968. The relationship between immunologic function and oncogenesis. In R. A. Good and D. Bergsma (eds.). Immunologic Deficiency in Man. Birth Defects Original Article Series, vol. 4. National Foundation Press, New York, pp. 443–458.

43. DiGeorge, A. M. 1965. Discussion of Cooper et al. J. Pediat. 67:908.

44. DiGeorge, A. M. 1968. Congenital absence of the thymus and its immunologic consequences: Concurrence with congenital hypoparathyroidism. In R. A. Good and D. Bergsma. (eds.). Immunologic Deficiency Diseases in Man. Birth Defects Original Article Series, vol. 4. National Foundation Press, New York, pp. 116–121.

45. Doak, P. B., J. Z. Montgomerie, J. D. K. North and F. Smith. 1968. Reticulum cell sarcoma after renal homotransplantation and azothioprine-prednisone therapy. Brit. Med. J. 4: 746–748.

46. Editorial: Immunosuppression and cancer. Lancet 1: 505–506, 1969.

47. Finstad, J. and R. A. Good. Unpublished observations.

48. Frommel, D., R. A. Good and R. Hong. 1969. Immunoglobulin levels and protracted hematopoietic malignancy. Helv. Paediat. Acta. Suppl. XIX.

49. Fulginiti, V. A., G. H. Kempe, W. E. Hathaway, D. S. Pearlman, O. F. Sieber, Jr., J. J. Eller, J. J. Soyner, Sr., and A. Robinson. 1968. Progressive vaccinia in immunologically deficient individuals. In R. A. Good and D. Bergsma (eds.). Immunologic Deficiency Diseases in Man. Birth Defects Original Article Series, vol. 4. National Foundation Press, New York, pp. 129–145.

50. Gajl-Peczalska, K., A. J. Fish and H. J. Meuwissen. 1969. Localization of C'3 in germinal centers of human lymph nodes. (Abstract.) Fed. Proc. 28:364.

51. Gajl-Peczalska, K., A. J. Fish, H. J. Meuwissen, D. D. Frommel and R. A. Good. Localization of immunologic complexes fixing B1C (C'3) in germinal centers of lymph nodes. J. Exp. Med. In press.

52. Gatti, R. A. and R. A. Good. Unpublished observations.

53. Gatti, R. A. and R. A. Good. Aging, immunity and malignancy. Geriatrics. In press.

54. Gatti, R. A., H. J. Meuwissen, H. D. Allen, R. Hong and R. A. Good. 1968. Immunologic reconstitution of sex-linked lymphopenic immunological deficiency. Lancet 2:1366–1369.

55. Gewurz, H. 1967. The immunologic role of complement. Hosp. Prac. 2:45–56.

56. Gitlin, D. and J. Craig. 1963. The thymus and other lymphoid tissues in congenital agammaglobulinemia. I. Thymic alymphoplasia and lymphocytic hypoplasia and their relation to infection. Pediatrics 32:517–530.

57. Gitlin, D., C. A. Janeway, L. Apt, and J. M. Craig. 1959. Agammaglobulinemia. In H. S. Lawrence (ed.). Cellular and Humoral Aspects of the Hypersensitivity States. Hoeber-Harper, New York, p. 375.

58. Glick, B., J. S. Chang and R. C. Jaap. 1956. The bursa of Fabricius and antibody production. Poultry Sci. 35:224–225.

59. Good, R. A. 1964. Discussion of paper by Warner et al. *In* R. A. Good and A. E. Gabrielsen (eds.). Thymus in Immunobiology. Hoeber-Harper, New York, p. 413.

60. Good, R. A. 1968. Discussion of paper by DiGeorge. *In* R. A. Good and D. Bergsma (eds.). Immunologic Deficiency Diseases in Man. Birth Defects Original Article Series, vol. 4. National Foundation Press, New York, pp. 122–123.

61. Good, R. A. 1969. Immunologic reconstitution: The achievement and its meaning. Hosp. Prac. *4:*41–47.

62. Good, R. A. and W. A. Cain. Relationship between thymus-dependent cells and humoral immunity. Submitted to Nature.

63. Good, R. A., W. A. Cain, D. Y. Perey, P. B. Dent, H. J. Meuwissen, G. E. Rodey and M. D. Cooper. 1969. Studies on the nature of germinal centers. *In* L. Fiore-Donati and M. G. Hanna (eds.). Lymphatic Tissue and Germinal Centers in Immune Response. Adv. in Exp. Med. and Biol., Vol 5. Plenum Press, New York, pp. 33–47.

64. Good, R. A., A. P. Dalmasso, C. Martinez, O. K. Archer, J. C. Pierce and B. W. Papermaster. 1962. The role of the thymus in development of immunologic capacity in rabbits and mice. J. Exp. Med. *116:*773–796.

65. Good, R. A. and J. Finstad. 1967. The phylogenetic development of the immune responses and germinal center system. *In* H. Cottier, N. Odartchenko, R. Schindler and C. C. Congdon, (eds.). Germinal Centers in Immune Responses. Springer-Verlag, Berlin, pp. 4–27.

66. Good, R. A. and J. Finstad. 1968. The Gordon Wilson Lecture: The development and involution of the lymphoid system and immunologic capacity. Trans. Am. Clin. Climat. Assoc. *79:*69–107.

67. Good, R. A. and J. Finstad. 1968. The association of lymphoid malignancy and immunologic functions. *In* C. J. D. Zarafonetis (ed.). Proceedings of International Conference on Leukemia-Lymphoma. Lea & Febiger, Philadelphia, pp. 175–197.

68. Good, R. A. and J. Finstad. An essential relationship between the lymphoid system, immunity and malignancy. J. Nat. Cancer Inst. In press.

69. Good, R. A. and J. Finstad. Immunologic deficiency, malignancy and lymphoid deficits— an essential relationship. Proceedings of M. D. Anderson Hospital, March 5, 1969. *In* Genetic Concepts in Neoplasia. In press.

70. Good, R. A., J. Finstad, H. Gewurz, M. D. Cooper and B. Pollara. 1967. The development of immunological capacity in phylogenetic perspective. Am. J. Dis. Child. *114:*477–497.

71. Good, R. A., R. A. Gatti, R. Hong and H. J. Meuwissen. 1969. Graft treatment of immunological deficiency. Lancet *1:*1162.

72. Good, R. A., W. D. Kelly, J. Rotstein and R. L. Varco. 1962. Immunological deficiency diseases, agammaglobulinemia, hypogammaglobulinemia, Hodgkin's disease and sarcoidosis. *In* P. Kallos and B. H. Waksman (eds.). Progress in Allergy. vol 6. Karger, New York, pp. 187–319.

73. Good, R. A., C. Martinez and A. E. Gabrielsen. 1964. Progress toward transplantation of tissue in man. Adv. Pediat. *13:*93–127.

74. Good, R. A., R. D. A. Peterson and A. E. Gabrielsen. 1964. The thymus and central lymphoid tissue in immunobiology. Bull. Rheum. Dis. *15:*351–356.

75. Good, R. A., R. D. A. Peterson, D. Y. Perey, J. Finstad and M. D. Cooper. 1968. The immunological deficiency diseases of man: Consideration of some questions asked by these patients with an attempt at classification. *In* R. A. Good and D. Bergsma (eds.). Immunologic Deficiency Diseases in Man. Birth Defects Original Article Series, vol. 4. National Foundation Press, New York, pp. 17–39.

76. Good, R. A., P. G. Quie, D. B. Windhorst, A. R. Page, G. E. Rodey, J. White, J. J. Wolfson and B. H. Holmes. 1968. Fatal (chronic) granulomatous disease of childhood: A hereditary defect of leukocyte function. Seminars Hemat. *5:*215–254.

77. Good, R. A. and R. L. Varco. 1955. Clinical and experimental study of agammaglobulinemia. J.-Lancet *75:*245–271.

78. Gorer, P. A. 1958. Some reactions of the $H_2$ antibodies *in vitro* and *in vivo*. Ann. N.Y. Acad. Sci. *73:*707–721.

79. Hellstrom, I., K. E. Hellstrom, G. E. Pierce and A. H. Bill. 1968. Demonstration of cell-bound and humoral immunity against neuroblastoma cells. Proc. Nat. Acad. Sci. *60:*1231–1238.

80. Heremans, J. H. and P. H. Crabbé. 1968. IgA deficiency: General considerations and relation to human disease. *In* R. A. Good and D. Bergsma (eds.). Immunologic Deficiency Diseases in Man. Birth Defects Original Article Series, vol 4. National Foundation Press, New York, pp. 298–307.

81. Higashi, O. 1954. Congenital gigantism of peroxidase granules. Tohoku J. Exp. Med. *59:*315–332.

82. Hitzig, W. H. 1968. Swiss type of agammaglobulinemia. *In* R. A. Good and D. Bergsma

(eds.). Immunologic Deficiency Diseases of Man. Birth Defects Original Article Series, vol. 4. National Foundation Press, New York, pp. 82–87.

83. Hitzig, W. H., Z. Biró, H. Bosch and H. J. Huser. 1958. Agammaglobulinämic und Alymphocytose mit Schwand des lymphatischen Gewebes. Helv. Paediat. Acta *13*:551–585.

84. Holmes, B., A. R. Page and R. A. Good. 1967. Studies of the metabolic activity of leukocytes from patients with a genetic abnormality of phagocytic function. J. Clin. Invest. *46*: 1422–1432.

85. Holmes, B., P. G. Quie, D. B. Windhorst and R. A. Good. 1966. Fatal granulomatous disease of childhood: An inborn abnormality of phagocytic function. Lancet *1*:1225–1228.

86. Hong, R., R. A. Gatti and R. A. Good. 1968. Hazards and potential benefits of blood transfusion in immunologic deficiency. Lancet *2*:388–389.

87. Hong, R., H. E. M. Kay, M. D. Cooper, H. J. Meuwissen, M. J. G. Allan and R. A. Good. 1968. Immunological restitution in lymphopenic immunological deficiency syndrome. Lancet *1*:503–506.

88. Hoyer, J. R., M. D. Cooper, A. E. Gabrielsen and R. A. Good. 1968. Lymphopenic forms of congenital immunologic deficiency diseases. Medicine *47*:201–226.

89. Hoyer, J. R., M. D. Cooper, A. E. Gabrielsen and R. A. Good. 1968. Lymphopenic forms of congenital immunologic deficiency: Clinical and pathologic patterns. *In* R. A. Good and D. Bergsma (eds.). Immunologic Deficiency Diseases in Man. Birth Defects Original Article Series, vol. 4. National Foundation Press, New York, pp. 91–103.

90. Ishizaka, K. and T. Ishizaka. 1967. Identification of gamma-E antibodies as a carrier of reaginic activity. J. Immunol. *99*:1187–1198.

91. Jankovic, B. D., B. H. Waksman and B. O. Arnason, 1962. Role of the thymus in immune reactions in rats. I. The immunologic response to bovine serum albumin (antibody formation, Arthus reaction and delayed hypersensitivity) in rats thymectomized and splenectomized at various times after birth. J. Exp. Med. *116*:159–176.

92. Johansson, S. G. O.: 1967. Raised levels of a new immunoglobulin class (IgND) in asthma. Lancet *2*:951–953.

93. Kaplan, E. L., T. Laxdal and P. G. Quie. 1968. Studies of polymorphonuclear leukocytes from patients with chronic granulomatous disease of childhood: Bactericidal capacity for streptococci. Pediatrics *41*:591–599.

94. Kellum, M. J., D. E. R. Sutherland, E. Eckert, R. D. A. Peterson and R. A. Good. 1965. Wasting disease, Coombs positivity and amyloidosis in rabbits subjected to central lymphoid tissue extirpation and irradiation. Int. Arch. Allerg. *27*:6–26.

95. Kelly, W. D., R. A. Good and R. L. Varco. 1958. Anergy and skin homograft survival in Hodgkin's disease. Surg. Gynec. Obst. *107*:565–570.

96. Kelly, W. D., D. L. Lamb, R. L. Varco and R. A. Good. 1960. Investigation of Hodgkin's disease with respect to the problem of homotransplantation. Ann. N.Y. Acad. Sci. *87*: 187–202.

97. Klebanoff, S. J. and L. R. White. 1969. Iodination defect in the leukocytes of a patient with chronic granulomatous disease of childhood. New Eng. J. Med. *280*:460–466.

98. Kretschmer, R., B. Say, D. Brown and F. S. Rosen. 1968. Congenital aplasia of the thymus gland (DiGeorge syndrome). New Eng. J. Med. *279*:1295–1301.

99. Krivit, W. and R. A. Good. Unpublished observations.

100. Kulneff, N., R. O. Pederson and J. Waldenstrom. 1955. Drei Falle von Agammaglobulinämie: ein klinischer, genetischer und physikalischchemischer Beitrag zur Kenntnis des Protein-Stoffwechsels. Schweiz. Med. Wschr. *85*:363–368.

101. Lamb, D. L., F. Pilney, W. D. Kelly and R. A. Good. 1962. A comparative study of the incidence of anergy in patients with carcinoma, leukemia, Hodgkin's disease and other lymphomas. J. Immunol. *89*:555–558.

102. Lemmel, E. M., M. D. Cooper and R. A. Good. Improved responses of neonatally thymectomized mice to sheep red blood cells. To be published.

103. Lischner, H. W., H. H. Punnett and A. M. DiGeorge. 1967. Lymphocytes of extra thymic origin from an infant with congenital absence of the thymus: behavior in vitro. Nature (Lond.) *214*:580–582.

104. Mackaness, G. B. 1969. The influence of immunologically committed lymphoid cells on macrophage activity in vivo. J. Exp. Med. *129*:973–992.

105. Mackaness, G. B. and W. C. Hill. 1969. The effect of anti-lymphocyte globulin on cell-mediated resistance to infection. J. Exp. Med. *129*:993–1012.

106. Marchelonis, J. J. 1967–68. Phylogeny of Immunity: Evolutionary studies of antibody structure in the Queensland lungfish, Neoceradotus forestare. Annual Report Walter and Eliza Hall Institute for Medical Research.

107. Marchelonis, J. J. and G. M. Edelman. 1968. Phylogenetic origins of antibody structure.

III. Antibodies in the primary immune response of the sea lamprey, Petromyzon marinus. J. Exp. Med. *127*:891–914.

108. Martinez, C., J. Kersey, B. W. Papermaster and R. A. Good. 1962. Skin homograft survival in thymectomized mice. Proc. Soc. Exp. Biol. Med. *109*:193–196.

109. McKelvey, Z. M. and J. L. Fahey. 1965. Immunoglobulin changes in disease; quantitation on the basis of heavy polypeptide chains IgG (gamma G), IgA (gamma A) and IgM (gamma M) and of light polypeptide chains type K (I) and type L (II). J. Clin. Invest. *44*:1778–1787.

110. McKhann, C. F.: Primary malignancy in patients undergoing immunosuppression for renal transplantation. Transplantation. In press.

111. McKneally, M. F., M. J. Kellum and D. E. R. Sutherland. 1966. Functional studies of thymectomized and appendectomized rabbits. (Abstract.) Fed. Proc. *24*:613.

112. McKneally, M. F., D. E. R. Sutherland and R. A. Good. The central lymphoid tissues of rabbits: II. Functional and morphologic studies in adult rabbits. Submitted to Surgery.

113. Merigan, T. C., Jr. 1969. Interferon and interferon inducers: The clinical outlook. Hosp. Prac. *4*:42–49.

114. Meuwissen, H. J., R. A. Gatti, P. I. Terasaki, R. Hong and R. A. Good. Long-lasting reconstitution of lymphopenic hypogammaglobulinemia and bone marrow aplasia by transplantation of allogeneic marrow: Crucial role of histocompatibility matching. New Eng. J. Med. In press.

115. Meuwissen, H. J., P. J. Van Alten, M. D. Cooper and R. A. Good. 1969. Dissociation of thymus and bursa function in the chicken by phytohemagglutinin. *In* W. O. Rieke (ed.). Proceedings of the Third Annual Leucocyte Culture Conference. Appleton-Century-Crofts, New York, pp. 227–234.

116. Meuwissen, H. J., P. J. Van Alten and R. A. Good. 1969. Decreased lymphoid cell multiplication in the post-thymectomy state. Transplantation *7*:1–11.

117. Miller, D. G. 1962. Patterns of immunological deficiency in lymphomas and leukemias. Ann. Int. Med. *57*:703–716.

118. Miller, J. F. A. P. 1961. Immunological function of the thymus. Lancet *2*:748–749.

119. Miller, J. F. A. P., G. F. Mitchell and N. S. Weiss. 1967. Cellular basis of the immunological defects in thymectomized mice. Nature (Lond.) *214*:992–997.

120. Mosser, G., R. A. Good and M. D. Cooper. The immune responses and lymphoid tissues of neonatally thymectomized x-irradiated mice. Submitted for publication.

121. Mueller, A. P., H. R. Wolfe and W. P. Cote. 1964. Antibody studies in hormonally and surgically bursectomized chickens. *In* R. A. Good and A. E. Gabrielsen (eds.). Thymus in Immunobiology. Hoeber-Harper, New York, pp. 359–373.

122. Nossal, G. J. V., A. Cunningham, G. F. Mitchell and J. F. A. P. Miller. 1968. Cell to cell interaction in the immune response. III. Chromosomal marker analysis of single antibody-forming cells in reconstituted irradiated or thymectomized mice. J. Exp. Med. *128*:839–853.

123. Oort, J. and J. L. Turk. 1965. A histological and autoradiographic study of lymph node during development of contact sensitivity in the guinea pig. Brit. J. Exp. Path. *46*:147–154.

124. Ortega, L. G. and B. K. Der. 1964. Studies on agammaglobulinemia induced by ablation of the bursa of Fabricius. (Abstract.) Fed. Proc. *23*:546.

125. Page, A. R. and R. A. Good. 1960. Plasma cell hepatitis with special attention to steroid therapy. A.M.A. J. Dis. Child. *99*:288–314.

126. Page, A. R., A. E. Hanson and R. A. Good. 1963. Occurrence of leukemia and lymphoma in patients with agammaglobulinemia. Blood *21*:197–206.

127. Parrott, D. M., M. A. B. deSoussa and J. East. 1966. Thymus-dependent areas in the lymphoid organs of neonatally thymectomized mice. J. Exp. Med. *123*:191–203.

128. Perey, D. Y. E., M. D. Cooper and R. A. Good. 1967. Normal second set wattle homograft rejection in agammaglobulinemic chickens. Transplantation *5*:615–623.

129. Perey, D. Y. E., M. D. Cooper and R. A. Good. 1968. Lymphoepithelial tissues of the intestine and differentiation of antibody production. Science *161*:265–266.

130. Perey, D. Y., M. D. Cooper and R. A. Good. 1968. The mammalian homologue of the avian bursa of Fabricius. I. Neonatal extirpation of Peyer's patch-type lympho-epithelial tissues in rabbits. Methods and inhibition of development of humoral immunity. Surgery *64*:614–621.

131. Peterson, R. D. A., M. D. Cooper and R. A. Good. 1965. The pathogenesis of immunological deficiency diseases. Am. J. Med. *38*:579–604.

132. Peterson, R. D. A., M. D. Cooper and R. A. Good. 1966. Lymphoid tissue abnormalities associated with ataxia-telangiectasia. Am. J. Med. *41*:342–359.

133. Peterson, R. D. A. and R. A. Good. 1968. Ataxia-telangiectasia. *In* R. A. Good and

D. Bergsma (eds.). Immunologic Deficiency Diseases in Man. Birth Defects Original Article Series, vol. 4. National Foundation Press, New York, pp. 370–377.

134. Peterson, R. D. A., W. D. Kelly and R. A. Good. 1964. Ataxia-telangiectasia: its association with a defective thymus, immunological deficiency disease and malignancy. Lancet 1:1189–1193.

135. Pollara, B., W. A. Cain, J. Finstad and R. A. Good. The amphibian as a key step in the evolution of lymphoid tissue and diverse immunoglobulin classes. Proceedings of the Amphibian Tumor Symposium. In press.

136. Pollara, B., J. Finstad and R. A. Good. 1969. Specific immunoglobulin synthesis in lower vertebrates lacking germinal centers. In L. Fiore-Donati and M. G. Hanna (eds.). Lymphatic Tissues and Germinal Centers in Immune Response. Adv. in Exp. Med. and Biol., Vol. 5. Plenum Press, New York, pp. 1–8.

137. Pollara, B., A. Suran, J. Finstad and R. A. Good. 1968. N-terminal amino acid sequences of immunoglobulin chains in Polyodon spathula. Proc. Nat. Acad. Sci. 59:1307–1312.

138. Rodey, G. E., B. H. Park, D. B. Windhorst and R. A. Good. 1969. Defective bacterial activity of monocytes in fatal granulomatous disease. Blood 33:813–820.

139. Salvin, S. B., R. D. A. Peterson and R. A. Good. 1965. The role of the thymus in resistance to infection and endotoxin toxicity. J. Lab. Clin. Med. 65:1004–1022.

140. Schier, W. W., A. Roth, G. Ostroff and M. H. Schrift. 1956. Hodgkin's disease and immunity. Am. J. Med. 20:94–99.

141. Seligmann, M. M., H. G. Fudenberg and R. A. Good. 1968. A proposed classification of primary immunological deficiencies. Am. J. Med. 45:817–825.

142. Sidky, Y. A. and R. Auerbach. 1968. Tissue culture analysis of immunological capacity of snapping turtles. J. Exp. Zool. 167:187–196.

143. Silverstein, A. Development of antibody production in fetal lambs subjected to complete extirpation of the bowel. In preparation.

144. Simonsen, M. 1962. Graft-vs-host reactions. Their natural history and applicability as tools of research. Prog. Allergy 6:349–467.

145. Sinclair, N. R. St. C. and E. V. Elliott. 1968. Neonatal thymectomy and the decrease in antigen sensitivity of the primary response and immunological memory systems. Immunology 15:325–333.

146. South, M. A., M. D. Cooper, R. Hong and R. A. Good. 1967. The IgA local antibody system. In A. Monroy and A. A. Moscona (eds.). Current Topics in Developmental Biology. vol. 2. Academic Press, New York, pp. 191–222.

147. South, M. A., M. D. Cooper, R. Hong, F. A. Wollheim and R. A. Good. 1968. Secretory IgA and the immunologic deficiency. In R. A. Good and D. Bergsma (eds.). Immunologic Deficiency Diseases in Man. Birth Defects Original Article Series, vol. 4. National Foundation Press, New York, pp. 283–291.

148. Southam, C. E. 1967. Cancer immunology in man. In Busch, H. (ed.). Methods in Cancer Research. vol. 2. Academic Press, New York, pp. 1–42.

149. Starzl, T. E., C. G. Groth, P. I. Terasaki, C. W. Putnam, L. Brettschneider and T. L. Marchioro. 1968. Heterologous antilymphocyte globulin, histocompatibility matching and human renal homotransplantation. Surg. Gynec. Obst. 126:1023–1035.

150. Stutman, O., E. J. Yunis and R. A. Good. 1969. Reversal of post-thymectomy wasting in mice with immuno-competent cells: influence of histocompatibility differences. J. Immunol. 102:87–92.

151. Stutman, O., E. J. Yunis and R. A. Good. Tolerance induction with thymus grafts in neonatally thymectomized mice. J. Immunol. In press.

152. Stutman, O., E. J. Yunis, C. Martinez and R. A. Good. 1967. Reversal of post-thymectomy wasting disease in mice by multiple thymus grafts. J. Immunol. 98:79–87.

153. Suran, A. A., M. H. Tarail and B. W. Papermaster. 1968. Immunoglobulins of the leopard shark. J. Immunol. 99:679–686.

154. Sutherland, D. E. R., O. K. Archer and R. A. Good. 1964. The role of the appendix in development of immunologic capacity. Proc. Soc. Exp. Biol. Med. 115:673–676.

155. Sutherland, D. E. R., O. K. Archer, R. D. A. Peterson, E. Eckert and R. A. Good. 1965. Development of "autoimmune processes" in rabbits subjected to neonatal removal of central lymphoid tissue. Lancet 1:130–133.

156. Sutherland, D. E. R., M. F. McKneally, M. J. Kellum and R. A. Good. A definition of thymic-dependent areas in the peripheral lymphoid tissue of rabbits. Int. Arch. Allerg. In press.

157. Teague, P. E., E. J. Yunis, G. E. Rodey, A. J. Fish, O. Stutman and R. A. Good. Autoimmune phenomena and renal disease in mice: Role of thymectomy, aging and involution of immunologic capacity. Submitted to Lab. Invest.

158. Ten Bensel, R. W., E. M. Stadlan and W. Krivit. 1966. The development of malignancy in the course of the Aldrich syndrome. J. Pediat. 68:761–767.

159. Thieffry, S., M. Arthuis, J. Aicardi and C. Lyon. 1961. L'ataxie-télangiectasie (7 observations personnelles). Rev. Neurol. *105*:390–405.

160. Thorbecke, G. J., M. W. Cohen, E. B. Jacobson and J. D. Wakefield. 1967. The production of memory cells by the white pulp of the spleen in rabbits. *In* H. Cottier, N. Odartchenko, R. Schindler and C. C. Congdon (eds.). Germinal Centers in Immune Responses. Springer-Verlag, Berlin, pp. 259–269.

161. Tobler, R. and H. Cottier. 1958. Familiäre Lymphopenie mit Agammaglobulinämie und schwerer Moniliasis: die essentialle Lymphocytophthise als besondere Form der frühkindlichen Agammaglobulinämie. Helv. Paediat. Acta *13*:313–338.

162. Turk, J. 1967. Cytology of the induction of hypersensitivity. Brit. Med. Bull. *23*:3–8.

163. Turk, J. L. and S. H. Stone. 1963. Implication of cellular changes in lymph nodes during development inhibition of delayed hypersensitivity. *In* B. Amos and H. Koprowski (eds.). Cell-Bound Antibodies. Wistar Institute Press, Philadelphia, p. 51.

164. Uphoff, D. E. and L. W. Law. 1959. An evaluation of some genetic factors influencing irradiation protection by bone marrow. J. Nat. Cancer Inst. *22*:229–241.

165. Van Alten, P. J., W. A. Cain, R. A. Good and M. D. Cooper. 1968. Gamma globulin production and antibody synthesis in chickens bursectomized as embryos. Nature *217*:87–89.

166. Waksman, B. H., B. G. Arnason and B. D. Jankovic. 1962. Role of the thymus in immune reactions in rats. III. Changes in the lymphoid organs of thymectomized rats. J. Exp. Med. *116*:187–206.

167. Warner, N. L. and A. Szenberg. 1964. Immunologic studies on normally bursectomized and surgically thymectomized chickens: dissociation of immunologic responsiveness. *In* R. A. Good and A. E. Gabrielsen (eds.). Thymus in Immunobiology. Hoeber-Harper, New York, pp. 395–411.

168. Warner, N. L., A. Szenberg, and F. M. Burnett. 1962. The immunological role of different lymphoid organs in the chicken. I. Dissociation of immunological responsiveness. Aust. J. Exp. Biol. Med. Sci. *40*:373–387.

169. Windhorst, D. B., J. G. White, P. B. Dent, J. Decker and R. A. Good. 1968. Defective defense associated with genetic disease of subcellular organelles. *In* R. A. Good and D. Bergsma (eds.). Immunologic Deficiency Diseases in Man. Birth Defects Original Article Series, vol. 4. National Foundation Press, New York, pp. 424–432.

170. Windhorst, D. B., A. S. Zelickson and R. A. Good. 1966. Chediak-Higashi syndrome: Hereditary gigantism of cytoplasmic organelles. Science *151*:81–83.

171. Young, R. R., K. F. Austen and H. W. Moser. 1964. Abnormalities of serum gamma 1–A globulin and ataxia-telangiectasia. Medicine *43*:423–433.

172. Yunis, E. J., H. R. Hilgard, C. Martinez and R. A. Good. 1965. Studies on immunologic reconstitution of thymectomized mice. J. Exp. Med. *121*:607–632.

173. Zinneman, H. H. and W. A. Hall. 1954. Recurrent pneumonia in multiple myeloma and some observations on immunological responses. Ann. Int. Med. *41*:1152–1163.

# Chapter 5

# PEDIATRIC IMMUNIZATION AS A DEVELOPING MIRROR OF NATURE

JOSEPH STOKES, JR.

*Emeritus Professor of Pediatrics, School of Medicine, University of Pennsylvania and the Henry Phipps Institute, Philadelphia, Pennsylvania*

The phylogenetic developments responsible for the defenses of the body against pathogenic microorganisms in the higher forms of life remain but poorly understood. In contrast, the often brilliant studies illuminating the ontogenetic developments of such defenses and their enhancement in these higher forms, and particularly in man, present some of the most distinctive and dramatic advances in all of history. The unbalancing of world ecology in favor of man by virtue of his enhancing these defenses stands as a prime cause of overpopulation—a problem second to none in its serious consequences in the world today. This demographic imbalance originating in the biological sciences is also dramatically paralleled by the lack of balance of the historians in recording both wars and population movements and fluctuations with little reference to man's diseases.

The ecologic problems involved in man's defenses as related to his pathogenic parasites have been enormously complicated by the rapidly increasing facility of travel. Even with the slow access to the Western Hemisphere by sailing vessels in the sixteenth and seventeenth centuries, it is now well recognized that two parasites apparently new to the American Indians, smallpox and measles viruses, far exceeded the small bands of settlers in their power of conquest—a fact almost entirely neglected in historical writings.[102]

With the extension of rapid access to all parts of the world and with the increasing contact by air travel of man with parasites endemic to a variety of regions and in a variety of animals and vectors, together with extreme variations in sanitation, the ecologic balance is subjected to great and often overwhelming challenges, as repeatedly demonstrated in many regions and in the splendid work and studies of the World Health Organization, the Rockefeller Foundation, and many others.

An exceptional example of the attainment of ecologic balance to a parasite, for which a balance had already been attained in one part of the world, Brazil, was demonstrated in Australia upon the introduction of myxomatosis virus to the rabbit population. The rabbit was a virgin soil for the virus, as well as an extraordinarily destructive pest for the pasture lands and therefore for sheep farming, one of Australia's major industries. At first only an occasional rabbit survived the infection, but with time a balance is being slowly established between the pest and the parasite, although as yet the balance is much in favor of the parasite.[19]

The specific factors responsible for such a balance differ considerably among the enormous variety of parasites as well as with respect to the host. An excellent example of the variability of a host factor has been demonstrated in West Africa where the mortality rate in all epidemics of measles in the past has approximated 25 per cent as a result of the protein malnutrition in the children with the accompanying poverty of antibody.[73] The natural measles virus, although it can be attenuated, has not provided evidence of increase in virulence and would not in itself account for this. Fortunately, the recently developed attenuated measles virus vaccine has wiped out a majority of these deaths. But this in turn has reduced the quality of life in that area by flooding the West African countries with persons whose nutrition can even less readily be maintained.

It was first noted by Pasteur about 1870[63] that nonpathogenic microorganisms could replace certain pathogenic bacteria by interference, a finding that was most dramatically confirmed by Fleming in his studies on *Penicillium notatum* in 1929.[21]

Avirulent staphylococci, saprophytic in nature, when seeded extensively over the skin of the newborn, have been shown not only to inhibit but to displace the virulent pathogenic staphylococci that have been of etiological importance in severe nursery staphylococcal epidemics[77]—a type of symbiosis with, and protection of, man for which there may well be a number of other examples. If the usual flora of the intestinal tract is reduced by an antibiotic, such as neomycin, the customary balance may be disturbed sufficiently to permit the active, and often dangerous, growth of fungi in the intestine.[76, 96] The balance produced by nonpathogenic *Escherichia coli* in usually preventing growth of fungi may not necessarily be of additional benefit to the host. Thus animals raised without access to microorganisms actually grow larger and apparently are healthier and live longer than the bacteria-populated animals of the same strain,[66] but obviously nonpathogenic enteric organisms have some protective value against fungi.

Only rather recently has a symbiosis or even a synergism been established between bacteria and viruses, such as occurs between a bacteriophage and the diphtheria bacillus[29] or between a bacteriophage and the β-hemolytic streptococcus.[101] In epidemic influenza, such as that occurring in 1918, influenza virus apparently acts in synergism with the staphylococcus, *Haemophilus influenzae*, and other bacteria.[92] Such microbiologic complexities are briefly mentioned in the present discussion for the purpose of indicating the enormous variety of problems presented to the body's defenses.

## THE IMAGE OF IMMUNIZATION

It is of particular interest that man's raising of the mirror to nature in developing his defenses precedes any knowledge of microorganisms, whether pathogenic or nonpathogenic. This image was thus raised long before Pasteur. As an astute observer of nature, Jenner[41] initiated a method of challenging man that was a reflection of nature's own method of arousing defensive mechanisms. The story of the milkmaids and cowpox is so great a classic as to warrant no further elaboration of it here.* However, it clearly represents the primary offering by nature of a virus that may well have been, and probably was, the first attenuated virus vaccine, possibly transmitted from man to animal and perhaps later from animal to man. Whichever way the original transmission occurred, or even if transmission was from a prior host, the result was a mild lesion in man that protected him for a considerable period of years from a far more virulent and yet antigenically closely related disease, smallpox. The calf lymph used for vaccinia has always been a crude preparation, usually with some bacterial contamination. Recently the bacteria-free tissue culture vaccinia virus is proving more suitable, particularly when eczema, herpes, or other skin lesions are present.*

It is of great interest also that this natural immunity was discovered not only before bacteria or viruses were known, but even long before man had any suggestion of the variety of defense mechanisms of his body. The biologist, the medical scientist, and the practitioner had to wait three-quarters of a century before the larger microorganisms, bacteria, were described by Pasteur and Koch, and again many years before Iwanowski[39] demonstrated the passage of pathogenic viruses through porcelain filters. Pasteur, without extensive knowledge of the causative agent of rabies, had attempted to immunize against the disease with injections of dried spinal cord of rabbits after serial intracerebral passage in rabbits that resulted in loss of pathogenicity for dogs.[62] It was many years before rabies virus was more completely characterized and more adequate attenuated vaccines were developed. As bacteria have been cultured on artificial media, as viruses have been grown first in the chick embryo and its membranes and finally in a variety of tissue cultures,[18] as the defensive mechanisms of the body have been more fully understood, and as dead and living vaccines have been augmenting those defenses, an increasing degree of similarity between artificial and natural exposure in pediatric immunization has been attained. With the further characterization of these organisms and the immunological responses of a considerable technological variety that have been developed for the serum and cells of the host, an increasingly close paral-

---

* See Chapter 21, Smallpox, by Allan W. Downie.

lelism, a mirror image, has become more clearly visible between resistance obtained by vaccination and resistance resulting from natural disease, together with a frequent mitigation by such vaccines of the more severe reactions of the natural diseases.

The present discussion outlines first the similarity of defense to both types of challenge, artificial and natural, and later, in several examples of the newer studies on pediatric immunization, the approach that seems to be of increasing importance at the present time.

The striking reason that pediatric immunization in this era presents increasingly an image of the ecologic balance of nature is the rapidly increasing biologic knowledge of a considerable group of viral diseases that usually attack in childhood, that each contains antigenically but a single entity, and that almost invariably produce permanent immunity. An exception, poliomyelitis, is represented by three such entities (Types I, II, and III) that are antigenically different and yet produce usually permanent immunity.* The influenza viruses may be excluded from consideration in the discussion of pediatric immunization owing to their antigenic lability, at least in Type A, and the absence of prolonged immunity to epidemic influenza in man as a result of such lability.

In the second historical position to Jenner's mimicry of nature stands Theiler's mutant virus,[95] the 17D strain of yellow fever virus, which when injected in precisely the same manner as the *Aedes aegypti* mosquito injects it produces apparently an even more solid and permanent immunity to yellow fever than vaccinia virus does to smallpox. This is the only live arbovirus that has been used successfully for long-term immunization, and because of geographic limitation of its vector and therefore of the disease to relatively few and restricted areas, it need not be considered as a significant factor in pediatric immunization in the so-called developed countries.

Before those viruses related to pediatric immunization are discussed in greater detail, brief mention should be made of the general defenses of the body to such viral invasion—their nature and uses, and some of the factors responsible for their enhancement and for the decrease in their effectiveness.

The general protective properties of the skin and mucous membranes, together with the tears, saliva, sebaceous secretions, and sweat, are well known and will not be reviewed here. The attack of poliomyelitis, measles, mumps, rubella, varicella, infectious mononucleosis, and epidemic hepatitis concerns more specifically the internal organs and it is to this area that the general defenses are particularly related. The functions of the macrophages, small and large lymphocyte, reticulum cell, plasma cell, and polymorphonuclear leukocyte are discussed elsewhere in this book.† By means of the immune globulins, IgA, IgG, and IgM, produced in final effective form in the lymph structures, neutralizing antibodies to all of the viruses just listed are formed. These antibodies persist in varying amounts throughout life and, except for the transplacental antibodies of the first 10 to 12 months of life, they represent evidence of experience, either apparent or inapparent, with each specific patho-

---

*See Chapter 22, Poliomyelitis (Infantile Paralysis), by John R. Paul.

†See Chapter 2, Cellular Immunity, by G. B. Mackaness and R. V. Blanden, Chapter 3, The Mechanism of Macrophage Activation, by G. B. Mackaness, and Chapter 4, Bulwarks of the Bodily Defense, by R. A. Good, J. Finstad, and R. A. Gatti.

genic virus. Not only may they be used as evidence of previous experience with each virus, but their curve of elevation and decrease permits a rough estimate of the timing of the specific infection as well as evidence of the degree of resistance of the host. The body's experience with pathogenic microorganisms is by no means always reflected in circulating antibodies, but is almost universally reflected in the anamnestic response, when the memory of the lymph structures is restimulated by the same antigen. Exceptions to such a response and the absence of antibodies to the primary stimuli are discussed by Good in Chapter 4.

The first workers to use convalescent human serum in any disease for prevention or modification—in this case measles—were Nicolle and Conseil[57] in France. Remarkably small amounts were required, thus suggesting that measles virus was blood-borne. Later McKhann and Chu[51, 52] utilized successfully placental extract pooled from human placentas for such prevention, and finally the cold ethanol fractionation of pooled human blood plasma by the method of Cohn and Oncley[9] furnished an immune human globulin that has had many applications. Dr. Baird Hastings recounts an interesting story of the early World War II period when Walter Cannon and he were discussing in Cannon's office the limitations of acacia for shock in World War I and the similar problems raised by the new conflict. Hastings suggested that the two should visit Edwin Cohn in a laboratory just above them for suggestions in this area. As they told Cohn of the dilemma he leaned back in his chair and pulled from the shelf a bound volume of his papers on the cold ethanol fractionation of blood plasma—a remarkable example of studies in basic science without apparent practical application at the time they were carried out and yet which resulted in the albumin fraction used so extensively during the second world war and up to the present time. Albumin can be heated at 60°C. for 10 hours without denaturation, thus inactivating any serum hepatitis virus from the pooled plasma used, as demonstrated in volunteers by joint studies conducted by the Harvard group and our group at the University of Pennsylvania.*[25] At that time the gamma globulin fraction was considered by Edwin Cohn as a by-product without known value. However, he wisely insisted that the plasma protein fractions, other than albumin, be preserved for further study of their possible usefulness. Janeway's group at Harvard,[59] jointly with our group at the University of Pennsylvania,[88] demonstrated in studies on the prevention and attenuation of measles that the serum hepatitis virus was destroyed in the more severe handling of the globulin fraction in the process of fractionation.

---

* The blood products Cohn and Oncley developed and the studies based on their work cover many pages of modern reference books that make no mention either in text or index of their origin, just as the many pages devoted to types and modifications of viral tissue cultures permit the initiator of tissue culture work, Harrison, at times to remain unnoticed, and for many almost forgotten. No one today can point to the human originator of the wheel, or of the brick—perhaps chiefly because no written language was available to permit their adequate descriptions by the inventors. But the presence of such historical vacua is no reason for omitting essential rungs in descriptions of the remarkable ladders of medical advances. Perhaps one might leave such descriptions entirely to the medical historians, but if this were done, a major portion of students in the biologic sciences and medicine would fail to grasp the cultural continuity of their field of interest. Thus all up-dating should be an opportunity for *brief recapitulation* in so far as the author is able—the firm establishing of such cultural continuity.

This reassurance concerning the sterility of the gamma globulin fraction, as well as its efficacy, made it available not only for the control of infectious diseases but later for use in agammaglobulinemia and for many other conditions in which the globulin has been of value.[40] In the earlier studies it could be administered only by intramuscular injection owing to the severe febrile reactions following intravenous injection, but as indicated later, further treatment of the globulin has made it available for effective intravenous therapy.

Antibody remains the only "magic bullet" yet available to strike specifically at a single antigen or viral particle. This specific defense of the body used artificially furnishes the mirror image of the natural protection from challenge by the pathogenic virus. Not only has its protective value been demonstrated in measles and epidemic hepatitis in dosages (for the globulin from large pools of human plasma) which are remarkably similar,[89] but it also was the first method demonstrated jointly by Dr. Hammon's group in Pittsburgh and by our group in Philadelphia to be effective for the prevention of poliomyelitis for a period of at least five weeks. The significance of this demonstration resided not in the fact that it suggested the virus was blood-borne but rather in the fact that the protection by an almost unmeasurable trace of antibody in the blood clearly pointed to the probability that any measurable antibody in the blood produced by vaccine, whether dead or living, in all probability would be protective.[34] Thus the protection of passive immunization in poliomyelitis fortunately could soon be superseded first by the dead vaccine of Salk based on the cornerstone of Enders, Weller, and Robbins' remarkably successful growth of the polioviruses in tissue culture, and later by the successive studies of Koprowski[46] and Sabin[69] on attenuation of the three types of virus and the oral use of all three types of poliovirus in active immunization. The development of attenuated polioviruses in tissue culture and, by means of this, the replication of the challenge of the natural disease, followed by apparently permanent immunity to the infecting virus, was historically the third example of a modified natural exposure similar to the first example, vaccinia, and the second, yellow fever.[94]

With respect to epidemic hepatitis, the relatively long incubation period, usually ranging from 25 to 35 days, made possible the study of a variety of dosages of human gamma globulin for control of the clinical symptoms. At the same time, if exposure to the natural virus occurred during the asymptotic curve of disappearance of the globulin, a permanent protection, termed passive-active immunization, was found to ensue.[84, 87] Owing to the long half-life of human globulin, as compared to that of heterologous globulin,[81] the period over which such a method of immunization could be attained accorded with the amount of globulin injected[49] if the globulin was obtained from sufficiently large pools of plasma or serum. Thus the larger the amount of globulin, the longer was the period, and in general 0.06 ml. of globulin per pound of body weight would permit passive-active immunization over a six-month period —namely, for each 0.01 ml. added, one additional month could be added to the period during which such immunization was possible. Wherever the epidemic hepatitis virus is endemic, in regions with fewer sanitation measures, natural exposure of susceptibles entering such regions, as in work camps, the Peace Corps, or the armed forces, may well be taken for granted. Thus the injection of human gamma globulin in persons entering such regions in effect amounts to active immunization for a major portion of the persons involved. Actually, infective plasma in extremely small quantities from acute cases could be utilized for oral immunization if the globulin in amounts of 0.01 ml. per pound of body weight were injected at the same time or within a few days after the orally administered virus. This method of immunization has not been tested in extensive outbreaks or in institutions where the virus has been endemic—a situation that may well permit such immunization.

Because evidence suggests that epidemic hepatitis causes a permanent immunity, active immunization, such as it is hoped may be possible with a tissue culture vaccine, is being further pursued by a number of workers. The fact that extremely small doses of globulin are capable of controlling the epidemic disease strongly suggests that, as in measles, the etiological virus is antigenically of a single type which usually produces a permanent immunity.

Because the protection afforded by gamma globulin is less clear in serum hepatitis,[85] and because whenever it has been effective it has required much larger doses[12, 30] than in epidemic hepatitis, the relation of such usage to serum hepatitis may be determined only by appropriate characterization of the etiological viral agents, which may well be several in number.

The recent encouraging studies of Blumberg et al.[3, 53] on the Australia (Au) antigen and its localization in the blood and in the liver by fluorescent antibody and by electron microscopy strongly suggest that it represents at least one, or perhaps the definitive, viral agent responsible for serum hepatitis (SH) and its carrier state in man. Thus far these studies in Philadelphia, as well as in other centers, suggest that it may have no antigenic relation to epidemic hepatitis (IH).

But the story that started with the use of the natural "magic bullet," the specific antibody to a viral antigen or particle, was greatly augmented by the combining of a method of plasmapheresis—obtaining every week a unit of plasma, about 210 to 220 ml., by bleeding a donor, separating the red cells, retaining the plasma, and within about 15 minutes returning the red cells through the same needle[80]—with the use of plasma having high antibody levels produced by natural disease, attenuated viruses, or hyperimmunization with the appropriate antigen. This combined method initiated by Smolens and Stokes[80, 91] and shown to be safe for repetition every other week in the same person over long periods, has become standard for a number of serum products. Three of such hyperimmune products relate to the three bacterial antigens (i.e., D.P.T.) now used for routine pediatric immunization. These three antigens for active immunization were developed in a massive attack on the prevention and treatment of diphtheria, pertussis, and tetanus over a period of many years and need not be reviewed again here. Human immune globulin for tetanus has become a routinely available and most effective product, free of the allergic or anaphylactic reactions occurring in a large percentage of persons receiving horse serum tetanus antitoxin. Schofield and his co-workers[70] have demonstrated that in New Guinea active immunization of the mother against tetanus during pregnancy could furnish protection to the newborn by transplacental antibodies, and this might find application where neonatal tetanus is a real problem, as in Haiti and Brazil.

McGuinness, Armstrong, and Felton[50] conducted studies which suggested that large doses of hyperimmune human serum were effective in the prevention and treatment of pertussis. They hoped that human gamma globulin might be more convincingly protective. When this was tested later by Morris and McDonald[56] no protection was demonstrated, a finding that may represent a loss of a specific protective fraction against *H. pertussis* in the process of cold ethanol or cold ether (Kekwick and Mackay) fractionation. This requires further investigation in monkeys (*Macaca cyclopsis*) that have a susceptibility to the disease[8] and in which hyperimmune serum apparently afforded a fairly solid passive protection. Presumably antibodies to *H. pertussis*, a gram-negative organism, would be found in the 19S globulin fraction, of which only a small amount remains in the gamma globulin resulting from ethanol fractionation.

There has been no opportunity to determine the preventive or curative effect of such an immune globulin in diphtheria, although unreported studies of Ipsen* in Denmark during a severe outbreak of diphtheria in 1945 clearly suggested that serum from recently immunized adults was as effective in therapy as much larger doses of antitoxic serum of horses, used in controls. Aside from tetanus immune globulin, industry hesitates to produce any quantity of the other immune globulins, owing to the paucity of patients requiring such therapy.

Vaccinia immune globulin is an important human biological produced by the American National Red Cross from donors convalescent from a primary vaccinia,[43] as demonstrated by Kempe and his co-workers. It has been useful for preventing or modifying smallpox when given within 24 hours following exposure.[44] For extensions of its uses see Chapter 21, Smallpox, by Allan W. Downie.

More recently an advance has been made in the preparation of immune globulin that should add immeasurably to the usefulness of the combination of plasmapheresis and convalescent or hyperimmune globulin, namely, the marked reduction of its pyrogenic properties for the purpose of permitting its intravenous use.[2, 71, 74] This has been accomplished chiefly by reduction in serum anticomplementary activity that apparently has been primarily responsible for the marked febrile or, on occasion, shock-like reactions from intravenous use.

| Prognostic classification | Horse serum | Human serum |
|---|---|---|
| Severe | 7/31 | 1/4 |
| Very severe | 9/14 | 3/5 |
| Highly toxic, "bullneck" | 7/7 | 3/7 |
| Total | 23/52 (44%) | 7/16 (44%) |

Unpublished data from the State Serum Institute and Blegdams Hospital, Copenhagen (Johannes Ipsen and Esther Ammundsen); furnished by Dr. Johannes Ipsen, Henry Phipps Institute, Philadelphia, Pennsylvania.

---

* In 1945 serum was drawn from adults recently immunized against diphtheria. The pool contained 20 antitoxin units per milliliter. The treatment dose was 100 to 400 ml. while controls were treated with 100,000 to 200,000 antitoxin units in horse serum. Only severe cases were selected for human serum treatment. The results (number of deaths per number treated) were as follows:

The possible usefulness of large amounts of a variety of immune globulins injected intravenously is sufficiently obvious as hardly to warrant emphasis. Yet the availability and testing of such important applications of basic findings has been lagging far behind other areas of clinical investigation. An example of such a lag is in the development and use of antirabies hyperimmune human globulin. In the only controlled human studies of the relative values of antirabies horse serum, as compared to antirabies vaccine alone, that were carried out in Iran, the serum plus vaccine appeared to be greatly superior to the vaccine. In animal studies, the usefulness of antirabies serum has been clearly demonstrated.[47] The evidence suggests that it should always be injected immediately after the bite of a rabid animal. The less reactive human immune antirabies globulin can be obtained from veterinary students, who must be vaccinated against the disease with the duck embryo vaccine owing to their possible exposure to rabid dogs or to other rabid animals. Immediate use of such globulin intravenously would appear to be a vital extension of prophylactic measures.[1] This developmental problem is to a major extent a financial one. Although it involves a lethal disease, the small number of cases in the more developed areas of the world militates against an extensive industrial outlay. Such a development must be supported by public funds that are less frequently applied to clinical applications of this type. In less well developed areas of the world in comparison with developed countries the need for control of rabies is far greater, but apparently less urgent than, for example, family planning.

The wide range of immune human globulins for prophylaxis or therapy or both by the intravenous route could well extend over tetanus, pertussis, possibly diphtheria, rabies, malaria, measles, rubella, mumps, varicella, smallpox, vaccinia, poliomyelitis, epidemic hepatitis, and possibly infectious mononucleosis, in some of which it clearly could be effective and in others of which it deserves a thorough clinical investigation. Antistaphylococcal human immune globulin by intravenous administration may well be useful in the future for serious staphylococcal infections that do not respond to antibiotics.[20, 60]

Passive immunization or treatment with immune globulins in the diseases mentioned and by either the intramuscular or intravenous route may remain as a defensive measure to be held in reserve or to be used experimentally in therapy, as for example in severe zoster and in malaria (for which suggestive positive evidence has been available). Nevertheless, of far greater significance in the control of these diseases is the natural resistance that can be attained by active immunization. In addition to the advantage previously mentioned, that the causative agents of these diseases in almost all instances are single antigenic types which with natural infection usually produce permanent immunity, a new reason recently has appeared for using attenuated viruses rather than inactivated viral vaccines. This new reason followed the application by Enders and Peebles[17] of the chick tissue culture method used by Enders in growing the polioviruses to the growing of measles virus and its inactivation by formalin solution 1:4000 for use as a dead vaccine. The moderate antibody response to the dead vaccine, whether in single or multiple doses, tended to diminish rather rapidly following vaccination, but of far greater importance was the not infrequent febrile response when a vaccinated person was exposed to natural measles or to attenuated measles virus vaccine.[67] Accompanying the marked febrile reactions caused by exposure were urticarial and often vesicular skin lesions, together at times with angioneurotic edema. Such responses can be extremely disturbing to the parents of the patient and often persist for a number of days.

Reactions of this type tend to counterbalance the hesitation felt by many workers concerning the use of living tissue cultures with live viruses for vaccines. There was little concern about possible contaminating or oncogenic agents in the work of Jenner on vaccinia or of Theiler on yellow fever virus because such agents were unknown at that time. More recently, when the leukosis virus of chickens was found to be almost constantly endemic in the fertile hens' eggs, and particularly after evidence became available of oncogenic properties of the simian virus 40[93] from monkey kidneys when administered to newborn hamsters, the use of such tissue cultures for live virus vaccines raised doubts in the minds of some workers concerning contaminating viral agents. In addition to preference for dead rather than live virus, this has resulted, for example, in the restriction of poliomyelitis vaccination to dead poliovirus vaccines administered parenterally, with apparent success in nationwide eradication of the disease, in Sweden.[23] However, the unnatural response resulting from the use of dead measles virus vaccine may well cause concern lest injections of a variety of inactivated antigens produce excessive immune responses characteristic of so-called autoimmune reactions when the multiply vaccinated person is exposed to the natural diseases. If new antigens are to be added to the toxoids, diphtheria and tetanus, and to the pertussis antigen, it would thus seem appropriate for them to approximate milder types of natural infections. Because attenuated live viruses resemble most closely the balance that nature establishes between those single-type viruses naturally producing permanent immunity and their natural host, man, there would appear to be little, if any, chance of abnormal responses or autoimmune reactions occurring in the present developing program of pediatric immunization. Also, because the yellow fever live virus vaccination program with the use of the 17D strain of virus in the chick embryo was initiated in the 1930's, and because these embryo materials, almost without question, were contaminated with chicken leukosis virus, unknown until rather recently, any oncogenic effects in the millions of persons receiving this embryo vaccine would have been evident by the present time. Review of such persons thus far has not revealed evidence of an excess incidence of malignancy beyond the expected rate. Great care is taken at the present time to use leukosis-free flocks of chickens for production of chick tissue culture vaccines.

Tissue cultures of monkey kidneys (*Macaca mulatta*) are being used for the production of live poliovirus vaccines. These vaccines are not injected parenterally but are administered orally, which furnishes a certain element of safety in avoiding direct exposure of the body tissues and circulation to any possible contaminating viral agent. We should emphasize that if one wishes in immunization to develop for the child a mirror of nature, in the manner that nature exposes children successively under natural conditions, as mentioned, it would be well to use tissue cultures of animals more distantly related to man than those of other primates. Serious accidental infections have occurred in persons working with green monkey kidneys (*Circopithecus aethiops*),[45, 78] and in such primates complete assurance of the absence of oncogenic agents is difficult. The use of tissues for vaccines from animals more distantly related phylogenetically to man would appear to furnish greater assurance of the absence of oncogenic viral agents.

The three newer attenuated virus vaccines whose use in early life seems likely to provide permanent protection are measles, mumps, and rubella in that respective order of development. The combination of these three recently characterized viruses with the first crudely studied virus, vaccinia of Jenner, in a single jet-gun injection, may be a milestone in the field of pediatric immunization. This method of combined virus vaccines has already been tentatively considered by Buynak, Hilleman, and Whitman at the Merck Institute for Therapeutic Research, together with Weibel and Stokes at the University of Pennsylvania,[7] with some evidence of success. Obviously there is much to recommend it, if the combined vaccines can be desiccated in a single vial from the frozen state and kept at −4°C. until reconstituted for immediate use. Meyer et al.[54] have reported responses in Upper Volta children to inoculation of combined live measles, smallpox, and yellow fever vaccines.

## MEASLES

The early efforts at cultivation of measles virus (a myxovirus) were plagued by the same problems that plagued studies on mumps, epidemic hepatitis, and other viruses, namely, that chick embryo and its membranes were inadequate media for growth of the viruses. Suggestive evidence of growth of the virus in the early passages on the chick chorioallantoic membranes was obtained by Plotz[65] and by Shaffer, Rake, Stokes, and O'Neil,[75] but these studies were always defeated by the extremely rapid attenuation of the virus on such a medium. Infection in children from the early-passage virus was at times clearcut and at other times questionable. There was no certainty, as had previously been demonstrated by Goldberger and Anderson[27] and by Blake and Trask,[3] that the *Macaca mulatta* monkey was a susceptible host. When exposed to the natural disease the rate of "takes" was low and the evidence of clinical disease in the "takes" was minimal, with a faint and evanescent rash and few other symptoms. It was later demonstrated by Enders, using serological studies, that the *Macaca mulatta* monkeys, though usually susceptible at the time of capture in India, subsequently, because of contact with man and herding in cages under a variety of conditions, were exposed to measles virus and thus inapparently infected. For the early workers, lacking serological tests, the monkey was an uncertain experimental animal for the study of measles, and exposure of the susceptible child was the only means of detecting the presence of virus. When children were immunized with early-passage measles virus grown on the chorioallantois,[90] only a relatively small percentage of them were immune on later natural exposure, and the use of the chick embryo membranes was therefore abandoned. With the advent of the newer methods of tissue culture developed by Enders, Weller, and Robbins for the polioviruses, Enders and his co-workers[15, 17] applied similar methods of chick tissue cultures to the cultivation of the measles virus, and this resulted in the development of the Edmonston strain of attenuated virus and immediately opened a fresh prospect for the possible control of measles.

The rationale for the use of attenuated measles virus vaccine has been reviewed sufficiently so that only a few observations concerning its present status and the reasons for its inclusion in pediatric immunization are warranted. Measles has always been one of the major causes of mental crippling resulting from complicating meningoencephalitis, which, although not as frequent a complication as meningoencephalitis in mumps, has a far greater degree of severity with greater residual damage to the brain. The psychological tests that have been carried out by Byers and Meyer[7a] before and after mild measles encephalitis have shown, even when clinical recovery was apparently complete, evidence of a decrease in mental acuity. Owing to the varying degrees of protein deprivation in the developing countries and to an extent in the United States, not only the high fatality rate mentioned previously but also the residual spectrum of mental crippling in natural measles is a serious problem. Because measles so often occurs at an early age, usually before intelligence quotients can be accurately determined, the slight retardation or inability to advance as well as other children in school may be unsuspected or considered as more of a genetic or environmental phenomenon characteristic of the ghetto. Of course the effects of measles encephalitis may also be superimposed on environmental or genetic problems.

The second serious complication of measles, which causes comparatively many more deaths than encephalitis and yet on recovery is usually far less crippling, is bronchopneumonia. This can be primarily the result of the measles virus per se, but secondarily invading bacteria, the staphylococcus, *H. influenzae*, the pneumococcus, and the $\beta$-hemolytic streptococcus, are more apt to be responsible. The rash of measles is frequently noted in the larynx and reaching down well into the trachea, with the result of far greater susceptibility to the pathogenic bacteria acting as secondary invaders. The antibiotic treatment accords with the susceptibility of the bacterium, as determined in cultures from the nasopharynx or sputum. All of the usual complications related to bronchopneumonia may ensue but they will not be considered here.

The Edmonston strain of attenuated measles virus results in markedly modified measles; approximately 30 to 40 per cent of children experience fever (rectal temperature over 103°F.) beginning about the sixth postinoculation day and lasting two to four days.[42] Approximately 30 to 60 per cent of such vaccinees have a modified rash over the face, trunk, and upper arms, often not extending to or barely reaching the legs. Conjunctivitis, coryza, and cough are minimal. In some of the early studies of this vaccine, because of the relative severity of response, human immune globulin, 0.022 ml. per kg., was injected at the same time into the opposite arm. This reduced the incidence of temperature elevation over 103°F. to about 15 to 18 per cent, with a marked reduction in severity and length of occurrence of symptoms and the rare appearance of an evanescent rash. Another means of reducing the severity of response was sought by Schwarz[72] in the further attenuation of the Edmonston strain by low-temperature passage of the virus. Success was attained in reducing reactions to a point approximately equal to that occurring with the combination of the Edmonston strain and human immune globulin administered in opposite arms.[97] Even with use of the Edmonston strain unmodified by human immune globulin, the reactions experienced are far less severe than those seen in the natural disease and in at least 50 children tested by Gibbs[26] at the height of their response there was no evidence of electroencephalographic changes. This evidence would appear to rule out the type of inflammatory changes demonstrated by routine electroencephalography during natural clinical measles.

The attenuated measles virus vaccine apparently also will eliminate the likelihood of occurrence of the rare cases of subacute sclerosing panencephalitis. This is a degenerative chronic inflammatory infection of the central nervous system, apparently caused by latent measles virus, and producing intellectual deterioration in children and adolescents and convulsive seizures with motor abnormalities. The presence of measles virus in brain tissue of such cases has been determined by electron microscopy, by demonstration of measles antigen by fluorescent antibody, and finally by propagation of the measles virus from brain biopsies of such cases.[7b]

Because the attenuated measles virus vaccine does not produce any encephalitis, as suggested by the normal electroencephalograms, it would be extremely improbable that the attenuated virus would remain latent in the central nervous system.

A total of millions of doses of the Edmonston, of the more attenuated Edmonston (Moraten), and of the Schwarz strains of live virus vaccine have been used throughout the world. The question as to whether they are equivalent, or almost equivalent, in the degree and permanence of the immunity they produce remains unanswered. The neutralizing antibody titer following the use of all three viruses parallels the response occurring in natural measles but at a considerably lower level, irrespective of the use of human immune globulin. The curve of antibody response to the Schwarz strain decreases more rapidly in a straight-line descent than the curve of Edmonston antibody or of Moraten antibody but antibody remains measurable by the Norrby[58] technique using the ether-soluble antigen. There appears to be little doubt that immunity from the Edmonston strain of virus accords with the continuing elevation of neutralizing antibody, as readily measurable by the usual technique. Immunity from the Schwarz strain apparently has persisted solidly in this country for a period somewhat shorter than that demonstrated for the Edmonston strain, whereas questions have been raised both in Great Britain and in West Africa concerning a number of "breakthroughs" that have occurred following use of the Schwarz strain. Because "breakthroughs" have not been seen in the United States, it appears possible that the method of preparation, preservation, or handling of the Schwarz vaccine may have been responsible, rather than a deficiency in the original Schwarz strain of virus itself. The accumulating data concerning the efficacy of these strains should soon afford clear-cut answers to these problems. The use of the Moraten strain of virus has been for a shorter period, but the curve of antibody for at least one year has paralleled that of the Edmonston strain and at a slightly lower level.

The obvious precautions of avoiding use of such vaccines in leukemia, in the presence of other malignancies, during febrile illness, and in the presence of active or even quiescent tuberculosis should be carefully observed. Inasmuch as natural measles has been well recognized as having an unfavorable effect on both latent and active tuberculosis, one of the interesting problems, as yet unresolved, is whether live attenuated measles virus vaccine produces a somewhat similar effect. In this connection one interesting phenomenon is the anergy produced by the live measles virus vaccine in the tuberculin test.[53] A markedly positive tuberculin test will usually change to a negative one following injection of measles virus vaccine and will at times remain negative for a number of weeks. The reason for this change in delayed hypersensitivity is unknown. However, it emphasizes the importance of preceding the measles vaccination with a tuberculin test if there is any possibility of prior infection or exposure to tuberculosis because for a considerable period after measles vaccination a negative tuberculin test has no significance.

Because of the occasional severe response to natural measles or to live measles vaccine in children previously injected with dead vaccine, as mentioned previously, dead vaccine should not be used for immunization either alone or in combination with other vaccines or with live measles vaccine. As a result of these severe responses manufacture of dead measles vaccine has ceased.

There may be a rare use for human convalescent measles globulin prepared for injection intravenously in natural measles at the time Koplik's spots afford the earliest clinical evidence of disease, usually 2 to 3 days before the rash appears—if by chance a child or young person has not been vaccinated and proves to be susceptible. Suggestive evidence has been obtained that with intramuscular human immune globulin in considerable amounts the natural disease may be aborted and either no rash or only an evanescent rash may appear.[88] Only the globulin well prepared for intravenous injection should be used in such therapy—a type of product that can rarely be made available. On occasion the Koplik's spots and rash may appear almost simultaneously, in which case it is too late for intravenous therapy to be effective.

The timing of injection of attenuated measles virus vaccine depends primarily upon the disappearance of the mother's antibodies in the newborn infant; the final traces of the asymptotic curve probably disappear in 10 to 12 months. Disappearance can be gauged by the fact that on occasion the live virus vaccine will not immunize if given during the last two months of the first year of life. Thus the optimal time for such vaccination is at one year.

## MUMPS

Mumps immunization, like measles immunization, came into prominence also in the early 1940's and particularly during World War II when the control of these diseases in the Armed Services of the United States was more urgent. Although intramuscular injection of convalescent mumps immune globulin reduced the rate of mumps orchitis quite effectively when injected at the beginning of the acute parotitis,[24] other studies showed that even large doses of convalescent serum (200 ml.) failed to prevent the disease. Enders and his co-workers infected the *Macaca mulatta* by injecting Stensen's duct with mumps virus from patients with acute parotitis.[13] Typical mumps was produced in the salivary glands and a mumps skin test[16] that was similar in significance to the tuberculin test and read in the same manner was developed from tissue of the injected parotid gland. From the same tissue complement fixation, hemagglutination-inhibition, and neutralization tests were developed.[13, 14] The mumps virus was also soon adapted to the chick embryo and could be obtained in large amounts from the allantoic fluid.[14] The most disturbing characteristic of its growth on the chick embryo was the rapidity of attenuation on passage, to the point that it no longer produced parotitis although there appeared to be no diminution in the quantity of virus. Following inactivation by ether or by ultraviolet light, such virus was used successfully by Stokes et al.,[86] by Habel,[31, 32] and by the Henles et al.[35] for vaccination of man and monkey. However, as in measles, the adaptation of the mumps virus to chick tissue cultures has permitted remarkable advances in effecting a mimicry of nature.[33] The Henle group at the Children's Hospital of Philadelphia separated out a soluble (S) antigen and a viral (V) antigen from the mumps virus that permitted determination of a serological difference between recent and former infection. The anti-S antibody appears somewhat more rapidly in the clinical disease and both increases and later decreases more rapidly than the anti-V antibody. Thus the titer of the anti-S antibody, in comparison with the titer of anti-V antibody in the same specimen of serum, furnishes a fairly accurate picture of the time relation of the clinical disease to the time of obtaining the serum specimen. The Henle group also initiated studies on active immunization in susceptible children with attenuated virus from chick embryos, spraying the virus into the nasopharynx and around Stensen's duct to mimic nature's method of immunization, but with a less virulent viral antigen that produced no clinical disease. It was difficult to gauge the amount of virus used by this method or to place such vaccine material on a regular production basis. From this work it was predicted by W. Henle[36] that somewhere between the tenth and thirtieth passage tissue culture material would probably be appropriate for attaining adequate protection against clinical mumps.

At this time Smorodintsev and his co-workers[82] in Leningrad contributed an important step to the vaccination procedure by using the attenuated chick tissue culture mumps virus parenterally rather than by the natural route of the oropharynx or respiratory tract. This assured a constant quantity of virus reaching the tissues and apparently also permitted greater certainty of producing immunity. Smorodintsev, Klyachko, and their co-workers[83] have vaccinated many thousands of persons in the Soviet Union with this vaccine with a good immune response of neutralizing antibody and without any evidence of local or general reaction. The slow loss of resistance of these vaccinated persons over the years following vaccination is shown in Table 1, and although protection continues in a fairly high percentage of the vaccinees, Smorodintsev has suggested that they should be vaccinated again in about five years. This slow reduction in resistance demonstrated upon exposure to natural mumps, as well as the failure to provide complete protection as shown in Table 1, raised some question as to the wisdom of vaccinating in childhood and protecting only temporarily a considerable number of persons who after puberty might be susceptible to a more severe parotitis and its attendant complications.

Because the number of passages in tissue cultures has been shown to have

TABLE 1.   *Effectiveness of Mumps Vaccine in the U.S.S.R.**

| PERIOD POST VACC. (MONTHS) | ATTACK RATE PER 10,000 | | PER CENT EFFECTIVENESS |
|---|---|---|---|
| | *Vaccinees* | *Controls* | |
| 1–6 | 32 | 346 | 91 |
| 7–12 | 28 | 311 | 91 |
| 13–18 | 21 | 306 | 93 |
| 19–24 | 28 | 221 | 87 |
| 25–30 | 59 | 357 | 83 |

* From Smorodintsev et al. 1967. *In:* First International Conference on Vaccines against Viral and Rickettsial Diseases of Man. Pan American Health Organization, Washington, D. C. Publication No. *147*:422–429.

a direct relation to the degree of attenuation of the mumps virus, and owing to the fact that Smorodintsev and his co-workers used virus from about the twenty-fifth passage for preparation of the mumps vaccine, this may well account for the slow loss of protection mentioned. More recent efforts for protection appear to have been more successful because earlier-passage virus has been used. Buynak and Hilleman[5] developed the Jeryl Lynn strain of mumps virus on chick tissue cultures from leukosis-free chickens, early passages (twelfth) of which caused mild mumps in efforts at immunization. Together with Weibel, Stokes, and Whitman,[38] they conducted extensive tests by parenteral injection of the seventeenth passage of such chick tissue culture virus in large numbers of susceptible children in homes, schools, and institutions. Whereas early-passage attenuated virus was excreted from the throat or salivary glands at the time of infection, there was no evidence of continuing excretion of virus when the seventeenth chick tissue culture passage was used, nor was there an increase in serum amylase during the period of infection. Large-scale vaccination studies in seronegative children one to 11 years of age with vaccine of this passage demonstrated a satisfactory increase in neutralizing antibody in 98 per cent of the vaccinated group, as shown on Table 2, without spread of virus to susceptible contacts either in the home or in the school environment. In this first large group during the eight month period following vaccination, when considerable exposure to natural mumps occurred, there was a rate of protection of 96 per cent, as shown in Table 3. The excellent degree of protection in those vaccinees exposed at home, compared with the relatively high rate of natural mumps in the control children at home, was particularly striking.

There is a considerably greater amount of neutralizing antibody following natural mumps than following vaccine mumps, as shown in Table 4, whereas

TABLE 2.   *Serologic Response Rates in Children Given Jeryl Lynn Live Attenuated Mumps Vaccine and in Their Contact Controls**

| | DEVELOPING ANTIBODY | |
|---|---|---|
| | *No./Total* | *Per cent* |
| Vaccinated | 355/362 | 98 |
| Unvaccinated | 0/365 | 0 |

* From Weibel et al. 1967. New Eng. J. Med. *276:*245–251.

TABLE 3. *Protective Efficacy of Jeryl Lynn Live Attenuated Mumps Vaccine in the First 8 Months Post Vaccination**

| | No. AT RISK † | Mumps CASES ‡ | RATE (PER CENT) | PROTECTIVE EFFICACY |
|---|---|---|---|---|
| Vaccinated | 113 | 3 | 2.7 | 96 |
| Unvaccinated | 129 | 80 | 62 | — |

\* From Hilleman et al. 1967. New Eng. J. Med. *276:*252–258.
† Only homes or classrooms in which mumps appeared.
‡ Includes both laboratory and clinically diagnosed cases.

the difference between the titers of the hemagglutination-inhibiting antibody is not a striking one.

The most important fact this seventeenth-passage mumps virus vaccine has demonstrated serologically is that thus far, after three years, as of mid-1968, the neutralizing antibody of the vaccinee parallels the neutralizing antibody of the person who has had natural mumps. This parallelism of neutralizing antibody exists with another myxovirus, measles, in which the titer resulting from the vaccine also is lower but parallel to the antibody curve resulting from natural measles. In mumps not only does the neutralizing antibody continue to be elevated over the third year (to the present writing) following vaccination but the effective protection has been 100 per cent, as shown in Tables 5 and 6. As noted, sufficient cases of mumps occurred among the susceptible controls to assure significance of the results with respect to protection.

Unlike measles vaccine, mumps vaccine does not cause local or general reactions. Booster doses, widely separated in years from the original immunization, could assure anamnestic responses if the neutralizing antibody fell off toward zero, suggesting a recurrence of susceptibility.

However, if mumps attenuated virus vaccination became a routine procedure, similar to poliomyelitis vaccination, it too should so alter the ecological balance that natural mumps virus, like poliovirus, would disappear, or practically disappear, at the end of the first year. In such case the older male would no longer need to worry about the complications of adult mumps and children would no longer be subjected to the quarantine of summer camps or the slow and uncomfortable progress of the natural disease through the lower schools. In this connection it should be emphasized that mumps is not a disease to be

TABLE 4. *Geometric Mean Antibody Titers After Vaccination and After Natural Mumps**

| ANTIBODY | NATURAL MUMPS | VACCINE MUMPS |
|---|---|---|
| Neutralizing | 1:60 | 1:9 |
| Hemagglutination-inhibiting † | 1:9 | 1:5 |

\* From Weibel et al. 1967. *In:* First International Conference on Vaccines against Viral and Rickettsial Diseases of Man. Pan American Health Organization, Washington, D. C. Publication No. *147:*430–437.
† Using whole virus antigen. Tween-ether-treated antigen gives titers two to four times higher in both groups.

TABLE 5.  *Cases of Natural Mumps Which Occurred 18 to 32 Months Following the Time of Vaccination in Families**

| | VACCINATED CHILDREN AT RISK | | NONVACCINATED CHILDREN *No. of Clinical Cases of Mumps* | | | INTERVAL BETWEEN VACCINATION AND OCCURRENCE OF THE FIRST CASE IN THE FAMILY |
|---|---|---|---|---|---|---|
| *Family No.* | *No. Vaccinated* | *No. of Cases of Mumps* | *No. of Controls at Risk* | *Laboratory Proved* | *Clinical Diagnosis Only* | |
| 1† | 1 | 0 | 2 | 2 | — | 25, ? mo.‡ |
| 37† | 1 | 0 | 3 | — | 1 | 19 mo. |
| 43 | 1 | 0 | 2 | 1 | — | 22 mo. |
| 44 | 1 | 0 | 2 | 2 | — | 23, 24 mo. |
| 45 | 1 | 0 | 2 | 1 | — | 28 mo. |
| 46 | 1 | 0 | 3 | 3 | — | 27, 28, 28 mo. |
| 47 | 1 | 0 | 1 | 1 | — | 29 mo. |
| 48 | 1 | 0 | 2 | 2 | — | 29, 29 mo. |
| 49 | 1 | 0 | 1 | 1 | — | 29 mo. |
| 50 | 1 | 0 | 2 | 2 | — | 29, 30 mo. |
| 51 | 1 | 0 | 1 | 1 | — | 30 mo. |
| 52 | 2 | 0 | 4 | — | 1 | 22 mo. |
| 53 | 1 | 0 | 2 | 2 | — | 26, 27 mo. |
| 54 | 1 | 0 | 2 | 1 | — | 30 mo. |
| 55 | 1 | 0 | 2 | 2 | — | 31, 31 mo. |
| 56 | 1 | 0 | 1 | — | 1§ | 32 mo. |
| 57 | 1 | 0 | 3 | 1 | — | 32 mo. |
| Total | 18 | 0 | 35 | 22 | 3 | 19–32 mo. |
| Rates | 0/18 = 0% | | 25/35 = 71% | | | — |
| Protective efficacy | | | 100% | | | 19–32 mo. |

* From Weibel et al. 1969. J. A. M. A. *207*:1667–1670.
† One case of mumps had occurred in each of these families previously.
‡ Inapparent infection.
§ This child was also a member of a classroom and was included in Table 6.

considered lightly. Sterilization is rare in the adult male and probably does not occur in the female but the inflammatory lesions of the gonads are extraordinarily painful. According to the Communicable Disease Center of the United States Public Health Service, about 50 deaths have occurred yearly from mumps encephalitis in the United States from 1958 to 1968. Thus the meningoencephalitis, though less severe than that of measles, can still be a severe complication. No one can be certain how much damage to the pancreas occurs, or of the possible relation of mumps to diabetes mellitus. Perhaps one of the most urgent reasons for controlling the natural mumps virus by vaccination is the prevention of the unilateral nerve deafness. Because it is often difficult for parents to distinguish unilateral deafness in very young children, the etiological relation of mumps may be overlooked. Otolaryngologists feel its relation to unilateral deafness is of considerably greater importance than has usually been estimated.

Additional strains of attenuated mumps virus vaccine are being studied, such as that developed by Deinhardt[11] in Chicago. Confirmatory work concerning the value of the Jeryl Lynn strain of attenuated mumps virus is being

Table 6.  *Natural Mumps Among Children in Classrooms During 1967–1968 School Year\**

| School | 1967–68 Classroom | VACCINATED GROUP | | NONVACCINATED CHILDREN | | |
|--------|-------------------|------------------|---|---------------------|---|---|
| | | *No. of Children* | *No. of Cases of Mumps* | *No. of Children* | *No. of Cases of Mumps Study†Children* | *Others‡* |
| 02 | 1G2 | 1 | 0 | 1 | — | 1 |
| 19 | 2G1 | 1 | 0 | 3 | — | 1 |
| 19 | 2G2 | 3 | 0 | 3 | — | 1 |
| 21 | 2G | 1 | 0 | 2 | — | 2 |
| 22 | 2G | 2 | 0 | 3 | — | 2 |
| 30 | 1G1 | 3 | 0 | 4 | 2§ | 2 |
| 30 | 1G2 | 1 | 0 | 4 | — | 4 |
| 30 | 1G3 | 2 | 0 | 4 | 1 | 3 |
| 30 | 1G4 | 2 | 0 | 3 | — | 3 |
| 30 | 2G | 2 | 0 | 8 | 2 | 6 |
| 31 | 2G | 2 | 0 | 2 | — | 2 |
| 32 | 2G | 1 | 0 | 3 | — | 2 |
| 33 | 1G | 1 | 0 | 2 | — | 2 |
| 33 | 2G | 1 | 0 | 4 | — | 2 |
| 34 | 2G1 | 3 | 0 | 1 | 1 | — |
| 34 | 2G2 | 1 | 0 | 2 | 2 | — |
| 35 | 2G | 5 | 0 | 3 | — | 1 |

| Mumps rates | 0/32 at risk | 42/52 of susceptibles at risk |
|---|---|---|
| Protective efficacy | 100% during the third mumps year | |

\* From Weibel et al. 1969. J. A. M. A. *207*:1667–1670.
† All cases confirmed by laboratory diagnosis.
‡ Clinical diagnosis only.
§ One child was also a member of a family and was included in Table 5.

conducted in a number of other laboratories and in many thousands of children in other clinical studies, all of which studies apparently are in general accord with the data given here. A complete review of the disease is not appropriate in a discussion oriented, as is the present one, to the background of immunization.

## RUBELLA

A fourth antigen, rubella, is also appropriate for pediatric immunization, partly because of the single type of its antigen and its permanently immunizing capability, but primarily because of its severe teratogenic effect during the early months of pregnancy. The alert interest of a clinical ophthalmologist, Gregg[28] in Australia, about 28 years ago suddenly brought to light the relation between cataracts of the newborn and rubella during early pregnancy. From that time the list of confirmed congenital defects and the problems related to rubella during pregnancy and in the newborn have been steadily expanding in number. The congenital lesions may be listed in accordance with the organs involved. They demonstrate a tragic assortment of problems for the family.

*Blood*
Hypogammaglobulinemia
Megakaryocyte inhibition
Lymphadenopathy
Normocytic anemia

*Liver*
Giant cell hepatitis
Biliary cirrhosis

*Bones*
Osseous rarefaction

*Central nervous system*
Encephalitis
Microcephaly
"Cerebral palsy"
Retardation

*Lungs*
Interstitial pneumonia

*Development*
Esophageal atresia
Hypospadias
Growth retardation

*Heart*
Patent ductus
Pulmonary stenosis and coarctation
Myocardial necrosis

*Eye*
Cataracts, chorioretinitis
Glaucoma
Microphthalmia

*Ear*
Cochlear degeneration
Stapes fixation

The approach to control of the disease received its initial stimulus from the joint efforts of Weller and Neva[99] and Parkman, Buescher, and Artenstein[61] in cultivating the virus. After many failures in obtaining characteristic cytopathic changes in tissue cultures that would be useful for titration of serological neutralizing antibodies, they devised a method of interference that confirmed the presence of active rubella virus in the tissue culture cells. By means of exposing the cells to a second virus at a suitable time interval—in the original work echovirus 11 was used—the presence of active rubella virus could be determined by the resultant failure of the echovirus to produce its characteristic cytopathic changes in the cells. Neutralizing antibody could then be titrated by determination of the highest dilution at which interference no longer occurred. This method of culturing rubella virus and of obtaining the titer of antibody by means of interference and neutralization of the interference poses two major problems, first that it requires the simultaneous, careful, and quantitative cultivation in tissue cultures (preferably monkey kidney cells) of two viruses, rubella and echovirus 11, and second, that neutralizing antibodies to echovirus 11 may already be present in the serum of the person being tested. There is no present method of avoiding the first problem of using interference of one virus, rubella, with a second virus that provides a clear-cut cytopathic effect in the tissue culture cells. The second problem can best be avoided by using such a virus, as Bunyamwera (an arbovirus), against which neutralizing antibodies are never, or almost never, found in the United States population and yet that produces a highly characteristic cytopathic effect in the monkey tissue culture cells if they have not been infected with rubella virus. Later it was found that serum antibodies could best be titrated by means of the hemagglutination-inhibiting test, which is far simpler to perform and quite accurate in determining susceptibility and resistance.

Thanks to the ability to determine both the presence of rubella virus and the susceptibility or immunity of the human host, it was found that the infected newborn sheds the virus for months or even several years—actually an indefinite period. Also it was found by serological tests that approximately 17 per cent of the women in the United States in the fertile age range are susceptible to the disease. Women in the fertile age range are often unaware of their susceptibility to rubella, as well as of their pregnancy, and therefore the long period of shedding of the virus from the infected and congenitally defective newborn may well place an unknown number of pregnant women at risk. The problem is compounded by the difficulty in the differential diagnosis of the disease from the other infectious diseases of childhood that so often are mistaken for rubella. Thus the mother may have a sense of security as a result of a false belief that she has had rubella in childhood. Or, because of the frequently evanescent nature of the disease, she may have extreme anxiety concerning her susceptibility when she actually is immune.[4] For these reasons a premarital serologic test for rubella antibodies in the bride is at present far more important than a serologic test for syphilis, although both tests should be done. Many far-sighted parents have deliberately exposed their female children to rubella prior to puberty. With such exposure the child must be carefully quarantined from women in the fertile age range during both the incubation period and the period of symptoms. Such difficulties in exposing females emphasize the importance of serologic tests for all females between puberty and marriage for the purpose of revealing their serologic status and their possible future need for rubella vaccine. Most of these problems may well be solved by the rapidly expanding knowledge of rubella virus vaccines.

Five groups of workers have been making the most active progress in using a variety of cell-virus systems for propagation and attenuation of rubella virus. These are briefly outlined in Table 7 and all represent strains of attenuated virus that might well be acceptable for vaccines. In addition to producing little, if any, clinical response, as well as permanent immunity, vaccine must be noncontagious to susceptible contacts and must be grown in a safe and acceptable type of tissue culture cell. Studies previously were conducted on purified and concentrated *killed* rubella virus vaccine[6] which on human trial proved ineffective in withstanding challenge by live viruses. Also, in view of the previous experience of sharp reactions when a killed myxovirus, measles, was followed by the natural disease or by live attenuated measles virus, it seems unwise to pursue further the use of such dead virus vaccines.

TABLE 7. *Principal Cell Cultures and Virus Strains Used to Prepare Rubella Vaccines**

| CELL CULTURE† | VIRUS STRAIN |
| --- | --- |
| Duck embryo | Merck |
| | HPV-77 |
| Grivet monkey kidney | HPV-77 & 120 |
| Dog kidney | HPV-77 |
| Rabbit kidney | Cendehill |
| WI-38 (diploid human cell strain) | RA 27/3 |

* From Weibel et al. 1967. New Eng. J. Med. *276*:245–251.
† All primary cell cultures except WI-38.

In studying the type of cell to be used for attenuation it was evident that the rubella virus grew inadequately in chick embryo cell cultures and also became attenuated too rapidly. The suitability of the other cells mentioned in Table 7 would appear to accord with their descending phylogenetic relation to man. Thus the closest to man, monkey kidney, is the least suitable for parenteral use of living tissue; duck embryo appears to be the most suitable. Although monkey kidney has been used for attenuated poliovirus vaccines, such vaccine is given orally, by which route it may well be suitable for immunizing purposes. However, many viral diseases are common to man and monkey. Extremely few clinical diseases common to man and duck have been described and the Pekin ducks used for preparation of the rubella vaccine rarely develop spontaneous neoplasms. The WI-38 cell mentioned in Table 7 has not been licensed for use in the United States because of the presumed slight possibility of the cell serving in successive generations as a vertical carrier of an oncogenic genome. The objectives of all the attenuated vaccines have been to produce no clinical disease (i.e., no local or general reaction), to produce no infection in susceptible contacts, to produce relatively high antibody titers, and at the same time to effect a permanent immunity.

Table 8 indicates the influence of cell culture passage of rubella virus on virulence and immunogenicity as demonstrated by the studies of Hilleman, Buynak, Weibel, and Stokes.[37] It will be noted that A level, of early passage, permitted typical clinical rubella in the contact controls whereas further-passage virus, while permitting excretion of attenuated virus in the throat, did not infect the susceptible contact controls.

Table 9 illustrates an additional vaccination study with the HPV strain rubella virus in duck embryo cell culture among children in families. It can be seen that rubella virus, although excreted in the throat, caused no contact infections. A second study with B-level Merck strain rubella virus in duck embryo cell culture was conducted among children in an institution. Eight months after vaccination natural rubella occurred in the single large ward

TABLE 8.  *Influence of Cell Culture Passage of Rubella Virus on Virulence and Immunogenicity*\*

| VIRUS STRAIN | Level | ATTENUATION Passages grivet kidney | duck embryo | CLINICAL RESULT Rubella Illness (%) | Pharyngeal Virus Recovery (%) | HI-ANTIBODY RESPONSE Vaccinated conversion rate (%) | geometric mean | Contact Controls conversion rate (%) | DATES OF TESTS |
|---|---|---|---|---|---|---|---|---|---|
| Merck† | A | 11 | 10 | 86 | 100 | 100 | 156 | 86 | 1/25/65 |
|  | B | 19 | 20 | 0 | 67‡ | 100 | 323 | 0 | 1/14/66 |
|  | C | 11 | 20 | 0 | 25‡ | 92 | 39 | 0 | 6/30/66 |
|  |  |  |  |  |  |  |  |  | 6/13/67 |
|  | D | 11 | 25 | 0 | 41 | 83 | 14 | 0 | 6/13/67 |
|  | E | 11 | 30 | 0 | 0 | 65 | 9 | 0 | 3/17/67 |
|  |  |  |  |  |  |  |  |  | 5/11/67 |
| HPV-77 | — |  | 77 | 5 | 0 | 100 | 100 | 64 | 0 | 6/13/67 |

\* From Hilleman et al. 1968. New Eng. J. Med. *279*:300–303.
† Also passed one time in embryonated eggs.
‡ Possibly low owing to insensitivity of cultures used to detect virus.

TABLE 9.  *Hemagglutination-Inhibiting (HI) Antibody Titers of Sera Taken From Vaccinees and Contacts in Families Two Months After Vaccination (Study 153)\**

| GROUP | SEROLOGIC STATUS FOR RUBELLA PRIOR TO VACCINATION | | HI ANTIBODY TITER VS. RUBELLA AFTER VACCINATION AMONG THOSE WHO WERE SERONEGATIVE PRIOR TO VACCINATION | | | | | | | | *Sero-con-version Rate* | *Recip-rocal of Geo-metric mean HI titer* |
|---|---|---|---|---|---|---|---|---|---|---|---|---|
| | *Positive* | *Negative* | *No. of Subjects With Titer Of* | | | | | | | | | |
| | | | <8 | 8 | 16 | 32 | 64 | 128 | 256 | 512 | | |
| Rubella vaccinated | 4 | 265 | 9 | 8 | 17 | 51 | 99 | 71 | 9 | 1 | 97% | 53.2 |
| Unvaccinated sibling† contacts (controls) | 4 | 262 | 262 | — | — | — | — | — | — | — | 0 | <8 |
| Unvaccinated maternal contacts (controls) | 222 | 34 | 34 | — | — | — | — | — | — | — | 0 | <8 |

\* From Weibel et al. 1968. J. A. M. A. *205:*554–558.
† These children received trivalent parainfluenza virus vaccine.

under study in this institution. Twenty-six susceptible control children had typical rubella and rubella virus was isolated in the nasopharyngeal secretions. Final serologic tests of the entire ward following the epidemic and thus including both clinically apparent and inapparent cases, demonstrated that 36 of the 41 controls, or 88 per cent, were infected, while none of the 17 vaccinated children had either apparent or inapparent infection—an efficacy of 100 per cent. Serologic tests fully confirmed these findings.

Meyer and Parkman and their colleagues[55] conducted similar tests in children with their HPV-77 virus grown in cell cultures of grivet monkey kidney with quite similar results to those already described. In a challenge study of the vaccinated group, 10 children were exposed to an intranasal spray of virulent rubella virus of human origin—five had been vaccinated and five were susceptible controls. All of the controls but none of the vaccinated children suffered typical rubella.

Peetermans and Huygelen[64] in Belgium have used the rabbit kidney cell, fifty-first passage, mentioned in Table 1 (Cendehill strain) with similar antibody responses and apparent lack of contact infection, although antibodies in the contact controls were not obtained at two months. There was no report on the excretion of virus. The objectives of the present groups working on attenuated rubella vaccines have been to control the next extensive rubella outbreak, which is expected within two to three years. The outbreak in 1964 was responsible for congenital defects in about 20,000 infants in the United States[10] and for probably about the same number of fetal deaths. Whether the curve of antibody response and the parallelism of antibodies to those in natural rubella will be similar to those curves seen in measles and mumps cannot be determined until considerable time has elapsed.

That antibody titers will demonstrate the parallelism between natural infection and infection with attenuated virus vaccine, as previously shown in measles and mumps, has been clearly suggested by the studies in Philadelphia and by the antibody levels reported by Meyer, Parkman, et al.[54a] The latter workers followed for three years the antibody titers of 30 children vaccinated with HPV-77 (grivet monkey kidney tissue culture) and the somewhat higher titers from 16 children with natural rubella. Both groups showed little decline in antibody levels over this three year period.

A field trial of three rubella virus vaccines was conducted in Taiwan in 1957 to 1958 by Grayston, Detels, et al.[27a] in the face of an extensive outbreak of rubella. The three vaccines were from the grivet monkey kidney tissue culture (HPV-77 and three additional passages in the same medium), the duck embryo tissue culture (HPV-77 and five duck), and the dog kidney tissue culture (HPV-77 and 12 dog), and inactivated polio virus vaccine (Salk) was used as a placebo control. Boys (3259) in grades one through four in two schools each in Taipei and Taichung received vaccine, while 2735 boys in the same grades received the placebo—all by a suitably randomized method of selection. Within two to three weeks from the date of vaccination a sharp drop in incidence of rubella occurred in the boys who received the live virus vaccine. Beginning three weeks after vaccination comparison with the rates among the placebo controls demonstrated an efficacy of 93 to 94 per cent for all three vaccines, in view of overall attack rates in the controls and uninoculated of 50 per cent in Taipei and 20 per cent in Taichung. While three boys receiving the dog kidney vaccine demonstrated rather shock-like reactions shortly after the injections, outward reactions were not noted from the other two vaccines. Sensitivity to dog kidney could not be demonstrated in any of the three reactors and the cause of the reactions remained obscure.

The solid protection found at eight months after vaccination as mentioned before offers some suggestion that the elevation of antibody and protection will remain.

The continued successful reports of the duck embryo tissue culture vaccine by Hilleman et al., by McCollum et al., and by a number of other workers, together with the reports of extensive studies of the rabbit kidney tissue culture rubella vaccine (Cendehill strain) by Prinzie et al., and by a number of other workers, at the International Conference on Rubella Immunization at Bethesda, Maryland, February 18–20, 1969, have afforded considerable optimism that effective vaccines shortly will be available for worldwide use. If reactions can be eliminated, the dog kidney tissue culture vaccine may also become available.

In view of the fairly constant (three per cent) rate of anomalies in newborns among the general population and the present lack of knowledge concerning the possible transplacental transmission of the attenuated virus from rubella vaccines, it appears essential to limit such rubella virus vaccines almost entirely to children below the age when pregnancy may occur. Because children vaccinated with the attenuated virus do not infect susceptible contacts, the reservoir of natural rubella virus among school children in all probability could be eliminated by such childhood vaccination. By this means, pregnant females no longer would be exposed to the natural disease. On occasion, high-risk adult women should be permitted rubella live virus vaccine with adequate warning concerning pregnancy. In view of the present capability of determining high-titer rubella human serum or gamma globulin, it would be well to have available a biological for passive protection of an exposed and pregnant susceptible until widespread protection of the population by vaccination has been achieved.

# VARICELLA

Varicella, or chickenpox, for many years was the subject of controversy concerning its possible relation to zoster. Much epidemiological evidence linked the two clinical conditions with a single viral etiology. In such a linkage varicella is considered the primary clinical attack of the virus and zoster is a clinical syndrome representing the reactivation of a latent varicella virus that has survived over a varying number of years since the primary clinical attack of varicella. Not infrequently in the primary clinical attack the acute vesicular eruption extends with considerable pain along the area supplied by a posterior nerve root, suggesting a favored site of inflammatory activity of the virus. Reactivation of a susceptible site or of a possible latent varicella virus may be caused by exposure of an adult to an acute case or an epidemic of chickenpox despite an earlier varicella infection in childhood with resultant general resistance. The gradual senescent decrease in general resistance is a well recognized phenomenon in infectious diseases. Many other posterior nerve root irritants—cold, injury, leukemia, tumor, and so forth—or such drugs as steroids that reduce resistance may initiate reactivation of the varicella-zoster virus.

This strong epidemiological evidence, which had accumulated for a long time, was fully confirmed by the studies of Weller, Witton, and Bell,[100] who first grew the varicella virus in tissue cultures. In such cultures the virus is unusual in that passages cannot be accomplished unless a sufficient number of infected cells are transferred. The virus extends by contact with contiguous cells and not readily by means of the surrounding fluid media. The serological studies of Weller and his colleagues fully confirmed the epidemiological evidence that varicella and zoster represent two clinical aspects of a single disease process.

Much work is proceeding at present toward the development of an attenuated varicella-zoster virus in tissue culture that may provide, as mentioned in the discussions of measles, mumps, and rubella, a natural image of developing immunity in the absence of severe clinical symptoms of the natural disease. Convalescent varicella gamma globulin, when given in large amounts prior to the acute attack, has been shown to lessen the severity of the disease, as demonstrated by accurate counts of the numbers of vesicles in the injected group as compared to the controls.[68]

Epidemic hepatitis virus requires but brief mention in the category of agents that usually produce permanent immunity and that occur more frequently in the younger age groups. It has not as yet been adapted to either tissue or organ cultures, but, on the other hand, can be relegated to the category of inapparent infections by means of human immune globulin from pooled plasma injected intramuscularly at the proper time and in suitable amounts.[89] Persons changing their habitat from areas of adequate sanitation to areas of relatively poor sanitation can acquire a passive-active immunization if the epidemic hepatitis virus is superimposed on the slowly waning protection of a previous intramuscular injection of human immune globulin, as mentioned previously. In this way immunization of probably a permanent nature has been acquired by large numbers of persons who travel into areas where this virus is endemic. Also, apparently, if the newborn is exposed under primitive environmental conditions to the virus during the slowly descending curve of transplacental antibody protection, a natural mode of immunization is effected. For this natural mode of infection, the passive-active immunization described above provides a mirror image of nature.

Perhaps one of the most encouraging developments in the ecology of man and viruses as related to pediatric immunization, which has been mentioned briefly earlier, has been the favorable results obtained in 1967–1968 by Merck and the University of Pennsylvania group of workers with the combined polyvalent (measles, mumps, and rubella) and bivalent (measles and mumps) attenuated vaccines.[7] Each of these combined vaccines has been administered by means of a single injection. For certain groups of children the vaccines were mixed and frozen prior to the field trial, desiccated from the frozen state, and then reconstituted at the time of vaccination. For other groups of children the original mixture of the vaccines for injection was carried out at the time of vaccination. The serological responses of both groups, together with those of the monovalent vaccine control groups studied simultaneously, are shown in

TABLE 10.  Serological* Responses Among Initially Seronegative Children Given Combined Polyvalent or Monovalent Control Live Virus Vaccines

| STUDY | VACCINE Kind | $TCID_{50}$† Per dose | HOMOLOGOUS ANTIBODY RESPONSE Seroconversion Rate | % | Titer‡ Range | G.M.§ |
|---|---|---|---|---|---|---|
| 159 Trivalent (Field Mix) | | | | | | |
| Moraten measles[37a] | 14,000 | 28/28 | 100 | 10–160 | 51 |
| Jeryl Lynn mumps | 6,000 | 26/28 | 93 | 1–128 | 8 |
| HPV-77 rubella | 700 | 28/28 | 100 | 8–512 | 134 |
| 154 Bivalent (Premix) | | | | | | |
| Moraten measles[37a] | 4,000 | 37/38 | 97 | 5–640 | 69 |
| Jeryl Lynn mumps | 3,000 | 37/38 | 97 | 1–64 | 7 |
| Monovalent (controls) | | | | | | |
| Moraten measles[37a] | 4,000 | 7/7 | 100 | 20–160 | 54 |
| Jeryl Lynn mumps | 9,000 | 29/29 | 100 | 2–128 | 7 |
| 92 Bivalent (Premix) | | | | | | |
| Enders' measles | 1,600 | 13/13 | 100 | 20–640 | 61 |
| Jeryl Lynn mumps | 1,600 | 10/13 | 77 | 1–32 | 5 |
| Monovalent (controls) | | | | | | |
| Enders' measles | 10,000 | 29/29 | 100 | 20–160 | 63 |
| Jeryl Lynn mumps | 9,000 | 22/22 | 100 | 1–16 | 6 |

  * Recipients of trivalent vaccine were initially seronegative to all three viruses and those receiving bivalent vaccine were seronegative to the two viruses.
  † Fifty per cent tissue culture infectivity doses of virus.
  ‡ Measles = HI titer; mumps = neutralizing; rubella = HI.
  § G.M. = geometric mean.

Table 10. The excellent antibody responses to these vaccines suggest that inter-ference among the viruses is not a problem, although the elevation of antibodies to the attenuated mumps virus apparently is slightly delayed beyond that usually experienced with monovalent mumps vaccine. For the combined vac-cine the height of antibodies to each virus is similar to that resulting from its monovalent counterpart. In the absence of reactions to both the monovalent mumps and the rubella vaccines, the only reactions to the polyvalent vaccines accorded with the expected amount of reaction to the measles component of the combined attenuated viruses, and there was no evidence of a potentiation of such reactions to the measles virus as a result of the presence of the other components.

It is to be hoped that the stimulating newer developments in the area of nonspecific or general resistance of body cells, such as may well be accomplished by endogenous production of interferon,* and the genetic engineering en-visioned in the studies of Kornberg and his associates[48] may extend and greatly modify the image of nature man is slowly fashioning with the building blocks furnished by nature.

# References

1. Bahmanyar, M. 1966. Success and failure of sero-vaccination as prophylactic treatment of individuals exposed to rabies. International Symposium on Rabies, Tailloires 1965. Symposia Series in Immunobiological Standardization. Vol. 1. Karger, New York, pp. 307–312.
2. Barundun, S., P. Kistler, F. Jeunet, and H. Isliker. 1962. Intravenous administration of human γ-globulin. Vox Sang. 7:157–174.
3. Blake, F. G., and J. D. Trask, Jr. 1921. Studies on measles. I. Susceptibility of monkeys to the virus of measles. II. Symptomatology and pathology in monkeys experimentally infected. J. Exp. Med. 33:385–422.
3a. Blumberg, B. S., A. I. Sutnick, and W. T. London. 1968. Hepatitis and leukemia: their relation to Australia antigen. Bull. N.Y. Acad. Med. 2nd series 44:1566–1586.
4. Brody, J. A., J. L. Sever, and G. M. Schiff. 1965. Prevention of rubella by gamma globulin during an epidemic in Barrow, Alaska, in 1964. New Eng. J. Med. 272:127–129.
5. Buynak, E. B., and M. R. Hilleman. 1966. Live attenuated mumps virus vaccine. I. Vaccine development. Proc. Soc. Exp. Biol. Med. 123:768–775.
6. Buynak, E. B., M. R. Hilleman, R. E. Weibel, and J. Stokes, Jr. 1968. Live attenuated rubella virus vaccines prepared in duck embryo cell culture. I. Development and clinical testing. J.A.M.A. 204:195–200.
7. Buynak, E. B., R. E. Weibel, J. E. Whitman, Jr., J. Stokes, Jr., and M. R. Hilleman. 1969. Combined live measles, mumps and rubella virus vaccines. J.A.M.A. 207:2259–2262.
7a. Byers, R. K., and E. Meyer. 1952. Measles encephalitis: a follow-up study of 16 patients. Amer. J. Dis. Child. 84:543–579.
7b. Chen, T. T., I. Watanabe, W. Zeman, and J. Mealey, Jr. 1969. Subacute sclerosing panencephalitis: Propagation of measles virus from brain biopsy in tissue culture. Science 63:1193–1194.
8. Chiang Huang, C., P. Mein Chen, J. Kui Kuo, W. Hsung Chiu, S. Tien Lin, H. Shing Lin, and Y. Ching Lin. 1962. Experimental whooping cough. New Eng. J. Med. 266:105–111.
9. Cohn, E. J., J. L. Oncley, L. E. Strong, W. L. Hughes, Jr., and S. H. Armstrong, Jr. 1944. Chemical, clinical and immunological studies on the products of human plasma frac-tionation. I. The characterization of the protein fractions of human plasma. J. Clin. Invest. 23:417–431.
10. Cooper, L. Z. 1966. German measles. Sci. Amer. 215:30–37.

* See Chapter 26, Interferon Induction and Utilization, by M. R. Hilleman.

11. Deinhardt, F. 1967. Discussion. First International Conference on Vaccines against Viral and Rickettsial Diseases of Man. Pan American Health Organization, Washington, D.C. Publication No. 147.

12. Drake, M. E., J. A. Barondess, W. J. Bashe, G. Henle, W. Henle, J. Stokes, Jr., and R. B. Pennell. 1953. Failure of convalescent gamma globulin to protect against homologous serum hepatitis. J.A.M.A. *152:*690–693.

13. Enders, J. F., L. W. Kane, S. Cohen, and J. H. Levens. 1945. Immunity in mumps. I. Experiments with monkeys (Macacus mulatta). The development of complement-fixing antibody following infection and experiments on immunization by means of inactivated virus and convalescent human serum. J. Exp. Med. *81:*93–117.

14. Enders, J. F., L. W. Kane, E. P. Maris, and J. Stokes, Jr. 1946. Immunity in mumps: correlation of presence of dermal hypersensitivity and resistance to mumps. J. Exp. Med. *84:*341–364.

15. Enders, J. F., S. L. Katz, M. V. Milovanovic, and A. Holloway. 1960. Studies on effects of attenuated measles-virus vaccine. I. Development and preparation of the vaccine: Techniques for assay of vaccination. New Eng. J. Med. *263:*153–184.

16. Enders, J. F., J. H. Levens, J. Stokes, Jr., E. P. Maris, and W. Berenberg. 1946. Attenuation of virulence with retention of antigenicity of mumps virus after passage in the embryonated egg. J. Immun. *54:*283–291.

17. Enders, J. F., and T. C. Peebles. 1954. Propagation in tissue cultures of cytopathogenic agents from patients with measles. Proc. Soc. Exp. Biol. Med. *86:*277–286.

18. Enders, J. F., T. H. Weller, and F. C. Robbins. 1949. Cultivation of the Lansing strain of poliomyelitis virus in cultures of various human embryonic tissues. Science *109:*85–87.

19. Fenner, F., and F. N. Ratcliff. 1965. Myxomatosis. Cambridge University Press, London.

20. Fisher, M. W., and M. C. Manning. 1958. Studies on the immunotherapy of bacterial infections. I. The comparative effectiveness of human gamma globulin against various bacterial species in mice. J. Immun. *81:*291.

21. Fleming, A. 1946. Penicillin. Its Practical Application. Blakiston, Philadelphia.

22. Francis, T. 1956. Approaches to the prevention of poliomyelitis. Seventh Annual Don W. Gudakunst Memorial Lecture. Univ. Michigan Med. Bull. *22:*433–445.

23. Gard, S. 1967. Inactivated poliomyelitis vaccine—present and future. First International Conference on Vaccines against Viral and Rickettsial Diseases of Man. Pan American Health Organization, Washington, D.C. Publication No. 147.

24. Gellis, S. S., A. C. McGuinness, and M. Peters. 1945. Study of prevention of mumps orchitis by gamma globulin. Amer. J. Med. Sci. *210:*661–664.

25. Gellis, S. S., J. R. Neefe, J. Stokes, Jr., L. E. Strong, C. A. Janeway, and G. Scatchard. 1948. Chemical, clinical and immunological studies on the products of human plasma fractionation. XXXVI. Inactivation of the virus of homologous serum hepatitis in solutions of normal human serum albumin by means of heat. J. Clin. Invest. *27:*239–244.

26. Gibbs, F. A., E. L. Gibbs, and I. M. Rosenthal. 1961. Electroencephalographic study of children immunized against measles with live attenuated virus vaccine. New Eng. J. Med. *264:*800–801.

27. Goldberger, J., and J. F. Anderson. 1911. An experimental demonstration of the presence of the virus of measles with mixed buccal and nasal secretions. J.A.M.A. *57:*476–478.

27a. Grayston, J. T., R. Detels, K. P. Chen, L. Gutman, K. S. W. Kim, J. L. Gale, and R. P. Beasley. 1969. Field trial of live attenuated rubella virus vaccine during an epidemic on Taiwan. J.A.M.A. *207:*1107–1110.

28. Gregg, N. M. 1941. Congenital cataract following German measles in the mother. Trans. Ophthal. Soc. Aust. *3:*35–46.

29. Groman, N. B. 1953. Evidence for the induced nature of the change from nontoxigenicity to toxigenicity as a result of exposure to specific bacteriophage. J. Bact. *66:*184–191.

30. Grossman, E. B., S. G. Stewart, and J. Stokes, Jr. 1945. Post transfusion hepatitis in battle casualties and study of its prophylaxis by means of human immune serum globulin. J.A.M.A. *129:*991–994.

31. Habel, K. 1951. Vaccination of human beings against mumps: Vaccine administered at the start of an epidemic. I. Incidence and severity of mumps in vaccinated and control groups. Amer. J. Hyg. *54:*295–311.

32. Habel, K. 1951. Vaccination of human beings against mumps: Vaccine administered at the start of an epidemic. II. Effect of vaccination upon the epidemic. Amer. J. Hyg. *54:*312–318.

33. Habel, K. 1945. Cultivation of mumps virus in the developing chick embryo and its application to studies of immunity to mumps in man. Public Health Rep. *60:*201–212.

34. Hammon, W. M., L. L. Coriell, P. F. Wehrle, and J. Stokes, Jr. 1953. Evaluation of Red Cross gamma globulin as a prophylactic agent for poliomyelitis. 4. Final report of results based on clinical diagnoses. J.A.M.A. *151:*1272–1285.

35. Henle, G., J. Stokes, Jr., J. S. Burgoon, W. J. Bashe, C. F. Burgoon, and W. Henle. 1951. Studies on the prevention of mumps. IV. The effect of oral spraying of attenuated active virus. J. Immun. *66:*579–594.

36. Henle, W. 1960. Problems in the prevention of mumps. Quart. Rev. Pediat. *15:*90–93.

37. Hilleman, M. R., E. B. Buynak, R. E. Weibel, and J. Stokes, Jr. 1968. Live attenuated rubella virus vaccine. New Eng. J. Med. *279:*300–303.

37a. Hilleman, M. R., E. B. Buynak, R. E. Weibel, J. Stokes, Jr., J. E. Whitman, Jr., and M. B. Leagus. 1968. Development and evaluation of the Moraten measles virus vaccine. J.A.M.A. *206:*587–590.

38. Hilleman, M. R., R. E. Weibel, E. B. Buynak, J. Stokes, Jr., and J. E. Whitman, Jr. 1967. Live attenuated mumps-virus vaccine. 4. Protective efficacy as measured in a field evaluation. New Eng. J. Med. *276:*252–258.

39. Iwanowski, D. 1892. Uber die Mosaikrankheit der Tabakspflanze. Bull. Acad. Imp. Sci. St. Petersbourg (n.s.) *3:*67–70.

40. Janeway, C. A., and F. S. Rosen. 1966. The gamma globulins. IV. Therapeutic uses of gamma globulins. New Eng. J. Med. *275:*826–831.

41. Jenner, E. 1798. An inquiry into the causes and effects of the variolae vaccinae, a disease discovered in some western counties of England, particularly in Gloucestershire, and known by the name of cowpox. Reprinted by Cassell and Company, Ltd., available in pamphlet vol. 4232, Army Medical Library, Washington, D.C., 1896.

42. Katz, S. L., C. H. Kempe, F. L. Black, M. L. Lepow, S. Krugman, R. J. Haggerty, and J. F. Enders. 1960. Studies on an attenuated measles-virus vaccine. VII. General summary and evaluation of the results of vaccination. New Eng. J. Med. *263:*180–184.

43. Kempe, C. H., T. O. Berge, and B. England. 1956. Hyperimmune vaccinal gamma globulin. Source, evaluation and use in prophylaxis and therapy. Pediatrics *18:*177–188.

44. Kempe, C. H., C. Bowles, G. Meiklejohn, T. O. Berge, L. St. Vincent, B. V. Sundura Babu, S. Govindarajan, N. R. Ratnakannan, A. W. Downie, and V. R. Murphy. 1961. The use of vaccinia hyperimmune gamma globulin in the prophylaxis of smallpox. Bull. WHO *25:*41–48.

45. Kissling, R. E., R. Q. Robinson, F. A. Murphy, and S. G. Whitfield. 1968. Agent of disease contracted from green monkeys. Science *160:*888–890.

46. Koprowski, H., G. A. Jervis, and T. W. Norton. 1952. Immune responses in human volunteers upon oral administration of a rodent-adapted strain of poliomyelitis virus. Amer. J. Hyg. *55:*108–126.

47. Koprowski, H., J. van der Scheer, and J. Black. 1950. Use of hyperimmune antirabies serum concentrates in experimental rabies. Amer. J. Med. *8:*412–420.

48. Kornberg, A. 1968. The synthesis of DNA. Sci. Amer. *219:*64–68.

49. Krugman, S., and R. Ward. 1961–1962. Infectious hepatitis: current status of prevention with gamma globulin. Yale J. Biol. Med. *34:*329–339.

50. McGuinness, A. C., J. G. Armstrong, and H. M. Felton. 1944. Hyperimmune whooping cough serum. J. Pediat. *24:*249–258.

51. McKhann, C. F. 1937. The prevention and modification of measles. J.A.M.A. *109:*2034–2038.

52. McKhann, C. F., and F. T. Chu. 1933. Antibodies in placental extracts. J. Infect. Dis. *52:*268–277.

53. Mellman, W. J., and R. Wetton. 1963. Depression of the tuberculin reaction by attenuated measles virus vaccine. J. Lab. Clin. Med. *61:*453–458.

53a. Millman, I., V. Zavatone, B. J. Gerstley, and B. S. Blumberg. 1969. Australia antigen detected in the nuclei of liver cells of patients with viral hepatitis by the fluorescent antibody technique. Nature *222:*181–184.

54. Meyer, H. M., Jr., D. D. Hoestler, Jr., B. C. Bernheim, N. G. Rogers, P. Lambin, A. Chassary, R. Labusquiere, and J. E. Smadel. 1964. Response of Volta children to jet inoculation of combined live measles, smallpox and yellow fever vaccines. Bull. WHO *30:*783–794.

54a. Meyer, H. M., Jr., P. D. Parkman, T. E. Hobbins, H. E. Larson, W. J. Davis, J. P. Simsarian, and H. E. Hopps. 1969. Attenuated rubella viruses: Laboratory and clinical characteristics. Abstract. International Conference on Rubella Immunization. Bethesda, Maryland. p. 64.

55. Meyer, H. M., Jr., P. D. Parkman, and T. C. Panos. 1966. Attenuated rubella virus. II. Production of experimental live virus vaccine and clinical trial. New Eng. J. Med. *275:*575–580.

56. Morris, D., and J. C. McDonald. 1957. Failure of hyperimmune gamma globulin to prevent whooping cough. Arch. Dis. Child. *32:*236–239.

57. Nicolle, C., and E. Conseil. 1911. Reproduction expérimental de la rougeole chez le Bonnet

Chinois. Virulence du sang des malades 24 heures avant le début de l'éruption. C. R. Acad. Sci. (Paris) *153*:1522–1524.

58. Norrby, E. 1966. Present status of killed measles vaccines. First International Conference on Vaccines against Viral and Rickettsial Diseases of Man. Pan American Health Organization, Washington, D.C. Publication No. 147.

59. Ordman, C. W., C. G. Jennings, Jr., and C. A. Janeway. 1944. Use of concentrated normal human serum gamma globulin (human immune serum globulin) in the prevention and attenuation of measles. J. Clin. Invest. *23*:541–549.

60. Painter, R. H., J. C. W. Weber, and A. C. Wardlow. 1968. Antitoxic and antiviral antibodies in Cohn fractions of human plasma. Clin. Exp. Immun. *3*:179–187.

61. Parkman, P. D., E. L. Buescher, and M. S. Artenstein. 1962. Recovery of rubella virus from Army recruits. Proc. Soc. Exp. Biol. Med. *111*:225–230.

62. Pasteur, L. 1885. Méthode pour prévenir la rage après morsure. C. R. Acad. Sci. (Paris) *101*:765–772.

63. Pasteur, L. 1880. Sur les maladies virulentes, et en particulier sur la maladie appelée vulgairement choléra des poules. C. R. Acad. Sci. (Paris) *90*:239–248.

64. Peetermans, J., and C. Huygelen. 1967. Attenuation of rubella virus by serial passage in primary rabbit kidney cell cultures. I. Growth characteristics in vitro and production of experimental vaccines at different passage levels. Arch Ges. Virusforsch. *21*:133–143.

65. Plotz, H. 1938. Culture "in vitro" du virus de la rougeole. Bull. Acad. Méd. Paris *119*:598.

66. Proceedings of the Second Symposium on Gnotobiotic Technology. University of Notre Dame, Notre Dame, Indiana. May 8 and 9, 1959. Cosponsored by National Institutes of Health, Office of Naval Research, and Institute for Laboratory Animal Resources.

67. Rauh, L. W., and R. Schmidt. 1965. Measles immunization with killed virus vaccine: serum antibody titers and experience with exposure to measles epidemic. Amer. J. Dis. Child. *109*:232–237.

68. Ross, A. H. 1962. Modification of chickenpox in family contacts by administration of gamma globulin. New Eng. J. Med. *267*:369–376.

69. Sabin, A. 1956. Pathogenesis of poliomyelitis (reappraisal in light of new data). Science *123*:1151–1157.

70. Schofield, F. D., V. M. Tucker, and G. R. Westbrook. 1961. Neonatal tetanus in New Guinea: effect of active immunization in pregnancy. Brit. Med. J. *2*:785–789.

71. Schultze, H. E., and G. Schwick. 1962. Uber neue Möglichkeiten intravenoser Gamma-globulin Applikation. Deutsch. Med. Wschr. *87*:1643–1650.

72. Schwarz, A. J. F., P. A. Boyer, L. W. Zirbel, and C. J. York. 1960. Experimental vaccination against measles. I. Tests of live measles and distemper vaccine in monkeys and two human volunteers under laboratory conditions. J.A.M.A. *173*:861–867.

73. Scrimshaw, N. S., C. E. Taylor, and J. E. Gordon. 1959. Interactions of nutrition and infection. Amer. J. Med. Sci. *237*:367–403.

74. Sgouris, J. T. 1966. Stability of immunoglobulin G preparations. Fed. Proc. *25*:726.

75. Shaffer, M. F., G. Rake, J. Stokes, Jr., and G. C. O'Neil. 1941. Studies on measles. II. Experimental disease in man and monkey. J. Immun. *41*:241–257.

76. Sheldon, W. H., and H. Bauer. 1962. The role of predisposing factors in experimental fungus infections. Lab. Invest. *11*:1184–1191.

77. Shinefield, H. R., J. C. Ribble, H. F. Eichenwald, M. Boris, and J. M. Sutherland. 1963. Bacterial interference: its effect on nursery acquired infection with Staphylococcus aureus. V. An analysis and interpretation. Amer. J. Dis. Child. *105*:683–688.

78. Siegert, R., H-L. Shur, W. Slenczka, D. Peters, and G. Muller. 1967. Zur Ätiologie einer unbekannten von Affen ausgegangenen menschlichen Infectionskrankheit. Deutsch. Med. Wschr. *92*:2341–2343.

79. Smolens, J., and J. Stokes, Jr. 1956. The safety and feasibility of biweekly plasmapheresis on the same human donors and its effect on antibody levels. Tenth Conference on the Plasma Proteins and Cellular Elements of the Blood. Cambridge, Mass., pp. 63–70.

80. Smolens, J., J Stokes, Jr., E. McGee, and V. Hunter. 1956. Feasibility and safety of frequent plasmapheresis of the same human donors. Proc. Soc. Exp. Biol. Med. *91*:611–614.

81. Smolens, J., A. B. Vogt, M. N. Crawford, and J. Stokes, Jr. 1961. The persistence in the human circulation of horse and human tetanus antitoxins. J. Pediat. *59*:899–902.

82. Smorodintsev, A. A., and N. S. Klyachko. 1958. Live anti-mumps vaccine. Acta Virol. (Praha) *2*:137–144.

83. Smorodintsev, A. A., N. S. Klyachko, M. N. Nasibov, and E. S. Shickina. 1967. Experience with live mumps vaccine in the USSR. First International Conference on Vaccines against Viral and Rickettsial Diseases of Man. Pan American Health Organization, Washington, D.C. Publication No. *147*:422–429.

84. Stokes, J., Jr. 1956. Passive-active immunization in certain viral diseases that produce

permanent immunity. Third Kenneth D. Blackfan Memorial Lecture, Children's Hospital Medical Center. New Eng. J. Med. *255*:943–949.

85. Stokes, J., Jr., M. Blanchard, J. R. Neefe, S. S. Gellis, and G. Wade. 1948. Methods of protection against homologous serum hepatitis: Studies on protective value of gamma globulin in homologous serum hepatitis SH virus. J.A.M.A. *138*:336–341.

86. Stokes, J., Jr., J. F. Enders, E. P. Maris, and L. W. Kane. 1946. Immunity in mumps. VI. Experiments on vaccination of human beings with formolized mumps virus. J. Exp. Med. *84*:407–428.

87. Stokes, J., Jr., J. D. Farquhar, M. E. Drake, R. B. Capps, C. S. Ward, Jr., O. Mills, and A. W. Kitts. 1951. Infectious hepatitis. Length of protection by immune serum globulin (gamma globulin) during epidemics. J.A.M.A. *147*:714–719.

88. Stokes, J., Jr., E. P. Maris, and S. S. Gellis. 1944. Use of concentrated normal human serum gamma globulin (human immune serum globulin) in the prophylaxis and treatment of measles. J. Clin. Invest. *23*:531–540.

89. Stokes, J., Jr., and J. R. Neefe. 1945. The prevention and attenuation of infectious hepatitis by gamma globulin. Preliminary note. J.A.M.A. *127*:144–145.

90. Stokes, J., Jr., G. C. O'Neil, M. F. Shaffer, G. Rake, and E. P. Maris. 1943. Studies on measles: Results following inoculation of children with egg passage measles virus. J. Pediat. *22*:1–16.

91. Stokes, J., Jr., and J. Smolens. 1957. Repeated plasmapheresis in the same person—a rationale for modern blood-letting. Proc. Amer. Phil. Soc. *101*:330–335.

92. Stokes, J., Jr., and I. J. Wolman. 1940. Probable synergism of human influenza virus and Staphylococcus aureus in rapidly fatal respiratory infection. Int. Clin. *1*:115–123.

93. Sweet, B. H., and M. R. Hilleman. 1960. The vacuolating virus, S.V. 40. Proc. Soc. Exp. Biol. Med. *105*:420–427.

94. Theiler, M. 1951. The virus. *In* Strode G. K. (ed.): Yellow Fever. McGraw-Hill Book Co., New York, pp. 39–136.

95. Theiler, M., and H. H. Smith. 1937. The use of yellow fever virus modified by in vitro cultivation for human immunization. J. Exp. Med. *65*:787–800.

96. Torack, R. M. 1957. Fungus infections associated with antibiotic and steroid therapy. Amer. J. Med. *22*:872–881.

96a. Weibel, R. E., E. B. Buynak, J. Stokes, Jr., J. E. Whitman, Jr., and M. R. Hilleman. 1967. Evaluation of live attenuated mumps virus vaccine, strain Jeryl Lynn. First International Conference on Vaccines against Viral and Rickettsial Diseases of Man. Pan American Health Organization, Washington, D.C. Publication No. *147*:430–437.

97. Weibel, R. E., E. B. Buynak, J. E. Whitman, Jr., M. B. Leagus, J. Stokes, Jr., and M. R. Hilleman. 1969. Durable immunity for three years following Jeryl Lynn strain live mumps virus vaccine. J.A.M.A. *207*:1667–1670.

98. Weibel, R. E., R. Halenda, J. Stokes, Jr., M. R. Hilleman, and E. B. Buynak. 1962. Administration of Enders' live measles virus vaccine with human immune globulin. J.A.M.A. *180*:1086–1094.

98a. Weibel, R. E., J. Stokes, Jr., E. B. Buynak, J. E. Whitman, Jr., and M. R. Hilleman. 1967. Live attenuated mumps virus vaccine. 3. Clinical and serological aspects in field evaluation. New Eng. J. Med. *276*:245–251.

98b. Weibel, R. E., J. Stokes, Jr., E. B. Buynak, J. E. Whitman, Jr., M. B. Leagus, and M. R. Hilleman. 1968. Live attenuated rubella virus vaccines prepared in duck embryo cell culture. II. Clinical tests in families and in an institution. J.A.M.A. *205*:554–558.

99. Weller, T. H., and F. A. Neva. 1962. Propagation in tissue culture of cytopathic agents from patients with rubella-like illness. Proc. Soc. Exp. Biol. Med. *111*:215–225.

100. Weller, T. H., H. M. Witton, and E. J. Bell. 1958. The etiologic agents of varicella and herpes zoster. Isolation, propagation and cultural characteristics in vitro. J. Exp. Med. *108*:843–868.

101. Zabriskie, J. B. 1964. The role of temperate bacteriophage in the production of erythrogenic toxin by Group A streptococci. J. Exp. Med. *119*:761–780.

102. Zinsser, H. 1935. Rats, Lice and History. Little, Brown & Co., Boston.

# Chapter 6

# THE PATHOGENESIS OF FEVER

W. BARRY WOOD, Jr.

*Department of Microbiology, School of Medicine,*
*The Johns Hopkins University, Baltimore, Maryland*

Normal body temperature is maintained by a complex series of "feedback" mechanisms controlling the dissipation and production of body heat. These mechanisms are regulated by the hypothalamus in response to stimuli from two sources: the *superficial thermoreceptors* of the skin, which respond to changes in ambient temperature; and the *deep receptors*, which lie in, or near, the hypothalamus and respond to minute changes in blood temperature.[1-3]

During fever the hypothalamic "thermostat" behaves as though its "set point" had been raised.[4-7] The principal factor in disease that raises the set point appears to be an endogenous pyrogen derived from leukocytes.[8-11]

## INTRAVENOUS INJECTION MODELS

The experimental evidence supporting this concept is based primarily on studies of fever models produced by intravenous injections of bacterial endo-toxins,[12-15] viruses,[16-21] or whole bacteria[22, 23] into normal rabbits, or by the injection of bacterial antigens (e.g., tuberculin) into sensitized rabbits[24-27] (Table 1).* All of these agents act as *exogenous pyrogens;* that is, they are all

TABLE 1.  *Intravenous Injection Fever Models*

---

Normal rabbits:
  Endotoxin[13-15]
  Myxo- or Coxsackie virus[17-21]
  Bacteria[22,23]
Sensitized rabbits:
  Sensitizing antigen[25,26]

---

* Some similar studies have been made in cats,[28] dogs,[29] and guinea pigs.[27]

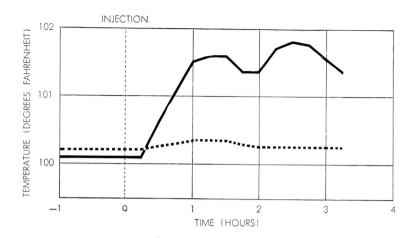

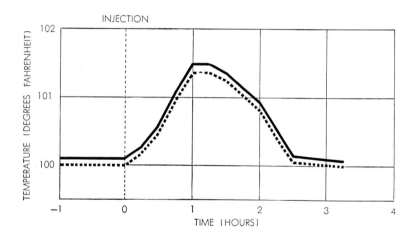

*Figure 1.* Upper curves show comparative responses of normal and tolerant rabbits to bacterial endotoxin. Note that response to endotoxin is suppressed in tolerant animals (dotted line). In contrast, lower curves indicate that fever-producing effect of granulocytic (endogenous) pyrogen is uninfluenced by tolerance. (From Fever, by W. B. Wood, Jr. Copyright 1957 by Scientific American, Inc. All rights reserved.)

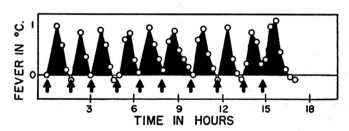

*Figure 2.* Response of a single rabbit to repeated injections of granulocytic pyrogen. (From Petersdorf et al. J. Exp. Med. *106*:787, 1957.)

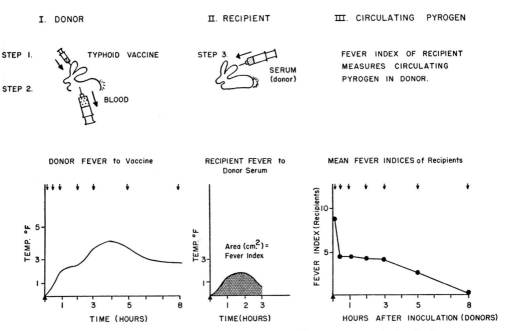

*Figure 3.* Passive transfer method used to detect the presence of circulating pyrogen. Note that fever index (area in square centimeters beneath the fever curve) of the recipient measures the amount of circulating pyrogen present in the serum of the donor at the time of transfer. (From Atkins and Wood. J. Exp. Med. *102:*499, 1955.)

foreign and they all cause fever when injected intravenously. The resulting fevers, however, have been found to correlate quantitatively with the presence in the circulation of very different kinds of pyrogens, termed *endogenous pyrogens.*[13–15] Because their action is indistinguishable from that of a pyrogenic substance that can be extracted from polymorphonuclear leukocytes,[30–32] the endogenous pyrogens are believed to come, at least partially, from granulocytes (see Monocytic Pyrogen) of the injected rabbits.[8–11]

# THE PRIMARY ROLE OF ENDOGENOUS PYROGENS

This relation between exogenous and endogenous pyrogens was first demonstrated in the bacterial endotoxin model.[14, 15] Here it is possible to distinguish between these two kinds of pyrogens by the fact that repeated intravenous injections of bacterial endotoxin (exogenous pyrogen) induce a state of refractoriness, known as *tolerance,* in which the febrile response is markedly suppressed (Fig. 1, upper graph),[33, 34] whereas similar injections of granulocytic (or endogenous) pyrogen continue to cause a full response (Fig. 2).[35] Also, rabbits made tolerant to exogenous pyrogen remain fully responsive to endogenous pyrogen (Fig. 1, lower graph).[31, 34] The amount and kind of pyrogen circulating in the blood of the endotoxin-inoculated rabbit may therefore be measured by a passive transfer method (Fig. 3) in which samples of its serum, drawn at various time intervals after inoculation, are injected into other normal and other tolerant rabbits.[15] The febrile responses of both donors and recipients are conventionally recorded in arbitrary *fever index* (or FI) units (Fig. 3), representing the areas under the fever curves.[36]

By these methods it can be shown that in the bacterial endotoxin model, as indicated in Figure 4, most of the injected endotoxin (labelled injected pyrogen) is cleared from the blood before the endogenous pyrogen can be detected. Furthermore, the concentration of endogenous pyrogen in the serum is roughly proportional to the height of the fever.[15]

That the endogenous pyrogen in the endotoxin model comes, in part, from circulating granulocytes is suggested by the observation that in rabbits made granulocytopenic with nitrogen mustard less fever develops and less endogenous pyrogen is produced than in normal rabbits given the same dose of endo-

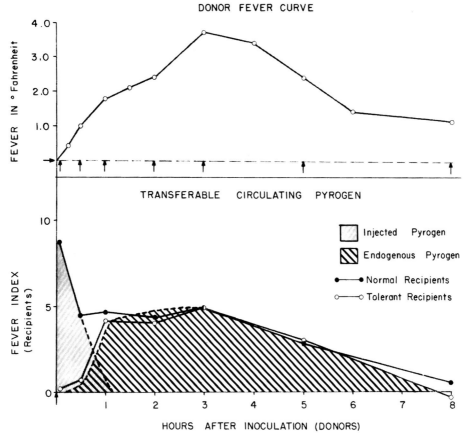

*Figure 4.* Relation of mean fever curve of seven donor rabbits receiving typhoid vaccine (upper chart) to concentrations of circulating endotoxin and endogenous pyrogen respectively, as measured by passive transfer (Fig. 3) to normal and tolerant recipients (lower chart). Fever index refers to area under fever curve (Fig. 3) of recipients and is a measure of both the height and the duration of the fever produced. Whereas endotoxin is rapidly cleared, endogenous pyrogen persists throughout the febrile response, its concentration being approximately proportional to the height of the fever. (From Atkins and Wood. J. Exp. Med. *102*:499,1955.)

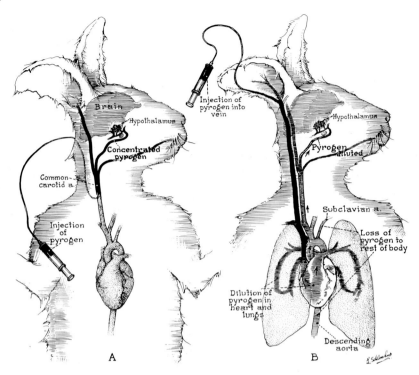

*Figure 5.*   Diagram of experimental method employed to compare sites of action of endotoxin and leukocytic pyrogen. (From King and Wood. J. Exp. Med. *107*:291, 1958.)

toxin.[37,38] The transient granulocytopenia that regularly follows the injection in normal rabbits[12] also suggests that the granulocytes are affected.[39]

Finally, when the endogenous pyrogen is introduced into the carotid artery, leading directly to the hypothalamic centers (Fig. 5), it causes a more prompt and a greater febrile response than when administered intravenously. The endotoxin, on the other hand, elicits the same response when given by either route.[39] These findings are in keeping with the hypothesis that the endogenous pyrogen acts directly on the hypothalamus (see below) and that the endotoxin (or exogenous pyrogen) acts on the circulating leukocytes, which in turn release endogenous pyrogen (see Fig. 6).[15, 34]

The same relationship between the fever and the presence of endogenous pyrogen in the circulation has also been demonstrated in the viral,[17, 20] the bacterial,[22, 23] and the hypersensitivity models.[25]

## GRANULOCYTIC PYROGEN

If the theory is correct that all of the exogenous pyrogens in these intravenous injection models act by causing circulating granulocytes (and possibly other cells*) to release endogenous pyrogen, it should be possible to produce

---

* See Monocytic Pyrogen.

| Injected | | Injury of | | Release of | | Stimulation of | | |
|----------|--|-----------|--|------------|--|----------------|--|--|
| Pyrogen | → | Cells | → | Endogenous | → | Thermoregulatory | → | Fever |
| (Exogenous) | | (Leukocytes) | | Pyrogen | | Centers of Brain | | |

*Figure 6.* Postulated mechanism of endotoxin-induced fever. (From Fever, by W. B. Wood, Jr. Copyright 1957 by Scientific American, Inc. All rights reserved.)

endogenous pyrogen *in vitro* by merely interacting granulocytes and exogenous pyrogen under proper conditions. This too has been accomplished with each of the model systems. For example, when blood granulocytes from rabbits sensitized by intravenous injection of BCG are incubated at 37°C. with tuberculin, a pyrogen indistinguishable from granulocytic pyrogen appears in the supernatant fluid.[40] The same is true when normal granulocytes are incubated with endotoxin,[41, 42] virus,[43] or bacteria.[23] In the bacterial system the cells first phagocytize the organisms and then release pyrogen, suggesting that phagocytosis somehow triggers the release process. When phagocytosis is blocked by a chemical inhibitor, such as sodium fluoride, no pyrogen is generated.[23]

Collectively, the foregoing results leave little doubt that granulocytic pyrogen is a critical "messenger" substance in these injection forms of experimental fever.

## EXPERIMENTAL INFECTION MODELS

It must be admitted, however, that the intravenous injection models are extremely artificial, for each involves a relatively large "bolus" injection of a toxic exogenous pyrogen. Much more meaningful evidence has been obtained from studying experimental bacterial infections of the peritoneal cavity[44] or skin.[45] With these more natural models it has been possible to demonstrate that endogenous pyrogen is formed in the granulocytic exudate of the lesion[44] and is thence transported via the lymphatics[44] to the blood.[45] When the infection is suppressed by penicillin therapy, the endogenous pyrogen disappears from the lesion and lymph, and the fever subsides.[44]

## MONOCYTIC PYROGEN

More recently it has been shown that cells of the rabbit monocyte-macrophage system will also generate endogenous pyrogen that is biologically indistinguishable from rabbit granulocytic pyrogen.[46, 47] Whether it is chemically the same remains to be determined (see below). This finding not only provides a plausible explanation for the fevers observed in diseases in which mononuclear cells dominate the pathological lesions (e.g., agranulocytosis, tuberculosis, and other granulomatous diseases),[48] but it also raises the possibility that the small amounts of pyrogen that have been found in normal rabbit tissues[49] may come from tissue macrophages rather than from parenchymal cells.

## STUDIES IN HUMANS

Although fewer experiments have thus far been performed in man, there is good reason to believe that endogenous pyrogens derived from leukocytes[50-52] play much the same role in analogous human fevers as they do in experimental animal fevers. The recent finding that human endogenous pyrogens can be assayed by intravenous injection into rabbits[53] has greatly facilitated the study of human fevers and has led to the demonstration that human monocytes,[52] as well as granulocytes, are capable of generating endogenous pyrogen. Furthermore, sterile extracts of human granulocytic exudates obtained from patients with febrile illnesses have been shown to cause fever when injected intravenously into the same patients after their original fevers have subsided.[54] Although attempts to demonstrate circulating endogenous pyrogen in the blood of such patients during their original fevers were unsuccessful,[55] it seems possible, from analogous studies in animals,[45] that the amounts of blood transferred (see Fig. 3) were insufficient to detect the circulating pyrogen.

## HORMONAL FEVERS

One form of experimental fever can be produced in man[56-58] but not in rabbits.[59] It results from the intramuscular injection of the naturally occurring hormonal metabolite, etiocholanolone ($3\alpha$-hydroxy-etiocholane-17-one). An acute inflammatory reaction regularly develops at the site of injection.[60] Other closely related end products of androgen metabolism, sharing the $5\beta$ configuration, have the same effect.[61] There is a delay of approximately six hours before the febrile response begins, and it often lasts for more than 12 hours (cf. Fig. 1).[57] None of these steroids consistently produces fever when injected *intravenously*.[57]

*In vitro*, etiocholanolone causes leukocytes from human blood (but not rabbit blood) to release endogenous pyrogen, provided the cells are exposed to its action for about six hours.[62] Since pyrogenic steroids, like etiocholanolone, cause the release of lysosomal enzymes from suspensions of leukocyte granules and liver lysosomes,[63] it seems probable that they act on cell membranes. Their failure to cause fever when injected intravenously may merely be due to their being conjugated and excreted[64] before having enough time to interact with the circulating leukocytes. At the intramuscular sites of injection they presumably remain in contact with inflammatory cells much longer.

Because certain forms of periodic fever in man seem to be associated with abnormalities in steroid metabolism, the suggestion has been made that they are "steroid fevers."[65, 66] Evidence supporting this hypothesis, however, is not conclusive.[62, 64] Likewise, the precise mechanisms involved in other forms of "hormonal fevers" (e.g., ovulation, thyrotoxicosis) have not been fully elucidated.[3, 11]

## MOLECULAR PATHOLOGY

It should be evident from the foregoing discussion that the pathogenesis of most forms of fever will not be understood in molecular terms until each of the following questions can be answered:

1. What metabolic factors control the release of endogenous pyrogen from granulocytes and monocytes?
2. What is the chemical nature of the endogenous pyrogen molecules?
3. How do they act on thermoregulatory neurons in the hypothalamus?

## CELLULAR RELEASE OF PYROGEN

The original method of obtaining endogenous pyrogen from exudate granulocytes involved direct extraction in the cold.[30, 31] Later it was learned that greater yields could be achieved by incubating the cells with exogenous pyrogens at 37°C.,[67] as already described in the *in vitro* models.[23, 41] In the cold (i.e., at 0°C.) no detectable pyrogen is released into the supernatant.[67] These facts suggest: (1) that more than mere leakage of preformed pyrogen through a damaged cellular membrane is involved in the release process; and (2) that either new pyrogen is synthesized in the cells during incubation in the *in vitro* models, or else inactive preformed "propyrogen" is converted to active pyrogen and then released from the cells.

The most efficient way of stimulating pyrogen release from exudate granulocytes is to incubate the cells in isotonic NaCl.[67–69]* The mechanism of this highly unphysiological stimulus is of interest.

If potassium chloride is added to the sodium chloride, the release of pyrogen is inhibited (Fig. 7). At physiological concentrations of potassium (i.e., 5 meq.) the inhibition is approximately 95 per cent. When calcium ions are also added, at physiological concentrations, the inhibition is even greater.[69] These facts indicate how unphysiological the sodium chloride stimulus really is. It is due, not to the sodium ions, but rather to the absence of potassium and calcium ions —particularly the potassium. For, as shown in Figure 7, if ouabain is added to the sodium-potassium system, to suppress the transfer of potassium through the cell membrane,[70] the inhibitory effect of the potassium is blocked.[69] The stimulus, then, depends upon *potassium deprivation,* either in the cell or in its membranes.

Extensive electrolyte studies have revealed that shifts in cellular potassium (or sodium) levels do not account for the potassium deprivation stimulus.[71] An illustration of this is shown in Table 2.

---

* Blood leukocytes are less responsive to this stimulus (i.e., 0.15 M NaCl) than exudate granulocytes,[67] unless previously incubated in four hour peritoneal exudate fluid;[68] and the responsiveness of exudate granulocytes is depressed by preincubation in serum or plasma.[68] Blood leukocytes, on the other hand, produce more pyrogen than exudate granulocytes when incubated with endotoxin.[41, 42]

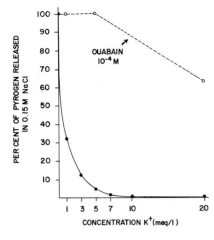

*Figure 7.* Blocking effect of ouabain (o----o) on K⁺-induced inhibition of pyrogen release from rabbit granulocytes (●———●). (From Berlin and Wood. J. Exp. Med. *119*:697, 1964.)

TABLE 2. *Lack of Correlation of Pyrogen Release and Changes in Cellular K⁺ and Na⁺* [*]

| MEDIUM | $K^+$[†] | $Na^+$[†] | $FI_{120}$[‡] |
|---|---|---|---|
| Ionic-inorganic: sodium chloride (0.15 M) | −4.4 | +12.8 | 16.4 |
| Ionic-organic: choline chloride (0.15 M) | −6.0 | −19.0 | 10.0 |
| Nonionic: inulin (0.3 M) | −8.4 | −19.0 | 2.5 |
| Ionic "pump" inhibitor: sodium chloride (0.1 M) + Veronal (0.05 M, pH 6.5) | −5.6 | +14.4 | 1.1 |

[*] From Hahn et al.[71]
[†] μeq. per 3.5 × 10⁸ cells.
[‡] $FI_{120}$ = fever index of febrile response followed for 120 minutes. Response was produced by supernatant from 3.5 × 10⁷ exudate granulocytes, incubated for two hours at 37°C.

Here exudate granulocytes have been incubated for two hours in four different media. It will be noted that in all four the intracellular potassium level fell, whereas the sodium level rose in the first and the fourth medium, and fell in the second and the third. In only the first two (the sodium chloride and choline chloride) were significant amounts of pyrogen released. In these ionic media the ionic pump of the cells may be assumed to have been active, since choline ions seem to be handled in the same manner as sodium ions in the cationic transport system of the cell membrane.[72] In the nonionic inulin medium, on the other hand, in which there were no extracellular ions to pump, and in the sodium chloride-Veronal medium, in which the electrolyte transport system is believed to be impeded by the Veronal,[73] little if any pyrogen was released, despite the fall in cellular potassium. Furthermore, other enzyme inhibitors that block glycolysis also inhibit pyrogen release in the potassium deprivation system (Tables 3 and 4),[74, 75] whereas exposure of the cells to cyanide or to anaerobiosis has no such suppressive effect.[69] Thus it is evident that neither the intracellular potassium nor the intracellular sodium levels *per se* are critical factors in the release process.

One additional observation is of interest. When the gaseous conditions that obtain *in vivo* are roughly simulated by aeration of the medium with 5 per cent carbon dioxide in nitrogen, exudate granulocytes incubated in peritoneal exudate fluid release pyrogen. Under aerobic conditions, on the other hand, the potassium in the exudate fluid suppresses the pyrogen release (Table 5).[79]

Together these results suggest that potassium deprivation may activate pyrogen release, either by stimulating glycolysis and thus lowering intracellular pH, or by somehow affecting the functional integrity of the cell membrane. Although glycolysis in granulocytes is known to be stimulated by endotoxin[76] and by phagocytosis[77] and pinocytosis,[77] no increased accumulation of lactic acid (indicative of accelerated glycolysis) results from potassium deprivation.[75] At present, therefore, it appears that the deprivation of potassium probably acts on the cell membrane.

TABLE 3. *Effect of Sulfhydryl-reactive Enzyme Inhibitors on Release of Pyrogen from Exudate Granulocytes Incubated in 0.15 M NaCl*[*]

| INHIBITOR ($2 \times 10^{-4}$ M) | PYROGEN RELEASED [†] |
|---|---|
| None (control) | 22.8 ($\pm 2.53$) (4) |
| Arsenite | 2.1 ($\pm 0.56$) (6) |
| Iodoacetate | 2.3 ($\pm 2.12$) (2) |
| p-Chloromercuribenzoate | 3.1 ($\pm 1.13$) (2) |
| N-Ethylmaleimide | 0.5 ($\pm 0.71$) (4) |

[*] From Kaiser and Wood.[74]
[†] Mean febrile responses ($FI_{120}$) of rabbits receiving supernatants from $3.5 \times 10^8$ cells incubated for four hours at 37°C. Figures in first parentheses = standard deviation; those in second parentheses = number of observations on which mean values were based.

TABLE 4. *Inhibitory Effect of NaF on Release of Pyrogen from Exudate Granulocytes Incubated in 0.15 M NaCl*[*]

| CONCENTRATION OF NaF | PYROGEN RELEASED [†] |
|---|---|
| None (control) | 1.09 ($\pm 0.12$) (8) |
| $7 \times 10^{-4}$ | 1.06 ($\pm 0.07$) (3) |
| $7 \times 10^{-3}$ | 0.63 ($\pm 0.17$) (3) |
| $1.4 \times 10^{-2}$ | 0.35 ($\pm 0.08$) (3) |
| $7 \times 10^{-2}$ | 0.15 ($\pm 0.06$) (9) |

[*] From Hahn and Wood.[75]
[†] Mean febrile responses ($+\Delta T$) of rabbits receiving supernatant from $1.75 \times 10^7$ cells incubated for two hours at 37°C. The cells were first kept at 4°C. for two hours to permit uptake of NaF. Figures in first parentheses = standard error of mean; those in second parentheses = number of observations from which mean values were calculated. Analysis of variance reveals the differences to be highly significant at the 1 per cent level.

TABLE 5. *Release of Pyrogen from Exudate Granulocytes Incubated in Early Exudate Fluid (4 Hours)*[*]

| CONDITIONS OF INCUBATION [†] | $FI_{120}$ [‡] |
|---|---|
| Aerobic | 0.7 ($\pm 0.3$)[§] |
| 5% $CO_2$ — 95% $N_2$ | 8.5 ($\pm 0.7$) |

[*] From Cheuk and Wood.[79]
[†] For two hours at 37°C.
[‡] From $1.75 \times 10^8$ cells.
[§] Standard error of mean.

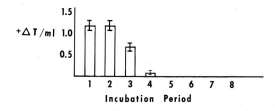

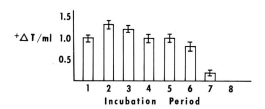

*Figure 8.* Comparative kinetics of pyrogen release from granulocytes (upper graph) and monocytes (lower graph), incubated for successive one hour periods in 0.15 M NaCl. Both types of cells were pre-incubated in four hour exudate fluid to maximize their responsiveness to the potassium deprivation stimulus (see text). Brackets indicate ± S. E. of mean. (From Hahn et al. J. Exp. Med. *126:*385, 1967.)

Most studies of the release process have been done with granulocytes, since only recently has it been known that monocytes generate pyrogen.[46, 47, 52] An important difference, however, has already emerged from comparative experiments with both types of cells. When granulocytes are incubated repeatedly for one hour periods in potassium-free saline, most of the pyrogen is released during the first two hours; whereas from monocytes appreciable amounts of pyrogen are released during the fifth and sixth hours (Fig. 8).[47] Thus the two release processes differ in their kinetics. In addition, the release of monocytic pyrogen has been blocked with puromycin ($10^{-4}$ M),[46] whereas attempts to suppress pyrogen release from exudate granulocytes with comparable concentrations of puromycin have been unsuccessful.[75]

## CHEMICAL CHARACTERISTICS OF GRANULOCYTIC PYROGEN

The known chemical characteristics of granulocytic pyrogen are summarized in Table 6.[80–83] It will be seen that the pyrogen molecule is a rather small protein with a molecular weight of about 14,000,[82, 83] i.e., approximately the size of the enzyme ribonuclease (Fig. 9).[83]

The fact that it is soluble in 66 per cent methanol[82] suggests that it may be a lipoprotein. The only lipid solvent yet shown to inactivate it, however, is acid isooctane,[82, 83] and there is no guarantee that this reagent will not inactivate a labile protein.

The pyrogenic activity of the molecule is destroyed by exposure to cupric ions, periodate, iodoacetate, *p*-chloromercuriphenylsulfonic acid, and *N*-ethylmaleimide at neutral pH and to alkaline media at pH levels above 8.5.[82, 83] The alkaline inactivation and the inactivation by *p*-chloromercuriphenylsulfonic acid both can be prevented, and even reversed, by sulfhydryl reducing agents such as mercaptoethanol and dithiothreitol,[83] suggesting that the molecule contains one or more essential sulfhydryl groups.

TABLE 6. *Chemical Properties of Granulocytic Pyrogen*

Nondialyzable (M.W. = 14,000 by sucrose gradient
   centrifugation and sephadex chromatography)[82, 83]
Heat labile (90°C. for 30 minutes)[80]
Removed by extraction with phenol[80]
Precipitated by perchloric acid (0.3 M)[80]
Soluble in 66% methanol[82]
Inactivated by:
   trypsin and pepsin[80]
   diisopropyl fluorophosphate (3 × 10⁻³ M)[74]
   dinitrofluorobenzene (5 × 10⁻⁴ M)[74]
   acid isooctane[82]
   periodate (7 × 10⁻³ M)[82]
   iodoacetate (1 × 10⁻² M)[74]
   cupric ions (1 × 10⁻² M)[82]
   *p*-chloromercuriphenylsulfonic acid (1 × 10⁻² M)[83]
   *N*-ethylmaleimide (1 × 10⁻² M)[83]
   pH 8.5[82, 83]
Alkaline inactivation reversed by:
   mercaptoethanol (1 × 10⁻² M)[83]
   dithiothreitol (1 × 10⁻² M)[83]
Not inactivated by extraction with:
   isooctane (neutral)[73]
   butanol[83]
   *n*-heptane[83]
   ethanol-ether (3:1)[83]

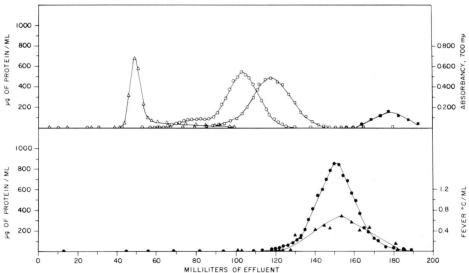

*Figure 9.* Chromatography of pyrogen and of proteins of known molecular weight on Sephadex G–200. The column was 40 × 2.5 cm. Pyrogen and the other proteins were individually applied and eluted from the column at 4°C. with 0.1 M sodium phosphate (pH 6.8) in saline. Pyrogen was assayed by injecting an aliquot of each fraction into a single rabbit. The other proteins were measured by the Folin procedure. Elution of blue dextran was determined by absorbance at 700 mμ, and glycine was detected by the ninhydrin reaction.

Upper figure: △———△, blue dextran (mol. wt. 2,000,000); 0———0, bovine serum albumin (mol. wt. 67,000); □———□, ovalbumin (mol. wt. 45,000); and ■———■, glycine (mol. wt. 61). Lower figure: ▲———▲, pyrogen; and ●———●, ribonuclease (mol. wt. 13,700). From Kozak et al. J. Exp. Med. *127*:341, 1968.

The present evidence, therefore, indicates that granulocytic pyrogen is a small, fairly labile protein, which may or may not possess a lipid moiety. Very recently, it has been separated from contaminating proteins by acrylamide gel electrophoresis.[83] The purified product is now being used for further chemical analysis, radiolabelling, and immunochemical studies.

Comparison of the chemical properties of monocytic pyrogen with those of granulocytic pyrogen should be of great interest.

## ACTION ON HYPOTHALAMUS

The observation, already mentioned, that granulocytic pyrogen when injected into the carotid artery causes a prompter and a greater fever response than when injected intravenously[39] indicates that it acts on the central nervous system, presumably in the hypothalamus. A crude preparation of granulocytic pyrogen labelled with [131]I has also been reported to label the hypothalamus when injected intravenously,[84] but in this experiment there was no way of telling whether the pyrogen molecule was labelled.

Fairly precise localization of the hypothalamic centers responsive to granulocytic pyrogen has recently been established in cats by direct injection of pyrogen through stereotactically localized microcannulae.[85] The sensitive fever centers thus localized lie in the anterior hypothalamus, on either side of the midline, just behind and below the anterior commissure (Fig. 10). Each of the two centers occupies no more than 4.5 cu. mm. Similar studies have been done in rabbits.[78]

Elucidation of the precise mode of action of the pyrogen on the target cells in these areas must await further definition of the pyrogen molecule. The availability of radiolabelled purified pyrogen and of antipyrogen antibody

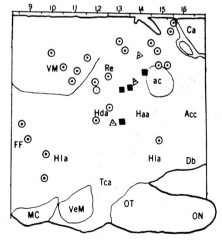

*Figure 10.* Schematic diagram of sagittal section of cat hypothalamus, 1.9 mm. lateral of midline (redrawn by Jackson[85] from atlas of Bleier)[86], showing loci (■) where injections of 2 to 5 μl. of granulocytic pyrogen caused immediate fevers of more than 0.7°C (as in Fig. 1, lower graph). Circles indicate negative loci where injections elicited no fever, and triangles represent sites of equivocal responses (0.5 to 0.7°C). Abbreviations: *ac,* anterior commissure; *Acc,* nucleus accumbens; *Ca,* caudate nucleus; *Db,* nucleus of the diagonal band of Broca; *Hla,* lateral hypothalamic area, *Haa,* anterior hypothalamic area; *Re,* reticular nucleus of thalamus; *Hda,* dorsal hypothalamic nucleus; *Tca,* area of tuber cinereum; *VM,* ventromedial nuclear group of thalamus; *FF,* nucleus of the fields of Forel; *MC,* mammillary body; *VeM,* ventromedial nucleus of hypothalamus; *OT,* optic tract; *ON,* optic nerve.

may eventually permit identification of the critically sensitive neurons in the hypothalamic "thermostat."

## CODA

In the 20 years since Beeson's discovery of granulocytic pyrogen, it has been demonstrated that the primary messenger molecules acting on the brain in experimental fevers are derived from granulocytes, monocytes, and macrophages. Although disease-induced fevers in humans have not been studied as extensively as experimental fevers in rabbits, there is reason to believe that they too, with few exceptions, are caused by the same kinds of leukocytic pyrogens. The recent isolation of granulocytic pyrogen in a relatively pure state has greatly facilitated the study of its chemistry. The mechanisms involved in its release from inflammatory exudates have already been partially defined, and methods are being developed for studying its action on the hypothalamus. The prospects of understanding the pathogenesis of fever in molecular terms are, therefore, promising.

## *References*

1. Cooper, K. E.: Temperature regulation and the hypothalamus. Brit. Med. Bull. 1966, *22:*238.
2. Hardy, J. D.: Physiology of temperature regulation. Physiol. Rev. 1961, *41:*521.
3. Cranston, W. I.: Temperature regulation. Brit. Med. J. 1966, *2:*69.
4. Cooper, K. E., Cranston, W. I., and Snell, E. S.: Temperature regulation during fever in man. Clin. Sci. 1964, *27:*345.
5. Palmes, E. D., and Park, C. R.: The regulation of body temperature during fever. Arch. Environ. Health 1965, *11:*749.
6. MacPherson, R. K.: The effect of fever on temperature regulation in man. Clin. Sci. 1959, *18:*281.
7. Nakayama, T., Hammel, H. T., Hardy, J. D., and Eisenman, J. S.: Thermal stimulation of electrical activity of single units of the preoptic region. Amer. J. Physiol. 1963, *204:*1122.
8. Wood, W. B., Jr.: Studies on the cause of fever. New Eng. J. Med. 1958, *258:*1023.
9. Atkins, E., Pathogenesis of fever. Physiol. Rev. 1960, *40:*580.
10. Wood, W. B., Jr.: Pathogenesis of fever. *In:* Physiologie und Pathophysiologie des vegetativen Nervensystems. (M. Monnier, ed.) Hippokrates-Verlag, Stuttgart, 1963.
11. Atkins, E., and Snell, E. S.: Fever. *In:* The Inflammatory Process. (B. W. Zweifach, L. Grant, and R. T. McCluskey, eds.) Academic Press, New York, 1965.
12. Bennett, I. L., Jr., and Beeson, P. B.: The properties and biologic effects of bacterial pyrogens. Medicine 1950, *29:*365.
13. Grant, R., and Whalen, W. J.: Latency of pyrogen fever: appearance of fast-acting pyrogen in blood of febrile animals and in plasma incubated with bacterial pyrogen. Amer. J. Physiol. 1953, *173:*47.
14. Atkins, E., and Wood, W. B., Jr.: Studies on the pathogenesis of fever. I. Presence of transferable pyrogen in the blood stream following injection of typhoid vaccine. J. Exp. Med. 1955, *101:*519.
15. Atkins, E., and Wood, W. B., Jr.: Studies on the pathogenesis of fever. II. Identification of endogenous pyrogen in the blood stream following injection of typhoid vaccine. J. Exp. Med. 1955, *102:*449.
16. Wagner, R. R., Bennett, I. L., Jr., and LeQuire, V. S.: The production of fever by influenza viruses. I. Factors influencing the febrile response to single injections of virus. J. Exp. Med. 1949, *90:*321.
17. Atkins, E., and Huang, W. C.: Studies on the pathogenesis of fever with influenzal viruses. I. The appearance of endogenous pyrogen in the blood following intravenous injection of virus. J. Exp. Med. 1958, *107:*383.

18. Atkins, E., and Huang, W. C.: Studies on the pathogenesis of fever with influenzal viruses. II. Effects of endogenous pyrogen in normal and virus-tolerant recipients. J. Exp. Med. 1958, *107*:403.

19. Atkins, E., and Huang, W. C.: Studies on the pathogenesis of fever with influenzal viruses. III. The relation of tolerance to the production of endogenous pyrogen. J. Exp. Med. 1958, *107*:415.

20. King, M. K.: Production of fever in rabbits with extracts of tissue culture cells infected with Coxsackie virus. J. Lab. Clin. Med. 1962, *59*:986.

21. King, M. K.: Pathogenesis of fever in rabbits following intravenous injection of Coxsackie virus. J. Lab. Clin. Med. 1964, *63*:23.

22. Atkins, E., and Freedman, L. R.: Studies in staphylococcal fever. I. Responses to bacterial cells. Yale J. Biol. Med. 1963, *35*:451.

23. Berlin, R. D., and Wood, W. B., Jr.: Studies on the pathogenesis of fever. XIII. The effect of phagocytosis on the release of endogenous pyrogen by polymorphonuclear leucocytes. J. Exp. Med. 1964, *119*:715.

24. Farr, R. S., Campbell, D. H., Clark, S. L., Jr., and Proffitt, J. E.: The febrile response of sensitized rabbits to the intravenous injection of antigen. Anat. Rec. 1954, *118*:385.

25. Hall, C. H., Jr., and Atkins, E.: Studies on tuberculin fever. I. The mechanism of fever in tuberculin hypersensitivity. J. Exp. Med. 1959, *109*:339.

26. Moses, J. M., and Atkins, E.: Studies on tuberculin fever. II. Observations on the role of endogenous pyrogen in tolerance. J. Exp. Med. 1961, *114*:939.

27. Uhr, J. W., and Brandress, M. W.: Delayed hypersensitivity. IV. Systemic reactivity of guinea pigs sensitized to protein antigens. J. Exp. Med. 1958, *108*:905.

28. Bard, P., and Woods, J.: Central nervous region essential for endotoxin fever. Trans. Amer. Neurol. Assoc. 1962, *87*:37.

29. Petersdorf, R. G., and Bennett, I. L., Jr.: Studies on the pathogenesis of fever. VIII. Fever-producing substances in the serum of dogs. J. Exp. Med. 1957, *106*:293.

30. Beeson, P. B.: Temperature-elevating effect of substance obtained from polymorphonuclear leukocytes. J. Clin. Invest. 1948, *27*:524.

31. Bennett, I. L., Jr., and Beeson, P. B.: Studies on the pathogenesis of fever. I. Effect of injection of extracts and suspensions of uninfected rabbit tissues upon body temperature of normal rabbits. J. Exp. Med. 1953, *98*:477.

32. King, M. K., and Wood, W. B., Jr.: Studies on the pathogenesis of fever. III. Leucocytic origin of endogenous pyrogen in acute inflammatory exudates. J. Exp. Med. 1958, *107*:279.

33. Beeson, P. B.: Tolerance to bacterial pyrogens: role of reticuloendothelial system. J. Exp. Med. 1947, *86*:39.

34. Wood, W. B., Jr.: Fever. Sci. Amer. 1957, *196*:62.

35. Petersdorf, R. G., Keene, W. R., and Bennett, I. L., Jr.: Studies on the pathogenesis of fever. IX. Characteristics of endogenous serum pyrogen and mechanisms governing its release. J. Exp. Med. 1957, *106*:787.

36. Bornstein, D. L., Bredenberg, C., and Wood, W. B., Jr.: Studies on the pathogenesis of fever. XI. Quantitative features of the febrile response to leucocytic pyrogen. J. Exp. Med. 1963, *117*:349.

37. Herion, J. C., Walker, R. I., and Palmer, J. G.: Endotoxin fever in granulocytopenic animals. J. Exp. Med. 1961, *113*:1115.

38. Gillman, S. M., Bornstein, D. L., and Wood, W. B., Jr.: Studies on the pathogenesis of fever. VIII. Further observations on the role of endogenous pyrogen in endotoxin fever. J. Exp. Med. 1961, *114*:729.

39. King, M. K., and Wood, W. B., Jr.: Studies on the pathogenesis of fever. IV. The site of action of leukocytic and circulating endogenous pyrogen. J. Exp. Med. 1958, *107*:291.

40. Atkins, E., and Heijn, C., Jr.: Studies on tuberculin fever. III. Mechanisms involved in the release of endogenous pyrogen *in vitro*. J. Exp. Med. 1965, *122*:207.

41. Collins, R. D., and Wood, W. B., Jr.: Studies on the pathogenesis of fever. VI. The interaction of leucocytes and endotoxin *in vitro*. J. Exp. Med. 1959, *110*:1005.

42. Snell, E. S., and Atkins, E.: Interactions of Gram-negative bacterial endotoxin with rabbit blood *in vitro*. Amer. J. Physiol. 1967, *212*:1103.

43. Atkins, E., Cronin, M., and Isacson, P.: Endogenous pyrogen release from rabbit blood cells incubated *in vitro* with parainfluenza virus. Science 1964, *146*:1469.

44. Bennett, I. L., Jr.: Studies on the pathogenesis of fever. V. Fever accompanying pneumococcal infection in the rabbit. Bull. Johns Hopkins Hosp. 1956, *98*:216.

45. King, M. K., and Wood, W. B., Jr.: Studies on the pathogenesis of fever. V. Relation of circulating endogenous pyrogen to fever of acute bacterial infections. J. Exp. Med. 1958, *107*:305.

46. Atkins, E., Bodel, P., and Francis, L.: The release of endogenous pyrogen *in vitro* from rabbit mononuclear cells. J. Exp. Med. 1967, *126*:357.

47. Hahn, H. H., Char, D. C., Postel, W. B., and Wood, W. B., Jr.: Studies on the pathogenesis of fever. XV. The production of endogenous pyrogen by peritoneal macrophages. J. Exp. Med. 1967, *126*:385.

48. Wood, W. B., Jr.: Editorial. New Eng. J. Med. 1967, *276*:1036.

49. Snell, E. S., and Atkins, E.: The presence of endogenous pyrogens in normal rabbit tissues. J. Exp. Med. 1965, *121*:1019.

50. Cranston, W. I., Goodale, F., Jr., Snell, E. S., and Wendt, F.: The role of leukocytes in the initial actions of bacterial pyrogens in man. Clin. Sci. 1956, *15*:219.

51. Snell, E. S., Goodale, F., Jr., Wendt, F., and Cranston, W. I.: Properties of human endogenous pyrogen. Clin. Sci. 1957, *16*:615.

52. Bodel, P., and Atkins, E.: Release of endogenous pyrogen by human monocytes. New Eng. J. Med. 1967, *276*:1002.

53. Bodel, P., and Atkins, E.: Human leucocyte pyrogen producing fever in rabbits. Proc. Soc. Exp. Biol. Med. 1966, *121*:943.

54. Snell, E. S.: An examination of the blood of febrile subjects for pyrogenic properties. Clin. Sci. 1961, *21*:115.

55. Snell, E. S.: Pyrogenic properties of human pathological fluids. Clin. Sci. 1962, *23*:141.

56. Kappas, A., Hellman, L., Fukushima, D. K., and Gallagher, T. F.: The pyrogenic effect of etiocholanolone. J. Clin. Endocr. 1957, *17*:451.

57. Kappas, A., Glickman, P. B., and Palmer, R. H.: Steroid fever studies: Physiological differences between bacterial pyrogens and endogenous steroid pyrogens of man. Trans. Assoc. Amer. Physicians 1960, *73*:176.

58. Kappas, A., and Palmer, R. H.: Selected aspects of steroid pharmacology. Pharmacol. Rev. 1963, *15*:123.

59. Palmer, R. H., Ratkovits, B., and Kappas, A.: Steroid pyrogen studies in laboratory and domestic animals. J. Appl. Physiol. 1961, *16*:345.

60. Glickman, P. B., Palmer, R. H., and Kappas, A.: Steroid fever and inflammation. Arch. Intern. Med. 1964, *114*:46.

61. Kappas, A., Soybel, W., Glickman, P., and Fukushima, D. K.: Fever-producing steroids of endogenous origin in man. Arch. Intern. Med. 1960, *105*:701.

62. Bodel, P., and Dillard, M.: Studies on steroid fever. I. Production of leucocyte pyrogen *in vitro* by etiocholanolone. J. Clin. Invest. 1968, *47*:107.

63. Weissmann, G.: Studies of lysosomes. VI. The effect of neutral steroids and bile acids on lysosomes *in vitro*. Biochem. Pharmacol. 1965, *14*:525.

64. Wolfe, S. M., Kimball, H. R., Perry, S., Root, R., and Kappas, A.: The biological properties of etiocholanolone. Clinical Staff Conference. Ann. Intern. Med. 1967, *67*:1268.

65. Bondy, P. K., Cohn, G. L., and Castiglione, C.: Etiocholanolone fever: A clinical entity. Trans. Assoc. Amer. Physicians 1960, *73*:186.

66. Bondy, P. K., Cohn, G. L., and Gregory, P. B.: Etiocholanolone fever. Medicine 1965, *44*:249.

67. Kaiser, H. K., and Wood, W. B., Jr.: Studies on the pathogenesis of fever. IX. The production of endogenous pyrogen by polymorphonuclear leucocytes. J. Exp. Med. 1962, *115*:27.

68. Berlin, R. D., and Wood, W. B., Jr.: Molecular mechanisms involved in the release of pyrogen from polymorphonuclear leucocytes. Trans. Assoc. Amer. Physicians 1962, *75*:190.

69. Berlin, R. D., and Wood, W. B., Jr.: Studies on the pathogenesis of fever. XII. Electrolytic factors influencing the release of endogenous pyrogen from polymorphonuclear leucocytes. J. Exp. Med. 1964, *119*:697.

70. Johnson, J. A.: Influence of ouabain, strophanthidin, and dihydrostrophanthidin on sodium and potassium transport in frog sartorii. Amer. J. Physiol. 1956, *187*:328.

71. Hahn, H. H., Cheuk, S. F., Tomasulo, P., and Wood., W. B., Jr.: To be published.

72. Fatt, P., and Katz, B.: Conduction of impulses in Crustacean muscle fibers. J. Physiol. 1951, *115*:45.

73. Thesleff, S.: The effect of anesthetic agents on skeletal muscle membrane. Acta Physiol. Scand. 1956, *37*:335.

74. Kaiser, H. K., and Wood, W. B., Jr.: Studies on the pathogenesis of fever. X. The effect of certain enzyme inhibitors on the production and activity of leucocytic pyrogen. J. Exp. Med. 1962, *115*:37.

75. Hahn, H. H., and Wood, W. B., Jr.: Unpublished data.

76. Cohn, Z. A., and Morse, S. I.: Functional and metabolic properties of polymorphonuclear leucocytes. II. The influence of lipopolysaccharide endotoxin. J. Exp. Med. 1960, *111*:689.

77. Karnovsky, M. L.: Metabolic basis of phagocytic activity. Physiol. Rev. 1962, *42*:143.

78. Cooper, K. E., Cranston, W. I., and Honour, A. J.: Observations on the site and mode of action of pyrogens in the rabbit brain. J. Physiol. 1967, *191*:325.
79. Cheuk, S. F., and Wood, W. B., Jr.: Unpublished data.
80. Rafter, G. W., Collins, R. D., and Wood, W. B., Jr.: Studies on the pathogenesis of fever. VII. Preliminary chemical characterization of leucocytic pyrogen. J. Exp. Med. 1960, *111*:831.
81. Wood, W. B., Jr., Bornstein, D. L., and Rafter, G. W.: Studies on experimental fever with particular reference to the pathogenetic role and chemical properties of leucocytic pyrogen. Proc. Nat. Acad. Sci. 1960, *46*:1248.
82. Rafter, G. W., Cheuk, S. F., Krause, D. W., and Wood, W. B., Jr.: Studies on the pathogenesis of fever. XIV. Further observations on the chemistry of leucocytic pyrogen. J. Exp. Med. 1966, *123*:433.
83. Kozak, M. S., Hahn, H. H., Lennarz, W. J., and Wood, W. B., Jr.: Studies on the pathogenesis of fever. XVI. Purification and further chemical characterization of granulocytic pyrogen. J. Exp. Med. 1968, *127*:341.
84. Allen, I. V.: The cerebral effects of endogenous serum and granulocytic pyrogen. Brit. J. Exp. Path. 1965, *46*:25.
85. Jackson, D. L.: A hypothalamic region responsive to localized injection of pyrogens. J. Neurophysiol. 1967, *30*:586.
86. Bleier, R. M.: The Hypothalamus of the Cat. Johns Hopkins Press, Baltimore, 1961.

# INFECTIONS
# BY
# GRAM-POSITIVE
# PATHOGENS

# Chapter 7

# PREVENTION OF PNEUMOCOCCAL PNEUMONIA BY IMMUNIZATION WITH SPECIFIC CAPSULAR POLYSACCHARIDES*

COLIN M. MacLEOD
*Vice President for Medical Affairs, Commonwealth Fund, New York, New York*

The title of this essay is the same as that of a paper published in 1945 with Drs. Hodges, Heidelberger, and Bernhard.[8] To some it may seem like raking over old bones and perhaps it is, although in this case it may be that "these bones will rise again" as times change and as satisfaction with past accomplishments gives way to appreciation of current realities.

Let us put the situation in a modern perspective and then go back to describe our epidemiological experiments of 25 years ago and their relevance to pneumococcal pneumonia as it occurs today.

One recalls vividly the introduction in the late 1930's of the sulfonamide drugs, which promptly supplanted the use of specific antiserum for the therapy of pneumococcal pneumonia. Specific antipneumococcal serum treatment was remarkably curative provided one had the technical resources to apply it effectively; however, such resources existed in only a handful of institutions in the United States and its impact upon the death rate from lobar pneumonia, therefore, was minor when looked at nationally. To achieve throughout the United States the level of technical competence required for effective serum

---

* This essay formed the substance of the James D. Bruce Memorial Award Lecture of the American College of Physicians, Chicago, April 21, 1969.

treatment of lobar pneumonia seemed an almost hopeless task. The sulfonamides were welcomed with relief and serum therapy was abandoned forthwith
even in those citadels of sophistication where its use had been brought to a
high level of effectiveness. Concurrently, the serological typing of pneumococci
responsible for disease was likewise given up except in a few university centers
where pneumococcophiles existed.

Experience with the sulfonamides in animals and in man was not long
in showing the limitations of these bacteriostatic compounds. It became apparent very early that an active immune response by the host is necessary for
the sulfonamides to be effective.[6] In infections caused by certain pneumococcal
types, especially type 3, which give a poor immune response, the sulfonamides
were correspondingly inadequate in therapy. In addition, pneumococci acquire
resistance to the sulfonamides readily so that their effect upon the complications
of pneumococcal pneumonia, in particular empyema, was unsatisfactory.
Bacteria isolated from empyemic pus were usually found to be sulfonamide-
resistant.[7]

Despite such limitations the sulfonamide drugs reduced significantly the
mortality from lobar pneumonia and there was general satisfaction in this
great step forward. The therapy of pneumonia was much better than it had
been and as a result there occurred a general relaxation in the study of the
disease.

Introduction of penicillin in the mid 1940's yielded another large dividend
in therapy. Penicillin has a more bactericidal action upon pneumococci, and
dependence upon an immune response by the host is correspondingly decreased,[9] although the need for it is not entirely eliminated. Penicillin has the
added advantage that under natural conditions pneumococci do not have the
capacity to develop a significant degree of resistance to it and therefore it is
effective in preventing the chronic suppurative complications of pneumococcal
pneumonia.

Why are we once again concerned about pneumococcal pneumonia when
there is available in penicillin such a remarkable antipneumococcal agent?
The fact is that there still occurs significant mortality from pneumococcal
pneumonia in patients who are treated with theoretically effective amounts of
this chemotherapeutic agent or who are treated with other antibiotics to which
pneumococcus is sensitive.

Robert Austrian[1] has shown through study of a large series of bacteremic
patients in hospitals in New York City and in Philadelphia that although the
mortality from penicillin-treated, bacteremic pneumococcal pneumonia is 7
per cent in persons between the ages of 12 and 49 years, it rises to 28 per cent
in patients more than 50 years of age. Furthermore, patients with preexisting
disease of the cardiovascular system or the respiratory tract, or those who have
endocrine disorders, kidney disease, or malignancies have a mortality rate of
30 per cent from bacteremic pneumococcal pneumonia as compared to a mortality rate of 7 per cent among those without preexisting disease. In short,
mortality in patients with bacteremic pneumococcal pneumonia increases
dramatically in the older age groups and in those who have certain preexisting
diseases. The point of therapeutic "no return" is reached earlier among these
groups of patients than in the young and healthy.

On the basis of these observations on this common disease, Austrian has suggested that consideration be given once again to specific antipneumococcal immunization of people who are at greatest risk—those in the older age groups and those with preexisting diseases that predispose to a high mortality rate. It is satisfying to report that Austrian's initiative and perseverance have led to a large-scale program administered by the National Institutes of Health which has the aim of determining whether immunization with pneumococcal polysaccharides will give a measure of protection to the large segment of our population that is at high risk from pneumococcal infections.

## STUDIES ON PNEUMOCOCCAL IMMUNIZATION

The background for the present studies on immunization derives from work carried on in the 1930's and 1940's. There is good evidence from our studies during World War II that immunization of healthy young men with purified pneumococcal capsular polysaccharides is effective in preventing the disease.[8] These studies, which provide the basis for the present decision to reinvestigate the use of these immunizing agents, will be briefly reviewed.

There is a multitude of pneumococcal types that parasitize and infect man. The number is beyond 80 at the latest count. However, among this very large number of types, only a small number are responsible for most human disease. Type specificity is determined by the chemical and immunological character of the complex polysaccharides that form a mantle or capsule around the cells. This capsule is also responsible for the pathogenicity and, as far as we know, the virulence of the microorganisms. Antibodies directed against the capsular polysaccharide protect animals against experimental infection.

Studies in man on the antigenicity of pneumococcal polysaccharides were initiated by Thomas Francis and William Tillett[2] at the Hospital of the Rockefeller Institute in New York; these investigators reported in 1930 that injection of small amounts of the isolated polysaccharides in man resulted in the production of specific antibodies. This observation set the stage for the work to be reviewed here.

In the early 1940's under the auspices of the Commission on Pneumonia of the Army Epidemiological Board, Michael Heidelberger and I carried out a series of studies on immunization of volunteers with polysaccharides of a number of types, singly and in combination.[4] We found that amounts on the order of 30 to 60 micrograms of as many as six different polysaccharides gave a good immune response when injected subcutaneously at the same time in the same water-clear solution. Because the materials were purified the reactions observed were mild, consisting, when they appeared, of local soreness. It seems likely that reactions can be further reduced by more extensive purification if that appears to be necessary.

Following subcutaneous injections of the polysaccharides in man, mouse-protective antibodies can be demonstrated in the blood serum within 6 to 9 days.[8] The peak titer is reached within 6 weeks. Presumably because the polysaccharide antigens are not destroyed in the body, antibodies to them in man are very persistent. Levels as high as one-third to one-half of the original maximum level were still present after 1 to 2 years in most subjects and were significantly elevated as long as 5 years after injection. Presumably immunity to the disease would be similarly enduring, although the longest period of observation of men at risk from epidemic pneumonia was 6 months. Six months can be set as the minimum period of immunity: the likelihood is that it is much longer because of the very long persistence of antibody levels in the blood serum.

The opportunity to test whether immunization of man with capsular polysaccharides protects against the common natural infection, pneumococcal pneumonia, arose during World War II in an Army Air Force Base in South Dakota. Pneumococcal pneumonia was epidemic in this Air Force Technical School over three winter seasons with but six of the many serological types (types 1, 2, 4, 5, 7, and 12) causing most of the disease. More than 1600 patients with pneumococcal pneumonia were hospitalized early in the course of their disease during this period, and all were treated with sulfonamides without a single death. These were healthy young adult males.

Richard Hodges and I, with the assistance of William Bernhard,[5] were able to study the epidemiology of the epidemic or series of epidemics during this period and finally, with Michael Heidelberger,[8] to intervene by immunizing half the troops with purified polysaccharides from four of the six types that were causing most of the disease. The remaining troops, who received injections of saline, served as controls. The results were dramatic. Within 2 weeks pneumococcal pneumonia caused by the types against which we had immunized (types 1, 2, 5, and 7) ceased in the half of the population that was immunized but continued to occur in the nonimmunized population, although at a much lower rate than was expected on the basis of the experience of the preceding two years of observation. In the case of the types against which we did not immunize there was no effect. The incidence of pneumonia caused by these types was unaffected. These points will be considered later in this discussion.

Figure 1 depicts the interval between immunization and development of pneumonia in the immunized and nonimmunized subjects. Pneumonia caused by the types in the vaccine (types 1, 2, 5, and 7) ceased in the immunized group within 11 days and there were no further cases in this group for the duration of the experiment. In the nonimmunized half of the population, pneumonia caused by these types continued to occur, but at a lower rate than expected, as mentioned previously.

The design of this extensive experiment enabled us to draw a number of conclusions that are of considerable epidemiological interest. As noted earlier, the incidence of pneumonia caused by types 1, 2, 5, and 7 in the control or nonimmunized group was lower than expected on the basis of the experience of the two preceding years. The admission rates for these types are shown in Figure 2, together with the rates for the other two epidemic types against which immunization was not practiced, namely type 12 and type 4. Inspection of this figure indicates that in 1944–45 pneumonia caused by types 1, 2, 5, and 7 in the total population was reduced much more than was expected on the basis of immunization of only one-half of the population against these types. It can also be seen from Figure 2 that there was no reduction in the incidence of infection with types 12 and 4 in the year of immunization (1944–45); this fact demonstrates that conditions conducive to epidemic pneumonia still prevailed.

The consistent behavior of types 12 and 4 in each of the three years provided a means for calculating the reduction in the incidence of pneumonia caused by types 1, 2, 5, and 7 among the nonimmunized which was brought about by immunizing one-half the population. Figure 3 shows the expected and observed incidence of types 1, 2, 5, and 7 for 1944–45, the year of immunization against these infections. The observed incidence was only 17.6 per cent of

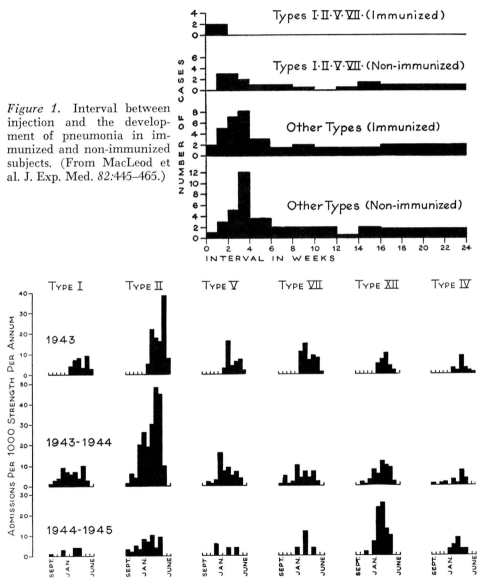

*Figure 1.* Interval between injection and the development of pneumonia in immunized and non-immunized subjects. (From MacLeod et al. J. Exp. Med. *82:*445–465.)

*Figure 2.* Admission rates for pneumococcal pneumonia caused by types I, II, V, VII, XII, and IV during 1942–43, 1943–44, and 1944–45. (From MacLeod et al. J. Exp. Med. *82:*445–465.)

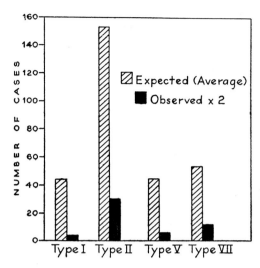

*Figure 3.* Expected and observed incidence of pneumococcal pneumonia caused by types I, II, V, and VII for 1944–45. The observed incidence for 1944–45 has been multiplied by two since the non-immunes comprised only one-half the population. (From Mac-Leod et al. J. Exp. Med. *82:*445–465.)

that expected as calculated from the behavior of types 12 and 4 in each of the two preceding years.

It seems, therefore, that immunization of one-half the population against types 1, 2, 5, and 7 greatly reduced the incidence of disease caused by these types in the rest of the population. The most likely explanation for this striking effect stems from our observation that immunization of half the population against types 1, 2, 5, and 7 caused a decrease in the carrier rates for these types in the immunized population whereas the carrier rates for other types were unaffected. The decrease in the number of cases of pneumonia in the immunized group would, in addition, decrease the number of case-contact carriers. With the thorough mixing of the immunized and nonimmunized subjects in the population, the chances would be that in every other one of its man-to-man transfers, the pneumococci would fall on infertile ground, either because the person was protected against pneumonia or because his ability to carry pneumococci in his throat was decreased by immunization. The net result would be a lowering of carrier rates for types 1, 2, 5, and 7 in the whole population, and this in turn could account for the marked decrease in pneumonia caused by these types not only in the immunized portion of the population but in the nonimmunized as well.

Reduction in the carrier rates of pneumococci following immunization thus appears to provide a second means for determining the effectiveness of the immunizing procedure, that is, in addition to the observed reduction in cases of pneumonia.

It seems likely that observations on carrier rates in other epidemic diseases might provide evidence of the effectiveness of immunization. An example that comes to mind is meningococcal infection, in which the incidence of pharyngeal carriage of the bacteria may be very high although the incidence of overt disease, meningococcemia or meningitis, may be very low and unpredictable. If, as is the case with pneumococci,[8] immunization of man reduces the carrier rate, then it should affect also the incidence of the disease. In the case of meningococcal disease, for which there is no useful experimental model in animals, measurement of carrier rates in immunized and nonimmunized populations may thus provide an indication of the efficacy of an immunizing procedure.

With the evidence that has been gathered on the effectiveness of immunization by means of pneumococcal polysaccharides in preventing pneumonia among troops, it is reasonable to believe that it will be effective also in protecting others in the population, such as older people and those afflicted with diseases which predispose them to severe infections. The opinion has been expressed that the evidence at hand is sufficient to warrant general use of these antigens in the high-risk population without the necessity for further epidemiological study. However, it should be emphasized that our experiment of 25 years ago was carried out among healthy young males in a military installation where pneumonia was epidemic and where high carrier rates prevailed for the infecting types. Although there is no reason to believe that the antibody response among older people will be any less active than among healthy young men, one cannot assume that protection will be as effective. Because of differences in the nature of the populations, it is possible that in older people and in the sick the protective effect will not parallel the antibody response. For these reasons it seems important to investigate the usefulness of these antigens in the populations in which they will be used.

In addition, because of the changed epidemiological pattern of the disease, particularly the marked decline in the incidence of type 2 infections since World War II, it is necessary to define precisely on a nation-wide basis the types of pneumococci that are causing disease, so that the appropriate mixture of polysaccharide antigens can be used to immunize the target population. For example, since the once-common type 2 disease has now become uncommon there is little point in including type 2 polysaccharide in a vaccine at this time.

Immunization against pneumococcal pneumonia by means of specific capsular polysaccharides may provide an additional means for reducing the mortality which is still considerable. It should be recalled that "pneumonia and influenza" is the only category of infectious disease remaining among the ten leading causes of death in the United States. Moreover, death from influenza is almost always caused by bacterial pneumonia for which the viral infection has paved the way, and among bacteria, pneumococci are by far the commonest causes of pneumonia.

Immunization against influenza has been recommended for the population groups at greatest risk from it, which are of course precisely the same as those at risk from pneumococcal pneumonia. Although immunization against influenza has been beset by many problems, especially the sudden appearance of new epidemic strains which then sweep over the world at the speed of jet airplanes, I have full confidence that much better immunizing materials will become available if we do not slacken our research on these frustrating tribes of viruses. The author's prejudice is that the more effective influenza antigens of the future will not be composed of intact virus particles but will consist of defined chemical fractions in appropriate mixture representing the significant protective antigens from strains with epidemic potential.

Even when greatly improved influenza vaccines become available and come into general use, the desirability of possessing effective antipneumococcal vaccines will not be lessened. Influenza is only one among a number of viral infections of the respiratory tract that predispose to severe and fatal pneumococcal pneumonia. During years when influenza is epidemic, as in 1957 or 1968, there is always a sharp increase in deaths from pneumonia, generally spoken of as "excess pneumonia mortality." But in other years deaths from pneumonia remain high and relatively unchanged except for the familiar seasonal fluctuations. It is against this, the largest, portion of the iceberg of disease that antipneumococcal immunization is likely to have its largest impact year in, year out.

Even though antipneumococcal immunization comes to be widely used, and, one hopes, effective, we will continue to be hampered in our approaches to the disease until the factor or factors produced by the bacteria which cause the severe clinical manifestations and death are understood. This is a mystery. None of the known substances produced by pneumococci during growth or upon autolysis can be incriminated and no one has found any clues from the signs and symptoms of pneumococcal infections in man or animals that might incriminate a particular class of toxic substances. It seems implausible that the presence of the bacteria themselves, in the absence of some toxic product or effect, is responsible for the manifestations of this disease. Compared to the mass of the invaded host that of the bacteria is trivial even at the time of death. It seems more likely that an elusive, perhaps ephemeral, toxic substance is produced. Presumably the young and healthy are more resistant to its malignant effects and the aging and otherwise ill, less so. The point of "no return" from the effects of this putative toxin apparently is reached much sooner in the old and infirm, and therefore antibacterial therapy is less effective among them even though, as commonly happens, their blood and tissues have been sterilized of pneumococci.

We are all aware of fads and fashions in research, which constitute one of the banes of the scientific life. An investigator announces a significant discovery, whereupon squads of research workers abandon what they were doing and move in to mop up. This common tactic stems from psychological insecurity, the fear of being alone in the ocean of scientific ignorance, with all the self-doubt this engenders. Much better to be hunting with the pack or, as it is put, "to be in the forefront of scientific advances." Because of these fears and uncertainties important scientific fields remain untended. Nowhere has this phenomenon been more apparent than in the case of pneumococcus. Studies of the epidemiology and pathogenesis of the disease, difficult and never very popular, were virtually abandoned in the rush from serum therapy to the sulfonamides and thence to penicillin and other antibiotics, and the result was popular but relatively superficial research. It should be apparent that what we are most in need of at the present time is a return to the study of the obscure biological phenomena that dictate the behavior of this common disease of man.

# References

1. Austrian, R. 1968. Current status of bacterial pneumonia with especial reference to pneumococcal infection. J. Clin. Path. *21*(Suppl. 2):93–97.
2. Francis, T., Jr., and W. S. Tillett. 1930. Cutaneous reactions in pneumonia. The development of antibodies following the intradermal injection of type-specific polysaccharide. J. Exp. Med. *52:*573–585.
3. Heidelberger, M. 1953. Persistence of antibodies in man after immunization. *In:* The Nature

and Significance of the Antibody Response. Edited by A. M. Pappenheimer, Jr. Columbia University Press, New York, pp. 90–101.

4. Heidelberger, M., C. M. MacLeod, and M. M. Di Lapi. 1948. The human antibody response to simultaneous injection of six specific polysaccharides of pneumococcus. J. Exp. Med. *88:*369–372.

5. Hodges, R. G., and C. M. MacLeod. 1946. Epidemic pneumococcal pneumonia. 1. Description of the epidemic. Am. J. Hyg. *44:*183–192. Hodges, R. G., and C. M. MacLeod. 1946. 2. The influence of population characteristics and environment. Am. J. Hyg. *44:*193–206. Hodges, R. G., C. M. MacLeod, and W. G. Bernhard. 1946. 3. Pneumococcal carrier studies. Am. J. Hyg. *44:*207–230. Hodges, R. G., and C. M. MacLeod. 1946. 4. The relationship of nonbacterial respiratory disease to pneumococcal pneumonia. Am. J. Hyg. *44:*231–236. Hodges, R. G., and C. M. MacLeod. 1946. 5. Final consideration of the factors underlying the epidemic. Am. J. Hyg. *44:*237–243.

6. MacLeod, C. M. 1939. Chemotherapy of pneumococcal pneumonia. J.A.M.A. *113:*1405–1410.

7. MacLeod, C. M. 1942. The antibacterial action of the sulfonamide drugs. Advances Intern. Med. *1:*83–101.

8. MacLeod, C. M., R. G. Hodges, M. Heidelberger, and W. G. Bernhard. 1945. Prevention of pneumococcal pneumonia by immunization with specific capsular polysaccharides. J. Exp. Med. *82:*445–465.

9. MacLeod, C. M., and E. R. Stone. 1945. Differences in the nature of antibacterial action of the sulfonamides and penicillin and their relation to therapy. Bull. N. Y. Acad. Med. *21:*375–388.

# Chapter 8

# UNSOLVED PROBLEMS OF THE NONSUPPURATIVE COMPLICATIONS OF GROUP A STREPTOCOCCAL INFECTIONS*

ANN G. KUTTNER†

*Associate Professor of Pediatrics, Emeritus,*
*New York University Medical Center,*
*New York, New York*

and

REBECCA C. LANCEFIELD

*Professor Emeritus, Microbiology, The*
*Rockefeller University, New York, New York*

## RHEUMATIC FEVER

In this chapter current knowledge of group A streptococci as related to rheumatic fever and acute glomerulonephritis is summarized. Only those aspects of these complicated microorganisms thought to be pertinent to the pathogenesis of these two diseases will be discussed. Some of the many un-

* This investigation was supported in part by the United States Public Health Service Grant No. HE 03919.
† Deceased May 19, 1968.

solved problems will be reviewed, and the need for further research with new techniques will be emphasized.

Streptococcal upper repiratory infections are extremely common in childhood. Even if they are not treated, most of these infections subside in a few days. At the present time severe toxic symptoms formerly associated with scarlet fever occur very rarely. Children with streptococcal pharyngitis, irrespective of the presence or absence of an erythematous rash, usually recover promptly. Since the advent of antibiotics, suppurative complications occur infrequently. Otitis media usually responds quickly to penicillin therapy and mastoiditis has virtually disappeared. Rheumatic fever, a nonsuppurative complication of streptococcal pharyngitis, on the other hand, is still a major concern of physicians because of the possibility that this disease may cause severe debilitating heart disease or death. It is now generally accepted that rheumatic fever never occurs except as a sequel to group A streptococcal pharyngitis. It required keen observations by clinicians and years of research by many different investigators to establish the importance of these organisms in this disease.

Beginning in 1865, clinicians first emphasized the relationship of rheumatic fever to scarlet fever and tonsillitis, and noted the asymptomatic latent period between the pharyngeal infection and the appearance of rheumatic symptoms.[30, 88] At that time, the science of bacteriology was just beginning to develop. Suitable culture media were not available and the dangers of bacterial contamination were not understood. A number of observers reported the isolation of *Streptococcus viridans* or of gamma streptococci from blood cultures and joint fluids obtained from rheumatic patients, and for many years these organisms were thought to be the cause of rheumatic fever. It was not until 1930–1932, as the result of studies by a number of English physicians,[7, 10, 23, 28, 72, 74] and by Coburn in the United States,[9] that it became apparent that only upper respiratory infections due to beta hemolytic streptococci are followed by rheumatic fever.

## GROUP A STREPTOCOCCI: GENERAL PROPERTIES

Beta hemolytic streptococci had been studied intensively because of the prevalence of streptococcal infections in schools and military centers. In 1933 Lancefield, on the basis of a group-specific carbohydrate detectable by a precipitin reaction, showed that strains of hemolytic streptococci isolated from human infections fall into a single group, designated group A.[44] It was found furthermore that group A streptococci contain numerous distinct serologic types, each characterized by a specific protein antigen, the M antigen. These types correspond with those identified by Griffith in England with the slide agglutination technique.[29] It is now generally accepted that infection with strains of any one of the 55 or more known serologic types may be followed by rheumatic fever.

## TYPE-SPECIFIC M ANTIGENS

In analyzing the relationship of individual strains of group A streptococci to rheumatic fever, the type-specific M antigens situated on the surface of the streptococcal cell wall are of special interest.[46, 71] In addition to being an important factor in the virulence of the organisms, they stimulate the production of type-specific antibodies best demonstrated in man by the so-called bactericidal test.[47] Because of these antibodies, which lead to the phagocytosis and destruction of homologous type streptococci, reinfection with the same type does not occur unless the immune response has been markedly suppressed by the early administration of penicillin.[53] Susceptibility to infection with other serologic types, however, remains unchanged.

Specific anti-M antibodies develop slowly, probably because each M antigen is unique and has not been previously encountered. Once these antibodies appear, they tend to persist and in some individuals remain demonstrable for decades.[47] Even in patients from whose sera "bactericidal" antibodies eventually have disappeared, these type-specific antibodies can be recalled by injection of relatively purified cell walls or M antigens of the same serologic type,[19, 61, 73, 93] but not by similar preparations obtained from heterologous types. This procedure caused the usual "booster" response which indicated that a basic tissue immunity had been present throughout the postinfection period as a result of the initial infection. In control experiments the injection of these immunizing antigens into individuals who had not experienced infections with these types previously did not result in the appearance of type-specific antibodies.

In rabbits, however, the injection of cell wall suspensions did result in the primary formation of type-specific protective antibodies. It seemed possible, therefore, that if solutions of M proteins or cell wall preparations containing M antigens could be purified and concentrated, the injection of such materials into man might also result in a primary response of type-specific antibodies. Both cell wall preparations containing M antigen but freed of the intracellular material and preparations of M protein in solution were injected into man by several different investigators. However, the antigenic response was disappointing and side reactions, though diminished, still occurred. Further studies of M antigen by a variety of different procedures are being continued and it seems likely that eventually an effective preparation of purified M antigens will be available as a means of producing type-specific immunity.[19, 80]

The fact that there are more than 55 known serologic types of these organisms is not considered an insurmountable difficulty for active immunization programs. A number of studies have shown that, in a given community over a period of years, five to six serologic types account for the majority of the acute pharyngeal infections.[51, 80] If effective M antigens could be prepared from these prevalent types, a combination of such antigens might be worth trying.

## CROSS REACTIVE ANTIGENS COMMON TO STREPTOCOCCI AND CARDIAC TISSUES

Studies by Kaplan in 1963, however, have raised the question of whether M vaccines of this kind, even if shown to be effective as a means of stimulating bactericidal protective antibodies, might possibly cause cardiac injury.[34] This investigator, with immunofluorescent techniques, first showed that M antigen preparations of certain serologic types of group A streptococci injected into rabbits produced antibodies which cross react with the myocardial fibers of normal cardiac tissue. This cross reacting antibody is considered to be distinct from the M antigen because it is not removed by absorption with M protein. Zabriskie and Freimer subsequently demonstrated an antigen present in protoplast membranes which also cross reacts with cardiac tissue.[100] Further studies suggested that this antigen was most probably glycoprotein in nature.

Another cross reacting antigen was demonstrated by Goldstein and his coworkers in 1967.[24] These investigators showed by precipitin reactions and immunofluorescent studies that sera of rabbits immunized with the group-specific group A carbohydrate gave cross reactions with glycoproteins present in cardiac valves. So far no data have been published to indicate that any of these antibodies actually cause cardiac lesions. Furthermore, despite many attempts to immunize man with a variety of streptococcal products, there is no evidence that these procedures produced either the symptoms of rheumatic fever or rheumatic heart disease.[22] Nevertheless it behooves anyone planning to immunize children with streptococcal vaccines to test the preparations for antigens which react with cardiac tissues to avoid the possibility of cardiac damage.

Although the importance of infection with group A streptococci as an essential factor in the etiology of rheumatic fever is no longer questioned, none of the findings so far described dealing with cellular components have served to explain how these organisms cause the clinical manifestations of this disease.

## Streptococcal Extracellular Products

Turning to the extracellular products so far identified, none of the many diverse and potent enzymes produced by streptococci is seriously incriminated. These enzymes attack a variety of substrates present in the tissues of the host, such as red blood cells, leukocytes, hyaluronic acid, and fibrin. However, with the exception of streptolysin S and hyaluronic acid, all these substances are antigenic. During the course of streptococcal infections, antibodies for many of these products develop which specifically inhibit their activity.[56] *In vivo*, therefore, there is nothing to suggest that these extracellular products play a part in the pathogenesis of rheumatic fever. There is no evidence to indicate that the antibody response to these enzymes in the rheumatic or nephritic patient differs from that in normal individuals.

## Diagnostic Value of Streptococcal Antibody Studies in Man

Aside from any possible value streptococcal antibodies may have in inactivating streptococcal enzymes, they are extremely useful in establishing the occurrence of a recent streptococcal infection. In many patients the preceding streptococcal pharyngitis may have been so mild as to be overlooked or forgotten by the time the rheumatic manifestations appear. In such cases, especially if the rheumatic symptoms are not entirely typical, significant elevations of the titers of one or more antistreptococcal antibodies is evidence of a recent streptococcal infection, a finding which tends to confirm the diagnosis of rheumatic fever.[71] In the absence of a significant rise in the titer of these antibodies, this diagnosis is unlikely.

The antistreptolysin O antibodies are determined most commonly because they can be measured easily and accurately. If, in addition to antistreptolysin O determinations, other antistreptococcal antibodies, such as antihyaluronidase or antistreptokinase, are measured, evidence of a preceding recent streptococcal infection can be obtained in virtually 100 per cent of rheumatic patients. Individuals who become carriers of group A streptococci without an infection developing do not show a rise in antistreptococcal antibodies. Antibody studies, therefore, are generally accepted as a means of distinguishing the streptococcal carrier from the infected patient.

In contrast to this point of view, Dunlap and Harvey have presented evidence suggesting that type-specific immunity not infrequently develops in streptococcal carriers who have never had a subclinical infection.[15] The occurrence of inapparent infections with group A streptococci, identified only by a significant rise in antistreptococcal antibodies, has been observed repeatedly. It must be emphasized, however, that it seems unlikely that the anti-M antibodies demonstrated by the long-chain reaction used by Dunlap and Harvey, indicative of type-specific immunity, differ from the other streptococcal antibodies and arise in the absence of infection merely as the result of the carrier state.

## STREPTOCOCCAL PHARYNGITIS PRECEDING THE FIRST RHEUMATIC ATTACK

The attack of streptococcal pharyngitis, which precipitates the initial episode of rheumatic fever, has no distinctive clinical features. It may be moderately severe or so mild as to be unrecognized by the child or his parents. The presence of pharyngeal exudate is not a reliable sign of a streptococcal infection since it occurs in viral as well as in bacterial infections. Strains with nephritogenic properties occur in only a few serologic types. Strains with "rheumatogenic" properties, on the other hand, are not associated with any special type, but may occur in any of the 55 known serologic types.[42, 85] Localization of the streptococci in the upper respiratory tract is essential. Skin infections due to group A streptococci are never, as far as is known, followed by rheumatic fever.[16] Strains isolated from patients with acute pharyngitis are frequently typable by the precipitin reaction with the available anti-M type-specific sera because they are rich in M protein. Usually typable strains evoke good antibody responses to the various streptococcal antigens. The most important single factor, which determines whether or not rheumatic sequelae will occur, is the magnitude of the rise in these antistreptococcal antibodies from the preinfection level, usually measured by sequential antistreptolysin O determinations.[85]

## CHARACTERISTICS OF EPIDEMIC STRAINS

Knowledge of the epidemiology of streptococcal upper respiratory infections and the subsequent development of rheumatic sequelae was greatly augmented by research studies carried out in military installations during World War II.[91] It was found that each outbreak was usually due to the spread of not more than two or three serologic types of group A streptococci. These strains were rich in M protein and therefore were readily typable by the precipitin reaction.

In addition to a high content of M antigen, typical epidemic strains often have large hyaluronic acid capsules. Hyaluronic acid is not antigenic, and the lack of antigenicity is usually attributed to the fact that this substance is an integral component of animal tissues.[13] Streptococcal hyaluronate is chemically identical with hyaluronate derived from such diverse sources as umbilical cord, mammalian connective tissue, and bovine and human synovial fluid. No antigenic stimulus occurs, therefore, when this substance is injected into animals.

## PHAGOCYTOSIS: ROLE OF HYALURONIC ACID CAPSULE AND M ANTIGEN

At present most observers agree that the hyaluronic acid capsule is a factor in the virulence of group A streptococci, but definitely of less importance than the M protein.[69] However, in laboratory tests, especially in the absence of M antigen, the presence of these capsules impedes phagocytosis somewhat; this probably occurs similarly in the human host.[57] Thus capsules surrounding group A streptococci may be presumed to facilitate the spread of these organisms and to favor their serial passage from one person to another.

The M antigen, which inhibits phagocytosis much more markedly, is localized on the outer surface of the streptococci. However, if homologous type-specific M antibodies are present, the specific antigenic sites are inactivated and the organisms are phagocytized and eliminated. Antibodies against other protein antigens, such as the T and R antigens, have no protective effect.

## HUMAN SERUM FACTOR IN PHAGOCYTOSIS

One of the most interesting findings to be derived from these studies of phagocytosis has been the observation that human blood is usually necessary for phagocytosis in *in vitro* bactericidal tests with streptococci. Rothbard showed that the essential factor is present in both human plasma and serum but not in the blood cells.[68] He found it is relatively thermostable, being destroyed at 70°C. but not at 56°C.

Stollerman and his coworkers also studied this phenomenon.[82] They reported that of 25 human sera tested, only two lacked this factor. In rabbits, on the other hand, this property is usually absent and is demonstrable only rarely. The activity of the factor is independent of complement. Its presence is, however, required for the phagocytosis of encapsulated streptococci. Although other organisms and inert particles are readily phagocytosed in its absence, Stollerman and his coworkers and Hirsch and Church agreed that the serum factor counteracted the antiphagocytic properties of the hyaluronic acid capsule.[32] The nature of this interesting constituent is not known and deserves further investigation.

### EPIDEMIC STREPTOCOCCAL PHARYNGITIS

Most outbreaks in the north temperate zone start in the winter months and continue into spring, subsiding in May or June. In closed communities new cases continue to occur until all the susceptible individuals have contracted the infection. Studies in military camps showed clearly that streptococci are transmitted directly from person to person by droplets. Although it was thought for many years that these infections were spread by means of blankets, dust, and other fomites, the work of Perry and his collaborators at Fort Warren Air Force Base, Wyoming, in 1957 refuted this concept.[60] Using human volunteers, these investigators were unable to cause infections with washings obtained from contaminated materials present in the patients' immediate environment.

It seems probable that rapid human passage during an epidemic might increase the M content of the strain. It is well known that in mice serial passage of streptococci usually increases the content of M antigen. These mouse-passaged strains used for the immunization of rabbits usually yield potent anti-M sera. Similarly, it seems possible that in epidemics in which streptococci are passed rapidly from person to person, the strain may acquire more M antigen and, therefore, be more likely to evoke a significant antibody response in the human host.

In individuals followed from the beginning to the end of their illness, strains isolated during the late carrier stage have been shown to contain less M antigen than those isolated earlier.[70] During epidemics a similar reduction in M antigen of the epidemic strain often occurs as the outbreak wanes. This change might be related to the decreasing number of human passages as well as to the effect of seasonal factors. Krause et al. investigated these possibilities during an epidemic occurring in a military installation situated in a northern zone. Some of the patients were sent to Florida for convalescence, and matched controls remained in the original cold climate.[39] With the passage of time most of the streptococci still being carried in both groups no longer gave a type-specific M precipitin reaction. However, when M antigen was restored to these late epidemic strains by laboratory passage through mice, it was found to be of the same serologic type as that of the strain which had caused the acute infection in these individuals, regardless of whether they had remained in the original cold environment or had been transported to Florida.

### ATTACK RATE

During outbreaks of streptococcal pharyngitis in military personnel, the attack rate of 3 per cent for rheumatic fever in different epidemics caused by different serologic types remained remarkably constant.[63] In civilian populations epidemics of streptococcal pharyngitis similar to those observed in military installations are uncommon except in boarding schools and similar closed populations.

A civilian epidemic of 18 cases of rheumatic fever did occur in a small, isolated, rural community in North Dakota.[102] The pattern of this outbreak was essentially the same as that of the epidemics observed among military personnel. In a follow-up report Zimmerman and Siegel outlined the conditions on the basis of which, in a given population, an epidemic of streptococcal pharyngitis and rheumatic fever might be predicted.[101] They therefore suggested that under these circumstances mass civilian prophylaxis should be considered.

In contrast to the high attack rate (3 per cent) of rheumatic fever following epidemics of streptococcal pharyngitis, the incidence of rheumatic fever following sporadic streptococcal upper respiratory infections is low. In a study of 519 Chicago school children with untreated streptococcal pharyngitis, Siegel et al. observed only two cases of rheumatic fever, an attack rate of 0.33 per cent, which is about one-tenth of the rate common under epidemic conditions.[75] Of the 519 strains of group A streptococci isolated, only 273, or 52 per cent, were typable by the precipitin technique. Among the typable strains approximately 50 per cent belonged to five different serologic types. The amount of M antigen in 48 per cent of the strains appeared to be low because the serologic types of these organisms could not be identified with the available diagnostic anti-M rabbit sera. The relative avirulence of the sporadic strains was also indicated by the weak antibody response elicited by these infections. Only 54 per cent of the patients showed a significant rise in titer of one or more antistreptococcal antibodies. Similar results under nonepidemic conditions were reported by Goslings et al.[26]

Because streptococcal infections are so common and yet the incidence of rheumatic fever in the general population is low (0.3 per cent), it was not surprising that for many years the role of group A streptococci in this disease was not generally accepted. It was not until it was clearly demonstrated that rheumatic recurrences could be prevented by maintaining rheumatic patients on continuous antistreptococcal prophylaxis that these organisms were generally accepted as an essential factor in the etiology of rheumatic fever.[94]

## PREVENTION OF RHEUMATIC FEVER

There is general agreement that once a diagnosis of rheumatic fever has been made, it is mandatory that the patient be placed on continuous antimicrobial prophylaxis to prevent subsequent streptococcal infections which might be followed by further rheumatic attacks and lead to progressive irreversible cardiac damage.[53] How long antistreptococcal prophylaxis should be maintained is controversial. Some observers are of the opinion that in rheumatic individuals, provided that the cardiac findings are entirely normal, prophylaxis may be safely discontinued at the age of 22 years, when college and military training have usually been completed. After puberty susceptibility to streptococcal infections appears to decline. Whether this is the result of immunity produced by infections caused by the serologic types prevalent in the community or due to an age factor is not known.[33] In individuals over

22 years with normal cardiac findings,[19] even if they should develop a rheumatic recurrence, it is unlikely that significant carditis would occur.[17] However, in patients with unequivocal evidence of rheumatic heart disease, a streptococcal infection, however mild, at any age, may precipitate a rheumatic recurrence. In such individuals prophylaxis should be continued throughout life. The decision to prescribe continuous drug prophylaxis for many years is a serious one. Active immunization against group A streptococci, if feasible, would be preferable and this possibility is being actively investigated at the present time.[19, 80]

The initial attack of rheumatic fever, as well as rheumatic recurrences, is preventable. Penicillin given in therapeutic doses maintained for 10 days in most instances eliminates streptococci from the nasopharynx. The crucial factor is the elimination of the streptococcal antigen from the tissues of the host.

Unlike many other diseases, an attack of rheumatic fever does not make the patient immune. The initial episode identifies the individual as a rheumatic subject prone to repeated rheumatic recurrences following subsequent infections with other rheumatogenic strains of group A streptococci.

It has been repeatedly observed that rheumatic individuals may have several intercurrent attacks of streptococcal pharyngitis without a rheumatic recurrence developing. Subsequently, however, following another streptococcal infection, a typical rheumatic attack may occur. Each of the streptococcal strains causing these infections is due to a different serologic type. No differences are apparent either in the clinical symptoms or in the immunologic responses to explain why the last of these successive infections is followed by a rheumatic recurrence.[41]

It seemed possible that special properties of the strains might determine whether or not a particular infection is followed by a rheumatic attack. It is well known that different strains of group A streptococci vary greatly in their cellular antigenic components and in their extracellular products. In most instances, what causes this variability of strains of group A streptococci is not known. Variations in erythrogenic toxin production by different strains has been repeatedly observed, but remained unexplained until the studies of Zabriskie.[98] This investigator showed that erythrogenic toxin production depends on infection of the strain with temperate bacteriophage. This finding indicated that a viral infection of group A streptococci might profoundly alter their synthetic processes. It was thought possible bacteriophage infection might also cause other changes in group A streptococci such as the property to precipitate rheumatic fever. This possibility was investigated by Kuttner (unpublished observations).

Kuttner studied bacteriophage infection in epidemic strains of Types 32 and 36 which had caused outbreaks of pharyngitis at Irvington House followed by a high incidence of rheumatic recurrences in this convalescent home for rheumatic children.[42] A Type 5 strain isolated from an epidemic of streptococcal pharyngitis occurring in nonrheumatic school children living in an isolated rural community, Dickinson, North Dakota, was also studied.[102] These strains were irradiated with ultraviolet light and then tested with three bacteriophage sensitive indicators without showing any evidence of bacteriophage infection. With the same technique, group A streptococci of six different serologic types isolated from sporadic cases of rheumatic fever were also tested. In only one instance was bacteriophage infection demonstrated, and this was in a Type 14 strain isolated from a mild case of rheumatic polyarthritis. The predominantly negative results may have been due to the lack of suitable indicator strains. The possible role of bacteriophage infection in inducing "rheumatogenic" properties deserves further study.

It appears, therefore, that the potency of different strains of group A streptococci to precipitate rheumatic sequelae may depend on unknown properties which so far have not been identified with temperate bacteriophage infection or with any known cellular components or extracellular products of these organisms. Nevertheless the concept of "rheumatogenic" strains is useful as a working hypothesis.

## Current Hypotheses Regarding the Pathogenesis of Rheumatic Fever

1. *Is rheumatic fever due to the persistence in the patient of group A streptococci or variants of these organisms?* Numerous attempts to isolate group A hemolytic streptococci from blood cultures, joint fluids, nodules, and cardiac tissues of rheumatic patients have been uniformly negative. During 1939 to 1940, however, several English pathologists reported the isolation of group A streptococci from the cardiac tissues of patients dying of acute rheumatic fever.[11, 28, 86] Interest in these findings was revived in 1950 when it was shown that the initial attack of rheumatic fever could be prevented if the preceding streptococcal infection was treated with therapeutic doses of penicillin maintained for 10 days sufficient to eradicate streptococci.[8]

To test the possibility that cardiac damage might be due to the persistence of streptococci, the administration of massive doses of penicillin continued for six weeks, was employed in a field trial in Chile: 49 children with an initial attack of rheumatic fever were given penicillin and 48 matched patients received no antimicrobial therapy.[58] No significant differences were observed either during the acute stage or in follow-up studies between the treated and untreated children. It seems possible, moreover, that the isolation of group A streptococci from cardiac tissues reported by the English pathologists may have been due to contamination from other infected sites such as lymph nodes. Watson et al. reported that if strict surgical technique was employed at the autopsy table, no streptococci were demonstrable in cardiac tissues.[92]

No systematic attempts to isolate L forms of group A streptococci from rheumatic fever patients have been reported. It seems unlikely, however, that the lesions of rheumatic fever are due to the persistence of L forms.

2. *Are cross reactions between group A streptococcal components and cardiac tissues a factor?* Further evidence that group A streptococci might play a direct role in causing cardiac lesions was suggested by the findings of Kaplan.[34] By immunofluorescent techniques he showed that antistreptococcal antibodies present in sera of rabbits immunized with streptococci as

well as in the sera of rheumatic patients caused antigen-antibody reactions on cardiac tissue slices. Similar observations were made by Zabriskie and Freimer.[100] The exact location of the streptococcal antigens responsible for these cross reactions has not been definitely established. Kaplan is of the opinion that these antigens are in the streptococcal cell wall, whereas Zabriskie and Freimer have presented evidence that there is a cross reactive antigen in the protoplast membranes. Several different antigens may be involved.

In addition, both groups of authors have described nonspecific antigens in heart muscle which give rise to antibodies, especially in postcardiotomy patients or in those with long-standing heart disease. These nonspecific antibodies can be absorbed from human sera only with muscle preparations or extracts.

On the other hand, antistreptococcal membrane antisera prepared in rabbits, as well as some human sera from rheumatic fever patients, contain no nonspecific heart-reactive antibodies. The antimembrane antibody, which is present, appears to be specific for streptococcal membranes and for the related membrane antigen present in the sarcolemma sheaths of heart muscle, and can be absorbed by preparations containing one or the other of these membrane antigens. Thus, purified streptococcal membranes and partially purified "sarcolemmal sheaths" absorbed these antibodies both from sera obtained from rheumatic fever patients and from sera of rabbits immunized with streptococcal membranes.

Zabriskie has presented evidence that the elevated titers of heart-reactive membrane antibody in patients with rheumatic fever may be of value in differentiating rheumatic patients from those with uncomplicated streptococcal infections or with unrelated arthritic or immunologic disorders. He presents a tentative hypothesis, as illustrated in his Figure 12, "that repeated streptococcal episodes (perhaps with subclinical symptoms of disease) are necessary to stimulate the production of heart-reactive antibodies, and only at a point when the titers are sufficiently elevated will the full-blown disease complex appear."[99] Zabriskie states that, as yet, there is no objective evidence to establish this hypothesis. It is tempting to speculate that perhaps the rheumatic recurrence would only occur if patients with elevated titers of heart-reactive antibodies contracted an infection with a "rheumatogenic" strain of group A streptococci (group A, Type 18, in Zabriskie's illustration).

In 1967 Goldstein and his coworkers reported observations which likewise suggested a direct link between streptococcal infections and rheumatic fever.[24] These investigators demonstrated cross reactions between antibodies against the group-specific carbohydrate of group A streptococci and the structural glycoproteins of cardiac valves. An antigen-antibody reaction occurring in the valvular connective tissue would probably prevent the valves from functioning efficiently and thus might cause mitral insufficiency, the cardiac lesion most commonly encountered in rheumatic children.

3. *Is rheumatic fever related to genetic factors leading to autoimmune hypersensitivity?* Rantz and his coworkers studied repeated streptococcal infections and the antistreptolysin O titers in children of different ages.[66] In infants less than 17 months of age, elevation in antistreptolysin O titers was absent or minimal, even in those with purulent complications such as otitis

media. In older children, as the result of repeated stimuli, the antistreptolysin O titer rose to the usual postinfection levels. In the opinion of these investigators, rheumatic fever is rare in children less than three years of age because it is only after several streptococcal infections have had time to occur that a significant immune response develops. In the absence of definite rise in the titer of antistreptococcal antibodies rheumatic fever does not occur.[85]

In the preprophylactic era, the initial attack of rheumatic fever was often followed by one or more rheumatic recurrences each of which was preceded by a streptococcal infection due to a different serologic type of group A streptococcus. In such patients the length of the latent period between the precipitating streptococcal infection and the appearance of rheumatic symptoms was approximately the same in the first and in subsequent attacks.[16, 64] Since rheumatic fever occurs only after the individual has had several streptococcal infections, the antibody response even in the initial rheumatic attack represents a secondary reaction to the antigen. In secondary responses, the length of time before the rise of antibodies occurs remains relatively constant. Therefore, it is not surprising that successive attacks do not lead to a shortening of the latent period in rheumatic patients. It is only with antigens not previously encountered that the length of the latent period after the second as compared to the first injection is markedly decreased, as is commonly observed with horse serum in serum sickness.

Hypersensitivity of the delayed type occurs in many different kinds of diseases of viral as well as bacteriologic origin. Exposure to group A streptococci is universal and, therefore, almost everyone becomes hypersensitive to these organisms and their products. With the crude antigens currently available, which contain a mixture of antigenic substances, the sensitivity of rheumatic patients does not appear to be more marked than that observed in normal individuals.

Knowledge of delayed hypersensitivity is based chiefly on data obtained from studies of the tuberculin reaction. At present positive tuberculin reactions in school children and young adults are observed less frequently than formerly. The number of individuals with positive tuberculin reactions is decreasing. This decline in positive reactions is considered to be due to the decreased exposure to the tubercle bacillus which is probably related to better diagnostic procedures and the widespread use of effective antituberculous therapy. Similar observations regarding streptococcal hypersensitivity have not been noted and there is nothing to suggest that a decline in the prevalence of group A streptococci has occurred. During the last 24 years the incidence of initial rheumatic attacks has shown no significant change.[55]

There is general agreement that following streptococcal pharyngitis, the individuals in whom rheumatic fever is most likely to develop are those who show a streptococcal antibody rise of significant magnitude above their preinfection level. Usually hypersensitivity reactions in man and in animals are accompanied by marked elevations of antibody titers.

The administration of penicillin in therapeutic dose for 10 to 14 days to patients with streptococcal upper respiratory infections is accepted as the best method currently available for preventing rheumatic sequelae. It seems likely that this therapeutic regimen is effective because the streptococci are eradicated from the tissues of the host. The antigenic stimulus is thereby curtailed so that a maximal antibody response does not occur.

A high familial incidence has been repeatedly observed and has led to the investigation of hereditary factors by several observers.[21, 27, 49, 78, 79, 96, 97] These studies indicate a probable hereditary predisposition. However, because of the difficulties of accurate diagnosis, the role of a genetic constitution in the onset of rheumatic fever is impossible to assess. There are differences in the penetrance and expressivity of the genotype. An unusual feature appears to be that the susceptibility to rheumatic fever is affected by hereditary factors which do not influence the frequency of streptococcal infections. In contrast, some investigators are of the opinion that an increased susceptibility to streptococcal infection is the important factor rather than a hereditary tendency to develop rheumatic fever.[12]

In addition to the marked variability of the clinical manifestations of rheumatic fever, another complicating factor is that a trigger mechanism of streptococcal infections is essential. Rheumatic fever, therefore, does not lend itself readily to accurate genetic analysis.

Nevertheless there is no doubt that the initial rheumatic episode serves as an indicator of the rheumatic genotype. Once an individual has had an attack of rheumatic fever, his response to subsequent upper respiratory infections caused by other potent "rheumatogenic" strains of group A streptococci is established, as shown by the fact that such infections are likely to be followed in 20 to 50 per cent of such patients by repeated rheumatic recurrences. In the normal individual, infections with such "rheumatogenic strains" are not followed by rheumatic fever. Moreover, the patient with acute glomerulonephritis, in contrast to the rheumatic individual, has a single attack following an infection with a nephritogenic strain and usually recovers completely.

It therefore is apparent that the genotype of the rheumatic subject differs both from that of the normal person and from that of the nephritic individual. So far no distinctive properties of "rheumatogenic" strains of group A streptococci have been identified. It may be that the decisive factors which determine the occurrence of rheumatic sequelae depend not on special characteristics of the precipitating "rheumatogenic" streptococcal strain, but on unknown or known streptococcal antigens which have been modified by host factors characteristic of the rheumatic genotype. These altered antigens could then give rise to antibodies capable of sensitizing various tissues of the host such as the joints, brain, skin, and heart.

## ACUTE GLOMERULONEPHRITIS

Acute glomerulonephritis, like rheumatic fever, is a nonsuppurative complication of group A streptococcal infections. How these bacteria cause the symptomatology characteristic of each of these two diseases is not known. It seems probable that the pathologic processes are basically different because the simultaneous occurrence of nephritis and rheumatic fever in the same patient is extremely uncommon.[77] In contrast to rheumatic fever, the overall prognosis of acute glomerulonephritis in children is excellent. Early in the attack in patients with hypertension, however, serious and sometimes fatal cerebral or cardiac complications may occur. The hypertension is considered to be due to generalized vasospasm caused by the production of hypertensive agents by the glomerular inflammation. Usually the hypertension subsides with bed rest. If, however, hypertension is marked or persists, it may be advisable to administer antihypertensive drugs. Recovery is complete without residual brain or cardiac damage.

## ETIOLOGY

It was known for many years that epidemics of scarlet fever were often followed by acute glomerulonephritis. It was noted, however, that in different outbreaks the attack rate of renal complications varied greatly.[63] This marked variability in the attack rate suggested to Rammelkamp that only certain serologic types of group A streptococci might have special nephritogenic properties. In 1953 Rammelkamp and Weaver reported that in a naval installation an outbreak of pharyngitis due to group A streptococcus Type 12 was followed by a high incidence of acute glomerulonephritis.[65] In contrast, upper respiratory infections, caused by three other serologic types occurring among patients hospitalized simultaneously with acute exudative pharyngitis, were not followed by renal complications. Furthermore, it was noted by these investigators that not every epidemic of Type 12 pharyngitis was associated with glomerulonephritis.[65]

In the same year as Rammelkamp's studies, Reed reported 21 cases of nephritis in children following pharyngitis due to Type 12 occurring in a small rural area of Nova Scotia.[67] Other studies showed that respiratory infections caused by Type 4 streptococci also were followed by nephritis. In 1954 Kleinman reported an epidemic of 63 cases of acute glomerulonephritis which occurred among Indian children at the Red Lake Indian Reservation in northern Minnesota.[36] During the summer months scarlet fever and impetigo were prevalent. Group A streptococci were isolated from the skin lesions and from the pharynx. It was shown by Updyke that these strains represented a new serologic type, designated Type 49.[89] Since 1954 in many different parts of the world Type 49 has been isolated from the throat and skin of patients with nephritis. It is associated with renal sequelae irrespective of whether it is localized in the skin or in the pharynx.[3, 54]

Ten years after the original outbreak of nephritis at Red Lake the bacteriology of pyoderma among the children on this Indian Reservation was again investigated.[3, 4] Only eight children had acute glomerulonephritis during 1964 to 1965. Type 49 was not isolated from these patients. However, in the summer and fall of 1966, acute glomerulonephritis developed in 26 children who had pustular skin lesions due to Type 49.[18] These patients had minimal symptoms of kidney involvement, but confirmation of the diagnosis of acute glomerulonephritis was obtained by renal biopsy in 21 children. The remaining patients were not available for biopsy.

In an outbreak of nephritis following pharyngitis in Prague, Šramek (1964) found strains which he could only identify as having a 14 T antigen without a detectable M antigen, although this was later identified as being Type 49.[76] Several other outbreaks in Europe were due to similar strains,[54] and Köhler noted that strains of the M Types 14, 35, 49, and 51 share a common T antigen.[37] Type 35, isolated at Irvington House in 1937,[42] has been found to be identical with Type 49 by several investigators and these strains are now included with Type 49 (Subcommittee on Streptococci and Pneumococci, 1967, Int. J. Syst. Bact.).

Maxted has recently reviewed the findings with regard to Type 49 and has described the preparation of specially absorbed antisera which gave type-specific agglutination of trypsin-digested suspensions of streptococci belonging to Types 14 and 49, respectively.[54] Apparently the antigens concerned were T antigens, and not M antigens, since they were unaffected by tryptic digestion. In Types 14 and 49 the presence of another T antigen, common to both, had caused confusion. This T antigen was previously unidentified in Type 49 and had been found only in Type 14 strains.

Only a few T antigens with the same type-specificity as the M antigen are known in other types: these occur in Type 6 and, with the exception of one strain (strain C203), in Type 1. Possibly further investigation might reveal type-specific T antigens in still other serologic types.

### STREPTOCOCCAL SKIN INFECTIONS

Clinicians for more than 25 years had noted the association of nephritis and skin infections.[20] In contrast to the streptococci isolated from the pharynx during streptococcal epidemics, usually the strains of group A streptococci isolated from impetiginous lesions could not be typed by the precipitin reaction, and therefore were frequently considered to be "untypable." With the slide agglutination technique, however, Parker et al. and Barrow showed that impetigo strains could be differentiated into a small number of distinctive patterns on the basis of T antigens.[5, 59] These T agglutination patterns were characteristic of group A streptococci isolated from skin lesions. The most commonly encountered patterns were: 3/13/B3264, 5/11/12/27/44, and 8/25/Imp.19. The findings of Parker and his coworkers and by Barrow on impetigo strains have led to renewed interest in studying skin infections. Their work has been confirmed by other investigators and extended to a study of the relationship of skin infections and glomerulonephritis.[14, 52]

In order to identify strains with distinctive T antigen patterns more precisely, Top and his coworkers, in 1967, immunized rabbits with strains of several different T antigen patterns.[87] With some of the strains of the various patterns these investigators obtained potent anti-M precipitating sera for three new serologic types (Types 52, 53, and 54). These findings were confirmed by bactericidal studies. At the same time Poon-King and his coworkers investigated an outbreak of acute glomerulonephritis among children living in southern Trinidad.[61] Strains of group A streptococci isolated from the skin and from the pharynx also showed the characteristic T antigen patterns associated with impetigo. Rabbits were immunized with these strains. In accord with Top's results, Potter found that strains in her series with the 3/13/B3264 T antigen pattern could be identified as the serologic Type 52 first isolated in Minnesota.

In addition, Potter found that other strains with the 8/25/Imp.19 pattern represent a new nephritogenic type, designated as serologic Type 55 (personal communication). So far, nephritogenic strains have been identified in five serologic types, Types 12, 4, 49, 52, and 55, and occasional strains in other types. It seems likely that as studies of outbreaks of acute glomerulonephritis are continued, other nephritogenic strains may be isolated among additional serologic types.

The difficulties encountered with Type 49 show that the finding of "new" types will not solve every typing problem. In addition to Type 49, other well recognized types such as Types 4 and 28 fail to evoke a strong anti-M antibody response in rabbits even if highly mouse-virulent strains (often successful with other types) are available as immunizing strains. The chemical basis for the marked differences in antigenicity of different M antigens is not known. Are the M antigens which usually do not give good precipitating antisera situated less superficially on the cell wall, or are these M antigens bound to some unknown substance or substances which interfere with antigenicity? One clue to these differences in antigenicity, which deserves further investigation, is suggested by the findings of Gooder[25] and Köhler.[37] They found that strains giving a poor antibody response were those which produced lipoproteinase. This finding might be useful in the much-needed solution of the problem of how to prepare potent antisera of all serologic types of group A streptococci. Whether improvement of our immunization procedures can best be achieved by more detailed studies of the chemical properties of the M proteins or by new methods for evoking a better immune response in the preparation of type-specific antisera is an area which deserves intensive research.

Other methods of study in addition to determining type-specificity have been employed by several investigators in attempts to differentiate nephritogenic from non-nephritogenic strains of streptococci. Hardin et al. studied strains of Types 12 and 4 isolated from patients with acute glomerulonephritis.[31] They tried to detect any possible differences between these strains and strains of group A streptococci isolated from rheumatic patients, from individuals with uncomplicated streptococcal pharyngitis, and from asymptomatic streptococcal carriers. They investigated streptolysin O and S production, streptokinase, hyaluronic acid, hyaluronidase, proteinase, and erythrogenic toxin. No significant differences were demonstrable.

Subsequent investigations of other properties, however, suggest that the nephritogenic types may have special characteristics. Wilson showed that 11 of 12 strains of Type 12 isolated from nephritic patients were leukotoxic for human leukocytes.[95] With Type 4 strains leukotoxicity was variable as it was with non-nephritogenic serologic types. Bernheimer, Lazarides, and Wilson noted a striking correlation between leukotoxicity and DPNase (diphosphopyridine nucleotidase) production in 22 strains of Types 12 and 4.[6]

Kuttner studied bacteriocines produced by group A and nongroup A streptococci.[40] Without exception 32 strains of Types 12, 4, and 49 isolated from nephritic patients produced bacteriocines. The majority of strains of Types 12 and 4 isolated from patients without renal complications also produced bacteriocines. The production of these substances by other serologic types of group A streptococci, and by streptococcal strains other than group A, was variable and occurred much less frequently.

Similar studies regarding special characteristics of the newly established nephritogenic Types 52 and 55 would be of interest. Eventually it may become possible to define what differentiates nephritogenic types or strains from other non-nephritogenic organisms.

## Pathogenesis

A current hypothesis to explain why the nephritogenic types cause acute glomerulonephritis postulates that these types contain a specific antigen which cross reacts with a special glomerular antigen characteristic of the "nephritis-prone" individual.[50] According to Markowitz and Lange, antibodies are formed during the course of streptococcal pharyngitis which unite first with the streptococcal nephritogenic antigen and then as an antigen-antibody complex unite with the special glomerular protein on the basement membrane of these nephritis-prone individuals. This reaction is accompanied by marked decrease in serum complement and an accumulation of polymorphonuclear leukocytes which conjointly may be responsible for the disease and is considered to be the cause of the renal lesion.

An alternate hypothesis has been advanced by Andres and his coworkers using immunofluorescent techniques.[2] They studied biopsy specimens obtained from patients with acute severe glomerulonephritis following group A Type 12 pharyngitis, and showed that Type 12 antistreptococcal antibodies bound to electron-dense deposits in the glomerular tissue of nephritic patients, but no binding was noted in the glomerular tissues obtained from normal individuals or from patients with other types of renal disease. With specific antisera prepared against gamma globulin, beta 1c globulin (complement 3'), and group A Type 12 streptococci, they demonstrated that all three of these substances were present in the antigen-antibody complexes. Antisera to streptococcal types other than Type 12 were nonreactive. These authors conclude that poststreptococcal nephritis is a result of glomerular damage from antigen-antibody complexes. However, they did not exclude the possibility of a cross reaction.

It would be of great interest to determine whether these findings regarding post-Type 12 glomerulonephritis are also valid in nephritis following Type 49. Biopsy material that confirmed the diagnosis of acute glomerulonephritis was obtained from 21 children during the 1967 outbreak of Type 49 infections at the Red Lake Indian Reservation. This material presents a unique opportunity to confirm and extend the hypothesis advanced for Type 12 nephritis. A serious technical obstacle, however, to such studies with Type 49 is the difficulty encountered by every investigator in the preparation of Type 49 antiserum.

It is possible that similar studies of the renal biopsy material obtained in Trinidad[61] from children with acute glomerulonephritis following infections with Types 52 or 55 might prove more satisfactory than those with Type 49 because the preparation of antisera to these two new types apparently presents no special difficulties.

Another aspect of acute glomerulonephritis, which urgently needs further investigation, is the variability of different strains of the known nephritogenic types in inducing renal sequelae. The attack rate of acute glomerulonephritis following outbreaks of pharyngitis due to Type 12 varies greatly, from 0 to 17 per cent.[90] During the last 20 to 30 years, upper respiratory infections due to group A streptococci Type 12 have been extremely common in many different parts of the world. These infections in some instances were followed by acute glomerulonephritis, whereas in others none of the patients developed renal sequelae.

Similar differences in nephritogenic properties of strains occurring in the newly identified Type 52 have also been observed. No cases of nephritis following skin infections due to Type 52 occurred in 1966 at Red Lake, Minnesota[3, 4] but in Trinidad, following infections due to this type, renal symptoms were frequently observed. Whether these differences are due to strain differences or host factors is not known.

## SUMMARY

Infection with group A streptococci is an essential factor in the etiology of both rheumatic fever and acute glomerulonephritis. Although both these diseases are nonsuppurative complications of streptococcal infections, there are important differences which are briefly outlined in Table 1.

Some of the differences listed in the table suggest that host factors rather than special characteristics of the streptococcal strains may explain why, in one

TABLE 1.   *Comparison of Rheumatic Fever and Acute Glomerulonephritis**

| | COMMON FEATURES | |
|---|---|---|
| Preceding infection | Group A streptococci | |
| Latent period | 7 to 21 days | |
| Lesions | No streptococci demonstrable | |

| | IMPORTANT DIFFERENCES | |
|---|---|---|
| | *Rheumatic Fever* | *Acute Glomerulonephritis* |
| Site of infection | Pharynx | Pharynx or skin |
| Prior sensitization | Essential | None |
| Infant < 2 yr. old | Rare | Not uncommon |
| Attack rate | Constant | Variable |
| Hereditary tendency | Present | Unknown |
| Family attacks | Staggered | Simultaneous |
| Repeated attacks | Common | None |
| Prophylaxis | Mandatory | Not needed |
| Serologic type | Any of 55 | Few, 5 of 55 |
| Immune response | Marked | Moderate |
| Complement | Normal | Decreased |
| Tissues affected | Joints, heart, brain, skin | Glomerulus |
| Residual lesions | Joints, brain, skin: none | Glomerulus: none |
| | Heart: chronic or none | |
| Prognosis | Heart: permanent damage or recovery | Complete recovery |

* Adapted from Wannamaker.[90]

individual, streptococcal infections are followed by rheumatic sequelae and in another by renal complications. In rheumatic subjects the hereditary tendency and the importance of prior sensitization indicate constitutional differences which are not apparent in the nephritic patient. In some rheumatic patients, chronic and continuing tissue reactions occur which are often exacerbated by successive streptococcal infections and may result in permanent cardiac damage.

The first rheumatic episode serves as an indicator which differentiates the rheumatic subject both from the normal and from the nephritic individual. Once an attack of rheumatic fever has occurred, the risk of repeated rheumatic recurrences subsequent to other infections due to "rheumatogenic" strains of group A streptococci is great.[41] The nephritic individual, on the other hand, has a single attack, the glomerular inflammation subsides, and recovery is complete. Repeated subsequent streptococcal infections with non-nephritogenic strains are not followed by renal complications. It is not known whether a second attack might occur following an infection with an effective strain of a known nephritogenic type other than the type that precipitated the original attack.

Occasionally acute glomerulonephritis and acute rheumatic fever may occur concurrently in the same patient.[77] Such cases are rare and usually data on the serologic types of the strains isolated from these patients are not available.

The concept that only certain strains of a small number of the 55 known serologic types of group A streptococci have special nephritogenic properties is generally accepted. Neither the basis for the nephritogenicity of certain serologic types nor the marked variation in nephritogenic properties from strain to strain of the recognized nephritogenic types is understood. As yet attempts to explain such data have yielded negative results; nevertheless these findings represent a point of departure for future research regarding the pathogenesis of acute glomerulonephritis.

In rheumatic fever, no special serologic types are associated with the streptococcal strains causing the respiratory infections which precipitate the initial rheumatic attack or subsequent rheumatic recurrences. Clinical observations, however, suggest that the same serologic type at different times, in different localities, may include some strains with marked "rheumatogenic" properties and others in which this property is entirely lacking. Such variations may be characteristic of the individual strains and do not appear to be directly related to host factors.

Recent current theories based on cross immunologic reactions between certain streptococcal antigens and human cardiac and glomerular tissues are discussed in relation to the pathogenesis of these diseases.

## References

1. Allison, V. D., and W. Gunn. 1932. Epidemiology of streptococcal infections. Proc. Roy. Soc. 25:927–944.
2. Andres, G. A., L. Accinni, K. C. Hsu, J. B. Zabriskie, and B. Seegal. 1966. Electron microscopic studies of human glomerulonephritis. Localization of antigen-antibody complexes

in glomerular structures of patients with acute glomerulonephritis. J. Exp. Med. *123:*399–412.

3. Anthony, B. F., E. L. Kaplan, S. S. Chapman, P. G. Quie, and L. W. Wannamaker. 1967. Epidemic acute nephritis with reappearance of Type 49 streptococcus. Lancet *2:*787–790.

4. Anthony, B. F., L. Y. Perlman, and L. W. Wannamaker. 1967. Skin infections and acute nephritis in American Indian children. Pediatrics *39:*264–279.

5. Barrow, G. I. 1955. Clinical and bacteriologic aspects of impetigo contagiosa. J. Hyg. *53:*495–508.

6. Bernheimer, A. W., P. D. Lazarides, and A. T. Wilson. 1957. Diphosphopyridine nucleotidase as an extracellular product of streptococcal growth and its possible relationship to leukocytoxicity. J. Exp. Med. *106:*27–37.

7. Bradley, W. H. 1932. Epidemic acute rheumatism in a public school. Quart. J. Med. *1:*79–98.

8. Catanzaro, F. J., C. A. Stetson, A. J. Morris, R. Chamovitz, C. H. Rammelkamp, Jr., B. L. Stolzer, and W. D. Perry. 1954. The role of the streptococcus in the pathogenesis of rheumatic fever. Amer. J. Med. *17:*749–756.

9. Coburn, A. F. 1931. The Factor of Infection in the Rheumatic State. The Williams & Wilkins Co., Baltimore.

10. Collis, W. R. F. 1931. Acute rheumatism and hemolytic streptococci. Lancet *1:*1341–1345.

11. Collis, W. R. F. 1939. Bacteriology of rheumatic fever. Lancet *2:*817–820.

12. Davies, H. M., and E. Lazarov. 1960. Heredity, infection and chemoprophylaxis in rheumatic carditis: an epidemiological study of a communal settlement. J. Hyg. *58:*263–276.

13. Dawson, M. H., and M. Olmsted. 1934. Mucoid phase of streptococcus hemolyticus. Science *80:*296–297.

14. Dillon, H. C., M. W. Moody, and W. R. Maxted. 1965. Epidemiologic and bacteriologic aspects of impetigo and its complications: specificity of streptococcal types. Southern Med. J. *58:*1578.

15. Dunlap, M. B., and L. S. Harvey. 1967. The carrier state and type-specific immunity in streptococcal disease. Amer. J. Dis. Child. *114:*229–243.

16. Earle, D. P., and D. Seegal. 1957. Natural history of glomerulonephritis. J. Chronic Dis. *5:*3–13.

17. Feinstein, A. R., M. Spagnuolo, H. F. Wood, A. Taranta, E. Tursky, and E. Kleinberg. 1964. Clinical features of streptococcal infections and clinical sequelae. Ann. Intern. Med. Suppl. 5. *60:*68–86.

18. Fish, A. J., R. C. Herdman, and R. A. Good. 1967. Investigation of 26 childhood cases of acute epidemic poststreptococcal glomerulonephritis. Program and abstracts. Thirty-Seventh Annual Meeting of the Society for Pediatric Research, Atlantic City, New Jersey, April 28–29, 1967.

19. Fox, E. N., M. K. Wittner, and A. Dorfman. 1966. Antigenicity of the M proteins of group A streptococci. III. Antibody responses and cutaneous hypersensitivity in humans. J. Exp. Med. *124:*1135–1151.

20. Futcher, P. H. 1940. Glomerular nephritis following infections of the skin. Arch. Intern. Med. *65:*1192–1210.

21. Gauld, R. L., and F. E. M. Read. 1940. Studies of rheumatic disease. III. Familial association and aggregation in rheumatic disease. J. Clin. Invest. *19:*393–398.

22. Gill, F. A. 1960. A review of past attempts and present concepts of producing immunity in humans. Quart. Bull. Northwest. Univ. Med. Sch. *34:*326–339.

23. Glover, J. A., and F. Griffith. 1930. An outbreak of scarlet fever at a preparatory school. Lancet *2:*815–817.

24. Goldstein, I., B. Halpern, and L. Robert. 1967. Immunological relationship between streptococcus A polysaccharide and the structural glycoprotein of heart valve. Nature *213:*44–47.

25. Gooder, H. 1961. Association of a serum opacity reaction with serologic type in *Streptococcus pyogenes.* J. Gen. Microbiol. *25:*347–352.

26. Goslings, W. R. O., H. A. Valkenburg, A. W. Bots, and S. C. Lorrier. 1963. Attack rates of streptococcal pharyngitis, rheumatic fever and glomerulonephritis in the general population. I. A controlled pilot study in one village. New Eng. J. Med. *268:*687–694.

27. Gray, F. G., R. W. Quinn, and J. P. Quinn. 1952. A long-term survey of rheumatic and non-rheumatic families with particular reference to environment and heredity. Amer. J. Med. *13:*400–412.

28. Green, C. A. 1939. Researches into the etiology of acute rheumatism. Rheumatic carditis: Postmortem investigation of nine consecutive cases. Ann. Rheum. Dis. *1:*86–98.

29. Griffith, F. 1934. The serological classification of streptococcus pyogenes. J. Hyg. *34:*542–584.

30. Haig-Brown, C. 1886. Tonsillitis in Adolescents. Bailliere, Tendoll and Cox, London.

31. Hardin, R. A., R. W. Quinn, and R. C. Avery. 1956. A survey of hemolytic streptococci

from patients with rheumatic fever, glomerulonephritis, pharyngitis and the carrier state. J. Infect. Dis. *99:*84–89.

32. Hirsch, J. G., and A. B. Church. 1960. Studies of phagocytosis of group A streptococci by polymorphonuclear leucocytes. J. Exp. Med. *111:*309–322.

33. Johnson, E. E., G. H. Stollerman, B. J. Grossman, and H. McCulloch. 1960. Streptococcal infections in adolescents and adults after prolonged freedom from rheumatic fever. New Eng. J. Med. *263:*105–111.

34. Kaplan, M. H. 1963. Immunologic reaction of streptococcal and tissue antigens. I. Properties of an antigen in certain strains of group A streptococci, exhibiting an immunologic cross reaction with human heart tissue. J. Immun. *90:*595–606.

35. Kaplan, M. H., and M. L. Suchy. 1964. Immunologic relation of streptococcal and tissue antigens. II. Cross-reactions of antisera to mammalian heart tissue with a cell wall constituent of certain strains of group A streptococci. J. Exp. Med. *119:*643–649.

36. Kleinman, H. 1954. Epidemic acute glomerulonephritis at Red Lake, Minnesota. Minnesota Med. *37:*479–483.

37. Köhler, W. 1963. Serum opacity reaction and the production of M antigen by *Streptococcus pyogenes.* Zbl. Bakt. [Orig.] *189:*275–281.

38. Krause, R. M., and C. H. Rammelkamp, Jr. 1962. Studies of the carrier state following infection with group A streptococci. II. Infectivity of streptococci isolated during acute pharyngitis and during the carrier state. J. Clin. Invest. *41:*575–587.

39. Krause, R. M., C. H. Rammelkamp, Jr., F. W. Denny, Jr., and L. W. Wannamaker. 1962. Studies of the carrier state following infection with group A streptococci. I. Effect of climate. J. Clin. Invest. *41:*568–574.

40. Kuttner, A. G. 1966. Production of bacteriocines by group A streptococci with special reference to nephritogenic type. J. Exp. Med. *124:*279–291.

41. Kuttner, A. G., and E. Krumwiede. 1941. Observations on the effect of streptococcal upper respiratory infections on rheumatic children. J. Clin. Invest. *20:*273–287.

42. Kuttner, A. G., and E. Krumwiede. 1944. Observations on the epidemiology of streptococcal pharyngitis and the relation of streptococcal carriers to occurrence of outbreaks. J. Clin. Invest. *23:*139–150.

43. Kuttner, A. G., and T. F. Lenert. 1944. The occurrence of bacteriostatic properties in the blood of patients after recovery from streptococcal pharyngitis. J. Clin. Invest. *23:*151–161.

44. Lancefield, R. C. 1933. A serological differentiation of human and other groups of hemolytic streptococci. J. Exp. Med. *57:*571–595.

45. Lancefield, R. C. 1940–1941. Specific relationship of cell composition to biological activity of hemolytic streptococci. Harvey Lectures. The Williams & Wilkins Co., Baltimore, Vol. 36, pp. 251–290.

46. Lancefield, R. C. 1954. Cellular constituents of group A concerned in antigenicity and virulence. *In:* McCarty, M. (Ed.). Streptococcal Infections. Columbia University Press, pp. 3–18.

47. Lancefield, R. C. 1959. Persistence of type-specific antibodies in man following infection with group A streptococci. J. Exp. Med. *116:*271–292.

48. Lancefield, R. C. 1962. Current knowledge of type-specific M antigens of group A streptococci. J. Immun. *89:*307–313.

49. Mallén, M. S., and F. Castillo. 1952. Istudios sabre la genética del rheumatisma cardioaricular. I. La hipótesis de un gene recesivo. Arch. Inst. Cardiol. Mex. *22:*136.

50. Markowitz, A. S., and C. F. Lange. 1964. Streptococcal related glomerulonephritis. J. Immun. *92:*565–575.

51. Markowitz, M. 1963. Studies on type-specific antibodies as indicators of previous streptococcal infections in rheumatic and non-rheumatic children. J. Clin. Invest. *42:*409–416.

52. Markowitz, M., H. D. Bruton, A. G. Kuttner, and L. E. Cluff. 1965. The bacteriologic findings, streptococcal immune response and renal complications in children with impetigo. Pediatrics *35:*393–404.

53. Markowitz, M., and A. G. Kuttner. 1965. Rheumatic Fever. Diagnosis, Management and Prevention. W. B. Saunders Co., Philadelphia.

54. Maxted, W. R., C. A. M. Fraser, and M. T. Parker. 1967. Streptococcus pyogenes, Type 49. A nephritogenic streptococcus with a wide geographical distribution. Lancet *1:*641–644.

55. Mayer, F. F., E. F. Doyle, L. Herrera, and K. D. Brownell. 1963. Declining severity of first attack of rheumatic fever. Amer. J. Dis. Child. *105:*146–152.

56. McCarty, M. 1964. Missing links in the streptococcal chain leading to rheumatic fever. Circulation *39:*488–493.

57. Morris, M., and C. V. Seastone. 1955. The relationship of M protein and resistance to phagocytosis in the beta hemolytic streptococci. J. Bact. *69:*195–203.

58. Mortimer, E. A., Jr., B. S. Vaisman, I. A. Vigneau, L. J. Guash, C. A. Schuster, L. Rakita, R. M. Krause, R. Roberts, and C. H. Rammelkamp, Jr. 1959. The effect of penicillin on acute rheumatic fever and valvular heart disease. New Eng. J. Med. 260:101–112.

59. Parker, M. T., A. J. H. Tomlinson, and R. E. O. Williams. 1955. Impetigo contagiosa: The association of certain types of Staphylococcus aureus and of Streptococcus pyogenes with superficial skin infections. J. Hyg. 53:458–473.

60. Perry, W. D., A. C. Siegel, C. H. Rammelkamp, Jr., L. W. Wannamaker, and C. E. Marple. 1957. Transmission of group A streptococci. I. The role of contaminated bedding. II. The role of contaminated dust. Amer. J. Hyg. 66:85–101.

61. Poon-King, T., I. Mohammed, R. Cox, E. V. Potter, N. M. Simon, A. C. Siegel, and D. P. Earle. 1967. Recurrent epidemic nephritis in South Trinidad. New Eng. J. Med. 277:728–733.

62. Potter, E. V., G. H. Stollerman, and A. C. Siegel. 1962. Recall of type-specific antibodies in man by injections of streptococcal cell walls. J. Clin. Invest. 41:301–310.

63. Rammelkamp, C. H., Jr. 1955–1956. Epidemiology of streptococcal infections. Harvey Lectures. Ser. 51, Academic Press, New York, 1957, pp. 113–142.

64. Rammelkamp, C. H., Jr., and B. L. Stolzer. 1961. The latent period before onset of acute rheumatic fever. Yale J. Biol. Med. 34:386–398.

65. Rammelkamp, C. H., Jr., and R. S. Weaver. 1953. Acute glomerulonephritis. The significance of the variation in the incidence of the disease. J. Clin. Invest. 32:345–358.

66. Rantz, L., A. M. Maroney, and J. M. DiCaprio. 1951. Antistreptolysin O response following hemolytic streptococcal infection in early childhood. Arch. Intern. Med. 87:360–371.

67. Reed, R. W. 1953. Epidemic of acute nephritis. Canad. Med. Assoc. J. 68:448–455.

68. Rothbard, S. 1945. Bacteriostatic effect of human sera on group A streptococci. II. Comparative bacteriostatic effect of normal whole blood from different animal species in the presence of human convalescent sera. J. Exp. Med. 82:107–118.

69. Rothbard, S. 1948. Protective effect of hyaluronidase and type-specific anti-M serum on experimental group A streptococcus infections in mice. J. Exp. Med. 88:325–342.

70. Rothbard, S., and R. F. Watson. 1948. Variation occurring in group A streptococci during human infection. Progressive loss of M substance correlated with increasing susceptibility to bacteriostasis. J. Exp. Med. 87:521–533.

71. Rothbard, S., R. F. Watson, H. F. Swift, and A. T. Wilson. 1948. Bacteriologic and immunologic studies on patients with hemolytic streptococcic infections as related to rheumatic fever. Arch. Intern. Med. 82:229–250.

72. Schlesinger, B. 1930. The relationship of throat infection to acute rheumatism in childhood. Arch. Dis. Child. 5:411.

73. Schmidt, W. D. 1960. Type-specific antibody formation in man following injection of streptococcal M protein. J. Infect. Dis. 106:250–255.

74. Sheldon, W. 1931. On acute rheumatism following tonsillitis. Lancet 1:1337–1341.

75. Siegel, A. C., E. E. Johnson, and G. H. Stollerman. 1961. Controlled studies of streptococcal pharyngitis in a pediatric population. New Eng. J. Med. 265:559–566.

76. Šramek, J. 1964. A contribution to the epidemiology of acute glomerulonephritis associated with group A streptococci different from Type 12. Zbl. Bakt. [Orig.] 196:56 (Symposium pp. 1–79).

77. Stetson, C. A., C. H. Rammelkamp, Jr., R. M. Krause, R. J. Kohen, and W. D. Perry. 1955. Epidemic acute nephritis: Studies on etiology, natural history and prevention. Medicine 34:431–450.

78. Stevenson, A. C., and E. A. Cheeseman. 1953. Heredity and rheumatic fever: A study of 462 families ascertained by affected child and 51 families by affected mother. Ann. Eugenics 17:177–210.

79. Stevenson, A. C., and E. H. Cheeseman. 1956. Heredity and rheumatic fever: Some later information about data collected in 1950–1951. Ann. Hum. Genet. 21:139–143.

80. Stollerman, G. H. 1967. Prospects for a vaccine against group A streptococci: The problem of the immunology of M proteins. Arthritis Rheum. 10:245–255.

81. Stollerman, G. H., and R. Ekstedt. 1957. Long chain formation by strains of group A streptococci in the presence of homologous antisera: A type-specific reaction. J. Exp. Med. 106:345–356.

82. Stollerman, G. H., F. S. Kantor, and B. D. Gordon. 1958. Accessory plasma factors involved in the bacteriocidal test for type-specific antibody to group A streptococci. I. Atypical behavior of some human and rabbit sera. J. Exp. Med. 108:475–491.

83. Stollerman, G. H., M. Rytel, and J. Ontiz. 1963. Accessory plasma cofactor(s) enhancing opsonization of encapsulated organisms. J. Exp. Med. 117:1–17.

84. Taranta, A., S. Torasdag, J. D. Metrakos, W. Jegier, and I. Ushida. 1959. Rheumatic fever in monozygotic and dizygotic twins. Circulation 20:778.

85. Taranta, A., H. F. Wood, A. R. Feinstein, R. S. Simpson, and E. Kleinberg. 1964. Relation of the rheumatic recurrence rate per streptococcal infection to the titers of streptococcal antibodies. Ann. Intern. Med. Suppl. 5. *60*:47–57.
86. Thomson, S., and J. Innes. 1940. Hemolytic streptococci in cardiac lesions of acute rheumatism. Brit. Med. J. *2*:733–736.
87. Top, F. H., L. W. Wannamaker, W. R. Maxted, and B. E. Anthony. 1967. M antigens among group A streptococci isolated from skin lesions. J. Exp. Med. *126*:667–685.
88. Trousseau, A. 1865. Clinique Médicale de Hôtel Dieu de Paris. 2nd ed. J.-B. Bailliere et fils, Paris, Vol. 1, p. 106.
89. Updyke, E. L., M. S. Moore, and E. Conroy. 1955. Provisional new type of group A streptococcus associated with nephritis. Science *121*:171–172.
90. Wannamaker, L. W. 1961. Theoretical and practical implications of the epidemiologic differences between acute rheumatic fever and acute nephritis. N. Carolina Med. J. *22*:485–492.
91. Wannamaker, L. W., C. H. Rammelkamp, Jr., F. W. Denny, W. R. Brink, H. B. Hauser, E. O. Hahn, and J. H. Dingle. 1951. Prophylaxis of acute rheumatic fever by treatment of the preceding streptococcal infection with various amounts of depot penicillin. Amer. J. Med. *10*:673–695.
92. Watson, R. F., G. K. Hirst, and R. C. Lancefield. 1961. Bacteriologic studies of cardiac tissues obtained at autopsy from eleven patients dying with rheumatic fever. Arthritis Rheum. *4*:74–85.
93. Wolfe, C. K. S., J. A. Hayashi, G. Walsh, and S. S. Barkulis. 1963. Type-specific antibody response in man to injections of cell walls and M protein from group A, Type 14 streptococci. J. Lab. Clin. Med. *61*:459–468.
94. Wood, H. F., A. R. Feinstein, A. Taranta, J. A. Epstein, and R. Simpson. 1964. Rheumatic fever in children and adolescents. III. Comparative effectiveness of three prophylaxis regimens in preventing streptococcal infections and rheumatic recurrences. Ann. Intern. Med. Suppl. 5. *60*:31–46.
95. Wilson, A. T. 1957. The leukotoxic action of streptococci. J. Exp. Med. *105*:463–482.
96. Wilson, M. G., and M. D. Schweitzer. 1954. Pattern of hereditary susceptibles in rheumatic fever. Circulation *10*:669–704.
97. Wilson, M. G., M. D. Schweitzer, and R. Lubschez. 1943. The familial epidemiology of rheumatic fever; genetic and epidemiologic studies; genetic studies. J. Pediat. *22*:468–581.
98. Zabriskie, J. B. 1964. The role of temperate bacteriophage in the production of erythrogenic toxin by group A streptococci. J. Exp. Med. *119*:89–92.
99. Zabriskie, J. B. 1967. Mimetic relationship between group A streptococci and mammalian tissues. Advances Immun. *7*:147–148
100. Zabriskie, J. B., and E. H. Freimer. 1966. An immunological relationship between group A streptococci and mammalian muscle. J. Exp. Med. *124*:661–678.
101. Zimmerman, R. A., and A. C. Siegel. 1966. A follow-up report of a streptococcal and rheumatic fever epidemic: Data confirming the epidemicity of the 1961 Dickinson, North Dakota, episode. Pediatrics *38*:578–584.
102. Zimmerman, R. A., A. C. Siegel, and C. P. Steele. 1962. An epidemiological investigation of a streptococcal and rheumatic fever epidemic in Dickinson, North Dakota. Pediatrics *30*:712–719.

# Chapter 9

# A SUCCESSFUL PARASITE: PARASITE-HOST INTERACTION IN INFECTION BY *STAPHYLOCOCCUS AUREUS*[*]

STUART MUDD

*U. S. Veterans Administration Hospital,*
*Philadelphia, Pennsylvania*

The association between *Staphylococcus aureus* and man is an ancient one. In the interest of species survival, both parasite and host have evolved complex arrays of capabilities for adaptation and defense. For the past ten years it has been the principal preoccupation of the team for which the writer is the spokesman to explore the more significant of these capabilities. Much was known and more has been learned, but a great deal remains obscure. The present chapter will attempt to recount the essentials of our exploration.

*S. aureus* and its infections are found in every continent. Indeed, the "Golden Horde" of *S. aureus* has been more successful than the Golden Horde of Genghis Khan in its world-wide invasiveness. Eradication is not a practical possibility within the foreseeable future. In its adaptation to parasitism in man staphylococcus has become one of the most successful, and certainly the most versatile, of pathogenic bacteria.

Theobald Smith[172] pointed out in his classic lectures on parasitism and disease that the successful parasite must gain lodgment on or in its host, must survive and multiply, must achieve egress from its host, and must find means

[*] This chapter is revised and expanded from a chapter by Stuart Mudd in *Topics in Medicinal Chemistry*, Joseph L. Rabinowitz and Ralph M. Myerson (eds.), Interscience Publishers, New York, 1968. The work of the author's group was supported by the U. S. Veterans Administration Central Office Research Service and by U. S. Public Health Service Grants E-2690 and A1-05473.

of conveyance to a new and susceptible host. The tubercle bacillus and *S. aureus* are pathogenic bacteria par excellence which have become adapted to the fulfillment of these requirements. The adaptation of the tubercle bacillus to parasitic coexistence with its host is singularly prefect, but the versatility of the golden coccus is without parallel.

## ANATOMY OF STAPHYLOCOCCUS AUREUS

### INTERNAL STRUCTURE

1. The staphylococcal cell is a spheroid of slightly less than 1 $\mu$ in diameter. Within the finely granular cytoplasm the electron microscope[193] reveals a complicated three-dimensional network of fibrils and interconnected denser granules which are probably microsomes, plus a convoluted skein of DNA fibrils, the nucleus. As in other bacteria, there is no nuclear membrane. Also within the cytoplasm are membranous organelles whose positions may be contiguous to the plasma membrane, to the septum between dividing cells, or to the nuclear area.

The cytoplasm is enveloped in a triple-layered "unit membrane,"[149, 179] about 70 Å in width. The membrane systems contiguous to the plasma membrane are continuous with the plasma membrane, from which they are thought to arise by infolding. The plasma membrane and cytoplasmic membrane systems have metabolic functions, including oxidation-reduction.[127, 179, 192, 193]

In close apposition to the plasma membrane is the bacterial cell wall, a structure with an outer electron-dense layer, a less dense middle layer, and an inner dense layer. In most electron micrographs the inner dense layer is not distinguishable from the outermost layer of the plasma membrane. Cell division is accomplished by centripetal growth of a complex structure comprising parts of the cell wall and of the plasma membrane. All of these morphologic features of *S. aureus* have been elegantly illustrated by Suganuma[179] and by Giesbrecht and Ruska.[43a]

2. The structures at the cell surface and immediately outside the surface are particularly significant in relation to host-parasite interaction. Capsulation and pseudocapsulation of *S. aureus* have, therefore, received special consideration.[123, 124] A true capsule may be defined operationally as an enveloping structure, outside the bacterial cell wall, which is regularly present under ordinary conditions of culture, and which can be demonstrated by negative staining.[124]

The Smith "diffuse" strain of *S. aureus* possesses a true capsule which can be demonstrated by negative staining,[92] by phase-contrast microscopy,[115] and by electron microscopy.[88] This capsule protects the Smith strain from phagocytosis and hence greatly enhances the virulence of the organism. Opsonization of this strain requires both heat-stable and heat-labile serum factors.[88, 102] Some 12 encapsulated Smith-type strains of *S. aureus* are known. A considerable amount of literature concerning this encapsulated staphylococcus has been summarized by Koenig and Melly.[88]

The Smith polysaccharide antigen has been characterized chemically by Morse,[115] and a polysaccharide antigen from a Smith-type strain has been studied by Haskell and Hanessian.[59] The capsular polysaccharide of the latter workers is described as composed of D-glucosaminuronic acid and L-alanine with O- and N-acetyl substitution.

3. Under somewhat special conditions of culture an ordinary strain of *S. aureus* can be caused to form an excess of extracellular material, which may accumulate about the staphylococcal cells. Since this extracellular accumulation does not conform to the operational definition of capsule, it is referred to as a pseudocapsule.[155] Under the special conditions referred to, this extracellular material is rich in soluble coagulase.[154] This material may be precipitated about the staphylococcal cells by cadmium salt, a precipitant for soluble coagulase.

A somewhat analogous phenomenon involving accumulation of extracellular material about staphylococcal cells has been described by Wiley, although he has consistently referred to the phenomenon as "capsulation."[196-200] Wiley's staphylococcus is a viscid strain isolated from a wound; the pericellular precipitate results from interaction with serum. This pseudocapsular phenomenon contrasts with true capsulation.[124] Wiley and Wonnacott[200] detected four serologically active components in the culture filtrate of the wound strain, but did not present thorough chemical characterization. The carbohydrate-peptide substances present in the culture filtrate of this viscid strain have been isolated and further characterized by Hisatsune et al.[62-64] Two electronegative and two electropositive components are found. The electronegative components give positive reactions for organic phosphorus, reducing sugar, amino sugar, and free $NH_2$ groups, and appear to be teichoic acids.[63] They are being further characterized by Hisatsune. One of the electropositive components has been characterized as the cell-wall peptide polymer.[64] This contains D-glutamic acid, D- and L-alanine, L-lysine, glycine, and ammonia in a molar ratio of 1:1:1:1:5:1 for Glu/L-Lys/D-Ala/L-Ala/Gly/$NH_3$. Alanine was identified as the N-terminal residue, and no significant free $NH_2$ groups other than that of alanine were detected. The peptide was strongly immunologically active in the precipitin reaction. The proposed structure is shown in Figure 1.

The cell-wall "mucopeptide" is believed to exist in the cell walls of all bacterial species as a "basal structure."[129, 156] It is largely responsible for the structural rigidity of the cell wall. This mucopeptide consists of two primary structural components; one component is the N-acetyl-glycosamine-N-acetyl-muramic acid polysaccharide backbone, and the other is the so-called "cell-wall peptide," which is linked to the carboxylic group of the muramic acid through a peptide linkage.[106] The cell-wall peptide has not previously been isolated as a polymer with serological activity. Some evidence suggests that the peptide is not exposed at the cell surface, at least in significant amounts[64, 117] (see Figures 2 and 3). However, using a strain of *S. aureus* which is unusually susceptible to the enzyme lysostaphin, Schuhardt et al.[157a] have been able to convert viable staphylococcal cells to spheroplasts and protoplasts by brief exposure to lysostaphin. This enzyme hydrolyzes the pentaglycine cross-linkages of the mucopeptide polymer of the cell wall.

To increase resistance to the invasiveness of the Smith-type encapsulated strains of *S. aureus* is a straightforward matter of producing opsonic antibodies

$$\overset{+}{N}H_3 \qquad\qquad \overset{+}{N}H_3 \qquad\qquad \overset{+}{N}H_3$$

```
    +                          +                          +
   NH₃                        NH₃                        NH₃
    |                          |                          |
  L-Ala                      L-Ala                      L-Ala
    |        α                 |        α                 |        α                     .
  D-Glut-(CONH₂)             D-Glut-(CONH₂)             D-Glut-(CONH₂)                    .
    |                          |                          |                              .
  L-Lys-NH                   L-Lys-NH                   L-Lys-NH                          .
    |      ε     \             |      ε     \             |      ε     \                  .
  D-Ala        (Gly)ₛ       D-Ala        (Gly)ₛ       D-Ala        (Gly)ₛ     D-Ala
    |              \           |              \           |              \                |
   CO              CO          CO              CO          CO              CO            CO
```

*Figure 1.*   Proposed structure of polypeptide polymer of cell wall. (From Hisatsune et al. Biochemistry, *6:*595–602.)

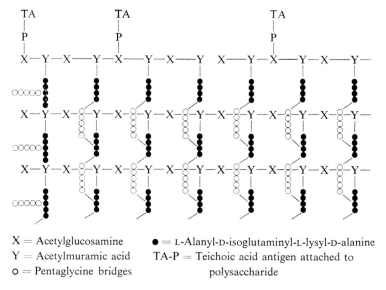

X = Acetylglucosamine         ● = L-Alanyl-D-isoglutaminyl-L-lysyl-D-alanine
Y = Acetylmuramic acid        TA-P = Teichoic acid antigen attached to
o = Pentaglycine bridges              polysaccharide

*Figure 2.*   Two-dimensional diagram of the relationship within the mucopolysaccharide–teichoic acid layer of the staphylococcal cell wall. (From Tipper et al. Biochemistry, *6:*906–920.)

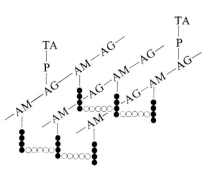

AG = Acetylglucosamine   AM = Acetylmuramic acid
o = Pentaglycine bridges
● = L-Alanyl-D-isoglutaminyl-L-lysyl-D-alanine
TA-P = Teichoic acid antigen attached to polysaccharide

*Figure 3.*   Diagram suggesting three-dimensional relationships in the mucopolysaccharide–teichoic acid layer of the staphylococcal cell wall. (From Tipper et al. Biochemistry, *6:* 906–920.)

to the carbohydrate capsule[88] (plus of course antibodies to the exotoxins). Unfortunately, however, the encapsulated staphylococci constitute only a negligibly small fraction of clinically infecting strains. The writer is not aware of any convincing evidence that clinically significant protection against *S. aureus* can be brought about by circulating antibodies against any *extracellular* products of the staphylococcus except the exotoxins.

## THE SUCCESSFUL PARASITE

The terms applied to the phenomena of parasitism are often quite misleading. The "aggressive factors" of the parasite are expressions neither of willful violence nor of aggression for aggrandizement. Rather they are mechanisms of survival, evolved through long adaptation to the parasitic habit by organisms which coexist with their host in a single ecosystem. What, then, are the products of *Staphylococcus* which have been recognized as involved in this adaptation to parasitism?

### LODGMENT UPON OR WITHIN ITS HOST

LIPASE, ESTERASE, AND SOME OTHER METABOLIC ENZYMES.   Of the necessary attributes of the successful parasite, the first cited by Theobald Smith was the ability to gain lodgment on or in its host. *S. aureus* is peculiarly well endowed to colonize the outer or inner surfaces of its human or animal hosts, or to survive in sites of injury or reduced resistance.[69, 101, 147, 165, 178]

All staphylococci possess lipase and esterase, enzymes which are uncommon in other pathogenic species. Colonization of the skin by staphylococci is "much more intense around sebaceous sites, and the fats and waxes of the skin are susceptible to lipolysis by the lipase-esterase complex of the organism which can, under partially anaerobic conditions, use fat as a main source of carbon . . . The possession of a powerful widely acting lipase is a characteristic of strains which are metabolically active and, in biochemical terms, versatile . . . The most pathogenic and drug-resistant strains fall into this category."[178]

*S. aureus* is also able to transport and oxidize amino acids[69] and metabolize carbohydrates. "This biochemical agility—quite unique in what is, after all, a highly specialized parasite—goes far to explain the adaptability of the organism to its changing environment."[178]

McKee and Braun[110] have also shown that digests of DNA can markedly stimulate the growth of *S. aureus in vitro* or in local infection sites.

SOLUBLE COAGULASE.   Pathogenic staphylococci are in practice distinguished from nonpathogenic strains by the secretion of soluble coagulase, although pathogenic *S. aureus* differs from nonpathogenic staphylococci in numerous compositional,[80, 117, 195] metabolic,[4, 69] and biological[34, 50] characteristics. Coagulase is a protein which, in combination with coagulase-reacting factor (CRF), clots blood plasma with striking similarity to thrombin clotting.[71, 183] Coagulase action has been very extensively investigated.[34, 183, 210] Production of fibrin deposits, limited proteolysis, and esterase activity are suggested as mechanisms by which coagulase may contribute to pathogenicity. In this regard Tager and Drummond write: "This in no sense allows the assignment of any assessable role in relation to the operation of other virulence factors of the staphylococcus, but merely indicates that coagulase may contribute to the total pathogenic effect."[183]

Suggestive evidence that staphylocoagulase may contribute to the pathogenesis of suppurative foci has been presented by Worms.[210]

CLUMPING FACTOR. A second factor usually present at the surface of virulent staphylococci has been conventionally known as "bound coagulase," but is better termed "clumping factor." This was shown by Duthie[33] to be quite distinct from soluble coagulase. Clumping factor is an antigenic protein which adsorbs fibrinogen, with resulting aggregation of the staphylcoccal cells. Kato and Omori[85] have extracted from a soluble coagulase-negative variant two fibrinogen-adsorbing substances, one of which could adsorb clumping factor-inhibiting antibody from antisera. Whether or not clumping factor is causally related to pathogenicity has not been established.

FIBRINOLYSIN (STAPHYLOKINASE). The majority of coagulase-positive human strains of *Staphylococcus* are fibrinolytic. The literature has been reviewed by Elek,[34] who found little evidence of importance of this enzyme in pathogenesis.

HYALURONIDASE OR SPREADING FACTOR. Nearly all coagulase-positive strains of staphylococci produce hyaluronidase, an enzyme capable of hydrolyzing the mucoid ground substance of the connective tissue. Elek,[34] after thorough review of the extensive literature on this spreading factor, concludes: "In view of the fact that both specific and nonspecific inhibitors of staphylococcal hyaluronidase are frequently found in normal human sera, it is unlikely that circulating spreading factor is of great clinical importance . . . If it plays a role at all it is likely to be in the initial stages of infection, since the earliest appearance of inflammation suppresses it."

## SURVIVAL WITHIN THE HOST. EXOTOXINS AND ANTITOXINS

The second necessary attribute of the successful parasite is the capability to survive and multiply upon or within its host. Ability to ward off the defensive cells of the host or to counteract the resistance of normal tissues to invasion by producing local injury obviously contributes to this capability.

$\alpha$-TOXIN. Of the "aggressive factors" of *S. aureus*, the most thoroughly studied is the $\alpha$-toxin,[9, 34, 45] a protein with a molecular weight of about 44,000 that is produced *in vitro* by pathogenic staphylococci and *in vivo* in the course of staphylococcal infection. It is dermonecrotic, hemolytic to the erythrocytes of most mammalian species, and lethal in sufficient dosage. $\alpha$-Toxin produces spasm and paralysis of both smooth and skeletal muscle and can destroy or damage a wide variety of tissue culture cells, as well as leukocytes, platelets, and lysosomes.[9, 182] $\alpha$-Hemolysin aggregates human and rabbit blood platelets, whereas sheep platelets are unaffected.[72] Human polymorphonuclear leukocytes are resistant, but human macrophages are susceptible to $\alpha$-toxin.[45] $\alpha$-Toxin is believed to be an enzyme whose primary action is on cell membranes but whose substrate has yet to be identified.[9, 40]

It seems probable that such a powerful enzyme, producing injurious changes in membrane permeability of a wide variety of cells, must have survival value to the parasitic staphylococcus in the tissues of its hosts. This is particularly true in view of the exceptional capacity of staphylococci to metabolize breakdown products of cells.

Taubler et al.[187] have investigated the role of α-toxin in lesion formation by *S. aureus* on sutures subcutaneously implanted in mice. Silk sutures impregnated with staphylococci were employed according to the technique of Elek and Conen,[35] as modified by James and MacLeod.[70] Evidence was obtained that α-hemolysin is essential for the development of purulent lesions by several strains of *S. aureus* thus adsorbed onto sutures and implanted in mice. Mouse polymorphonuclears and macrophages are both susceptible to α-toxin.[45] Active immunization with staphylococcal toxoid afforded significant protection and α-hemolysin-negative mutants were almost devoid of the ability to produce lesions by this route of infection. Human γ-globulin afforded some protection against such lesions.[190]

In man, fatal cases of staphylococcal septicemia are characterized by symptoms strongly suggestive of the action of α-toxin.[22, 27, 87, 144, 173] Antitoxin is reported to have therapeutic value in septicemia.[22, 27, 173] The aggressive action of α-toxin in such cases of systemic infection is clearly excessive, and has negative survival value for parasite as well as host.

PANTON-VALENTINE LEUKOCIDIN. A second exotoxin which undoubtedly serves to protect *S. aureus* against the defending leukocytes of the host was first described by the British investigators, Panton and Valentine.[144] Panton-Valentine (P-V) leukocidin has since been studied definitively by Gladstone and van Heyningen,[48] and in particular by A. M. Woodin.[205, 206] The leukotoxic action of this nonhemolytic leukocidin requires the synergistic action of two proteins, the F and S components. Both proteins have been crystallized and shown to have molecular weights of about 30,000. The only biological effects thus far observed are the cytotoxic symptoms developed in human and rabbit polymorphonuclear leukocytes and macrophages. No effects have been observed on cells in tissue culture.[90]

It appeared initially that the F and S components were adsorbed to the leukocyte surface.[207, 208] Later experiments showed that the interaction of leukocidin with the cell surface membrane is complex and involves interaction with phospholipids, in particular triphosphoinositide, in the granulocyte membrane.[206, 209] Various biochemical changes ensue. A striking morphologic change is the fusion of the lysosomal membranes of the polymorphonuclear leukocytes with the membrane of the cell surface, and the extrusion of the contents of the lysosomal granules from the cell.[207] Both components of leukocidin are highly antigenic in man.[75, 125] Gershon and Gladstone,[43] using fluorescent specific F and S antibodies, stained cells and areas between cells of colonies of staphylococci.

Intravenous injection in rabbits of 1 mg. per kilogram of body weight of highly purified leukocidin caused a reduction in the number of polymorphonuclear leukocytes and lymphocytes in the peripheral blood and bone marrow during the following eight hours.[181] A comprehensive review of the interaction of staphylococcal leukocidin and polymorphonuclear leukocytes has recently been published by Woodin.[206a]

β-Hᴇᴍᴏʟʏsɪɴ.   This exotoxin is produced predominantly by strains of *S. aureus* of animal origin, although many human strains may throw off β-producing variants. β-Hemolysin appears to be much less toxic than α-hemolysin.[45] A cytopathic action on platelets has been described by Bernheimer and Schwartz.[10] It appears that β-hemolysin is a sphingomyelinase and lysophospholipase.[28]

δ-Hᴇᴍᴏʟʏsɪɴ.   δ-Hemolysin has been obtained by Yoshida[211] as a crystalline protein of known amino acid composition and molecular weight of approximately 68,000. This is the least specific of the staphylococcal hemolysins. It produces hemolysis of the red cells of all species thus far tested, and is cytotoxic for a wide variety of cells in tissue culture. Human polymorphonuclear leukocytes, macrophages, and lymphocytes, as well as those of laboratory animals, are lysed by δ-toxin.[45] Gladstone[45] and Gladstone and Yoshida[49] have demonstrated that ribonuclease and β-hemolysin are present in small amounts in Yoshida's crystalline preparation of δ-toxin, but they showed that these contaminants alone were not responsible for the cytotoxic effect. The possibility, however, that β-hemolysin may have contributed to the cytotoxic action was not excluded. Wiseman and Caird[203] have shown that purified δ-hemolysin liberates organic phosphorus from phosphatidylinosotol and to a less extent from phosphatidylserine.

δ-Toxin is neutralized by normal serum and its α- and β-globulin fractions, but only to a small extent by γ-globulin. Injection of δ-toxin into laboratory animals was well tolerated. Gladstone[45] found no convincing evidence that δ-toxin is antigenic.

γ-Hᴇᴍᴏʟʏsɪɴ.   Marks[105] and Smith[170] demonstrated the existence of a hemolysin resembling α-toxin but differing from it antigenically. Gladstone[45] has recently found that a contaminant of his earlier preparations of P-V leukocidin was apparently γ-hemolysin.

Eɴᴛᴇʀᴏᴛᴏxɪɴ.   According to Casman[17] approximately one-third of clinical specimens of coagulase-positive staphylococci produce a toxin which causes food poisoning in man. This enterotoxin occurs in two antigenic types, A and B, and occasionally in other types. Clinical food poisoning is most commonly caused by ingestion of preformed enterotoxin associated with growth of coagulase-positive staphylococci in cooked meat.[111] Under certain circumstances, however, the symptoms of food poisoning may occur as the result of growth of the staphylococcus in the intestinal tract and conceivably elsewhere in the body.[17, 58, 86]

Aɴᴛɪᴛᴏxɪɴs.   The aforementioned are the recognized extracellular products of *S. aureus* which may contribute to the multifactorial pathogenicity of this most resourceful parasite. Fortunately for the host, the great majority of these exotoxins and metabolites are antigenic and capable of eliciting antibodies which, at least in part, neutralize their effects on the host. Thus, the activity of the lipase-esterase complex is to some extent neutralized in growing cultures by crude antitoxin.[147, 178] Ribonuclease is antigenic.[45] Soluble coagulase occurs in two or more distinct antigenic forms.[13, 146] Clumping factor is antigenic.[85] α-Toxin[22, 126] and both F and S components of Panton-Valentine leukocidin are strongly antigenic.[44, 125] Two antigenically distinct forms of β-hemolysin have been described, but only one is found in strains of human origin.[45] γ-Hemolysin[45] and hyaluronidase are antigenic.[34] Enterotoxin occurs in at least two antigenic forms, A and B.[17, 41, 58, 86]

The investigations of our group have been focused on the two exotoxins whose actions are most clearly related to the pathogenicity of *S. aureus*, and whose neutralizing antitoxins seem to offer most promise of clinical benefit, namely, α-toxin and P-V leukocidin. Immunization of human populations with representative examples of the staphylococcal toxoids commerically available showed that significant increments of anti-α-toxin titers were, indeed, elicited, but that no increments in antileukocidin titers were detected.[126]

We have therefore directed our efforts to producing a suitable immunizing agent for the F and S components of leukocidin. A leukocidin rendered nontoxic by formalin has been prepared and made available by Gladstone.[44] Administration of this toxoid to a small group of human subjects resulted in significant increments of titer against both F and S components. Accordingly the same toxoid was administered to a considerable group of patients with chronic staphylococcal osteomyelitis, together with Divasta (staphylococcal toxoid plus bacterial lysate, distributed by the Institut Pasteur, Paris) and Staphylococcal Bacteriophage Lysate (Delmont Laboratories, Swarthmore, Pennsylvania). Significant increments of titer against both F and S components of leukocidin and against α-toxin were elicited by this treatment, despite the fact that in most of the patients coagulase-positive staphylococci had been draining from the chronic lesions. Obviously, even patients with chronic infections were not making optimal immune response either to α-toxin or to staphylococcal leukocidin, and significant increments in response were elicited by dosages of toxoids which were quite feasible clinically.

In the article by Mudd et al.,[125] it was noted that in three years the toxoid, originally prepared in January, 1962, had become reduced in antitoxin-combining power, as estimated by Gladstone et al.,[47] to 31 per cent of the original combining equivalents for F, and to 67 per cent for S. Nevertheless, lacking a fresher preparation, we have continued administration of this toxoid to patients with chronic staphylococcal infections, and have been surprised to obtain patterns of response quite similar to those described previously.[125] This whole matter requires further investigation.

Also requiring further investigation are the local and sometimes systemic reactions following administration of leukocidin toxoid.[125] Gladstone[44, 45] has apparently traced these reactions to a slight contamination with γ-hemolysin, but attempts to eliminate the reactions by further purification or by the use of adjuvants have thus far been disappointing.[46] Efforts are continuing and recent results with a purer toxoid preparation are encouraging (G. P. Gladstone, unpublished).

Rabbits have also been immunized with leukocidin toxoid and challenged with virulent strains of staphylococci.[46, 174]

## SURVIVAL WITHIN THE HOST. SOMATIC FACTORS

Host resistance to staphylococcal infection falls within two broad categories: the elaboration of circulating antibodies to neutralize the exotoxins and other noxious metabolites, and anti-invasive resistance mediated in particular by polymorphonuclear and monocytic phagocytes and their accessory serum factors.

THE SINGULAR CASE OF PROTEIN A.    Verwey[194] in 1940 described a protein in strains of S. aureus which was "type-specific" in the sense of Julianelle and Wieghard, i.e., found in pathogenic but not in nonpathogenic staphylococci. Jensen[73] next studied this component, which he designated "antigen A," and found it to be precipitated by each one of 500 human sera. His interpretation was that "this must be due to the widespread occurrence of antigen A among the staphylococci and its powerful immunizing properties." Jensen's interpretation received rather wide acceptance.

Extensive studies by Lenhart, Mudd, Yoshida, and Li[93] and by Yoshida, Mudd, and Lenhart[214] yielded surprising results not in accord with Jensen's hypothesis. Staphylococci of the internationally recognized serotypes were found to be agglutinated by all human sera tested, although the agglutination titers were very different for the several serotypes. To our astonishment we found no significant differences in the titers against any given serotype, whether the sera tested were from healthy individuals, from patients with severe chronic staphylococcal infections, or from members of endemically infected populations. An appreciable increase in agglutination titers after immunization was found in rabbits, however. Martin, Crowder, and White,[107] more recently, studying human clinical cases, have also reported that "the concentration of antibodies against antigen A did not increase following staphylococcal infection."

This surprising lack of antibody response in human subjects to protein A has become more understandable through recent biochemical work of Löfkvist and Sjöquist[99] and of Forsgren and Sjöquist,[38, 39] who report that protein A is in fact not an antigen, but rather a nonspecific precipitant of γ-globulin. "Protein A was isolated from S. aureus and shown to precipitate about 45 per cent of a pooled normal γG-preparation. In addition it was demonstrated that protein A reacts with myeloma γG-globulin, H-chains from both normal and myeloma γG-globulins and the Fe fragment of normal γG-globulin. Thus the reaction is not a true antigen-antibody reaction." Working with guinea pig serum, Forsgren[37] has recently found that protein A precipitates both with γ1- and γ2-globulin, but not with γM-globulin.

Protein A was characterized by Yoshida et al.[214] as a basic protein of about 13,000 molecular weight. The molecular weight subsequently found by Grov[53] was 12,200.

Further chemical work, notably in Oeding's Institute, has indicated that crude protein A preparations are complex. The protein A preparation described by Oeding et al.[139] formed two precipitation lines in agar with rabbit antisera against the homologous strain, sensitized tanned sheep erythrocytes to agglutination, and inhibited agglutination of S. aureus strains. Of the two proteins in crude protein A only one (protein A) forms a precipitate with normal human serum. The second substance showing precipitating lines (protein B) gives no line against normal human serum, no sensitization of tanned sheep erythrocytes, and no effect on the bacterial agglutination. The only difference observed between protein A and protein B was the molar ratio of their neutral amino acids.

Grov[54] showed that the crude protein A preparation inhibited agglutination of *S. aureus* strains in rabbit antisera and normal human sera, and induced production of precipitins and agglutinins when injected into rabbits. The antiserum to crude protein A agglutinated 17 *S. aureus* strains but only Cowan 1 bacteria were agglutinated after absorption of antiserum by the other strains. Absorption with purified protein A or protein B did not affect the bacterial agglutination.

Grov concluded from his extensive experiments that the existence of specific agglutinogens in crude protein A had been demonstrated. "The agglutinogens are distinct from the other antigens in the preparation (protein A, protein B and sensitizing substance), are present in relatively small amounts, and were removed by separation and purification of the precipitinogens."

Martin and White[109] have shown that precipitins in human sera against antigen A prevent plaque formation and propagation of several staphylococcal bacteriophages. They present evidence suggesting both specific and nonspecific antigen A precipitins in human sera, and suggest that the specific and nonspecific antigen A precipitins in human sera may prevent the *in vivo* activity of staphylococcal bacteriophages which have been demonstrated previously in animals whose sera do not contain either specific or nonspecific antigen A precipitins.

A study of the component of protein A which sensitizes tanned sheep erythrocytes has recently been published by Live and Ranu.[98] They reported the reaction of this factor in the passive hemagglutination test with sera of normal human subjects and of six species of domestic animals.

TEICHOIC ACIDS AND OTHER ANTIGENS. It is of obvious survival value to the parasitic bacterium to have as a component of its cell surface some substance upon which the surface membranes of phagocytes cannot readily spread.[119] It is of obvious survival value to the host to be able to elaborate antibody to combine with and cover over the phagocytosis-resisting substances of the bacterial surface. The phagocytosis-resisting substances of the bacterial surface, in the majority of instances, are carbohydrates, e.g., the capsular polysaccharides of the pneumococci and of the Smith-type staphylococci. An exception is the M-protein of *Streptococcus pyogenes*.[91]

The teichoic acids of the cell wall of *S. aureus* are $N$-acetyl-glucosaminides of ribitol phosphate. D-Alanine in ester linkage is attached at position 2 or 3 of the ribitol. Teichoic acid occurs in two antigenically distinct forms, depending upon whether the $N$-acetylglucosamine is linked in $\alpha$- or $\beta$-configuration.[3, 157] Specific strains of *S. aureus* contain the teichoic acid polymer in different proportions, ranging from approximately 15 per cent of the $N$-glucosaminyl residue in $\alpha$-linkage and 85 per cent in $\beta$-linkage, to approximate equality of the two types of polymer, to 85 per cent in the $\alpha$-linkage and 15 per cent in the $\beta$-linkage.[66, 191] The individual teichoic acids may be separated by specific precipitation. Serum of healthy persons contains antibodies to the $\alpha$- and $\beta$-polymers in varying proportions, and the titers of each can be increased by immunization.[191] The teichoic acids produce skin tests of the immediate wheal and erythema type.[107] Human sera reacting to $\alpha$- and $\beta$-ribitol teichoic acids do not react with the glycerol-teichoic acid of *S. albus*.[107]

In a series of clinical cases Martin, White, et al.[23, 107, 108] found a very significant increment of antiteichoic acid antibodies in patients who had had clinical staphylococcal infections for 30 days or more. Healthy carriers of coagulase-positive staphylococci were not found to differ in such antibodies from noncarriers.

The sera of healthy human subjects promote the phagocytosis and killing of *S. aureus* by human polymorphonuclear leukocytes and macrophages. In a preliminary study Mudd et al.[128] found that the phagocytosis-promoting and killing action of fresh human serum could be wholly or partially removed by absorption with teichoic acid extracted from the cell walls or cells of the test strain of *S. aureus*.[212, 213] Inhibition of phagocytosis and killing was also found following absorption of fresh serum with $\alpha,\beta$-methyl-$N$-acetyl-D-glucosaminide. However, the absorbing amounts of teichoic acid used were relatively large, and the specificity of these effects with respect to $\alpha$- and $\beta$-configurations was not examined in detail.[128] Wolin, Archibald, and Baddiley have recently shown that the teichoic acid of certain mutants of *S. aureus* differs markedly from that of the parent strain.[204]

The effects of absorption of hyperimmune rabbit sera with homologous staphylococcal cell-wall teichoic acids of homologous, primarily $\alpha$-, $\beta$-, or $\alpha$-$\beta$-teichoic acids, have been quantitatively reviewed by M. G. Shayegani. It is found that in fact absorption with excessive amounts of teichoic acid may significantly decrease phagocytosis. However, when the absorbing teichoic acid is in concentration equivalent to the antiteichoic acid antibody (i.e., just sufficient to remove the relevant precipitation line on an Ouchterlony plate), no significant reduction in phagocytosis is found, when compared with the same serum without absorption. The interpretation of Mudd et al.[128] that combination of antibody with teichoic acid on the surface of *S. aureus* is critical for promoting phagocytosis is therefore not confirmed.[169a] It is an extraordinary, and to us surprising, fact that as of this writing (September, 1969) we cannot identify any specific circulating antibody (except, of course, in the case of Smith-type strains, the anticapsular antibody), which makes phagocytosis and intracellular killing of *S. aureus* more efficacious than does fresh normal serum (M. G. Shayegani, unpublished).

The surface of *S. aureus* also contains some 18 recognized factor-specific antigens[60, 137, 138] and a phage receptor site or sites.[52, 116, 117, 152] The relationship, if any, of these several surface antigens to phagocytosis and intracellular killing remains unknown.[52, 53, 56, 57, 66, 67]

Recent studies of the undigested, purified cell walls, as well as of intact cells, of *S. aureus* from Oeding's Institute have thrown additional light on the cell-wall composition. Grov and Rude,[56] after extraction of protein A and teichoic acids from undigested cell walls of the *S. aureus* strain Cowan 1, have found an unextractable material containing organic phosphorus, glucosamine, muramic acid, lysine, aspartic acid, serine, glycine, glutamic acid, alanine, smaller amounts of valine and leucine, and traces of proline and threonine. This unextractable material was found to have even higher agglutination titers against three *S. aureus* antisera than intact Cowan 1 cell walls.

Three teichoic acids are described as present in the cell walls of *S. aureus:* $N$-acetyl-glucosaminides of ribitol phosphate in $\alpha$- and $\beta$-configuration, and a glycerol teichoic acid containing glucose residues; Oeding's factor-specific agglutinogens are also present in the cell wall. The factor-specific antigens are present in very small amounts, are difficult to extract, and have not been characterized chemically. Recent evidence[55] indicates, however, that the factor-specific n-antigen is composed of two entities: a carbohydrate component and a polypeptide component.

The deep-seated mucopeptide is of course the principal source of structural rigidity of the cell wall.

PHAGOCYTOSIS AND INTRACELLULAR KILLING. Intracellular killing of *S. aureus* both by human and rabbit polymorphonuclear leukocytes and by monocytes of rabbits has been found to be significantly augmented by fresh serum in contrast to heated serum.[97, 169] Analysis of the heat-labile factors in human serum which significantly augment phagocytosis and intracellular killing showed that they correspond rather closely to the components of hemolytic complement.[95]

Melly et al.[111a] and Zucker-Franklin and Hirsch[215] have presented elegant demonstrations of the intracellular events following phagocytosis by polymorphonuclear leukocytes. The surface of the leukocyte spreads around the particle[50, 119] and pinches off, leaving the ingested particle in a tiny phagocytic vacuole. This vacuole moves toward the center of the cell. Membranes of the leukocytic granules (lysosomes) fuse with the membrane of the phagocytic vacuole and extrude their hydrolytic enzymes and phagocytin into this vacuole.[215]

Li and Mudd,[96] using the procedure of Cohn and Hirsch, have separated the lysosomes from human polymorphonuclear leukocytes and exposed staphylococci to these extracts in buffer at pH ranges from 6.0 to 4.8; survival was determined by plating out. It was found that staphylococci are largely capable of surviving in buffer at a pH range of 5.6 to 5.0, at which point killing by the lysosomal extract is demonstrated. Washed, untreated staphylococci are quite resistant to the leukocytic material, usually showing greater than 50 per cent survival after 90 minutes of incubation. The rate of killing may be significantly increased by pretreatment of the bacteria with fresh human serum, and the increase in killing following serum treatment is found to be correlated with the amount of serum used, as well as with the temperature and the duration of incubation with serum.

In our earlier experiments on phagocytosis[95, 97, 168] we did not detect intracellular killing in the absence of heat-labile components of fresh serum, and we stated, probably imprecisely, that killing did not occur under these circumstances. It now appears,[96, 169] however, that the difference between the killing of staphylococci by lysosomal contents without presensitization, with heated serum and with fresh serum, is quantitative only, killing increasing significantly in the order mentioned. This result is in agreement with recent work by Craig and Suter,[19] who use a quite different experimental technique.

Some light is thrown on the mechanism by which fresh serum sensitization augments the intracellular killing of staphylococci by the work of Shayegani.[167] He has observed that *S. aureus* cells, after sensitization with fresh serum and exposure to lysosomal extract, survive significantly longer in a hypertonic salt solution, or in L-form agar medium, than in isotonic buffer and agar medium. In this respect the sensitized staphylococci behaved like staphylococcal L-forms, suggesting that injury of the cell wall by the fresh serum components and lysosomal extract exposes the plasma membrane to the suspending medium. This interpretation is rendered the more likely by the observations of Borsos et al.[16] and Bladen et al.[11] Borsos et al. reported irregularly spaced "holes" in the membranes of erythrocytes subjected to Forssman antibody-complement hemolysis. The numbers of holes corresponded quite well with the numbers of sites of injury as predicted from titration of antibody and complement. Bladen et al. treated *Escherichia coli* cells with dilute antiserum and complement; negative staining of the spheroplasts among the bacteria thus treated and examined electron microscopically revealed lesions in the plasma membrane similar to those reported on erythrocyte membranes by Borsos et al. Spitznagel and Wilson[176] have recently demonstrated more drastic injury to the cell wall and plasma membrane of *E. coli* following exposure to fresh serum.

Downey and Kajima[29] have examined intracellular digestion of *S. aureus* by guinea pig granulocytes under the somewhat special condition that the granulocytes were allowed to ingest staphylococci in amounts approaching saturation numbers. They conclude: "Although normal (non-immune) serum stimulated the adsorption and ingestion of bacteria to a significant extent, it subsequently imposed an appreciable lag in the digestion of bacteria by the phagocyte. . . . It was concluded that serum places an additional burden on the digestive mechanism of the leukocyte by promoting the ingestion of more bacterial substance than can be digested by these cells."

Under experimental conditions in which granulocytes were allowed to ingest staphylococci in moderate numbers, Melly et al.[111a] concluded: "Phagocytosis of more than one pair of staphylococci by a single leukocyte appeared to act as a stimulus to bacterial destruction. Multiple ingestions of pathogenic staphylococci reduced the incidence of survival of the total microbial population contained within the cell."

We wish to stress the fact that intracellular killing of *S. aureus* both in polymorphonuclear leukocytes and in monocytes proceeds incompletely as compared with intracellular killing of other pyogenic cocci, such as pneumococci and streptococci. We believe that staphylococci may in some cases outlive the cells which have ingested them and may multiply extracellularly, thus setting up a state of smoldering infection,[169] and contributing to the chronicity of staphylococcal infection.

Olitzki and Gershon[140–142] have prepared an extract from murine spleen cells. This "splenocytin" is described as protecting *in vivo* against inoculations of *Salmonella typhi*, *Pasteurella pestis*, *S. aureus* and vaccinia virus.

According to Olitzki and Gershon,[142] "Lethal staphylococcal infections of white mice were produced by an intra-abdominal injection of $10^7$ staphylococci suspended in 5% mucin solution (pH 7.4), corresponding to 5 lethal doses. 100% of the animals survived when 10 mgm. of splenocytin were administered at varying time intervals (10 or 5 days, 20 or one hour) prior to the onset of infection. An intra-abdominal administration of 5 mgm. of splenocytin, at the same time intervals, effected a 93% survival, while by an administration of 1 mgm. 27% were protected." This phenomenon would certainly seem to merit further investigation.

## SURVIVAL WITHIN THE HOST. DELAYED HYPERSENSITIVITY

In a number of diseases in which the bacterial parasite is facultatively intracellular, a state of delayed hypersensitivity of the host may be induced. In these diseases active specific resistance is critically dependent upon the augmented capacity of the macrophages to ingest and destroy the bacterial pathogen. This crucial role of the macrophage has been demonstrated with particular clarity in tuberculosis of the rabbit by the classic studies of Lurie[100] and of Dannenberg.[20, 21] The crucial role of the macrophages of hypersensitive animals has been shown also for listeriosis and brucellosis by Mackaness,[103, 104] and for mouse salmonellosis by Blanden et al.[12]

*S. aureus* is more refractory to intracellular killing in polymorphonuclear leukocytes and macrophages than are the other pyogenic cocci. However, Kapral and Shayegani[84] were not able to demonstrate intracellular multiplication of staphylococci. It might be tempting to suppose, nevertheless, that resistance to *S. aureus* might follow the pattern of resistance to the facultatively intracellular pathogens mentioned above—tempting, but very dangerous! The supposition that resistance to *S. aureus* should follow the pattern of resistance to other pyogenic cocci has already cost much time of a number of investigators, including the writer. *S. aureus* as a pathogen has a resistance pattern all its own.

Bacterial allergy to staphylococci was demonstrated in earlier studies, and a considerable literature developed around it.[79, 81, 83, 143, 177, 180] More recent reports also have appeared indicating delayed hypersensitivity in animals infected with *Staphylococcus*.[14, 15, 18, 74, 78, 107] As astute an observer of infectious disease as Professor D. T. Smith has long treated staphylococcal infection with autogenous vaccine in the belief that he is desensitizing his patients.[171] Nevertheless, the whole subject of sensitivity as a significant factor in staphylococcal infection has been neglected in later years, and is in need of thorough reinvestigation both in animals and in man. Effects of various types of inflammation, including that of hypersensitivity, on local resistance to *S. aureus* have been reviewed by Cluff.[18]

Taubler has successfully demonstrated delayed hypersensitivity in mice. Mice were infected by the subcutaneous injection of $10^8$ viable staphylococci weekly for 6 to 8 weeks. Infected and normal mice were challenged by injection of the cytoplasmic contents of crushed staphylococcal cells into a hind foot pad; the opposite hind foot received a saline injection. When challenged with antigen the infected mice showed foot-pad swelling significantly greater than normal mice simultaneously challenged. The enhanced foot-pad swelling was transmissible to normal animals by suspensions of spleen cells but not by plasma or cell-free splenic extracts from hypersensitive mice.[184, 188]

Mice similarly infected with *S. aureus*, and a second population of mice rendered hypersensitive to tuberculin by subcutaneous injections of viable H37Ra tubercle bacilli, were used to test the specificity of inhibition of migration of cells from explanted fragments of spleen. Migration from explants from mice hypersensitive to staphylococci was specifically inhibited by critical concentrations of staphylococcal cytoplasmic extract but not by old tuberculin

(O.T.); migration from explants of tuberculin sensitive mice was specifically inhibited by critical concentrations of O.T. but not by staphylococcal extract.[185, 186, 189]

The feet of normal mice and of mice hypersensitive to staphylococci, injected with staphylococcal cytoplasmic extract, together with appropriate controls, have been examined histopathologically by Dr. J. Součková-Štěpánová. The dose of cytoplasmic extract injected in one hind foot was 200 gamma in 0.02 ml. volume of saline. Even in normal mice this extract of crushed staphylococcal cells produced acute inflammation, apparent after 30 minutes and increasing up to 24 hours after injection. The inflammatory picture after 24 hours is thus described by Součková-Štěpánová:[175]

"There was massive polymorphonuclear infiltration with formation of abscesses spreading into the muscular tissue. There were areas of necrosis, disintegration of muscle fibres, areas of suppuration showing the picture of myositis abscedens. In the deeper layers the massive polymorphonuclear infiltration extended focally to the periosteum in the form of periostitis abscedens. The vessels in affected regions were also infiltrated with polymorphonuclears and the endothelium of their intima was swollen. Although in some animals the response was milder, there were always foci and streaks of polymorphonuclear infiltration. In some places the inflammatory filtrate spread into the tendon sheaths. . . . After 48 hours the intensity of the inflammatory reaction somewhat decreased. In all phases there was predominance of polymorphonuclears in the inflammatory exudate and the mononuclear response was only minimal."

In hypersensitive mice similarly injected with extract of crushed staphylococci, there was also early acute inflammation, but this was followed by inflammation in which mononuclear cells predominated. The pictures at 24 and 48 hours post injection are thus described by Dr. Součková-Štěpánová.[175]

"Twenty-four hours after injection the inflammatory infiltration was mainly in the subcutis. The composition of the infiltrate varied from place to place. In some areas the inflammatory exudate was made up of mononuclears and polymorphonuclears as well, in other places, namely in deeper layers, mononuclear elements predominated. In all cases examined there was focal destruction of muscle fibres. The inflammatory infiltrate penetrated also into the muscular tissue, in some places up to the periosteum, up to the tendon sheaths or into the joint cavity producing exudation of fibrin. In the oedematous tissue of the corium and subcutis there were also foci of fibrinoid necrosis surrounded by inflammatory infiltrate.

"After 48 hours the macroscopical swelling of the feet is only mild. The oedema decreased and the corium was densely infiltrated by mononuclears which penetrated also into the muscles. In some places there were foci of massive mononuclear infiltration with destruction of muscular fibres. In the joint capsular tissue and in the synovial membrane there was mononuclear infiltration and macrophages were found also in the synovial fluid. In some cases the changes are less marked, only with focal mononuclear infiltrates in the corium and subcutis, spreading eventually into the surface layers of the skeletal muscular tissue."

The effects of hypersensitivity to *S. aureus* and to tuberculin on challenge of mice by subcutaneous injection in the neck of viable staphylococci are now under intensive study. Pending further progress of such studies, the following tentative conclusions can be drawn:

1. Hypersensitivity is certainly a factor in the pathogenesis of staphylococcal infection, and should be considered in the management of such infection.

2. The subject is very complex, and such factors as site of challenge, dosage, and timing can be critical.

A clinical study of hypersensitivity to *S. aureus* in human subjects is in progress.[6]

## SURVIVAL WITHIN THE HOST. ADAPTIVE GENETIC CHANGES IN THE PARASITE

One might suppose that the capabilities already cited which favor the survival of *S. aureus* as a parasite might exhaust its resources. Such is by no means the case. Several mechanisms exist by which the genetic constitution of staphylococci, in an environment which is inimical or is made inimical by the intervention of the physician, may be altered to favor the survival of the parasite.

TRANSDUCTION. Almost all strains of *S. aureus* are lysogenic; i.e., they carry prophages which may be induced to become lytic phages. These bacteriophages may lysogenize receptor strains of staphylococcus, and, in so doing, convey to them genetic determinants which may have been derived either from the chromosome or from an extrachromosomal plasmid of the donor strain.
[1, 112, 132–134, 136, 148]

Particularly significant observations have been made by Mitsuhashi and collaborators[89, 113, 114] who have found that the capacity to elaborate penicillinase, and hence resistance to penicillin, may be transduced jointly with resistance to macrolide antibiotics (erythromycin, oleandomycin, leucomycin, and spiramycin). The determinants of penicillinase production and resistance to macrolide antibiotics could be irreversibly eliminated by treatment with acriflavine or with ultraviolet light. It appears that these several determinants are controlled by a single genetic element which exists extrachromosomally, a plasmid.[113] Mixing the lysates from multiply resistant "epidemic strains" of staphylococci with nonresistant strains, Mitsuhashi et al. were also able to transduce resistance to tetracycline and to streptomycin, in some instances together with alterations in phage type. These authors propose[114] "that transduction and lysogenization by phages and the selection of these strains through extensive use of therapeutic agents are responsible for the wide distribution of multiply resistant staphylococci of restricted phage-typing pattern." Plasmid transduction in *S. aureus* has been further analyzed by Novick and Richmond, by Novick, and by Miller and Harmon,[112, 132–134, 136] and transduction of chromosomal fragments by Pattee et al.[145]

Novick and Morse[135] recently have demonstrated *in vivo* transfer between strains of *S. aureus* of genetic factors responsible for antibiotic resistance. Lysogenic strains that possessed extrachromosomal elements (plasmids) conferring erythromycin resistance or both erythromycin and penicillin resistance, and strains with presumably chromosomal mutations for streptomycin or both streptomycin and novobiocin resistance, were employed in these studies. Organisms with multiple resistance were isolated after double infection of mouse kidneys. The direction of transfer was from the plasmid-carrying strains to the plasmid-negative organisms. The authors conclude that "infectious transfer may play an important role in the occurrence and dissemination of strains of *Staphylococcus aureus* with multiple resistance."

Staphylococci of a single strain have been reported to exhibit striking differences in respiration[42] and in pathogenicity for laboratory animals,[8] when grown *in vitro* and when recovered from the body fluids of infected guinea pigs. Whether this difference between *in vitro* and *in vivo*-grown organisms rests upon temporary metabolic states or upon heritable change is not known.

MUTAGENESIS. Sevag and his collaborators have demonstrated another and very important mechanism by which the constitution of the bacterial parasite may be altered in such a way as to favor survival in an environment made inimical by the presence of an antibiotic. Sevag et al.[30, 161, 164] have demonstrated that antibiotics, in addition to acting as inhibitors of mechanisms of bacterial metabolism, are *mutagenic;* they induce heritable alterations in a percentage of cells exposed to them. In the continuing presence of the antibiotic, clones emerge which exhibit heritable alterations in metabolic characteristics, including specific resistance to the antibiotic in question.

Sevag reasoned that substances which form stable complexes with DNA might reduce or even abolish the frequency of such mutational events. Certain polyamines are known to complex in a stable fashion with DNA.[161] Indeed, it was found that cultures of bacteria exposed simultaneously to appropriate concentrations of antibiotic and spermine or spermidine died without producing clones of resistant mutants.[30, 164] In later work, with clinical applications in view, it was found that Atabrine[160, 162] and more recently phenothiazines and dibenzocycloheptenes[25, 61] exhibit similar antimutagenic effects. Whether the sites of mutagen-antimutagen action are upon chromosomal or extrachromosomal DNA has not yet been ascertained. Although this will be an interesting question for future investigation, from the point of view of the present discussion it does not matter whether the DNA is chromosomal or cytoplasmic (i.e., in plasmids). The mechanisms described above are obviously not in agreement with the view that strains resistant to antibiotics arise solely from spontaneous mutation and selection.[24, 26]

A point of critical importance for the clinical application of the work of Sevag and collaborators is that the antimutagens (e.g., Atabrine) act only to prevent the emergence of mutants. Bacteria which have already become resistant through exposure to a given antibiotic are not suppressed by the combination of Atabrine with that particular antibiotic.[161] In the presence of another antibiotic to which these bacteria are still susceptible, however, this antibiotic plus Atabrine does suppress the culture entirely.[25] Spermine and Atabrine have been shown to be antimutagenic also with respect to ultraviolet irradiation and caffeine.[76, 77]

Concerning the mechanism of action of Atabrine, Lerman[94] shows that DNA may be regarded as a rouleau of base pairs and that acridines may be intercalated into the stack. These alter the stability of the DNA molecule. Many acridines are mutagenic. In the special case of Atabrine, however, Lerman writes, "There seems to be no question that Atebrin [Atabrine] is intercalated, but it is one of the compounds that is very weakly mutagenic, even though the binding is strong."

Dr. Sevag and his many collaborators devoted some 20 years to exploration of the metabolic patterns of drug-resistant bacterial mutants, and to the quest for conditions which might prevent the emergence of such drug-resistant strains. Acceptance of this extensive work has been delayed by various factors, important among which is the impression that *mutation exclusively directed toward resistance* to each given anti-infectious agent was necessarily implied.

That this impression is not justified is indicated by the following passage by Dr. Sevag from *Origins of Resistance to Toxic Agents*, (Sevag, M. G., R. D. Reid, and O. E. Reynolds (eds.), 1955, Academic Press, New York): "There is not a single chemical entity that is not capable of exercising more than one affinity, particularly when in contact with a complex living system. As a consequence, a cell, on acquiring resistance, would experience several modifications, not all of which can be related directly to a single mode of action of a drug. However, multiplicity of action does not negate the specificity of action. It must be considered multispecific to varying degrees rather than a single specificity of action."

The present writer, who was the close associate of the late Dr. Sevag during these 20 years, takes the responsibility for reemphasizing that no such *exclusively directed mutation* need be implied, or, indeed, seems probable. It is obviously unlikely that each anti-infective agent could so alter the DNA molecule as to induce one exclusive metabolic pattern appropriate to resistance to that particular anti-infective agent. On the other hand, it seems less improbable that an anti-infective should induce a variety of mutations in one of which a phenotypic metabolic pattern appropriate to resistance should emerge. Under the conditions of growth obtaining, i.e., multiplication in the presence of the anti-infective agent, only those cells possessing a metabolic pattern viable in the given concentration of anti-infective would survive to form a resistant strain.

In a comprehensive review of "The Chemical Production of Mutations" by Charlotte Auerbach,[2] the following relevant statements occur:

"The mutated cell has to grow into a population of mutant cells. In mutation experiments on microorganisms, this last sieve has often to be passed in competition with a vast majority of nonmutant cells. . . .

"A chemical change in DNA is a necessary but not a sufficient condition for the production of an observable mutation. Intercalated between this primary change and the emergence of a population of cells with a new hereditary property is a whole series of cellular events, including a variety of repair mechanisms, transcriptions and translation of the new information, and growth of the mutant cell into a mutant population, often in the face of severe competition from non-mutant cells. These events act as so many sieves that screen out a proportion of potential mutations for realization."

The present writer then presumes to suggest the following modification of the interpretation of the comprehensive work of Dr. M. G. Sevag[163] and his collaborators:

1. That contact with sublethal concentration of sulfonamide or antibiotic induces changes in the DNA which are expressed phenotypically as altered patterns of metabolism. This is a fact attested to by a large body of experimental studies by Sevag and coworkers over a period of 15 years.

2. That in the "sublethal" concentrations of the primary exposure to anti-infective agent there is selection of such induced metabolic patterns as are compatible with growth in the inducing agent.

3. That subsequent exposure of the clones so produced to lethal concentrations of the homologous anti-infective plus Atabrine permits survival because no further mutations are required.

4. That exposure of the above induced clones to lethal concentrations of another anti-infective plus Atabrine yields no survival because the Atabrine, acting as antimutagen, prevents the requisite induced mutations.

A therapeutic trial of the above principles has been reported from the service of Michie at the Children's Hospital in Philadelphia. A combination of Atabrine and an antibiotic was used in a series of urinary tract infections. The combined therapy was reported as successful in eight of ten patients in whom previous treatment had failed.[166] A more extensive study of the efficacy of anti-infective agents, with and without Atabrine, in cases of nonobstructive uropathy is in progress.[68]

## Survival Within the Host. Going Underground

When grown in the presence of such a cell wall-inhibiting drug as penicillin or methicillin, S. aureus, as well as other bacteria, may grow as L-forms, which are very small protoplasmic bodies, having reduced or negligibly small amounts of cell wall substance. Such L-forms may revert to the parent bacterial morphology on withdrawal of the cell wall-inhibiting drug, or may persist in stable L-form. As such, it has been suggested[82] that they may become responsible for the "persister state" or of recurrent staphylococcal disease. Several reports have been made of the isolation of such L-forms from patients[82] with staphylococcal infections. It is noteworthy that L-forms are quite resistant to therapy with antibiotics whose action is on the cell wall (penicillins, cephalothin, vancomycin, bacitracin), but are susceptible to antibiotics which act upon the bacterial protoplasm.

## Survival Within the Host. Possible Action by Bacteriophage

Bartell, Thind, Orr, and Blakemore were able to reduce the effective dose in mouse intraperitoneal infection by homologous phage injected intravenously.[7] Gratia[51] many years ago described a phage of wide host range against S. aureus. A preparation including this phage is now in limited use clinically.[5] However, Martin and White[109] have reported recently that γ-globulin in human serum can inhibit the propagation of certain staphylococcal bacteriophages. In the author's judgment the case for or against polyvalent staphylococcal bacteriophage as a therapeutic agent under suitable conditions has never been either convincingly proved or disproved, and the possible efficacy of phage therapy deserves critical investigation.

## Egress From the Host and Transmission To New Host

*S. aureus* is a natural colonizer of skin and mucous membranes. Therefore a large proportion of human beings are carriers and shedders of staphylococci. Moreover, this microorganism tends to produce superficial infections and to drain from abscesses, sinuses, and fistulae in deeper tissues. A formidable literature has grown up around the epidemiology of staphylococcal infection, which is beyond the scope of the present chapter. Various useful reviews have been published.[120, 121, 130, 153, 201, 202, 216]

# HOST FACTORS IN RESISTANCE TO STAPHYLOCOCCUS

This chapter has been concerned primarily with the diverse capacities of a highly successful parasite. Obviously this parasite in infection is interacting with hosts possessing capabilities of defense which vary widely. In particular, the normal defensive mechanisms of the healthy host are subject to reduction by a variety of nutritional, metabolic, and traumatic conditions. Within the scope of the present chapter it is hardly practical to do more than cite works which can introduce the reader to the relevant literature. Such works are those of Dubos and collaborators[31, 32] and of Lurie. The monograph of Lurie,[100] *Resistance to Tuberculosis,* is possibly the most penetrating and comprehensive study that has ever been published on an experimental bacterial disease. Although it is not specifically related to staphylococcal infection, the guidelines established are of great general interest, particularly with respect to infections by facultatively intracellular parasites; however, these guidelines should not be carried over uncritically or without verification to other diseases.

Dubos and Schaedler[32] state: "The nutritional state can affect infectious processes through many unrelated mechanisms, modifying either the multiplication and activities of infectious agents, the susceptibility of the host to their toxic manifestations, or the immunologic and histochemical response to infection. On several occasions in the Bible, famine and pestilence are mentioned together and the two apocalyptic horsemen still continue to ride in association today. All over the world infectious diseases take their heaviest tolls in the less-privileged social classes and in the underdeveloped countries where malnutrition is most prevalent. Likewise, infectious diseases became a large problem in Europe during the last two wars wherever and whenever social disturbances resulted in severe food shortages. These epidemiologic findings are in accord with clinical experience. As is well known, infection is often a serious problem in malnourished individuals, whether malnutrition is the result of lack of certain food-stuffs as in kwashiorkor or of metabolic disorders as in diabetes or in cystic fibrosis of the pancreas."

Specific indications of the effect of predisposing factors in the host on the likelihood of staphylococcal infection are given by Farrer and MacLeod in a study of staphylococcal infections in a general hospital.[36] They state: "Approximately 80 percent of the patients with hospital-acquired staphylococcal infection suffered from chronic disease of one kind or another. The highest rate occurred among patients with diabetes mellitus: some 98 per thousand developed staphylococcal infection. A rate of 58.3 was found among patients with bone fractures, generally elderly persons in this institution. Likewise, high rates of infection were observed among patients with diseases of the nervous system, 30.1; diseases of the urinary system, 25.1; and diseases of the digestive system, 24.1 per thousand. Patients with malignant neoplasms comprised 27 percent of the infected group; the attack rate in this group was 49.0 per thousand. Patients with neoplasms of the breast, digestive system, and nervous system, almost all of which were brain tumors, composed an extremely high-risk group."

For more detailed discussion of the interaction of nutritional states and infection, see Scrimshaw.[158, 159]


## PROSPECT

Infectious diseases are complex interactions between parasite and host, each seeking survival within one ecosystem. An obligation of the physician is to intervene in this interaction in such ways as may maximize the probability of survival of the human host. Our examination of the successful parasite has disclosed lines of ongoing investigation which offer promise of leading to such useful interventions.

Patients with staphylococcal infection are found not to be making optimal immune response. A very impressive literature documents the therapeutic value of α-toxoid under appropriate conditions. There is evidence also that staphylococcal leukocidin toxoid appropriately administered, either prophylactically or therapeutically, can afford useful augmentation of resistance. Our efforts to provide leukocidin toxoid in acceptable form are continuing.

A more intimate understanding of the mechanisms of phagocytosis and intracellular killing of staphylococci certainly should afford means of improving anti-invasive resistance.

It should be mentioned here that one experienced investigator of staphylococcal infection, D. E. Rogers, has written that the attempt to increase human resistance to staphylococci by active immunization is unpromising.[150, 151] This view is based on the assumption that almost every human adult has developed about as much specific resistance against *Staphylococcus* as he is capable of. The writer certainly agrees that human adults do possess a considerable degree of resistance to staphylococci.

However, the fact has been documented in this chapter that human subjects, even with active staphylococcal infection, usually have not responded optimally in specific resistance and that significant increments in titers of antibodies against α-toxin and Panton-Valentine leukocidin may be elicited by inoculation of these antigens. Furthermore, it is well known that under favorable circumstances human resistance to staphylococci can fall far below optimal levels. It therefore seems to the writer that attempts to increase resistance in chronically infected patients therapeutically and prophylactically, under such circumstances as can attend elective surgery on mediastinum or joints, or childbirth under unhygienic conditions, are logical and do offer promise.

The existence and implications of hypersensitivity in staphylococcal infection, particularly hypersensitivity of the delayed type, have been strangely neglected. In view of the critical role of delayed hypersensitivity in tuberculosis and other diseases caused by facultatively intracellular parasites, the importance of more thorough exploration of this factor in staphylococcal disease is certainly long overdue.

The fact that the temperate bacteriophages carried by staphylococci may aid in adaptation to parasitism, in particular by the transduction of factors contributing to virulence, is becoming documented, and is causing considerable disquiet.

The possibility that lytic phages of sufficiently broad host range may have a place in therapy under suitable conditions is now largely ignored or disbelieved. In the writer's judgment, adequate documentation either for or against bacteriophage as a possible therapeutic agent has never been provided.

The emergence of strains resistant to antibiotics can be prevented *in vitro* by the appropriate use of an antimutagenic agent such as Atabrine. Animal experiments and thorough clinical trial may well support this laboratory evidence, and demonstrate very important new possibilities in antibiotic therapy.

Conditions in the host which predispose to staphylococcal infection may be nutritional, metabolic, or traumatic. Malnutrition is a particularly important predisposing factor. This consideration is of special significance at the present time, when food production per capita is actually falling in the developing countries of the world, because populations are growing faster than resources.[23a, 122, 131] For governments and other agencies to adopt anything less than all-out campaigns to correct this situation is to invite the apocalyptic horsemen, famine, pestilence, and indeed war, to ride again.

# References

1. Arber, W. 1967. Les facteurs de résistance à des antibiotiques. Point de vue de généticien moléculaire. Path. Microbiol. *30*:1007–1014.
2. Auerbach, C. 1967. The chemical production of mutations. Science *158*:1141–1147.
3. Baddiley, J. 1962. Teichoic acids and related compounds in bacteria. J. Roy. Inst. Chem. *86*:366–373.
4. Baird-Parker, A. C. 1965. Staphylococci and their classification. Ann. N. Y. Acad. Sci. *128*:4–25.
5. Baker, A. G. 1963. Staphylococcus bacteriophage lysate. Topical and parenteral use in allergic patients. Penn. Med. J. *66*:25–28.
6. Baker, A. G., J. H. Taubler, and S. Mudd. 1968. Delayed hypersensitivity to *Staphylococcus aureus* in mice and men. Bact. Proc., p. 100.
7. Bartell, P. F., I. S. Thind, T. Orr, and W. S. Blakemore. 1963. The *in vivo* interaction between staphylococcus bacteriophage and *Staphylococcus aureus*. J. Exp. Med. *118*:13–26.
8. Beining, P. R., and E. R. Kennedy. 1963. Characteristics of a strain of *Staphylococcus aureus* grown *in vivo* and *in vitro*. J. Bact. *85*:732–741.
9. Bernheimer, A. W. 1965. Staphylococcal alpha toxin. Ann. N. Y. Acad. Sci. *128*:112–123.

10. Bernheimer, A. W., and L. L. Schwartz. 1965. Effects of staphylococcal and other bacterial toxins on platelets *in vitro*. J. Path. Bact. *89:*209–223.

11. Bladen, H. A., R. T. Evans, and S. E. Mergenhagen. 1966. Lesions in *Escherichia coli* membranes after action of antibody and complement. J. Bact. *91:*2377–2381.

12. Blanden, R. V., G. B. Mackaness, and F. M. Collins. 1966. Mechanisms of acquired resistance in mouse typhoid. J. Exp. Med. *124:*585–600.

13. Boake, W. C. 1956. Antistaphylocoagulase in experimental staphylococcal infections. J. Immun. *76:*89–96.

14. Bodel, P. T., and E. Atkins. 1964. Studies in staphylococcal fever. IV. Hypersensitivity to culture filtrates. Yale J. Biol. Med. *37:*130–144.

15. Bøe, J. 1945. Investigations on the importance of bacterial allergy for the development of cutaneous infections due to staphylococci. Acta Dermatovener. *26:*111–136.

16. Borsos, T., R. Dourmashkin, and J. H. Humphrey. 1964. Lesions in erythrocyte membranes caused by immune haemolysis. Nature *202:*251–252.

17. Casman, E. P. 1965. Staphylococcal enterotoxin. Ann. N. Y. Acad. Sci. *128:*124–131.

18. Cluff, L. E. 1965. Cellular reactions in the pathogenesis of staphylococcal infection. Ann. N. Y. Acad. Sci. *128:*214–230.

19. Craig, C. P., and E. Suter. 1966. Extracellular factors influencing staphylocidal capacity of human polymorphonuclear leucocytes. J. Immun. *97:*287–296.

20. Dannenberg, A. M., Jr. 1968. Cellular hypersensitivity and cellular immunity in the pathogenesis of tuberculosis: specificity, systemic and local nature and associated macrophage enzymes. Bact. Rev. *32:*85–102.

21. Dannenberg, A. M., Jr., O. T. Meyer, J. R. Esterly, and T. Kambara. 1968. The local nature of immunity in tuberculosis, illustrated histochemically in dermal BCG lesions. J. Immun. *100:*931–941.

22. D'Antona, D. 1958. L'anatoxine staphylococcique en medicine humaine (bases doctrinales, préparation, contrôle et applications critiques). C. R. Quatrième Congrès International de Standardisation Biologique, Brussels, Ministère de la Santé Publique et de la Famille, pp. 3–71.

23. Daugharty, H., R. R. Martin, and A. White. 1967. Antibodies against staphylococcal teichoic acids and type-specific antigens in man. J. Immun. *98:*1123–1129.

23a. Davis, K. 1967. Population policy: Will current programs succeed? Science *158:*730–739.

24. De Courcy, S. J., Jr., and M. G. Sevag. 1966. Time study of emergence of drug resistance. Bact. Proc., p. 51.

25. De Courcy, S. J., Jr., and M. G. Sevag. 1966. Specificity and prevention of antibiotic resistance in *Staphylococcus aureus*. Nature *209:*373–376.

26. De Courcy, S. J., Jr., and M. G. Sevag. 1967. Population dynamics and results of fluctuation tests in a study of the role of atabrine as an antimutagen in preventing streptomycin resistance in *Staphylococcus aureus*. In: Antimicrobial Agents Chemotherapy—1966. pp. 235–244.

27. Dóbiás, G., T. Balló, and J. Keménynvári. 1965. Einige Laboratoriumsuntersuchungen im Zusammenhang mit Serumtherapie der Staphylokokken-Toxikose im Säuglingsalter. Z. Immun. Allergieforsch. *128:*436–450.

28. Doery, H. M., B. J. Magnusson, J. Gulasekharam, and J. E. Pearson. 1965. The properties of phospholipase enzymes in staphylococcal toxins. J. Gen. Microbiol. *40:*283–296.

29. Downey, R. J., and M. Kajima. 1967. Influence of serum on intracellular digestion of *Staphylococcus aureus* by polynuclear neutrophils from the guinea pig. J. Reticuloendothel. Soc. *4:*168–176.

30. Drabble, W. T., and M. G. Sevag. 1963. Prevention of the development of microbial resistance to drugs. In: Antimicrobial Agents Chemotherapy—1962. pp. 649–653.

31. Dubos, R. J. 1954. Biochemical Determination of Microbial Diseases. Harvard University Press, Cambridge, Mass.

32. Dubos, R. J., and R. W. Schaedler. 1959. Nutrition and infection. J. Pediat. *55:*1–14.

33. Duthie, E. S. 1954. Evidence for two forms of staphylococcal coagulase. J. Gen. Microbiol. *10:*427–436.

34. Elek, S. D. 1959. Staphylococcus pyogenes and Its Relation to Disease. Livingstone, Edinburgh.

35. Elek, S. D., and P. E. Conen. 1957. The virulence of *Staphylococcus aureus* for man. A study of the problem of wound infection. Brit. J. Exp. Path. *38:*573–586.

36. Farrer, S. M., and C. M. MacLeod. 1960. Staphylococcal infections in a general hospital. Amer. J. Hyg. *72:*38–58.

37. Forsgren, A. 1968. Protein A from *Staphylococcus aureus*. V. Reaction with guinea-pig γ-globulins. VI. Reaction with subunits from guinea-pig γ1- and γ2-globulin. J. Immun. *100:*921–930.

38. Forsgren, A., and J. Sjöquist. 1966. "Protein A" from S. aureus. I. Pseudo-immune reaction with human γ-globulin. J. Immun. 97:822–827.
39. Forsgren, A., and J. Sjöquist. 1967. "Protein A" from Staphylococcus aureus. III. Reaction with rabbit γ-globulin. J. Immun. 99:19–24.
40. Freer, J. H., J. P. Arbuthnott, and A. W. Bernheimer. 1968. Interaction of staphylococcal α-toxin with artificial and natural membranes. J. Bact. 95:1153–1168.
41. Friedman, M. E. 1968. Inhibition of staphylococcal enterotoxin B formation by cell wall blocking agents and other compounds. J. Bact. 95:1051–1055.
42. Gellenbeck, S. M. 1962. Aerobic respiratory metabolism of Staphylococcus aureus from an infected animal. J. Bact. 83:450–455.
43. Gershon, A., and G. P. Gladstone. 1968. Immunofluorescent demonstration of staphylococcal leucocidin components F and S. Brit. J. Exp. Path. 49:477–495.
43a. Giesbrecht, P., and H. Ruska. 1968. Über Veränderungen der Feinstrukturen von Bakterien unter der Einwirkung von Chloramphenicol. Klin. Wschr. 46:575–582.
44. Gladstone, G. P. 1965. Staphylococcal leucocidin toxoid. Brit. J. Exp. Path. 46:292–307.
45. Gladstone, G. P. 1966. Staphylococcal hemolysins. Postepy Mikrobiol. 5:145–161.
46. Gladstone, G. P. 1966. Discussion of Woodin's paper. Postepy Mikrobiol. 5:169–170.
47. Gladstone, G. P., S. Mudd, H. D. Hochstein, and N. A. Lenhart. 1962. The assay of antistaphylococcal leucocidin components (F and S) in human sera. Brit. J. Exp. Path. 43:295–312.
48. Gladstone, G. P., and W. E. Van Heyningen. 1957. Staphylococcal leucocidins. Brit. J. Exp. Path. 38:123–137.
49. Gladstone, G. P., and A. Yoshida. 1967. The cytopathic action of purified staphylococcal δ-haemolysin. Brit. J. Exp. Pathol. 48:11–19.
50. Goodman, J. R., R. E. Moore, and R. F. Baker. 1956. Electron microscopic study of phagocytosis of Staphylococcus by human leukocytes. J. Bact. 72:736–745.
51. Gratia, A. 1922. La lyse transmissable du staphylocoque, sa production; ses applications thérapeutiques. C. R. Soc. Biol. 86:276–278.
52. Grov, A. 1965. Studies on antigen preparations from Staphylococcus aureus. 1. The influence of modification of functional groups and enzymatic digestion on the serological activity of Protein A. Acta Path. Microbiol. Scand. 65:600–606.
53. Grov, A. 1967. Studies on antigen preparations from Staphylococcus aureus. 3. On the homogeneity and structure of protein A. Acta Path. Microbiol. Scand. 69:567–575.
54. Grov. A. 1968. Studies on antigen preparations from Staphylococcus aureus. 4. Separation and purification of protein A and a related precipitinogen. 5. Inhibition of bacterial agglutination by protein A preparations. Acta Path. Microbiol. Scand. 73:400–412.
55. Grov, A., B. Myklestad, and P. Oeding. 1966. Immunochemical studies on antigen preparations from Staphylococcus aureus. 3. The η antigen. Acta Path. Microbiol. Scand. 68:149–156.
56. Grov, A., and S. Rude. 1967. Immunochemical characterization of Staphylococcus aureus cell walls. Acta Path. Microbiol. Scand. 71:409–416.
57. Grov, A., and S. Rude. 1967. Immunochemical examination of phenylhydrazine-treated Staphylococcus aureus cell walls. Acta Path. Microbiol. Scand. 71:417–421.
58. Hallander, H. O., and G. Laurell. 1966. Enterotoxin-producing staphylococci—some aspects of diagnosis, frequency and types of infection. Postepy Mikrobiol. 5:421–428.
59. Haskell, H. T., and S. Hanessian. 1964. The purification and characterization of a new active immunizing polysaccharide prepared from Staphylococcus aureus. Biochim. Biophys. Acta 83:35–41.
60. Haukenes, G. 1967. Serological typing of Staphylococcus aureus. 7. Technical Aspects. Acta Path. Microbiol. Scand. 70:590–600.
61. Heller, C. S., and M. G. Sevag. 1966. Prevention of the emergence of drug resistance in bacteria by acridines, phenothiazines and dibenzocycloheptenes. J. Appl. Microbiol. 14:879–885.
62. Hisatsune, K., S. J. De Courcy, Jr., and S. Mudd. 1966. An immunologically active cell-wall peptide polymer of Staphylococcus aureus. Biochim. Biophys. Acta 121:210–212.
63. Hisatsune, K., S. J. De Courcy, Jr., and S. Mudd. 1967. Studies on the carbohydrate-peptide fraction of the centrifugal supernatants of Staphylococcus aureus cultures. Biochemistry 6:586–594.
64. Hisatsune, K., S. J. De Courcy, Jr., and S. Mudd. 1967. The immunologically active cell-wall peptide polymer of Staphylococcus aureus. Biochemistry 6:595–602.
65. Hofstad, T. 1964. Studies on the antigenic structure of the 80/81 complex of Staphylococcus aureus. 1. Agglutinogens. Acta Path. Microbiol. Scand. 61:558–570.
66. Hofstad, T. 1965. Studies on the antigenic structure of the 80/81 complex of Staphylococcus aureus. 4. Antigenic properties and chemical basis of serological reactivity of a purified polysaccharide. Acta Path. Microbiol. Scand. 63:422–434.

67. Hofstad, T. 1965. Studies on the antigenic structure of the 80/81 complex of *Staphylococcus aureus*. 7. Preparation and properties of cell walls from strain 263. Acta Path. Microbiol. Scand. *65:*151–160.

68. Horwitz, M. R., J. L. Eshelman, M. G. Sevag, S. J. De Courcy, Jr., S. Mudd, and W. S. Blakemore. 1968. The effect of combined atabrine-antimicrobial drug therapy on urinary tract infections: *in vitro* and *in vivo* studies. Surg. Forum *19:*532–534.

69. Ivler, D. 1965. Comparative metabolism of virulent and avirulent staphylococci. Ann. N. Y. Acad. Sci. *128:*62–80.

70. James, R. C., and C. M. MacLeod. 1961. Induction of staphylococcal infections in mice with small inocula introduced on sutures. Brit. J. Exp. Path. *42:*266–277.

71. Jeljaszewicz, J. 1966. Staphylococcal coagulases. Postepy Mikrobiol. *5:*171–183.

72. Jeljaszewicz, J., S. Niewiarowski, A. Poplawski, and L. Blawat. 1966. Platelet aggregation by staphylococcal toxins. Postepy Mikrobiol. *5:*203–207.

73. Jensen, K. 1944. A normally occurring staphylococcus antibody in human serum. Acta Path. Microbiol. Scandinav. *44:*421–428.

74. Johanovský, J. 1958. Role of hypersensitivity in experimental staphylococcal infections. Nature *182:*1454.

75. Johanovský, J. 1958. Die Bedeutung des Antileukozidins und Antitoxins bei der Immunität gegen Staphylokokken Infektionen. Z. Immunitätsforsch. *116:*318–328.

76. Johnson, H. G., and M. K. Bach. 1965. Apparent suppression of mutation rates in bacteria by spermine. Nature *208:*408–409.

77. Johnson, H. G., and M. K. Bach. 1966. The antimutagenic action of polyamines; suppression of the mutagenic action of an *E. coli* mutator gene and of 2-amino purine. Proc. Nat. Acad. Sci. *55:*1453–1456.

78. Johnson, J. E., L. E. Cluff, and K. Goshi. 1961. Studies on the pathogenesis of staphylococcal infection. I. The effect of repeated skin infections. J. Exp. Med. *113:*235–247.

79. Julianelle, L. A., D. Jones, and A. F. Hartmann. 1935. Experimental hypersensitivity to staphylococcus. Proc. Soc. Exp. Biol. Med. *32:*945–948.

80. Julianelle, L. A., and C. W. Wieghard. 1935. The immunological specificity of staphylococci. I. The occurrence of serological types. J. Exp. Med. *62:*11–21.

81. Julianelle, L. A., and C. W. Wieghard. 1935. The immunological specificity of staphylococci. III. Interrelationships of cell constituents. J. Exp. Med. *62:*31–37.

82. Kagan, B. M. 1965. Staphylococcal L-forms—Ecologic perspectives, and discussion of this paper. Ann. N. Y. Acad. Sci. *128:*81–91.

83. Kahn, M. C., H. S. Baldwin, B. R. Zeitlin, and M. Smart. 1951. Cutaneous reactions to staphylococcal polysaccharide, protein and an unfractionated extract in hypersensitive and normal individuals. J. Allergy *22:*237–248.

84. Kapral, F. A., and M. G. Shayegani. 1959. Intracellular survival of staphylococci. J. Exp. Med. *110:*123–138.

85. Kato, Y., and G. Omori. 1959. Extraction of bound coagulase from staphylococcal cells. Biken J. *2:*321–332.

86. Kienitz, M. 1966. Studies on staphylococcal enterotoxin. Postepy Mikrobiol. *5:*189–194.

87. Kleiger, B., and J. E. Blair. 1943. Role of toxin and use of antitoxin in systemic staphylococcic infections. Arch. Surg. *46:*548–554.

88. Koenig, M. G., and M. A. Melly. 1965. The importance of surface antigens in staphylococcal virulence. Ann. N. Y. Acad. Sci. *128:*231–250.

89. Kono, M., R. Ogawa, and S. Mitsuhashi. 1968. Drug resistance to staphylococci. VI. Genetic determinant for chloramphenicol resistance. J. Bact. *95:*886–892.

90. Korbecki, M., and J. Jeljaszewicz. 1965. Action of staphylococcal toxins in cell cultures. J. Infect. Dis. *115:*205–213.

91. Lancefield, R. C., and G. E. Perlmann. 1952. Preparation and properties of type-specific M antigen isolated from a Group A, Type 1, hemolytic streptococcus. J. Exp. Med. *96:*71–82.

92. Lenhart, N. A., I. W. Li, S. J. De Courcy, Jr., and S. Mudd. 1962. Nonmucoid mutant of the encapsulated Smith strain of *Staphylococcus aureus*. J. Bact. *83:*1165–1166.

93. Lenhart, N. A., S. Mudd, A. Yoshida, and I. W. Li. 1963. The common protein agglutinogen of *Staphylococcus aureus*. I. Distribution in international serotypes and corresponding antibody in human populations. J. Immun. *91:*771–776.

94. Lerman, L. S. 1964. Acridine mutagens and DNA structure. J. Cell. Comp. Physiol. *64:* Suppl. 1, pp. 1–18.

95. Li, I. W., and S. Mudd. 1965. The heat-labile serum factor associated with intracellular killing of *Staphylococcus aureus*. J. Immun. *94:*852–857.

96. Li, I. W., and S. Mudd. 1966. Serum effect on the killing of *Staphyloccus aureus* by human leukocytic extracts. J. Immun. *97:*41–45.

97. Li, I. W., S. Mudd, and F. A. Kapral. 1963. Dissociation of phagocytosis and intracellular killing of *Staphylococcus aureus* by human blood leucocytes. J. Immun. *90:*804–809.
98. Live, I., and R. S. Ranu. 1968. Serological activity of protein A of *Staphylococcus aureus:* the precipitinogen as an antigen for determining antibodies by the passive hemagglutination test. J. Bact. *96:*14–23.
99. Löfkvist, T., and J. Sjöquist. 1964. Immunological analysis of staphylococcal antigenic preparations. Int. Arch. Allerg. *24:*244–253.
100. Lurie, M. B. 1964. Resistance to Tuberculosis. Experimental Studies in Native and Acquired Defensive Mechanisms. Harvard University Press, Cambridge, Mass.
101. Macfarlane, M. G. 1962. Lipid components of *Staphylococcus aureus* and *Salmonella typhimurium*. Biochem. J. *82:*40–41.
102. Mackaness, G. B. 1960. The phagocytosis and inactivation of staphylococci by macrophages of normal rabbits. J. Exp. Med. *112:*35–53.
103. Mackaness, G. B. 1964. The immunological basis of acquired cellular resistance. J. Exp. Med. *120:*105–120.
104. Mackaness, G. B., and R. V. Blanden. 1967. Cellular immunity. Progr. Allerg. *11:*89–140.
105. Marks, J. 1951. The standardization of staphylococcal α-toxin with special reference to anomalous haemolysins including δ-lysin. J. Hyg. *49:*52–66.
106. Martin, H. H. 1966. Biochemistry of bacterial cell walls. Ann. Rev. Biochem. *35:*457–484.
107. Martin, R. R., J. G. Crowder, and A. White. 1967. Human reactions to staphylococcal antigens. A possible role of leukocyte lysosomal enzymes. J. Immun. *99:*269–274.
108. Martin, R. R., H. Daugharty, and A. White. 1966. Staphylococcal antibodies and hypersensitivity to teichoic acids in man. *In:* Antimicrobial Agents Chemotherapy—1965. p. 91–96.
109. Martin, R. R., and A. White. 1968. Prevention of staphylococcal bacteriophage activity by antigen A precipitins in human sera. J. Bact. *95:*2177–2181.
110. McKee, J. J., and W. Braun. 1962. Effects of enzymatic digests of DNA on staphylococci. Proc. Soc. Exp. Biol. Med. *109:*166–170.
111. McLean, R. A., H. D. Lilly, and J. A. Alford. 1968. Effects of meat-curing salts and temperature on production of staphylococcal enterotoxin B. J. Bact. *95:*1207–1211.
111a. Melly, M. A., J. B. Thomison, and D. E. Rogers. 1960. Fate of Staphylococci within human leukocytes. J. Exp. Med. *112:*1121–1129.
112. Miller, M. A., and S. A. Harmon. 1967. Genetic association of determinants controlling resistance to mercuric chloride, production of penicillinase and synthesis of methionine in *Staphylococcus aureus*. Nature *215:*531–532.
113. Mitsuhashi, S., H. Hashimoto, M. Kono, and M. Morimura. 1965. Drug resistance of staphylococci. II. Joint elimination and joint transduction of the determinants of penicillinase production and resistance to macrolide antibiotics. J. Bact. *89:*988–992.
114. Mitsuhashi, S., H. Oshima, U. Kawaharada, and H. Hashimoto. 1965. Drug resistance of staphylococci. I. Transduction of tetracycline resistance with phage lysates obtained from multiply resistant staphylococci. J. Bact. *89:*967–976.
115. Morse, S. I. 1962. Isolation and properties of a surface antigen of *Staphylococcus aureus*. J. Exp. Med. *115:*295–311.
116. Morse, S. I. 1962. Studies in the interactions between components of *Staphylococcus aureus* and staphylococcus bacteriophage. J. Exp. Med. *116:*247–251.
117. Morse, S. I. 1966. Biological and immunological properties of the staphylococcal cell walls. Ann. N. Y. Acad. Sci. *128:*191–213.
118. Morse, S. I. 1966. Biological and immunological properties of the staphylococcal cell wall. Postepy Mikrobiol. *5:*129–138.
119. Mudd, E. B. H., and S. Mudd. 1933. The process of phagocytosis. The agreement between direct observation and deductions from theory. J. Gen. Physiol. *16:*625–636.
120. Mudd, S. 1958. Staphylococcic infections in the hospital and community. J.A.M.A. *166:* 1177–1178.
121. Mudd, S. 1960. The practicability of enhancing specific resistance to staphylococcic infection. J.A.M.A. *173:*1360–1361.
122. Mudd, S. (ed.). 1964. The Population Crisis and the Use of World Resources. World Academy of Art and Science, II. Dr. W. Junk, Publishers, The Hague; Indiana University Press, Bloomington, Ind.
123. Mudd, S. 1965. Capsulation, pseudocapsulation, and the somatic antigens of the surface of *Staphylococcus aureus*. Ann. N.Y. Acad. Sci. *128:*45–58.
124. Mudd, S., and S. J. De Courcy, Jr. 1965. Interaction of viscid material of *Staphylococcus aureus* with specific immune serum. J. Bact. *89:*874–879.
125. Mudd, S., G. P. Gladstone, and N. A. Lenhart. 1965. The antigenicity in man of staphylococcal leucocidin toxoid, with notes on therapeutic immunization in chronic osteomyelitis. Brit. J. Exp. Path. *46:*455–472.

126. Mudd, S., G. P. Gladstone, N. A. Lenhart, and H. D. Hochstein. 1962. Titrations of anti-bodies against α-haemolysin and the components of staphylococcal leucocidin in human subjects following immunization. Brit. J. Exp. Path. *43*:313–319.

127. Mudd, S., T. Kawata, J. I. Payne, T. Sall, and A. Takagi. 1961. Plasma membranes and mitochondrial equivalents as functionally coordinated structures. Nature *189*:79–80.

128. Mudd, S., A. Yoshida, I. W. Li, and N. A. Lenhart. 1963. Identification of a somatic antigen of *Staphylococcus aureus* critical for phagocytosis by human blood leucocytes. Nature *199*:1200–1201.

129. Murray, R. G. E., P. Steed, and H. E. Elson. 1965. The location of the mucopeptide in sections of the cell wall of *Escherichia coli* and other gram negative bacteria. Canad. J. Microbiol. *11*:547–560.

130. Nahmias, A. J., M. J. Lepper, V. Hurst, and S. Mudd. 1962. Epidemiology and treatment of chronic staphylococcal infections in the household. Amer. J. Public Health *52*: 1828–1843.

131. Ng, L. K. Y., and S. Mudd (eds.). 1965. The Population Crisis, Implications and Plans for Action. Indiana University Press, Bloomington, Indiana.

132. Novick, R. P. 1965. The genetic determinant of staphylococcal penicillinase. Ann. N.Y. Acad. Sci. *128*:165–182.

133. Novick, R. P. 1966. Extrachromosomal inheritance of antibiotic resistance in *Staphylococcus aureus*. Postepy Mikrobiol. *5*:345–359.

134. Novick, R. P. 1967. Penicillinase plasmids of *Staphylococcus aureus*. Fed. Proc. *27*:29–38.

135. Novick, R. P., and S. I. Morse. 1967. *In vivo* transmission of drug resistance factors between strains of *Staphylococcus aureus*. J. Exp. Med. *125*:45–59.

136. Novick, R. P., and M. H. Richmond. 1965. Nature and interactions of the genetic elements governing penicillinase synthesis in *Staphylococcus aureus*. J. Bact. *90*:467–480.

137. Oeding, P. 1965. Antigenic properties of staphylococci. Ann. N.Y. Acad. Med. *128*:183–190.

138. Oeding, P. 1966. Antigenic structure of staphylococci. Postepy Mikrobiol. *5*:221–230.

139. Oeding, P., A. Grov, and B. Myklestad. 1964. Immunochemical studies on antigen preparations from *Staphylococcus aureus*. 2. Precipitating and erythrocyte-sensitizing properties of protein A (antigen A) and related substances. Acta Path. Microbiol. Scand. *62*:117–127.

140. Olitzki, A. L. 1966. The modifications of experimental infections by monocytin and splenocytin. Ninth International Congress for Microbiology, Moscow, Symposia, pp. 223–225.

141. Olitzki, A. L., and Z. Gershon. 1965. Splenocytin, a protective and curative product of murine spleen cells. Path. Microbiol. *28*:704–712.

142. Olitzki, A. L., and Z. Gershon. 1966. Prevention of lethal staphylococcal infections of mice by splenocytin. Ninth International Congress for Microbiology, Moscow, Abstracts of Papers, p. 405.

143. Panton, P. N., and F. C. O. Valentine. 1929. Staphylococcal infection and reinfection. Brit. J. Exp. Path. *10*:257–262.

144. Panton, P. N., and F. C. O. Valentine. 1932. Staphylococcal toxin. Lancet *1*:506–508.

145. Pattee, P. A., W. E. Kloos, J. B. Bodensteiner, and A. Zara. 1968. Homogeneity in a *Staphylococcus aureus* transducing fragment. J. Virology *2*:652–654.

146. Rammelkamp, C. H., M. M. Hezebicks, and J. H. Dingle. 1950. Specific coagulases of *Staphylococcus aureus*. J. Exp. Med. *91*:295–307.

147. Renshaw, E. C., and C. L. San Clemente. 1967. Lipase of *Staphylococcus aureus*, its purification and characterization. Developments Ind. Biol. *8*:214–226.

148. Richmond, M. H., and M. John. 1964. Co-transduction by staphylococcal phage of the genes responsible for penicillinase synthesis and resistance to mercury salts. Nature *202*:1360–1361.

149. Robertson, J. D. 1959. The ultrastructure of cell membranes and their derivatives. Biochem. Soc. Symp. *16*:3–43.

150. Rogers, D. E. 1966. Experimental observations on staphylococcal disease. Postepy Mikrobiol. *5*:279–296.

151. Rogers, D. E., and M. A. Melly. 1965. Speculations on the immunology of staphylococcal infections. Ann. N. Y. Acad. Sci. *128*:274–284.

152. Rosato, R. R., and J. A. Cameron. 1964. The bacteriophage receptor sites of *Staphylococcus aureus*. Biochim. Biophys. Acta *83*:113–119.

153. Rountree, P. M., M. A. Beard, J. Lowenthal, J. May, and S. B. Renwicke. 1967. Staphylococcal sepsis in a new surgical ward. Brit. Med. J. *1*:132–137.

154. Sall, T. 1962. Interrelationship of extracellular enzymes and pseudocapsulation in a strain of *Staphylococcus aureus*. J. Bact. *83*:1238–1243.

155. Sall, T., S. Mudd, and J. Taubler. 1961. Concerning the surfaces of cells of *Staphylococcus*

*pyogenes*. A pseudocapsulation phenomenon under certain experimental conditions. J. Exp. Med. *113*:693–700.

156. Salton, M. R. J. 1964. The Bacterial Cell Wall. Elsevier, Amsterdam, p. 133.

157. Sanderson, A. R., W. G. Juergens, and J. L. Strominger. 1961. Chemical and immunochemical structure of teichoic acid from *Staphylococcus aureus* (Copenhagen). Biochem. Biophys. Res. Commun. *5*:472–476.

157a. Schuhardt, V. T., T. W. Huber, and L. M. Pope. 1969. Electron microscopy and viability of lysostaphin-induced staphylococcal spheroplasts, protoplast-like bodies, and protoplasts. J. Bact. *97*:396–401.

158. Scrimshaw, N. S. 1961. Nutrition and infection. *In:* Brock, J. F. (ed.). Recent Advances in Human Nutrition. Little, Brown & Co., Boston.

159. Scrimshaw, N. S. 1966. Interactions of nutrition and infection: Synergistic and antagonistic interactions of nutrition and infection. Fed. Proc. *25*:1679–1681.

160. Sevag, M. G. 1964. Prevention of the emergence of antibiotic-resistant strains of bacteria by atabrine. Arch. Biochem. Biophys. *108*:85–88.

161. Sevag, M. G., and B. Ashton. 1964. Evolution and prevention of drug-resistance. Nature *203*:1323–1326.

162. Sevag, M. G., and B. Ashton. 1965. Prevention of antibiotic and sulfonamide resistance by atabrine. *In:* Antimicrobial Agents Chemotherapy—1964. pp. 410–414.

163. Sevag, M. G., and S. J. De Courcy, Jr. 1969. Biochemical events underlying the evolution and prevention of drug resistance in microorganisms. *In:* Oparin, A. I. (ed.). N. M. Sissakian Memorial Volume [in Russian].

164. Sevag, M. G., and W. T. Drabble. 1962. Prevention of the emergence of drug-resistant bacteria by polyamines. Biochem. Biophys. Res. Commun. *8*:446–452.

165. Shah, D. B., and J. B. Wilson. 1965. Egg yolk factor in *Staphylococcus aureus*. II. Characterization of lipase activity. J. Bact. *89*:949–953.

166. Sharda, D. C., D. Cornfeld, and A. J. Michie. 1966. Effect of mepacrine (atebrin) on the success of antibacterial treatment of urinary infections. Arch. Dis. Child. *41*:400–401.

167. Shayegani, M. G. 1968. Action of lysates of leukocytic granules on staphylococcal cell walls. J. Infect. Dis. *118*:402–410.

168. Shayegani, M. G., F. A. Kapral, and S. Mudd. 1964. Phagocytosis and intracellular killing of *Staphylococcus aureus* by human and rabbit blood leucocytes. J. Immun. *93*:88–93.

169. Shayegani, M. G., and S. Mudd. 1966. Role of serum in the intracellular killing of staphylococci in rabbit monocytes. J. Bact. *91*:1393–1398.

169a. Mudd, S., Zappasodi, P., and Taubler, J. H. 1969. Resistance to vaccinia in tuberculin-hypersensitive mice. Bact. Proc. 1969 M16.

170. Smith, D. D. 1956. α- and γ-lysin production by R variants of *Staphylococcus aureus*. Nature *178*:1060–1061.

171. Smith, D. T. 1968. *In:* Smith, D. T., Conant, N. F., and Overman, J. R. (eds.): Zinsser Microbiology. 14th ed. Appleton-Century-Crofts, New York, pp. 462–465.

172. Smith, T. 1963. Vanuxem Lectures on Parasitism and Disease. Princeton University Press, 1934 and 1963; reprinted by Hafner Publishing Co., New York, 1963.

173. Součková, J., and J. Johanovský. 1961. Experiences gained in the preparation and administration of staphylococcal toxoid in Czechoslovakia. Proceedings of the Seventh International Congress on Biological Standardisation, London.

174. Součková-Štěpánová, J., G. P. Gladstone, and R. Vaněček. 1965. The immunization of rabbits with staphylococcal leucocidin toxoid. Brit. J. Exp. Path. *46*:384–407.

175. Součková-Štěpánová, J., R. Vaněček. J. H. Taubler, and S. Mudd. 1969. Unpublished.

176. Spitznagel, J. K., and L. A. Wilson. 1966. Normal serum cytotoxicity for P32 labeled smooth Enterobacteriaceae. I. Loss of label, death and ultrastructural damage. J. Bact. *91*:393–400.

177. Stevens, F. A., and L. Jordani. 1936. Reactions to intracutaneous injections of nucleoproteins of the upper respiratory pathogenic bacteria in asthmatic patients. J. Allerg. *7*:443–450.

178. Stewart, G. T. 1965. The lipases and pigments of staphylococci. Ann. N. Y. Acad. Sci. *128*:132–151.

179. Suganuma, A. 1965. Fine structure of *Staphylococcus aureus*. Ann. N. Y. Acad. Sci. *128*:26–44.

180. Swineford, O., Jr., and J. Holman. 1949. Studies in bacterial allergy. J. Allerg. *20*:420–427.

181. Szmigielski, S., J. Jeljaszewicz, J. Wilczynski, and M. Korbecki. 1966. Reaction of rabbit leucocytes to staphylococcal (Panton-Valentine) leucocidin *in vivo*. J. Path. Bact. *91*:599–604.

182. Szmigielski, S., J. Jeljaszewicz, and C. Zak. 1967. Reaction of rabbit leukocytes to staphylococcal alpha hemolysin *in vivo*. J. Infect. Dis. *117*:209–214.

183. Tager, M., and M. C. Drummond. 1965. Staphylocoagulase. Ann. N. Y. Acad. Sci. *128:*92–111.

184. Taubler, J. H. 1966. Staphylococcal delayed hypersensitivity in mice. Bact. Proc., p. 62.

185. Taubler, J. H. 1966. *In vivo* and *in vitro* demonstration of delayed hypersensitivity in mice following infection with *Staphylococcus aureus.* J. Reticuloendothel. Soc. 3:367–368.

186. Taubler, J. H. 1968. Staphylococcal delayed hypersensitivity in mice. I. Induction and *in vivo* demonstration of delayed hypersensitivity. J. Immun. *101:*546–549.

187. Taubler, J. H., F. A. Kapral, and S. Mudd. 1963. Role of alpha-toxin in lesion formation by *Staphylococcus aureus* on sutures subcutaneously implanted in mice. J. Bact. *86:*51–57.

188. Taubler, J. H., N. A. Lenhart, and S. Mudd. 1966. Evidence of delayed hypersensitivity in staphylococcal infection. Ninth International Congress for Microbiology, Moscow, Abstracts of Papers, p. 405.

189. Taubler, J. H., and S. Mudd. 1968. Staphylococcal delayed hypersensitivity in mice. II. *In vitro* demonstration and specificity of delayed hypersensitivity. J. Immun. *101:*550–555.

190. Taubler, J. H., S. Mudd, and T. Sall. 1962. Partial protection of mice by human gamma-globulin against *Staphylococcus aureus* on subcutaneous sutures. Proc. Soc. Exp. Biol. Med. *109:*20–23.

190a. Tipper, D. J., J. L. Strominger, and J. C. Ensign. 1967. Structure of the cell wall of *Staphylococcus aureus*, strain Copenhagen. VII. Mode of action of the bacteriolytic peptidase from *Myxobacter* and the isolation of intact cell wall polysaccharides. Biochemistry *6:*906–920; Chem. Eng. News *45:*19, 1967.

191. Torii, M., E. A. Kabat, and A. E. Bezer. 1964. Separation of teichoic acid of *Staphylococcus aureus* into two immunologically distinct specific polysaccharides with α- and β-N-acetylglucosaminyl linkages, respectively. Antigenicity of teichoic acid in man. J. Exp. Med. *120:*13–29.

192. Vanderwinkel, E., and R. G. E. Murray. 1962. Organelles intracytoplasmiques bactériens et site d'activité oxydoréductrice. J. Ultrastruct. Res. *7:*185–199.

193. Van Iterson, W. 1965. Symposium on the fine structure and replication of bacteria and their parts. II. Bacterial cytoplasm. Bact. Rev. *29:*299–325.

194. Verwey, W. F. 1940. A type-specific antigenic protein derived from the Staphylococcus. J. Exp. Med. *71:*635–694.

195. Wieghard, C. W., and L. A. Julianelle. 1935. The immunological specificity of staphylococci. II. The chemical nature of the soluble specific substances. J. Exp. Med. *62:*23–30.

196. Wiley, B. B. 1961. A new virulence test for *Staphylococcus aureus* and its application to encapsulated strains. Canad. J. Microbiol. *7:*933–943.

197. Wiley, B. B. 1963. The incidence of encapsulated staphylococci and anticapsular antibodies in normal humans. Canad. J. Microbiol. *9:*27–32.

198. Wiley, B. B. 1964. Virulence and encapsulation in hospital strains of *Staphylococcus aureus.* Bact. Proc., p. 76.

199. Wiley, B. B., and N. H. Maverakis. 1968. Virulent and avirulent encapsulated variants of *Staphylococcus aureus.* J. Bact. *95:*998–1002.

200. Wiley, B. B., and J. C. Wonnacott. 1962. Isolation and partial characterization of a capsular material from *Staphylococcus aureus.* J. Bact. *83:*1169–1176.

201. Williams, R. E. O. 1966. Epidemiology of airborne staphylococcal infections. Bact. Rev. *30:*660–674.

202. Williams, R. E. O., R. Blowers, L. P. Garrod, and R. A. Shooter. 1960. Hospital Infection, Causes and Prevention. Year Book Medical Publishers, Chicago.

203. Wiseman, G. M., and J. D. Caird. 1968. Phospholipase activity of the delta hemolysin of *Staphylococcus aureus.* Proc. Soc. Exp. Biol. Med. *128:*428–430.

204. Wolin, M. J., A. R. Archibald, and J. Baddiley. 1966. Changes in wall teichoic acid resulting from mutations of *Staphylococcus aureus.* Nature *209:*484–486.

205. Woodin, A. M. 1965. Staphylococcal leucocidin. Ann. N.Y. Acad. Sci. *128:*152–164.

206. Woodin, A. M. 1966. Staphylococcal leucocidin. Postepy Mikrobiol. *5:*163–170.

206a. Woodin, A. M. 1968. The basis of leucocidin action. *In:* Bittar, E. C., and N. Bittar (eds.): The Biological Basis of Medicine. Vol. 2. Academic Press, New York.

207. Woodin, A. M., J. E. French, and V. T. Marchesi. 1963. Morphological changes associated with the extrusion of protein induced in polymorphonuclear leucocyte by staphylococcal leucocidin. Biochem. J. *87:*567–571.

208. Woodin, A. M., and A. A. Wieneke. 1966. The interaction of leucocidin with the cell membrane of the polymorphonuclear leucocyte. Biochem. J. *99:*479–492.

209. Woodin, A. M., and A. A. Wieneke. 1967. The participation of phospholipids in the interaction of leucocidin and the cell membrane of the polymorphonuclear leucocyte. Biochem. J. *105:*1029–1038.

210. Worms, R. 1966. On the physiopathology of staphylococcal infections associated with blood stream invasion. Postepy Mikrobiol. *5:*473–484.

211. Yoshida, A. 1963. Staphylococcal δ-hemolysin. I. Purification and chemical properties. Biochim. Biophys. Acta *71:*544–553.

212. Yoshida, A., and C.-G. Hedén. 1962. Some serological properties of staphylococcal cells and cell walls. J. Immun. *88:*389–393.

213. Yoshida, A., C.-G. Hedén, B. Cedergren, and L. Edebo. 1961. A method for the preparation of undigested bacterial cell walls. J. Biochem. Microbiol. Tech. Eng. *3:*151–159.

214. Yoshida, A., S. Mudd, and N. A. Lenhart. 1963. The common protein agglutinogen of *Staphylococcus aureus*. II. Purification, chemical characterization and serologic comparison with Jensen's antigen. J. Immun. *91:*777–782.

215. Zucker-Franklin, D., and J. G. Hirsch. 1964. Electron microscope studies on degranulation of rabbit peritoneal leukocytes during phagocytosis. J. Exp. Med. *120:*569–576.

216. Jessen, O., K. Rosendahl, P. Bülow, V. Faber, and K. R. Ericsen. 1969. Changing staphylococci and staphylococcal infections. A ten year study of bacteria and cases of bacteremia. New Eng. J. Med. *281:*627–635.

# Chapter 10

# TUBERCULOSIS: RETROSPECTS AND PROSPECTS

GARDNER MIDDLEBROOK

*Professor of International Medicine,*
*University of Maryland, Baltimore, Maryland*

On the occasion of a meeting of the National Tuberculosis Association of the United States, nearly 60 years ago, Dr. William Welch, that most distinguished physician of the Johns Hopkins University, said: "It may now be stated that while all of these problems relating to tuberculosis have not yet been solved, we have an amount of information which enables us to state positively that, if practical measures based upon this exact scientific knowledge are properly applied, the amount of tuberculosis can be reduced to a relatively small figure."[1]

And at another meeting of the same organization, one of its most outstanding founders, Dr. Lawrence Flick, of Philadelphia, said, "The measures by which tuberculosis is to be stamped out have been fully outlined and clearly defined."[2] He went on to list those measures, emphasizing "clean living" and isolation of active cases; he did not even mention the need for further research! Now, more than 60 years later there are about 50,000 new active cases of tuberculosis each year in this country at an estimated annual direct cost to the nation of $750 million; and the U.S. Public Health Service tells us that their estimate of the number of new cases to be anticipated in the year 1980 is 41,000, a reduction of only 9000 cases per year, with a total of 500,000 new cases between 1968 and 1980. If tuberculosis were a newly appearing disease, this present and future burden would indeed seem impressive.

Nevertheless, perhaps Drs. Welch and Flick were right, at least partly so. Tuberculosis, which was already declining epidemically at the time they spoke, has dramatically decreased since their day, in the United States and in Europe, though it is still rampant in the developing nations. And more than two-thirds of the new cases of the next decade, in the United States, will arise in individuals already infected with virulent tubercle bacilli. Therefore it seems worth-while to examine the scientific evidence available at the start of this century regarding the nature of tuberculosis in man, the evidence that was available to Drs. Flick and Welch and on which they based their convictions.

The germ theory of Pasteur and the bacteriologic discoveries of Koch had a unifying influence on scientific concepts relating to infectious diseases in general, and to tuberculosis in particular. Even before Koch's detection and artificial cultivation of tubercle bacilli, Villemin[3] in his animal investigations of more than 100 years ago demonstrated the transmissibility of a supposed "virus" of tuberculosis; and he concluded on the basis of limited observation and much speculation that the germs must be transmitted from man to man by the airborne route. Therefore, he recommended ventilation of living and sleeping quarters as the primary method of prevention of tuberculosis. At the same time Villemin expressed the hopeful conviction that an immunizing agency like Jenner's vaccination against smallpox would ultimately be discovered against tuberculosis. Undoubtedly Welch and Flick knew of and believed in these same approaches. The crusade which they participated in did not emphasize the importance of more fundamental research into the details of the pathogenesis of tuberculosis. It was based, like all crusades, on simplification of the problem, and action based upon this simplification achieved results. Perhaps the continuing decline in tuberculosis since their time is largely due to "cleaner living." Certainly it is due to better living and, in particular, to all of the many factors which have permitted, intentionally or unintentionally, greater and greater dilution of tubercle bacilli in the air that we breathe, and thus in a spectacular reduction in the number of new infections, year by year.

The one question that can fairly be asked now is: can we afford to wait until the next century for the predicted disappearance of tuberculosis in our country? The answer cannot be primarily humanitarian in nature: thanks to direct antimicrobial chemotherapy, very few persons suffer or die as a result of tuberculosis in the United States today. The response must be essentially economic, because effective as chemotherapy can be, its application is expensive: $750 million per year. Can further research reduce this burden?

One unequivocal lesson of the development of science and technology during the last 200 years is that scientific research, in addition to the gratification which it brings to the curiosity of individual investigators, is the principal handmaiden of economic benefit. If this be so, then is it not reasonable for the pharmaceutical houses to seek more effective chemotherapeutic agents for tuberculosis? Such would indeed be the case were it not for the most important obstacle in the chemotherapy of bacterial infections: The fundamental deficiency of therapeutic chemical antimicrobial agents acting directly on microbes is their ineffectiveness in sterilizing those few residual, resting, metabolically dormant microorganisms which serve as the seeds of relapse.[4] The sterilizing antimicrobial action of antiseptics, which are cellular poisons too nonspecific to be employed as systemic chemotherapeutics, are not shared by any of the chemotherapeutic agents for infectious processes. Thus one is forced to look for other than the classic chemotherapeutic agencies for the prevention of infection and of relapse of established infection into disease, except when very long-term administration of drugs is employed. And such long-term treatment is fraught with hazards and the obstinacy and forgetfulness of human beings. Therefore, one is forced to return to immunologic methods which obviate these deficiencies of chemoprophylaxis.

At the present time it is estimated that about $5 million is expended in the United States for all research on tuberculosis. This is only about 0.65 per cent of the total burden of the disease in our country. This can be contrasted to our expenditure of $18 billion for all research out of a gross national product of $800 billion, or 2.2 per cent. Thus, in this frame of reference, we are spending only one-third to one-fourth of what we should be spending for research on tuberculosis. How should the additional funds be spent and what promise is there that they would be productive of some new, practically applicable immunologic tools for the prevention or better control of tuberculosis? Indeed, why don't we use more widely the immunologic tool we already have, a living attenuated vaccine such as BCG? The reasons are clear:

1. BCG vaccination, as it is practiced today, confers tuberculin hypersensitivity on the vaccinated and it is not distinguishable from the tuberculin hypersensitivity of the natural infection. Thus it interferes with the epidemiologic monitoring of tuberculous infection and cannot be widely applied except in certain high risk groups.

2. BCG vaccination provides no protection against disease in those individuals who are already infected with *Mycobacterium tuberculosis*, and two-thirds of all new cases of tuberculosis in the United States today develop in those who are already infected.

It might be profitable at this point to return to Villemin's prediction that a living attenuated "virus" may someday find usefulness as a vaccine against tuberculosis.[3] Perhaps it is not too much of an exaggeration to state that only two important steps have been made in the direction suggested by Villemin: first, many attenuated mutant strains of *M. tuberculosis* and other related strains of mycobacteria as well, in living state, have been shown to be capable of immunizing against tuberculosis in experimental animals and in man; and, second, several killed vaccines have been shown also to be more or less effective—indeed, equally so, for a limited period of time, in some investigations. This second observation established the fact that a state of resistance can be elicited by one or several chemical components of the bacterial cells.

One of the most active fields of immunologic research during the past four decades, and one of the most fruitful in other fields, has been the analysis in chemical terms of the antigenic mosaic of microbial cells, the separation of its components and the determination of their chemical nature and of their biologic properties. However, in the chemical analysis of mycobacteria, this approach has been quite unproductive. And it seems worthwhile to inquire why this has been so. Before this is done, however, it might be appropriate to consider the continuing attempts to understand antituberculous immunity in biologic terms by studying the host-parasite relationship *in vitro* with macrophages and tubercle bacilli.

All of the investigations which have revealed an antibacterial effect of immune macrophages against tubercle bacilli have employed streptomycin in the fluid medium in order to prevent the confusing effect of extracellular proliferation of the bacilli, on the assumption that streptomycin did not affect the intracellular bacilli. More recent studies, however, have suggested that the streptomycin is *not* inactive against the intracellular bacilli in macrophages from immune and tuberculin-hypersensitive animals.[5] Indeed, one of the important properties of hypersensitive macrophages seems to be an increased permeability of their membranes for streptomycin and even much larger molecules—including proteins—when they are bearing an antigen to which they are "hypersensitive."[6] Thus the results of such experiments can no longer be fairly interpreted as evidence of a purely cellular immunity in tuberculosis. However, they do suggest that the increased permeability of "hypersensitive" macrophages may permit humoral factors to play a role against intracellular parasites, which can no longer be considered to be "protected" against humoral antibodies merely by virtue of their intracellular habitat.

Other evidences of what is probably an overemphasis on the purely biologic aspects of immunity, as a manifestation of frustration with failure of immunochemical approaches, are found in the contemporary preoccupation with what is called "cellular immunity." The expression "cellular immunity" itself implies a kind of immunity which denies a place for humoral antibodies. Yet, in spite of those elegant experiments[7] which have again emphasized that the final, common pathway for the antibacterial manifestations of immunity against intracellular parasites, such as mycobacteria, brucellae, and listeriae, is located within the macrophage, the nonspecific cross-immunity between these infections has been shown to persist for no longer than three weeks after appropriate stimulation. On the other hand, the species-specific immunity persists for many months or even years.[8]

It should also be pointed out that the discovery of, and enthusiasm for, lysosomes of phagocytic cells[9] has obscured the possibly greater importance of hydrogen peroxide and perhaps other peroxides in the metabolic economy of hypersensitive macrophages exposed to their specific allergens, as non-specific antibacterial agents in the final, common pathway of antibacterial immunity against such organisms as *M. tuberculosis*,[10] *Brucella abortus*,[11] and *Pasteurella pestis*.[12]

Another, though very worthwhile, endeavor, which is again at least in part a result of failures with the immunochemical approach to analysis of bacterial structures concerned in the immune process, has been the study of host variations, genotypic and phenotypic, in susceptibility to tuberculous infection and disease.[13] Important as these studies have been considered to be, they have not contributed to molecular explanations of mechanisms of immunity in tuberculosis.

Still another area of investigation has been considered a closed book by nearly all investigators,[7] namely, passive transfer of immunity with immune serum or its various fractions. This is not justified in view of the following. The few passive transfer experiments which have been reported have been performed either with guinea pigs, whose level of acquired immunity is poor at best, or, when successful,[14] with too few animals. On the other hand, experiments have been reported with rabbits which are known to be capable of mounting a strikingly effective, almost absolute, immunity against aerogenic tuberculous infection, even with *M. bovis*.[15] Furthermore, if it should be shown that humoral factors, especially specific antibodies, can only penetrate hypersensitive macrophages bearing parasites to which they are hypersensitive, then cellular hypersensitivity of the tuberculin type must also be considered essential for the successful transfer of immunity by antibodies.* Tuberculin hypersensitivity, without immunity, has been conferred on guinea pigs with the wax D fraction of *M. tuberculosis* along with tuberculoprotein in water-in-oil emulsion.[16] Thus the technical basis for more properly oriented experiments relating to the role of serum factors is at hand.

In summary, regarding these biologic aspects of immunity in tuberculosis, it seems appropriate to quote Max Lurie.[13] "The historical separation of cellular and humoral factors in acquired resistance to tuberculosis and other intracellular pathogens is hardly tenable in the light of the interdependence and integration of the processes which characterize the responses of the body to injury."

Before leaving the biologic aspects of the host-parasite relationship, it seems important to point to the chaotic state of opinions among contemporary investigators of immunity in tuberculosis regarding the proper experimental animal model to be employed for this purpose. One can find almost as many "models" as investigators. They vary with respect to animal species: there are the mouse, the guinea pig, the rabbit, and sometimes the monkey "enthusiasts." The routes of challenge employed as favored by one or the other groups range from intracorneal, to intravenous, to aerogenic, and many others. The evaluation of immunity varies from lung density measurements to crude gross observation of lesions, to bacterial counts by culture (called "microbial enumeration" by some sophisticates), to gross survival times after either small or large infective doses by the various routes.[17] And, what is most important, different "immunizing preparations," extracts and cell fractions, have widely different effects in this multiplicity of experimental models.[18]

Some two decades ago, as a result of the wealth of experimental observations relating "virulence antigens" to specific protective antibodies in a variety of acute bacterial infections, efforts were begun to identify some chemical substance(s) or biochemical properties of *M. tuberculosis* with "virulence." Thus it was observed that all virulent strains of *M. tuberculosis* grow *in vitro* in an impressively oriented pattern of "cords" or bacilli, serpentine in appearance, with the rods arranged in parallel along the long axis of the cord. On the other hand, all strains of *M. tuberculosis* which present a nonoriented microscopical arrangement of bacilli were observed to be attenuated in virulence.[19] That this phenomenon involved orientation of the virulent bacilli to each other during multiplication, and that it could be overcome by certain nontoxic surface-action agents, give some confidence this was a reflection of a "virulence factor" composing an important part of surface of each bacterial cell.

---

* The authors invited to contribute to this volume were carefully selected as being among the most experienced and knowledgeable in their respective fields. Certainly Professor Middlebrook is such an author. The Editor, however, would like to point out the highly hypothetical nature of this sentence, which seems to be rather essential to Professor Middlebrook's critical view of cellular immunity in tuberculosis. The Editor would point out: (1) that macrophages derived from normal animals are capable of engulfing their suspending fluids by pinocytosis, and (2) that the majority of attempts thus far to show protective action by antibodies to tubercle bacilli have been unsuccessful. One hopes that Professor Middlebrook's investigation of a new fraction in the antigène méthylique may prove more rewarding. Ed.

About the same time a cytochemical reaction was described which clearly distinguished between the cord-forming and the noncord-forming mutant strains of *M. tuberculosis*—the so-called neutral red test.[20] It seems likely that this cytochemical reaction was a reflection of the presence of some strongly acidic substance at or near the surface of the virulent bacterial cells. Several years later, by use of this cytochemical reaction on extracts of *M. tuberculosis* strains, a sulfolipid substance was isolated[21] which proved to contain a sulfuric acid bound in ester form to trehalose which was in turn esterified with two or more long-chain fatty acids. Further studies revealed this fraction to be extractable from a series of strains of *M. tuberculosis* of different degrees of virulence in amounts closely related to their infectivity.[22] A variety of serologic tests have failed to reveal the presence of antibodies against this sulfolipid material in a variety of sera from tuberculous animals or human beings. Thus it appears to be immunologically inert; and it has not proved to be especially toxic for mammalian tissues or cell cultures. Its possible role in the pathogenesis of tuberculosis is still obscure. Nevertheless, because of its close relationships to the morphologic phenomenon of cord formation and neutral red reaction of virulent strains of *M. tuberculosis*, it seems fair to consider it the "cord factor." The term "cord factor" was applied several years ago to a substance[23] which proved to be trehalose-6,6'-dimycolate without adequate justification for considering it responsible for the phenomenon of cord formation.[24] It has subsequently been shown that certain avirulent strains of *M. tuberculosis* are unable to synthesize trehalose[25] and are thus deficient in both trehalose-dimycolate and sulfolipid. However, sulfolipid has never been isolated from mycobacteria other than virulent *M. tuberculosis*, whereas trehalose-dimycolate has been found in significant amount in the saprophyte *M. phlei*.

In summary, as of this date, the studies of virulence of tubercle bacilli, as correlated with their morphologic or chemical properties, have been disappointing in terms of their yield of information relating to mechanisms of pathogenicity and immunity.

Boquet and Nègre,[26] in France, during the 1920's, were probably the first to claim that a relatively nontoxic, chemical fraction of tubercle bacilli as they are grown artificially in the laboratory could establish a significant degree of acquired resistance against experimental tuberculosis in animals. Their original observation has been confirmed by many subsequent investigations; but it was not until a very few years ago that the science and technology of chemistry could provide some tools which would permit the separation and study of the many different chemical substances in their crude fraction, the "antigène méthylique" of Boquet and Nègre.

Starting with chromatographic procedures which have recently been applied to this crude material by the well known lipid procedures and biochemists, Lederer[27] in Paris, Ballou[28] in Berkeley, California, and Pangborn[29] in Albany, New York, and using some new procedures of our own, as well as a hemagglutination test with human and animal sera, we have been able to isolate in much purer form a fraction which appears to us to be especially interesting at this time, for the following reasons:

1. The amount of antibodies against this material in the sera of mice appears in preliminary tests to be correlated with the degrees of immunity which

those animals manifest after aerogenic challenge with virulent tubercle bacilli. These antibodies are often of an "incomplete" type and they are present in quite low concentration in the sera of the immunized animals—indeed, so low and of such a nature, that it seems doubtful that they have been detected previously.

2. This material from methanol extracts of mycobacterial cells is a phosphoglycolipid which exists in two different forms, with the same immunochemical specificity, in such extracts. One form ("G") reacts readily with antibodies; the other ("K") does not, unless its aqueous solution is treated with a surface-active substance such as sodium desoxycholate or nonionic surface-active agents. The latter form predominates in extracts of virulent strains, and the former in attenuated (BCG) strains, according to present results.

3. By special hemagglutination inhibition techniques we have observed that the bacilli of leprosy have a substance of the same or very similar structure. This seems relevant to the fairly well documented observation that BCG vaccination can immunize human beings against tuberculoid leprosy,[30] and that BCG cell walls, specially prepared, can confer resistance against multiplication of *M. leprae* in the foot pads of mice.[31]

Finally, would it or should it be possible to immunize against tuberculosis and, perhaps, leprosy with this substance? Several investigators, immunologists, have tried to immunize experimental animals with the various subfractions of the crude extract of Boquet and Nègre, and been uniformly disappointed. Indeed, the entire history of the immunochemistry of tuberculosis is one of loss of vaccinating activity associated with separation and purification of the chemical substances of which the tubercle bacilli are constructed. This behavior is quite characteristic of the behavior of what immunologists have been wont to call haptens, although, of course, this is not the only possible explanation of the loss of activity of fractions. Nevertheless, this hypothesis was something which suggests a feasible new direction of work, namely, the chemical coupling or conjugation of this reasonable well purified, apparently haptenic, molecule to a protein molecule in efforts to endow the substance with powerful antigenic activity, to cause animals to produce serum antibodies against itself. This would permit examination, without the impossibly complicating interference of many other immunologic responses, of the role which this substance and antibodies against it might play in tuberculosis.

Suffice it to end by stating the conviction that recent and future progress in the general technology of chemistry and immunochemistry will someday provide us with better understanding and, perhaps, control of the mechanisms of immunity and vaccination against tuberculosis. Such information would doubtless have important implications for the mechanisms of pathogenesis of and immunity against other parasites, both "exogenous," as infectious agents, and "endogenous," as neoplastic cells.

# References

1. Welch, W. H. 1909. Address. Trans. Nat. Tuberc. Assoc. 5:34–36.
2. Flick, L. 1906. The relative value of home treatment of tuberculosis. Trans. Nat. Tuberc. Assoc. 2:442–458.

3. Villemin, J. A. 1868. Etudes sur la tuberculose. J. B. Baillière et Fils, Paris.

4. Middlebrook, G., W. F. Russell, and S. H. Dressler. 1956. Chemotherapy of tuberculosis. Advances Intern. Med. *8:*221–257.

5. Chang, Y. T. 1967. Suppressive activity on the growth of *Mycobacterium lepraemurium* in macrophage culture. J. Reticuloendothel. Soc. *4:*430.

6. Kochan, I., and L. Smith. 1965. Antimycobacterial activity of tuberculostatic factor on intracellular bacilli. J. Immun. *94:*220–227.

7. Mackaness, G. B. 1968. The immunology of antituberculous immunity. Amer. Rev. Resp. Dis. *97:*337–344.

8. Anacker, R. L., W. R. Barclay, W. Brehmer, C. L. Larson, and E. Ribi. 1967. Duration of immunity to tuberculosis in mice vaccinated intravenously with oil-treated cell walls of *Mycobacterium bovis* strain BCG. J. Immun. *98:*1265–1273.

9. Cohn, Z. A., and S. I. Morse. 1960. Functional and metabolic properties of polymorphonuclear leucocytes. II. The influence of a lipopolysaccharide endotoxin. J. Exp. Med. *111:*689–704.

10. Middlebrook, G. 1956. Diagnostic and biological problems of isoniazid-resistant tubercle bacilli. Bull. Int. Un. Tuberc. *26:*179–205.

11. Wilson, J. B., and B. L. Dasinger. 1960. Biochemical properties of virulent and avirulent strains of brucellae. Ann. N. Y. Acad. Sci. *88:*1155–1166.

12. Rockenmacher, M. 1949. Relationship of catalase activity to virulence in *Pasteurella pestis.* Proc. Soc. Exp. Biol. Med. *71:*99–101.

13. Lurie, M. B. 1964. Resistance to Tuberculosis. Harvard University Press, Cambridge, Mass., p. 104.

14. Neufeld, F., and B. Lange. 1922. Versuche einer passiven Übertragung der Tuberkuloseimmunität an Schafen. Z. Hyg. *98:*215–228.

15. Ratcliffe, H. L., and W. F. Wells, 1948. Tuberculosis of rabbits induced by droplet nuclei infection. II. Response to reinfection. J. Exp. Med. *87:*585–594.

16. Raffel, S. 1950. Chemical factors involved in the induction of infectious allergy. Experientia *6:*410–419.

17. Smith, D. W., A. A. Grover, and E. Wiegeshaus, 1968. Nonliving immunogenic substances of Mycobacteria. Advances Tuberc. Res. *16:*191–227.

18. Ribi, E., W. Brehmer, and K. Milner. 1967. Specificity of resistance to tuberculosis and to salmonellosis stimulated in mice by oil-treated cell walls. Proc. Soc. Exp. Biol. Med. *124:*408–413.

19. Middlebrook, G., R. J. Dubos, and C. Pierce. 1947. Virulence and morphological characteristics of mammalian tubercle bacilli. J. Exp. Med. *86:*175–184.

20. Middlebrook, G., and R. J. Dubos. 1948. Cytochemical reaction of virulent tubercle bacilli. Amer. Rev. Tuberc. *58:*698–699.

21. Middlebrook, G., C. M. Coleman, and W. B. Schaefer. 1959. Sulfolipid from virulent tubercle bacilli. Proc. Nat. Acad. Sci. *45:*1801–1804.

22. Gangadharam, P. R. J., M. L. Cohn, and G. Middlebrook. 1963. Infectivity, pathogenicity and sulpholipid fraction of some Indian and British strains of tubercle bacilli. Tubercle *44:*452–455.

23. Bloch, H. 1950. Studies on the virulence of tubercle bacilli: Isolation and biological properties of a constituent of virulent organisms. J. Exp. Med. *91:*197–217.

24. Dubos, R. J. 1955. Mechanisms of microbial pathogenicity. *In:* Symp. Soc. Gen. Microbiol. Cambridge University Press, London, pp. 103–125.

25. Goldman, D., and F. A. Lornitzo. 1962. Enzyme systems in the mycobacteria. XII. The inhibition of the transglycosidase-catalyzed formation of trehalose-6-phosphate. J. Biol. Chem. *237:*3332–3338.

26. Boquet, A., and L. Nègre. 1923. Sur les propriétés biologiques des lipoïdes du bacille tuberculeux. Ann. Inst. Pasteur. *37:*787–805.

27. Pigretti, M., E. Vilkas, and E. Lederer. 1965. Propriétés chimique et biologiques de fractions phosphatidiques isolées de "l'antigène méthylique" de *Mycobacterium tuberculosis.* Bull. Soc. Chim. Biol. *47:*2039–2046.

28. Ballou, C. E., E. Vilkas, and E. Lederer. 1963. Structural studies on the myo-inositol phospholipids of *Mycobacterium tuberculosis* (var. *bovis*, strain BCG). J. Biol. Chem. *238:*69–76.

29. Pangborn, M., and J. A. McKinney, 1966. Purification of serologically active phosphoinositides of *Mycobacterium tuberculosis.* J. Lipid Res. *7:*627–633.

30. Brown, J. A. K., and I. Sutherland. 1968. Studies of BCG vaccination against leprosy in Uganda. Ann. N. Y. Acad. Sci. *154:*237–243.

31. Shepard, C. C., and E. Ribi. 1968. Cell walls from *Mycobacterium tuberculosis* (BCG) as vaccine against *Mycobacterium leprae* infections in mice. Proc. Soc. Exp. Biol. Med. *127:*517–521.

# INFECTIONS
# BY
# GRAM-NEGATIVE
# PATHOGENS

# Chapter 11

# BORDETELLA PERTUSSIS —BACTERIAL AND HOST FACTORS IN THE PATHOGENESIS AND PREVENTION OF WHOOPING COUGH

MARGARET PITTMAN

*Chief, Laboratory of Bacterial Products, Division of Biologics Standards, National Institutes of Health, Bethesda, Maryland*

Pertussis (whooping cough) presents a number of anomalous features, clinical, pathological, epidemiological, and immunological, and the causative bacterium *Bordetella pertussis* possesses unique properties among pathogenic bacteria. This paper is directed toward the nature of the infection, natural and experimental, and immunological and reactive components of *B. pertussis* as they relate to the efficacy, safety, and control of pertussis vaccine. Special emphasis is placed on the properties of pertussis vaccine from the viewpoint of affording the child maximum protection against whooping cough with minimum untoward reaction. Deficiencies in information are noted. The paper is not a chronological review, and references cited will not necessarily be chronological or complete. Extensive literature citations appear in the reviews by Andersen,[6] Bradford,[20] Kind,[91] Kuwajima and Niwa,[96] Lapin,[100] Munoz,[129, 130] and Munoz and Bergman.[131] The human and animal responses to infection are presented at the beginning of the paper. Some readers may wish to begin with the later sections on General Description of *B. pertussis* and Cellular Components.

# HUMAN RESPONSE TO *BORDETELLA PERTUSSIS* INFECTION

Pertussis is a localized respiratory infection with specific manifestations of paroxysmal coughing, lymphocytosis, and neurological symptoms. The disease presents a number of unique symptoms and epidemiological features.[63] After an incubation period of 10 to 16 days,[36, 63, 101, 189] there is an undifferentiated catarrhal stage with low-grade fever which lasts one to two weeks. After the acute phase is largely past and the patient is afebrile, the characteristic symptom, paroxysmal coughing, is manifested. Coughing lasts for four to eight weeks and may persist for 20 weeks. The average duration of the disease is 50 to 60 days. The incidence of recovery of bacteria from the respiratory tract is highest in the acute stage and declines rapidly in the early stage of paroxysmal coughing and is low or nil after the second week of coughing. Nevertheless the coughing usually persists for several weeks after bacterial cultures are negative. The bacteria are not recovered from the blood.

## LUNG PATHOLOGY

Autopsy reports have shown considerable variation in pertussis pathology.[cf. 100] It is difficult to determine the initial pulmonary lesion because few cases come to autopsy, and in the later stages the lesions are often complicated by secondary infection. *B. pertussis* multiplies rapidly on the mucous membrane of the respiratory tract. It seems that initially there is a peribronchial lymphoid hyperplasia with a concomitant lymphoid hyperplasia of the tracheobronchial nodes. Subsequently there is a necrotizing inflammation of the bronchi, larynx, and nasopharyngeal cavity. As the infection extends to the deeper structures there results a diffuse bronchopneumonia with marked desquamation of the alveolar epithelium and lymphocytic infiltration of the peribronchial tissues and alveolar walls. There is little evidence of severe toxic necrosis. There may be numerous small areas of atelectasis, caused by obstruction of the lower airways with mucous plugs, and increased fibrous tissue about the bronchi with leukocytic infiltration. One distinctive feature is localization of the pertussis bacteria massed between the cilia of the epithelial cells of the respiratory tract. As the infection progresses the bacteria may appear in the alveoli.

## NEUROLOGICAL COMPLICATIONS

Pulmonary complications have overshadowed those of the nervous system, which are no less important. Lapin[100] and Litvak[107] cited more than 60 references on neurological complications. In hospital cases the incidence has ranged from 1.5 to 14 per cent, and among these, mortality ranged from 60 to 90 per cent.[135, 209] The neurological symptoms usually appear at the peak of the paroxysmal cough, sometimes after it subsides, and last for a few days to several weeks. The incidence is highest in infants and younger children with bronchopneumonia. Zellweger[209] reported that one-third recover without sequelae, one-third are left with varying neurological sequelae, and one-third remain incurable. In a followup of 35 hospitalized cases, Byers and Rizzo[25] found that 17 per cent had permanent damage. Schachter[185] studied 200 children after uncomplicated whooping cough and found that 27.5 per cent showed more or less significant retardation in school; a higher percentage showed character disorders.

The neurological complications concern the brain exclusively. The most common manifestations are convulsions, coma, paralysis in the form of hemiplegia, blindness, and psychic disturbances. Late sequelae are epilepsy, mental retardation, spastic paralysis, or other disturbances.[135] Zellweger[209] noted a familial susceptibility to encephalopathy. Among 23 families investigated in which a case of encephalopathy had occurred he found that 20 had an unusual incidence of neurological conditions. Other references on familial relationship are given by Wilson.[205]

Jochims[76] and Dolgopol[41] suggested the term "pertussis encephalopathy." Anoxemia due to circulatory stasis and toxic effects were said to account for most of the anatomical findings.[41, 209] With the introduction of regulated pertussis vaccine and its widespread use, pertussis has been largely controlled and reports of pertussis encephalopathy have been superseded by reports of rare cases of vaccine encephalopathy. The risk of vaccination is by far outweighed by the risk of the disease.[25, 29-31]

The incidence of the severe or fatal vaccine encephalopathy is not known. Muggleton[128] suggested one fatal reaction in about a million injections in England. My estimate is one in 5 to 10 million injections in the United States. The number of injections per year is not known but the distribution of 22.5 million doses of pertussis vaccine in 1966 and about the same number in the three preceding years (Biologics Surveillance, National Communicable Disease Center) provides an indirect measure of utilization. In 1966, 55 deaths from pertussis were reported.[123] At the 1940 to 1944 rate (84.7 per 100,000 population of those under the age of one year[154]) there would have been more than 3000 infant deaths, and several hundred would have been left mentally retarded or incompetent. Vaccination contributed significantly to the reduction in mortality as well as morbidity. Therefore, vaccination is in the public interest in spite of the tragic but rare cases of encephalopathy. Additional comments on this subject appear under the heading Sensitizing Factors and Provocation.

## Blood Disturbances

During the catarrhal stage of pertussis there is an increase in total leukocyte count. At the height of the paroxysmal stage, the lymphocytes rise to 60 to 80 per cent of the total and may not fall to normal for two to three months although decline usually coincides with the disappearance of *B. pertussis*.[cf. 100]

Reports of studies of blood chemistry in pertussis are few. Regan and Tolstoouhov[171] observed marked biochemical changes and suggested that these changes are associated with the characteristic and unusual symptomatology of the disease. Hydrogen ion concentration was decreased, inorganic phosphorus was moderately to markedly diminished, the carbon dioxide combining power was within normal limits, and there was a low-normal or subnormal blood sugar and an increase in uric acid. The hypoglycemia tended to last into con-valescence. The subnormal sugar level may be of particular significance. Pertussis vaccine induces hypoglycemia in animals,[145, 199] and pertussis vac-cine fetal wastage in mice is prevented by adding glucose to the drinking water.[204]

### ETIOLOGY OF CLINICAL MANIFESTATIONS

The cause of the paroxysmal cough and the other manifestations of the localized *B. pertussis* infection has remained an enigma. Before the isola-tion of the causative bacteria, Czerny[cf. 100] considered that the whoop was neurological. Beginning with Bordet and Gengou,[19] a toxin or endotoxin (so-called because it was demonstrable after bacterial lysis; it is different from the Boivin-type endotoxin) has been implicated as the cause of paroxysmal coughing and other clinical manifestations. Bordet and Gengou suggested that coughing was due to irritation of the nerve endings. Wiltgrube[cf. 100] and Soboleva[189] stressed the toxic element as the cause of injurious effects on the respiratory, lymphatic, and nervous systems.

Among the many proposed causes of the whoop, a neurological reaction is the most plausible. Paroxysmal coughing does not occur during the acute stage of the infection and the insult to the reactive mechanism(s) persists long after the causative organism disappears. It appears that the reaction is due not to an immediate response but to an altered enzymatic, hormonal, or pharmacological response which is slow in recovery. Current information on β-adrenergic blockade in mice by pertussis vaccine supports the hypothesis of a neurological effect. Reactive factors of *B. pertussis* are discussed in the section on Pertussis Vaccine.

### IMMUNITY TO PERTUSSIS

The nature of immunity to *B. pertussis* infection, which remains localized on the ciliated epithelium of the respiratory tract, is unknown. The disease is highly communicable and it has been frequently but erroneously assumed that one attack protects for life. There is ample evidence that after infection or vaccination with adequately potent vaccine[12, 81, 115, 117, 119] there is resistance to infection. However, duration of immunity even after infection is probably not as long as commonly believed. Mannerstedt[112] cited a number of reports of whooping cough in adults and observed in a two-month survey 29 infec-tions in adults coming into a juvenile pertussis clinic and also three cases in children, aged five, 12, and 15 years, with histories of previous pertussis. Symptoms are less severe than in primary cases of young children and are often atypical. Second attacks are often overlooked or ignored.

The lack of longtime protection afforded by vaccine is attested to by the current recommended immunization schedule[168, 173] of three injections in the first year of life followed by a reinforcing injection one year after the third injection and a fifth injection (booster) at age three to six years. More injections were recommended earlier.[172] Lambert[98] has shown that protection is directly related to interval since vaccination: in a local epidemic the infection rate was 21 per cent among those immunized within three years and 95 per cent when the interval was greater than 12 years. In two recent small epidemics[124, 125] 80 and 95 per cent of the infections were in persons over age 10 years.

In 1955, Ipsen and Bowen[73] noted that the incidence in persons aged 10 years and older had not declined with routine immunization of children and predicted that pertussis would become a disease of the older age. Eldering[43] noted a shift in age with more cases occurring in those aged 10 years or older. A similar shift has occurred in Russia.[208] Prolongation of immunity in children older than six years might be effected by boosters with less antigen than now used per single injection. This is supported by reports of Kendrick et al.[84] and Burian et al.[22] The use of less antigen would provide a lower risk of reactions.

Protection against the disease, in which the bacteria remain localized, is quite remarkable. How do the circulating antibodies reach the pertussis bacteria localized on the ciliated epithelium of the respiratory tract? The protection of mice against experimental pertussis infection, which is described later, may provide a clue. In the brain infection the bacteria remain localized on the ciliated ependymal cell layer of the ventricles. When vaccinated mice are challenged intracerebrally the bacteria multiply for several days and then rapidly disappear. The disappearance is associated with a change in the permeability of the brain barrier which permits the entrance of antibodies. Likewise, when the mice are challenged intranasally the bacteria multiply for several days and then rapidly disappear. The rapid disappearance suggests antibody action but there are no supporting data. It is postulated that *B. pertussis* multiplies on the epithelium of the human respiratory tract and causes a change in the permeability of the epithelium. If there are circulating antibodies the infection is arrested; if there are inadequate antibodies the infection progresses. This remains a subject for study.

Neither whooping cough itself nor vaccination against it provides lifelong immunity. However, previous experience with the disease does lessen symptoms and paroxysmal coughing may not develop.

### Response to Serum and Antibiotic Therapy

Both antiserum[cf. 100, 114] and broad-spectrum antibiotics[2, 13, 17, 67, 116, 136] are effective antibacterial agents against *B. pertussis* and may arrest or modify the course of the infection. Only when they are given early is the clinical response dramatic, with complete recovery following a few days of treatment. If paroxysmal coughing has developed, coughing will continue for three weeks or longer, the same as in the untreated case after the disappearance of the bacteria. This is illustrated in the result of the study on Aureomycin treatment by Bell et al.[13] When treatment was started two to 10 days after onset of the paroxysmal cough, duration was less than 20 days; when it was started 11 to 17 days after onset, duration was 20 to 40 or more days.

The lack of understanding of the nature of clinical pertussis has led to disappointing results and improper evaluation of antibacterial action. Nevertheless, the agents do stop the progression of the bacterial phase of the disease, thereby reducing acute toxicity and lessening the chance for pulmonary complications with other bacteria.

Whether or not pertussis antibodies have an effect other than antibacterial is not clear. Dr. F. Hansen (personal communication) has suggested that there is a decrease in histamine sensitivity in the treated child. There is very little information on the state of histamine sensitivity in the *B. pertussis*-infected child; Sanyal[180] has reported that it is increased. Man is normally very sensitive to histamine. In contrast to induction of histamine sensitization by pertussis vaccine in the mouse, which normally is insensitive, Stronk and Pittman[199] found that pertussis vaccine decreased slightly but significantly the histamine sensitivity of both guinea pigs and rabbits, which normally are sensitive to histamine. In the mouse antipertussis serum prevents the development of histamine sensitization if given concurrently with the vaccine but it does not prevent histamine shock in the sensitized mouse.[109, 110] The failure of antiserum to arrest paroxysmal coughing of the child may be analogous to its lack of effect in the mouse once sensitization has developed.

Antipertussis serum has been used effectively prophylactically and therapeutically.[cf. 100, 114] Continued use attests to the fact that it has some beneficial activity. Past results with antiserum have been based on treatments using sera without defined protective activity. With a prescribed unit of potency (anticipated to be in effect in the near future) for Pertussis Immune Globulin (Human) it may be possible to better evaluate human efficacy. However, with the low incidence of pertussis in the United States, results will be acquired slowly.

At one time antitoxin (heat-labile toxin) received considerable attention.[174, 198] Although it is effective against the lethal action of toxin in mice and rabbits, it has little influence on the experimental bacterial infection.[cf. 6] A combined antibacterial and antitoxic serum (rabbit) was available commercially several years ago but the efficacy of the antitoxin was not established. Antitoxin is now considered to be without great importance for immunity.[16]


## ANIMAL RESPONSE TO *BORDETELLA PERTUSSIS* INFECTION

*B. pertussis* is not a natural pathogen for animals. However, successful infection of a number of species—chimpanzee, monkey, dog, rabbit, mouse, ferret, and chick embryo—has been reported.[cf. 100, cf. 20] In early work much effort was directed toward the induction of a lethal infection. Positive results were complicated by the toxicity of large doses and negative results by lack of information about the characteristics of virulent strains. Only in the recent work by Chin et al.[28] has the monkey been used as a model to study immunity to *B. pertussis*. The method of infection, spraying the nares and pharynx, has failed in the hands of others.[cf. 100] The recent success may have been due to a peculiar susceptibility of the Taiwan monkey. Scattered bits of unpublished information indicate that *Macacus rhesus* is not susceptible to this infection.

The mouse has been studied more extensively than other species. Three routes of injection have been used: intraperitoneal (ip), intranasal or intra-tracheal (itn), and intracerebral (ic). The bacteria are rapidly killed or re-main localized, depending on the site of injection. Bacteremia does not occur but bacteria may spill over into the blood terminally.

### Intraperitoneal Toxemia

Injected ip, the bacteria are killed rapidly. After injection of about $2 \times 10^9$ bacteria the mouse dies of toxemia in one to three days.[64, 167] Without mucin there is no multiplication of the bacteria; with mucin there may be two or three generations of the slowly multiplying bacteria but in each case death is due to toxemia, not infection. Lethality by the ip route is inversely related to ic virulence. Strain 16945, used by J. F. Norton in the first and unpublished work on the ic mouse protection test of pertussis vaccine, required $10^5$ bacteria to induce a lethal ic infection when I received it. After many brain passages the lethal dose was less than $10^2$ bacteria. However, by the ip route more bacteria of the ic virulent culture were required to kill than of the original culture (Pittman, unpublished data). The latter culture, apparently more susceptible to lysis, provided a greater concentration of toxin in a shorter period than the more virulent culture. Standfast[195] showed that the ip $LD_{50}$ of the highly ic virulent strain 18323 was larger than the $LD_{50}$ of lesser ic virulent strains. Death from ip injection may be prevented by antitoxin but not by antibacterial serum.[cf. 6]

### Respiratory Infections

Itn injection causes infection of the lung of the mouse.[3, 4, 24, 35, 40, 151, 167, 197] If less than the lethal dose is given, the bacteria increase in number for seven to 14 days[35, 167] and then gradually decline, but infection may last three to four weeks.[4, 35, 151, 197] Duration of infection is similar to that in the child. Leukocytosis also occurs.[35] In the fatal lung infection of the mouse[24] and rat[70] there is patchy interstitial pneumonia with leukocyte infiltration, pro-liferation of bronchial epithelium, and other changes. The lesions are not unlike those seen in the fatal human infection.

The role of "toxin" in the itn infection has not been determined. Stand-fast[195] showed that the living bacteria, or "toxin," paralyze the cilia of the epithelium of sheep lung *in vitro*. The mouse has 10 to 100 times greater resistance to "toxin" by the itn route than by the ip route.[9] In contrast to the case in ip injection, mice are not protected against itn injection by anti-toxin but are protected by antibacterial serum.[9]

Of particular interest is the parallelism of the time of onset and duration of histamine sensitization in the lung-infected mouse and of paroxysmal coughing in the human infection, which was observed by Pittman.[151] The peak of sensitization was reached in 10 to 15 days and persisted for at least 50 days; the lung cultures were positive through 20 days but not at 30 days. Andersen[4] and Pittman[151] found that the mouse, after recovery from lung infection, was immune to ic infection. Cooper,[35] however, reported lack of ic immunity. The vaccinated mouse is protected against a progressive lung infection. After challenge large numbers of bacteria may be present for three to four days but the bacteria are usually absent by the seventh day.[7, 40] In contrast, the peak of infection in the nonimmune mouse occurs seven to 14 days after infection. Although the vaccinated mouse is protected against itn infection, the many attempts to use the itn challenge in quantitative assays of the potency of pertussis vaccine were not successful. Protective activity could not be measured by lethal and nonlethal response but had to be determined by culturing the lungs at the appropriate time.[3, 7] The procedure was time consuming, and the results were less accurate than by the ic challenge assay and did not correlate with human protection[6, 196]

Use of the mouse respiratory infection as a model for studying pertussis has not been fully exploited.

### INTRACEREBRAL INFECTION

Ic injection in the mouse causes a fatal infection. Relatively few strains of B. pertussis have high virulence (LD$_{50}$ of $10^2$ or fewer bacteria) by the ic route.[86, 195] The strain most widely studied and routinely used in potency assays is 18323.[82] Its serotype is 1.2.3.4.5.7.[47] It agglutinates poorly and may show variations in typing. In early developmental work, I used two highly virulent strains obtained by mouse brain serial passage (16945 and 17921). A mutant, 2-atox from 40103,[34] isolated by Andersen,[3] has been used experimentally by Andersen and Bentzon[7] and routinely for potency assay in Denmark (personal communication). 2-Atox has the unusual characteristic of causing bacteremia in mice.

After ic injection, the bacteria progressively multiply on the ventricle wall, intimately associated with the cilia. Secondarily, there is expansion of the ventricles caused by accumulation of exudate, meningitis, and degeneration of the parenchyma. The mouse usually dies within 10 days. There is no invasion of the bacteria in the brain substance.[14, 71, 72] With fluorescent antibody, the bacteria are found adhering to the wall of the ventricles or as detached colonies in the ventricles.[71] This localization is strikingly like the localization of the bacteria among the bronchial and tracheal cilia in the human infection, and like that in the experimental lung infection of animals and the chick embryo,[cf. 14] but in contrast to the invasion of the brain parenchyma by B. bronchiseptica and Salmonella typhosa following ic inoculation.[71] Further, the organisms do not multiply in the blood but may be present terminally.[14]

The adrenal glands of the ic-infected mouse show marked lipid depletion beginning about the fifth day and an increase in succinic dehydrogenase, nonspecific esterases, and acid phosphatase. There are terminal changes in the liver and atrophy of the lymphoid follicles of the spleen.[14]

In the immunized mouse, B. pertussis multiplies in the brain until the count reaches $10^5$ to $10^6$ in four to six days and then rapidly disappears.[14, 40] Disappearance is associated with an increase in the permeability of the brain barrier which has been demonstrated by use of dye[14, 68] and fluorescent tagged pertussis antibodies.[71] In view of the parallelism of the localization of the pertussis infection on the ciliated epithelium of the brain and the respiratory infection, the early criticism of the use of the so-called unnatural brain infection for potency assay of pertussis vaccine is no longer justified. Unlike the itn challenge, the ic challenge in the potency assay of pertussis vaccines provides relative values which correlate with human efficacy.[119] The intracerebral challenge is prescribed for the potency assay of pertussis vaccine[1, 206] and is used experimentally and proposed for the official assay of antipertussis serum (Pittman, unpublished data).

## GENERAL DESCRIPTION OF *BORDETELLA PERTUSSIS*

*B. pertussis* is a small gram-negative coccobacillus with a sheath or capsule[78, 101] which apparently does not swell in the presence of antiserum. It is aerobic, does not ferment carbohydrates, and attacks certain nitrogenous substance, resulting in alkalinity of medium, which may influence lysis of the bacteria or leaching or formation of toxic substances. Standfast[194] has reviewed the characteristics of freshly isolated strains.

Growth requirements are relatively simple but promotion of growth is complicated by interference of nutrients and inhibitors.[175, 176] Blood,[18] charcoal,[122, 161, 162] and ion-exchange resins[95, 170, 201] have been used to neutralize the inhibitors.

One of the most striking features of this bacterium is a great propensity to modulate culturally and serologically with alterations in the medium. Changes in propagation strains for vaccine production were the cause of some of the early immunization failures.

A significant contribution to vaccine production was made when Leslie and Gardner[103] observed the transition from smooth colony-forming bacteria (Phase I) to stable rough colony-forming bacteria (Phase IV) with intermediate Phases II and III and a concomitant change in nutrient requirements and in antigens, including protective antigen. Later, Lacey[97] effected antigenic modulations by alteration of the temperature of incubation and salt constituents of the medium. Unfortunately, the effect of modulation of the bacteria on protective activity was not observed. Even a growth factor for *B. pertussis*, nicotinic acid, in excessive concentration causes modulation in agglutinability, potency, and histamine-sensitizing factor (HSF).[169] Determination of the optimum medium and growth conditions for large-scale propagation of bacteria for potent vaccines with minimum untoward reactivity remains a fertile field for investigation.

## CELLULAR COMPONENTS

Many studies on cellular components have contributed to the understanding of the activity of *B. pertussis* in the infection and in the vaccine but the total remains to be revealed. Among the components are heat-labile dermonecrotic toxin (HLT), lipopolysaccharide (endotoxin), agglutinogen and serotypes, sensitizing substances including histamine-sensitizing factor (HSF), lymphocytosis-promoting factor (LPF), protective and adjuvant factors, hemagglutinin, and hemolysin (probably a metabolite). The literature has been reviewed by Munoz[129] and Kuwajima and Niwa.[96] The first five items are discussed here and the protective and adjuvant factors are presented in the section on Pertussis Vaccine.

### Heat-Labile Toxin (HLT)

The role of "toxin" in the *B. pertussis* infection has been the subject of considerable research. Toxic substances, designated endotoxin by early workers,[cf. 100] may be extracted from the bacteria or excreted in the culture medium.[cf. 96, cf. 129] HLT is dermonecrotic and antigenic and is inactivated at 56°C. within 15 minutes. The suckling mouse[79] provides the most sensitive method for detecting necrotic activity[6] (R. A. Gardner, unpublished data). Injected intravenously or intraperitoneally into mice, HLT causes death in 24 to 48 hours; injected intranasally the toxin is about 100 times less reactive.[9] Intravenous injection of HLT into rabbits causes hyperglycemia followed by hypoglycemia, convulsions, and death.[49] Much of the material studied has been crude in composition and has contained many reactive substances. Flosdorf and associates[cf. 6] studied a thermolabile toxin which induced subcutaneous infiltration but not necrosis. Billaudelle et al.[15, 16] separated from toxic preparations a lethal (neuro-) and an atoxic fraction. Both were dermonecrotic. Fractionation studies indicate that HLT is a protein.[cf. 96, cf. 129]

In spite of the dramatic demonstrations with animals, the role of HLT in human infection has not been clearly defined. Doubt of a role comes from the lack of antitoxin in convalescent serum,[9, 50] whereas the extracts of the bacteria induce antitoxin. Anderson and North[9] questioned whether toxin was an important or significant factor in the pathology of mouse lung infection and suggested that the toxin itself does not exist in the intact cell but is in the form of a precursor, and they cited Teisser's observation that the formalinized intact cell did not provoke antitoxin but disrupted formalinized cells did. An interstitial mononuclear pneumonia similar to that in human pertussis has been induced in rabbits with toxin[192] but the role of HLT alone cannot be isolated from that of other factors in the preparations used. The quantities given were greater than would be present in a natural infection.

A formalin-detoxified antigen afforded very low protection to children against pertussis.[37] Toxin does not protect against brain infection in the mouse.[202]

### Lipopolysaccharide (Endotoxin)

The heat-stable endotoxin obtained from the cell walls of *B. pertussis* by the Boivin procedure is similar to the endotoxins isolated from other gram-negative bacteria[cf. 129] and possibly has specific factors, depending on the extraction method.[96] The preparations are pyrogenic and may increase susceptibility of experimental animals to infection or provide nonspecific protection against infection, have adjuvant properties, and lack protective activity per se.[91, 96, 129, 155, 200] Characterization of endotoxins in general may be found in comprehensive reviews.[cf. 99]

## Agglutinogen and Serotypes

Agglutinogen was one of the earlier fractionated components of *B. pertussis*.[60, 188] The material elicits skin reactions in man and animals that have had previous experience with *B. pertussis*, pertussis vaccine, or agglutinogen,[53, 59, 188] and it induces agglutinins. It is distinct from the toxins, HSF, and protective antigen.[187] Andersen[6] reviewed the literature in 1958 and Munoz[129] in 1963.

Andersen[5] and Eldering et al.[48] showed that Phase I strains, i.e., strains with the so-called capsule, have a common heat-stable O antigen and one or more thermolabile K antigens. Serotype (or factor) 1 antigen is present in all strains but the presence of other serotype antigens differs between strains. In an epidemic, strains of a common antigenic pattern predominate, thereby providing an epidemiological tool for following contact cases. Recent findings have pointed up that strains of a common pattern seem to predominate throughout a country and that serotypes change. Preston[163, 164] called attention to the change in England from the dominant serotype 1.2.4 in the late 40's and mid 50's to 1.3 in the late 50's and early 60's. In 1963 to 1964, only 15 per cent of 132 strains had factor 2. In the United States, Dr. G. Eldering (unpublished data) has observed a decrease in the incidence of strains with factor 2. Among the typable strains in the Eldering-Kendrick collection factor 2 was present in 60 per cent of the 1938 to 1949 strains, in 25 per cent of the 1950 to 1955 strains, and in none of the 1962 to 1965 strains. Among 163 strains collected in 1966 to 1967 (150 from the United States and 13 from Canada), 10 per cent had factor 2, while 92.6 per cent had factor 3; 81.6 per cent were of serotype 1.3.6.[44]

Preston[164] suggested that the occurrence of 1.3 strains in Manchester[111] and other parts of England was due to a selective proliferation in a population of children vaccinated by 1.2 antigen vaccine, and that 1.2 antigen could not be expected to immunize against 1.3 infection. Similar claims have been reported from Canada[27] and Russia.[39] In no instance was the unitage of the vaccines used recorded.

Armitage and Perry[10] discussed the probability that the British Standard Pertussis Vaccine might be lower in potency than the field trial vaccine from which it was prepared. Recently, Muggleton[128] stated that the standard contained 5.3 protective units per ampule (50 × 10⁹ bacteria). Hence, a British vaccine equivalent in potency to the standard would have 6.4 units per prescribed 60 × 10⁹ bacteria per total human immunizing dose (THD). In the classic British trials,[119] vaccines containing 12 to 15 units provided 86 to 91 per cent protection against human exposure while with a vaccine having 7 units the attack rate was 29 per cent.[156] The Dutch experience also indicates that the epidemiological situation reflects the mouse protective potency of the vaccine.[33]

The shift in the antigen pattern of the pertussis strains in the United

States was not accompanied by a concomitant increase in reported cases and deaths. In fact there has been a decrease. From 1957 to 1966 morbidity dropped from 28,295 to 7717.[123] A recent analysis of the propagation strains used by the 12 United States licensed manufacturers of pertussis vaccine showed that a high percentage of the strains contained factor 3.[44] Sporadic local epidemics of pertussis continue to occur.[98, 124, 125] In the evaluation of the efficacy of pertussis vaccine cognizance must be taken of the fact that neither infection nor vaccine affords lifelong immunity.

With use of active mouse protection tests, Andersen and Bentzon[8] and Eldering et al.[46, 47] failed to show an influence of serotype on protection. Andersen and Bentzon used the sublethal intranasal challenge and found equal clearance of the bacteria from the lungs of mice vaccinated with strains of different serotypes and challenged with homologous and heterologous serotypes, respectively. Eldering et al. used active and passive intracerebral protection tests. Preston[165] and Preston and Garrity[166] showed the prime importance of factor 1 antiserum with the use of absorbed sera. Factor 1 antiserum afforded equal or better protection than factor 2 antiserum against 1.2 infection and likewise better than factor 3 antiserum against 1.3 infection. The factor 2 and factor 3 antiserum did provide significantly better protection than did normal serum. Failure of the bacteria to adsorb all of the protective activity is in agreement with Brown's finding[21] and suggests, as she pointed out, that protective activity is not due solely to the presence of agglutinins. Further, Munoz and Hestekin[132] have separated a protective antigen that is free of agglutinogen.

Of particular interest are the findings of Eldering et al.[45] that only B. pertussis antiserum containing factor 1 antibody was capable of positive fluorescent staining (FA) of B. pertussis. Absorbed sera specific for factors 2, 3, 4, or 5 gave negative FA reactions with all strains, irrespective of the serotype. On the other hand, each of the absorbed sera was capable of agglutinating the homologous strain.

Since factor 1 is present in all B. pertussis strains and required for the FA reaction, it is suggestive that the agglutinogen is primarily factor 1 and that the other factors are radicals on the factor 1 molecule. The propensity for the factor antigens to modulate could be due to an alteration in a factor radical(s). Certainly there is no evidence that serotypes of B. pertussis have immunological specificity like that of the capsular antigens of Diplococcus pneumoniae and Haemophilus influenzae. Whatever the role of the antigenic pattern in infection or in the protective activity of vaccine, the loss of a factor antigen during cultivation of a strain is evidence of modulation or mutation. Among the United States propagation strains, there were several cultures of strain 10536.[44] Three cultures were not agglutinated to titer in the anti-10536 serum and each had lost one or more factors. Decrease in agglutinability was not associated with loss of any particular factor. Cameron[26] observed a concurrent loss in protective activity, and also in HSF, with a loss of one or more factor antigens. Specific factor antisera provide a tool for surveillance of vaccine propagation cultures and also of the presence of the serotype antigens in the vaccine. It appears that a significant value to be derived from serotyping will be to determine that propagation strains have not modulated or mutated. This might be the end product of the controversial subject of the significance of serotypes and protective activity of pertussis vaccine.

Although evidence indicates that agglutinogens or serotype antigens are not the protective antigen, agglutinin[cf. 6] response to whole-cell vaccine does provide a very valuable tool for measuring response to whole-cell vaccine. Under certain conditions agglutinin titers parallel the protective response;[121, 178] a titer of 1:320 was accepted as consonant with clinical immunity.[cf. 20, 120] With the whole-cell vaccines used in the British trials there was general correlation between protection in the field and agglutinin response of children and of mice[119] except with the Pillemer[148] antigen. This antigen afforded good protection[119] but the agglutinin response was poor.[51] Failure was due to the test strain and not to inability of the antigen to induce agglutinins.[6, 32] The propagation strain P134 was of serotype 1.3 whereas the test strain had a different pattern. This instance provides further evidence that the serotype per se is not all-important in protective activity and that measurement of immunity by agglutinin titer at times may be misleading. In clinical trials of pertussis vaccine measurement of agglutinin titer is a useful tool for measuring human response, provided appropriate serotype strains are selected for the test.

## SENSITIZING FACTORS AND PROVOCATION

Pertussis vaccine has unique sensitizing properties which are manifested immunologically, physiologically, and pharmacologically. Eldering[42] observed that an isolated carbohydrate complex of *B. pertussis* rendered the mouse highly sensitive to ip challenge of *B. pertussis*. The mice could be desensitized with small amounts of the carbohydrate. Ospeck and Roberts[138] found that a toxoid prepared from a culture filtrate sensitized the mice to toxin challenge. Parfentjev et al.[142-144] showed that in mice and guinea pigs injected with pertussis vaccine fatal shock could be produced by challenge with denatured nucleoprotein from *B. pertussis* or with pertussis vaccine. The findings led to the observation of Parfentjev and Goodline[141] that pertussis vaccine increases the susceptibility of the mouse to histamine 50- to 100-fold and that shock could be prevented by an antihistaminic. Subsequently there have been many reports on altered reactions influenced by pertussis vaccine in experimental animals: increased susceptibility to histamine, serotonin, endotoxin, anaphylaxis, infection, reinjection of pertussis vaccine,[cf. 91, 129, 130, 155] and experimental allergic encephalomyelitis (EAE)[102, 105, 106] and delayed hypersensitivity.[65, 104, 177]

At this time it is not possible to ascribe a particular sensitizing reaction to a single component of *B. pertussis*. Parfentjev,[140] using a degraded nucleoprotein, showed differences between anaphylactic and histamine susceptibility. On the other hand, Kind[88] showed with pertussis vaccine-sensitized mice a parallelism between sensitivity to pertussis vaccine and to histamine. The potentiating effect on EAE has been demonstrated with fractions high in HSF content.[106] The delayed hypersensitivity, manifested by cutaneous reactions[177] and ascites, was induced by use of whole-cell vaccine.[65, 104] The unique HSF has received the greatest attention and it may be the prime factor in all of the sensitizing reactions. Its properties have been presented in several reviews, the most extensive of which is by Munoz and Bergman.[131] In brief, HSF is located in the cell wall or closely associated therewith and is part of or intimately associated with the mouse protective antigen. Recently, Sato and Nagase[181] and Nagel[134] claimed separation of the two factors. Fractions with high HSF activity have a high concentration of nitrogen and contain lipid. HSF is thermolabile at 80°C. for 30 minutes[90, 110] and is antigenic. Antiserum injected at the time of the vaccine prevents development of sensitization but it does not inhibit histamine shock after sensitization has developed.[110]

The early observations showed that certain antihistamines, Bromothen,[141] Thephorin,[139] Neo-Antergan,[87] and others, would prevent histamine shock but not the development of histamine sensitivity in the pertussis-vaccinated mouse, whereas some antihistaminics were without effect (Pittman, unpublished data). These results suggested a specific pharmacological mechanism of action. However, Schayer and Ganley[186] attributed histamine sensitization to an increase in histidine decarboxylase induced by the vaccine. Recent evidence indicates that the increased histidine decarboxylase activity is caused by the endotoxin and not the HSF component of the vaccine (S. Katsh and A. Szentivanyi, Abstracts, 24th Annual Meeting of the American Academy of Allergy, 1968, p. 34).

Kind[89] noted that Dibenzyline, an adrenergic blocking agent, inhibited the histamine shock in the sensitized mouse. Later, Fishel et al.[56] advanced the hypothesis that the pertussis-induced hypersensitivity is the result of functional imbalance between two types of adrenergic receptors or in the neural pathways leading to them. Subsequent work indicates that HSF blocks the β-adrenergic system functionally associated with the inhibition of muscle uptake of glucose[57] (A. Szentivanyi, S. Katsh, and R. G. Townley, Abstracts, 24th Annual Meeting of the American Academy of Allergy, 1968, pp. 34–35; C. W. Fishel and K. F. Keller, Fed. Proc. 27:267, 1968) and that β-adrenergic receptors of the pancreas are particularly involved (A. Gulbenkian and I. I. A. Tabacknick, Abstracts, 24th Annual Meeting of the American Academy of Allergy, 1968, pp. 35–36). It is tempting to infer that the vaccine through β-adrenergic blockade induces hypoglycemia which mediates a convulsive state in the child that may or may not lead to further neurological complications. The infant whose blood sugar level is influenced by food intake may be especially vulnerable to vaccine-induced hypoglycemia should a feeding be missed because of a feverish reaction following vaccination. Information on blood sugars of children following pertussis vaccination is nil so far as I am aware. During whooping cough the blood sugar does fall below normal.[171] As mentioned earlier, the vaccine induces hypoglycemia in mice and rabbits. Evans[49] found that glucose prevented the convulsive state in the rabbit following injection of crude HLT but did not prevent death or affect the time of death. On the other hand, glucose prevented fetal wastage in pertussis-vaccinated mice.[204]

Besides its relation to pertussis vaccination, HSF, as stated by Fishel et al.,[57] represents to the immunologist and the allergologist a unique analytical model for the investigation of nonimmunological acquired hypersensitivity to amine mediators of the allergic response. The phenomenon also is of interest to the neurophysiologist and the neuropharmacologist since it is the only known spontaneously acquired hypersensitivity to natural substances which may be regarded as the chemical organizers of neural integration. From the standpoint of this paper, which is directed toward host-bacteria relationship, the implications of the role of the HSF in the mechanism of the physiological, pathological, and neurological reactions of whooping cough are very attractive. In fact, the role of HSF in paroxysmal coughing and neurological reactions has been suggested by many workers. Mention was made previously of the parallelism of histamine sensitivity in the lung-infected mouse and the onset and duration of coughing in the human infection.[151] With a possible relation of HSF to the rare encephalopathy that follows pertussis immunization in the child as a basis, Levine et al.[106] studied the effect of fractions high in HSF activity on the "hyperacute" experimental allergic encephalomyelitis (EAE) induced in rats injected with pertussis vaccine and central nervous system material. Activity of HSF material was quantitative and not related to endotoxin. Although it acts as an adjuvant in the induction of EAE, there is no proof that the vaccine plays a specific role and that there is a relationship to human encephalopathy. In fact, the mechanism of the neurological sequelae to vaccination seems to be different from the demyelination type of encephalitis except in occasional cases.[cf. 205] The role of HSF, or of other factors with which it is combined, in EAE may be the same as that of *Mycobacterium tuberculosis*, which does not have a propensity to induce noninfectious encephalopathy.

Delayed hypersensitivity induced by whole-cell pertussis vaccine has been demonstrated by cutaneous reactions, ascites formation, and transfer with lymph nodes, but not with serum, to normal rats.[65, 104, 177]

Another reaction which may or may not be associated with HSF or delayed hypersensitivity is provocation. Provocation poliomyelitis paralysis in the pertussis vaccine-inoculated limb[118] and, likewise, experimental mouse encephalomyelitis (Theiler's virus) paralysis[38] have been reported. It is likely that in certain cases encephalopathy following pertussis vaccination is actually a viral infection which was in the incubation stage at the time of vaccination or was latent and was provoked by the vaccine. The rarity of the attacks suggests that the mechanism must depend upon some individual peculiarity or predisposition.[30]

In a review of 24 cases of infantile myoclonic seizures following illness or insult, Baird and Borofsky[11] noted that nine of the cases occurred after immunization with triple antigen containing diphtheria and tetanus toxoids and pertussis vaccine. The time of onset of the reactions after vaccination varied considerably: one was within 12 hours, four were two days after vaccination, and four were four to five days after vaccination. The lateness of the last four reactions suggests that a latent virus may have been present and that encephalopathy was provoked by the vaccine. Among the remaining 13 cases of myoclonic seizures, seven were associated with viral or bacterial encephalopathy (one was caused by *B. pertussis*), two were of unknown etiology, two were due to known trauma, and in four cases seizures developed at age four to seven months without known cause.

With advancements in viral diagnostic techniques, a viral cause of at least some cases of encephalopathy following pertussis vaccination will, no doubt, be found. Feldman and Schwartz[52] isolated cytomegalovirus from three of six infants with infantile spasms. The electroencephalograms of each of the six infants were compatible with hypsarhythmia. Had these infants with latent virus been vaccinated, there would have been a chance of provoking a severe or fatal reaction.

There remains the likelihood that pertussis vaccine does cause on rare occasions a neurological reaction in a child with an individual predisposition. The nature of the reactive factor is not known. The reaction occurs indifferently after the first, second, or third injection, and does not depend on the lot of vaccine. Whether the reaction is mediated through $\beta$-adrenergic blockade, hypoglycemia, delayed hypersensitivity, or other factors remains to be revealed.

### Lymphocyte-Promoting Factor

One of the diagnostic criteria of whooping cough is a relative lymphocytosis which appears with the paroxysmal coughing and declines with the disappearance of B. pertussis but may persist for two to three months.[cf. 100]

Leukocytosis occurs in lung-infected[35] and vaccinated mice. In the latter it lasts for at least two weeks (I. A. Parfentjev and E. E. Manuelidis, Fed. Proc. 15:607, 1957). The spleen increases in size and in direct relation to amount of vaccine injected (Pittman, unpublished data). On the other hand, there is a decrease in spleen size in the lethal ic infection.[14] Morse and Riester[126] have shown that lymphocytosis in the vaccinated mouse is due to an increase in circulation of preformed lymphocytes rather than an increase in newly formed cells, and they have contributed to an understanding of the mechanism of lymphocytosis in the mouse following injection of a specified number of bacteria of pertussis vaccine. (I assume the number injected was based on manufacturer's determination of opacity unitage and an interpretation that 10 opacity units equals $10 \times 10^9$ bacteria. The actual equivalent is about one-third less.[152]) The relation of lymphocytosis in the mouse to that in man has not been determined. Vaccine preparations are not constant in bacterial components, and published reports have not provided information on the specific component that induces lymphocytosis. Lawson[101] observed that an ether-soluble lipoid fraction induced leukocytosis with a relative increase in lymphocytosis whereas Phase IV bacteria caused a leukocytosis without a lymphocyte increase.

Recently, Ishida[74] and Kurokawa et al.[93] described a fraction which was designated as the lymphocytosis-promoting factor (LPF). LPF is different from HLT and endotoxin but it has HSF activity. The relationship to HSF is under investigation by the Japanese workers. LPF is thought to be the factor that causes slow weight gain and late deaths[94] in the mouse weight-gain toxicity test for pertussis vaccine. Since purified HSF has low toxicity for mice,[129] it might be assumed that LPF contains more than HSF. LPF is proteinaceous and may be similar to the lethal (neuro-) toxin of Billaudelle[16] or the degraded nucleoprotein fraction described by Parfentjev et al.[142-144] The Japanese work provides a new perspective for the study of the reactive factors of pertussis vaccine. Their work awaits repetition in other laboratories and a fuller understanding of the activity of LPF and its relation to and interplay with other described factors of pertussis vaccine, especially HSF.

# PERTUSSIS VACCINE

Pertussis vaccine was introduced shortly after Bordet and Gengou[18] isolated the causative organism of pertussis, but efficacy was not firmly established until many years later. The Felton and Willard review of 1944[55] relates the variable early results. The first encouraging report was from Denmark.[108] A number of successful studies followed in the United States[12, 81, 121, 178, 179, 182] but unfavorable reports came from England.[113] Advancements in knowledge pointed up reasons for successes and failures and methods for control: (1) phase changes of *B. pertussis* on artificial medium[103] and the use of freshly isolated strains by Sauer,[182] (2) the pioneer work of Kendrick and Eldering[80] that established the basic factors for the preparation of pertussis vaccine,[85] (3) the intracerebral mouse potency assay,[cf. 6, 43, cf. 154] and (4) the mouse weight-gain toxicity test.[152, 160]

Methods of production of pertussis vaccine differ between manufacturers, hence individual products may differ in quality. Even an individual manufacturer's product may show some variation from lot to lot. Although each lot meets the minimum requirements, the probability of variation between lots is not generally appreciated. There frequently appears in the literature the words "standard commercial vaccine." "Standard" is applicable only to national or international preparations with an accurately assayed property. Biological products cannot be produced with the constancy of a chemical solution. It would not be amiss to mention here that if two or more lots of vaccine are being compared, each should be carefully analyzed and any difference taken into account in interpretation of results. Two examples of lack of application follow: The Pillemer antigen was reported to be more reactive than the vaccine with which it was compared[119] but it was about three times more potent (Pittman, unpublished data). Haire et al.[66] noted that two lots of quadruple vaccine which contained *B. pertussis* cells grown on charcoal agar were less reactive than two lots prepared with cells grown in fluid medium. The difference was attributed to the medium. However, the former contained only one-half as many bacteria as the latter.

## POTENCY STANDARD AND EFFICACY

United States Minimum Requirements for Pertussis Vaccine were issued in 1949. At that time it was customary to express the human dose in numbers of bacteria, and the potency of the vaccine was measured by comparing the potency of the bacteria in a vaccine with the potency of the bacteria in the reference. Shortly afterward, the fallacy of this custom became apparent. Products varied in potency per total human immunizing dose (THD) as much as 6.2-fold.[153] In 1953 the potency requirement was revised relative to the THD and specified as 12 units. This unitage was assigned to that number of bacteria of the reference vaccine Lot 4 (96 × 10[9] bacteria), which was equivalent in potency to the average potency of the lots of vaccine prepared by the Michigan Department of Health and by the method developed by Kendrick and Eldering[80, 85] and used to prepare the vaccines for their successful field trial.[81] The number 12 was selected as it provided a whole number when divided by 2, 3, or 4, the number of single doses that were recommended for the primary THD. At present, three doses are recommended by all United States manufacturers except one state laboratory which recommends two doses.

Reference Lot 4 was diluted in Sörensen's phosphate buffer M/15, freeze-dried and designated as *the* United States Standard Pertussis Vaccine.[153] There was no loss during the drying. This Standard is held for standardization of potency of working standards which are distributed for the assay of potency of all lots of vaccine prior to their release in the United States. Only two Lots, 5 and 6, have been in distribution since 1953. The international and several national standards have been assayed against the Standard (Lot 4).

The classic British field trials of pertussis vaccine[119] showed a correlation between protection in children and protection in mice; and Pittman[156] showed that three vaccines which afforded 86 to 91 per cent protection against home exposure had 13 to 17 units per THD. Other field results confirmed these findings[33, 54, 207] and that low-unit vaccines were less effective.[75, 156]

Prior to the establishment of a standard of potency for pertussis vaccine, it was customary to specify a minimum of potency for biologicals. However, to reduce the risk of untoward reactivity with excessive amounts of antigen, a definite unitage for pertussis vaccine was established. Because of the biological variability of the potency assay, estimated values of no less than 8, 9.6, 10.4, and 12 units based on a one-, two-, three-, or four-test assay, respectively, are acceptable. In no case may the estimate be greater than 36 units.[1]

## PREPARATION

The secret of the preparation of pertussis vaccine with adequate potency and free from all untoward reactivity has not been fully revealed. Subsequent to the publication of the basic method for the manufacture of pertussis vaccine,[85] modifications have been made by many laboratories. How much the changes have contributed to quality cannot be answered, but they have simplified manufacturing procedures, especially the introduction of liquid medium by Hornibrook.[69] Changes include liquid and solid[122, 162] media without blood and detoxification by heating at 37°C. or 56°C. or by short exposure to formalin. The classic method includes Bordet-Gengou agar and detoxification with 0.02 per cent Merthiolate during several months storage at 4°C. I consider that 37°C. heating is a questionable procedure from the standpoint of stability.

Other factors that vary between laboratories are propagation culture strains, time and temperature of incubation of the culture, aluminum adjuvants, and the methods of precipitation or adsorption. Information is scarce on the influence of the different factors on potency, stability of potency, and untoward reactivity of the product.

Chemical separation of the various cellular components has been the subject of many studies for more than 20 years.[cf. 96, cf. 129] Nevertheless, the purification, concentration, and yield of the protective antigen (PA) have not been satisfactory to the point of commerical production. Two early fractionated preparations were efficacious in field trials. The noncellular antigen prepared by the method of Pennell and Thiele[146] was less reactive than the whole-cell control vaccine which was tested clinically by Felton and Verwey.[54] The Pillemer antigen[148] caused more reactions than the whole-cell vaccine with which it was compared[119] but it was more potent (48.3 vs. 16.3 units per THD; Pittman, unpublished data). Excessive antigen contributed to reactivity. Only one noncellular antigen is produced commercially in the United States. Whole cells are chemically extracted and the antigen is separated from the cell debris by centrifugation.[203] In the one published report[203] in which this antigen was compared with a whole-cell vaccine the antigen was less reactive. The potency of the respective products was not given.

It seems definite that the whole-cell vaccines will be in use for many years. However, the current studies directed toward analysis of production strains and assay of reactive components should lead to methods of preparation of stable, adequately potent vaccines with minimum reactivity.

The influence of preservatives and adjuvants on potency follows.


## PRESERVATIVES

For many years Merthiolate has been used as a killing and preservative agent in pertussis vaccines. Since the introduction of the intracerebral mouse potency assay, several studies have examined the influence of other chemical agents as well as physical treatments on the toxicity and potency. With a limited number of vaccine preparations, Pittman[152] found that potency stability was less in vaccines preserved with either formalin or phenol than with Merthiolate. Heating at 34°C. for longer than 24 hours was deleterious. Vaccine heated at 56°C. for 30 minutes and preserved with Merthiolate had the best stability. Heating at 56°C. was the most effective method for detoxification. Irradiation was unsatisfactory for detoxification or preservation of potency. Kendrick et al.[83] reported stability of potency of Merthiolate-preserved vaccine with or without heating at 56°C. Although they noted no deleterious effect of phenol or formalin on potency, these vaccines became dark in color and difficult to suspend after prolonged storage.

Others have reported the deleterious effect of formalin on antigenicity.[15, 77, 133] However, formalin treatment for 24 hours has been used by certain manufacturers[128, 207] for rapid detoxification, and also to prevent stringy aggregation which is difficult to disperse. Certainly if formalin is used, great caution must be taken.

Benzethonium chloride[62, 137] and parabens[62] also have been found to be deleterious to potency. Addition of cations prior to treatment with benzethonium chloride may inhibit deleterious action.[137]

Vaccine containing Merthiolate is more stable than vaccine without a preservative.[62] Besides stabilization of potency, Merthiolate has another significant effect, inhibition of reactivity. Severe shock in mice induced by formalin-treated vaccine was prevented by addition of Merthiolate.[128] The role of Merthiolate is not known. Its effect might be through the inhibition of *B. pertussis* enzyme action. In his fractionation studies, Billaudelle[16] used Merthiolate to inhibit enzyme action. The marked toxicity of lysed *B. pertussis*, as compared with intact cells, and the lack of antitoxin in convalescent serum led Anderson and North[9] to question the presence of HLT per se in the bacterial cell. Is HLT a product of enzyme action? A fertile but difficult field would be the investigation of the bacterial enzymes on toxicity and on potency of pertussis vaccines. Variations from lot to lot may occur without explanation.

Merthiolate remains the best preservative agent for pertussis vaccine.

### Adjuvants

Pertussis vaccines adsorbed or precipitated with aluminum salt compounds provide better and longer protection[120, 178, 179] and are less reactive[23, 184] than plain saline-suspended preparations. Using the criteria of an agglutinin titer of 1:320 or higher, Miller et al.[120] found that the responses to plain vaccine (80 × 10$^9$ bacteria) and adsorbed (40 × 10$^9$ bacteria) four to eight weeks after injection were 48.5 and 62.5 per cent and at 24 to 28 weeks 37.0 and 60.9 per cent, respectively. Bell[12] obtained significant protection with an adsorbed product containing only 20 × 10$^9$ bacteria per THD given in two injections.

With adsorbed and plain diphtheria and tetanus toxoids and pertussis vaccines, each prepared from the same antigens and containing 20 × 10$^9$ bacteria per single dose, Burland et al.[23] observed that the generalized reaction rates were 35 and 67 per cent and the persistent cry rates were 0.7 and 3.4 per cent, respectively. The adsorbed vaccine was less toxic in the mouse weight-gain test and significantly more potent in the mouse potency assay than the plain vaccine. Pittman[153] found that vaccines averaged 1.7 times more potency for the mouse after adsorption than before absorption.

There are insufficient comparative data to evaluate the relative merits of the three aluminum compounds, alum, aluminum hydroxide, and aluminum phosphate, from the standpoint of either potency or reactivity. In the early use of aluminum phosphate some difficulty with mouse toxicity was encountered but not with all products, and later observations have shown differences between the dose-response curves of individual products.[160] The differences probably were due to the antigen per se and not the adjuvant.

The aluminum adjuvants apparently do not affect (potentiate) the HSF activity of pertussis vaccine.[33, 150] If the HSF is reactive for human beings then adsorbed vaccines with fewer bacteria than plain vaccines have an additional advantage. This advantage would be lost if antigens low in potency were potentiated with an adjuvant. The HSF activity seems to be relatively higher in low-potency than high-potency antigens.[33, 158]

The adsorbed product is recommended by the Public Health Service Advisory Committee on Immunization Practices[168] and has been preferred by the Committee on the Control of Infectious Diseases of the American Academy of Pediatrics[173] since at least 1951 (the earliest report examined).[172] In 1943 the Academy[cf. 184] noted the greater risk of abscess formation with adsorbed than with plain vaccine. This reaction was eliminated by intramuscular injection of the vaccine.[183] Plain vaccine has been preferred in Great Britain because of interpreted findings that the adsorbed vaccine caused greater provocation poliomyelitis.[31] However, each product contained the same number of bacteria (Cockburn, personal communication). The maximum number of bacteria (opacity units) permitted in the United States is lower for the adsorbed product. When requirements were issued in 1949, maximum opacity unitages were 48 and 96 per THD; now they are 48 and 60 per THD[1] for adsorbed and plain products, respectively. Holland has used adsorbed vaccine (48 opacity units) since 1957.[33]

Pertussis vaccine in water-in-oil adjuvants causes marked local reactions probably due to delayed hypersensitivity.[127]

The vaccine has in addition to lipopolysaccharide endotoxin another adjuvant property. Pertussis vaccine potentiates the antitoxin response to diphtheria and tetanus toxoids[58, 190] and has been used as an immunological adjuvant in a number of experimental systems.[cf. 91, cf. 106, cf. 155] Although it is not proved, I am of the opinion that this adjuvant property acting on the protective antigen of pertussis vaccine is responsible for the wider variations observed in the potency assay of vaccines with 30 or more protective units per THD than of those vaccines with less than 12 units per THD.

## POTENCY ASSAY

In the section on response of animals to *B. pertussis*, it was related that potency of vaccines assayed by the intracerebral mouse protection test reflects the protective activity of the vaccine for children. The test[1] is recognized internationally as the one of choice and is specified in the international requirements for pertussis vaccine.[206] Potency estimates are influenced by mouse strain, challenge culture, and so forth. Therefore it is important to control each factor of the test and keep them constant between tests and the *same* as when assayed results were compared with clinical efficacy in the fifties. In the United States it has been necessary to change one factor, that is, the lot of the standard vaccine. The unitages of the field trial vaccines that were assayed in my laboratory were related to the Master United States Standard Pertussis Vaccine (Reference No. 4). Since then two working standards (Lots 5 and 6) have been issued. Although standardized against the Master, the effect of the two standards on potency titrations will remain unknown. However, routine tests have indicated no effect.

A strain of mouse that is free from endemic infection is fundamental. Our limited experience suggests that the best strain is one that is capable of being rendered highly sensitive to histamine by pertussis vaccine.[159] Such strains also have a relatively low susceptibility to toxic effects of the vaccine.[159] Vaccines that pass the toxicity test at the lower level of acceptability inhibit the immune response of some strains of mice more than others.[157] The NIH (NIH-BXS) and the CFW strains are the best we have studied. Satisfactory results have been obtained with other strains in other laboratories. The NIH strain used since 1944 was bred brother by sister until a few years ago when random breeding was inadvertently introduced. A new strain is being selectively bred out of the NIH strain for high HSF sensibility. The influence of gut microbial control on immunological response to pertussis vaccine is not known.

B. pertussis strain 18323 (serotype 1.2.3.4.5.7)[47] was introduced by Kendrick et al.[82] in the collaborative study of 10 laboratories which established the feasibility of the intracerebral test. It was used for the potency assay of field trial vaccines[54, 119] and is specified as the challenge strain by a number of national control laboratories. Other strains might be equally satisfactory or even better but there is scant or no information on whether they would provide relative potencies in the laboratory or in the field comparable to those obtained with 18323. Strain 353-Z (serotype 1) with the same virulence as 18323 influenced relative potencies divergent from those obtained with challenge strain 18323.[46] Strain 18323 tends to modulate and must be stored by a method that will assure retention of original characteristics. Storage on artificial medium at 4°C. does not provide this assurance.

Other influential factors of the test to be considered and kept constant are (1) temperature of the animal room, (2) sex[149] and randomization of mice in groups and in location of groups on shelves, (3) medium for cultivation of culture and a set time schedule for the transfers before use, (4) diluent for the challenge suspension, (5) a fixed time of day for the challenge (physiological rhythm makes a difference in response), (6) an experienced operator, and (7) discharge of each test by the same person from test to test.

When all variables are controlled, reproducible results can be obtained within and between laboratories. One or two tests are sufficient for routine assays and three or four tests are usually sufficient for a precise estimate.


## Toxicity

The untoward reactivity of pertussis vaccine is influenced by the presence of one or more reactive factors. No doubt the interplay of different factors confounds reactivity and its measurement in the laboratory. In 1965 Pittman and Cox[160] reviewed the literature on laboratory assessment of toxicity and the relation of animal response to human reactivity. The latter information was sparse. The mouse weight-gain test reflected best the human reactivity. The test, prescribed for United States licensed pertussis vaccines in 1949, was designed to prevent the presence of HLT.[152] It also reflects the presence of endotoxin by a 24-hour weight loss. The test revised in 1961 probably reflects the presence of a reactive amount of the so-called LPF, claimed to be the cause of late deaths in the seven-day test.[94] Weight gain and death after injection of LPF are slower than after HLT. Ishida[74] has shown that the slopes of the weight-gain response curves of HLT, LPF, and endotoxin are significantly different.

Muggleton[128] reported another type of reaction of the mouse characterized by early hypothermia and hypoglycemia which was maximum six to 12 hours after the injection of formalin-killed pertussis bacteria. The development of shock was inhibited when 1:7500 Merthiolate was added before injection. It is not known if this reaction in the mouse is a manifestation of the reactive factor of a quadruple antigen product that was reported by Haire et al.[66] to have caused persistent screaming and collapse in some children. Merthiolate was not listed among the ingredients of the product. Persistent screaming is not a commonly reported reaction to pertussis vaccine.

The recent Japanese work reported by Someya[191] failed to show a correlation between mouse toxicity as assayed in Japan at that time and clinical reactivity. Febrile responses reflected differences in the number of bacteria in the vaccines. On the other hand, Muggleton[128] reported a clear relationship between batches of vaccine that caused unfavorable weight gain of mice, assayed by the United States method, and those that caused a high incidence of reactions in children. The pertussis bacteria in the triple antigen batches were formalin-killed and Merthiolate-preserved. The flatter slope of the mouse weight curve of the more reactive vaccines resembles that of LPF. He also noted that storage temperature may affect reactivity. Certain batches (preservative not stated) caused an excessive number of sore arms. The samples, returned to the manufacturer, caused dermonecrosis in rabbits. Retention samples held at 4°C. were not dermonecrotic but became dermonecrotic after 37°C. storage for seven days. It is doubtful that Merthiolate was present in the product since Pittman[152] found that heating at 34°C. for one day in the presence of Merthiolate destroyed dermonecrotic toxin. A change in reactivity of United States licensed pertussis vaccine on the market has not been noted; all pertussis vaccine products contain Merthiolate.

A correlation between anaphylactic reactions in mice following a second injection of vaccine and clinical reactions was reported by Klimovitskya et al.[92]

Although tests other than the mouse weight-gain test have been proposed,[cf. 160] none has been accepted for routine testing except HSF titration in Holland.[33] Should fractionated protective antigen become available, it would be advisable to prescribe a limit for HSF to assure that the amount of HSF relative to protective antigen was not greater than in the whole-cell vaccine. The Dutch standard pertussis vaccine was assigned the same number of HSF units as protective units.[33]

Since the factor that contributes to the rare postvaccination encephalopathy is not known (see Cellular Components), it is not possible to prescribe a specific test to detect its presence. At present the only recourse is to assure that vaccines pass the prescribed test for freedom from toxicity while investigations are in progress to find more sensitive methods to detect specific reactive substances. If minor systemic reactions can be kept to a minimum, the likelihood of triggering a more severe reaction in the child with an individual idiosyncrasy will be reduced.

The strain of mouse has been a significant variable in the assay of toxicity. Piersma et al.[147] reported that the seven-day weight gain and mortality of different strains of mice injected with the same special vaccine ranged from 0 to 9.2 gm. and 4 to 43 per cent. In addition to similar results in my laboratory, Gardner et al.,[61] in a comparison of germ-free and conventional NIH-BXS mice, found that the germ-free mice were not sufficiently sensitive to be of practical use for toxicity testing. Preliminary results indicate that microbial-controlled NIH-BXS mice likewise are not sufficiently sensitive to detect toxic vaccines.

Progress is being made on methods of evaluating the specific reactivity factors of pertussis vaccine in the laboratory. The introduction of toxicity reference vaccine, now being used experimentally, will be helpful in selecting suitable mouse strains for the test and in determining the slope of the weight-gain curves relative to different reactive factors. The significance of the mouse weight-gain test and other tests must await clinical correlation obtained with the use of pertussis vaccines that have been analyzed in the laboratory. It is desirable that the quantitative clinical responses be measured as precisely and in depth as in the laboratory.

## SUMMARY

Pertussis is a distressing and dangerous disease of childhood. Both the infection and the causative bacterium *Bordetella pertussis* have many anomalous features. Although the bacteria remain localized in the respiratory tract, there are, besides respiratory symptoms, disturbances of the reticuloendothelial and the nervous systems. The unique symptom of paroxysmal whooping, probably neurological in nature, persists for several weeks after the bacteria can no longer be recovered. Antiserum and antibiotics are effective antibacterial agents but clinical effect on coughing depends on the time of initiation of therapy. Neither infection nor vaccination affords lifelong immunity.

Mice injected intranasally develop a respiratory infection similar to that in the child. The intracerebral infection is likewise similar in that the bacteria remain localized on the ciliated ependymal cells but dissimilar in that infection is usually lethal. Potency of vaccines assayed by the intracerebral protection test correlates with protection in children.

*B. pertussis* contains a number of reactive factors: heat-labile toxin, endotoxin (lipopolysaccharide), histamine-sensitizing factor, and lymphocyte-promoting factor or neurotoxin. The role of the individual factor or interplay of the factors in the infection is not clearly understood. It appears that the protective activity of vaccines is not dependent on the serotype composition of the propagation strains.

Preparation of adequately potent vaccine with no untoward reactivity presents a challenge. Merthiolate remains the preservative of choice. Vaccine adsorbed by an aluminum compound is less reactive and more potent than the plain vaccine from which it is derived. The mouse weight-gain toxicity test reflects best the reactivity of vaccines for children. Further study on the relation of reactive factors assayed in the laboratory to response of children is needed. The most distressing reaction is the rare vaccine encephalopathy. Its rarity indicates an individual idiosyncrasy or a predisposition such as a latent viral disease. The risk of vaccination is outweighed by risk of infection.

# References

1. Additional Standards: Pertussis vaccine. 1968. Federal Register *33:*8818–8819.
2. Ames, R. G., S. M. Cohen, A. E. Fischer, J. Kohn, A. Z. McPherson, J. Marlow, J. Rutzky, and H. E. Alexander. 1953. Comparison of the therapeutic efficacy of four agents in pertussis. Pediatrics *11:*323–327.
3. Andersen, E. K. 1952. Some observations made during experiments on mice inoculated with *H. pertussis.* Acta Path. Microbiol. Scand. *31:*546–560.
4. Andersen, E. K. 1953. Active pertussis immunity in mice after recovery from pulmonary infection or vaccination against *H. pertussis.* Acta Path. Microbiol. Scand., *32:*125–136.
5. Andersen, E. K. 1953. Serological studies on *H. pertussis, H. parapertussis* and *H. bronchisepticus.* Acta Path. Microbiol. Scand. *33:*202–224.
6. Andersen, E. K. 1958. Biological Standardization of Pertussis Vaccines. Nyt Nordisk Forlag Arnold Busck, Copenhagen, pp. 1–80.
7. Andersen, E. K., and M. W. Bentzon. 1958. Comparison between pertussis vaccine potency assays in mice challenged by the intracerebral route and mice challenged by the intranasal route (sublethal dose). Acta Path. Microbiol. Scand. *42:*333–356.
8. Andersen, E. K., and M. W. Bentzon. 1958. The failure to show correlation between type-specificity and protection in experimental pertussis in mice (sublethal intranasal challenge). Acta Path. Microbiol. Scand. *43:*106–112.
9. Anderson, G., and E. A. North. 1943. The relation of pertussis endotoxin to pertussis immunity in the mouse. Aust. J. Exp. Biol. Med. Sci. *21:*1–8.
10. Armitage, P., and W. L. M. Perry. 1957. British Standard for pertussis vaccine: its use in routine control of commercial vaccines. Brit. Med. J. *2:*501–505.
11. Baird, H. W., III, and B. G. Borofsky. 1957. Infantile myoclonic seizures. J. Pediat. *50:*332–339.
12. Bell, J. A. 1948. Pertussis immunization. Use of two doses of an alum-precipitated mixture of diphtheria toxoid and pertussis vaccines. J.A.M.A. *137:*1276–1281.
13. Bell, J. A., M. Pittman, and B. J. Olson. 1949. Pertussis and aureomycin. Public Health Rep. *64:*589–598.
14. Berenbaum, M. C., J. Ungar, and W. K. Stevens. 1960. Intracranial infection of mice with *Bordetella pertussis.* J. Gen. Microbiol. *22:*313–322.
15. Billaudelle, H. 1960. Observations on the stability of biologically active substances in *Bordetella pertussis.* Z. Immunitätsforsch. *120:*173–185.
16. Billaudelle, H., L. Edebo, E. Hammarsten, C.-G. Hedén, B. Malmgren, and H. Palmstierna. 1960. Studies on the chemical and immunological structure of *Bordetella pertussis.* Acta Path. Microbiol. Scand. *50:*208–224.
17. Bogdan, A. 1952. Terramycin in pertussis. Brit. Med. J. *2:*1186–1187.
18. Bordet, J., and O. Gengou. 1906. Le microbe de la coqueluche. Ann. Inst. Pasteur *20:*731–741.
19. Bordet, J., and O. Gengou. 1909. L'endotoxine coquelucheuse. Ann. Inst. Pasteur *23:*415–419.
20. Bradford, W. L. 1958. The pertussis group. *In:* Dubos, R. J. (ed.). Bacterial and Mycotic Infections of Man. J. B. Lippincott, Philadelphia, pp. 486–494.
21. Brown, A. M. 1958. Intracerebral infection in mice with *Haemophilus pertussis* and passive protection by hyperimmune rabbit sera. J. Gen. Microbiol. *18:*48–57.
22. Burian, V., B. Vysoká-Burianová, J. Mikulecký, J. Halík, and K. Maličký. 1966. [Vaccination against pertussis during school age.] Cesk. Epidem. *15:*141–146.
23. Burland, W. L., W. M. Sutcliffe, M. A. Voyce, M. L. Hilton, and P. W. Muggleton. 1968. Reactions to combined diphtheria, tetanus and pertussis vaccine: A comparison between plain vaccine and vaccine adsorbed on aluminum hydroxide. The Medical Officer *119:*17–19.
24. Burnet, F. M., and C. Timmins. 1937. Experimental infection with *Haemophilus pertussis* in the mouse by intranasal inoculation. Brit. J. Exp. Path. *18:*83–90.
25. Byers, R. K., and N. D. Rizzo. 1950. A follow-up study of pertussis in infancy. New Eng. J. Med. *242:*887–891.
26. Cameron, J. 1967. Variation in *Bordetella pertussis.* J. Path. Bact. *94:*367–374.
27. Chalvardjian, N. 1965. The content of antigens 1, 2 and 3 in strains of *Bordetella pertussis* and in vaccines. Canad. Med. Assoc. J. *92:*1114–1116.
28. Chin Chiang Huang, Pin Mein Chen, Jui Kui Kuo, Wen Hsung Chiu, Shou Tien Lin, Hua Shing Lin, and Yeng Ching Lin. 1962. Experimental whooping cough. New Eng. J. Med. *266:*105–111.
29. Christensen, C. N. 1963. More risky to give, or not to give? Letter to Editor. Amer. J. Dis. Child. *105:*417.

30. Clough, P. W. 1950. Encephalitis following vaccination against pertussis. Editorial. Ann. Intern. Med. *32:*343–348.
31. Cockburn, W. C. 1958. Incidents et accidents consécutifs à la vaccination anticoquelucheuse. Bull. WHO *19:*109–122.
32. Cohen, H. 1957. Een onderzoek naar bruikbaarheid van de "agglutinine produktie" proef voor de waardebepaling van kinkhoestvaccin. *In:* National Institute of Health Annual Report 1957, Utrecht, pp. 119–122.
33. Cohen, H. H. 1963. Development of pertussis vaccine production and control in the National Institute of Public Health in the Netherlands during the years 1950–1962. Antonie Leeuwenhoek *29:*183–201.
34. Cohen, S. M., and M. W. Wheeler. 1946. Pertussis vaccine prepared with Phase-I cultures grown in fluid medium. Amer. J. Public Health *36:*371–376.
35. Cooper, G. N. 1952. Active immunity in mice following the intranasal injection of sub-lethal doses of living *Haemophilus pertussis.* J. Path. Bact. *64:*65–74.
36. Court, D., H. Jackson, and G. Knox. 1953. The recognition of whooping-cough. Lancet *2:* 1057–1060.
37. Cravitz, L., and J. H. Cauley. 1945. Pertussis immunization program of the Boston Health Department. J.A.M.A. *129:*539–541.
38. Dean, D. J., S. M. Cohen, and G. Dalldorf. 1951. The effect of unrelated vaccines on the localization of paralysis in mouse encephalomyelitis. Proc. Soc. Exp. Biol. Med. *77:* 834–836.
39. Demina, A. A., L. I. Larina, and N. P. Devyatkina. 1968. [A change of the serological type of pertussis causative agent.] Zh. Mikrobiol. No. 2, pp. 13–17.
40. Dolby, J. M., D. C. W. Thow, and A. F. B. Standfast. 1961. The intranasal infection of mice with *Bordetella pertussis.* J. Hyg. *59:*191–204.
41. Dolgopol, V. B. 1941. Changes in the brain in pertussis with convulsions. Arch. Neurol. Psychol. *46:*477–503.
42. Eldering, G. 1942. A study of the antigenic properties of *Hemophilus pertussis* and related organisms. II. Protection tests in mice. Amer. J. Hyg. *36:*294–302.
43. Eldering, G. 1958. Whooping cough studies in Grand Rapids and Kent County. J. Mich. Med. Soc. 57:221–224, 232.
44. Eldering, G. 1967. Serotyping of *Bordetella pertussis* cultures. Contract PH43–66–552, Division of Biologics Standards, National Institutes of Health, Department of Health, Education and Welfare.
45. Eldering, G., W. C. Eveland, and P. L. Kendrick. 1962. Fluorescent antibody staining and agglutination reactions in *Bordetella pertussis* cultures. J. Bact. 83:745–749.
46. Eldering, G., J. Holwerda, and J. Baker. 1966. *Bordetella pertussis* culture having only species factor 1. J. Bact. *91:*1759–1762.
47. Eldering, G., J. Holwerda, and J. Baker. 1967. Mouse-protective properties of *Bordetella pertussis* serotypes in passive tests. J. Bact. *93:*1758–1761.
48. Eldering, G., C. Hornbeck, and J. Baker. 1957. Serological study of *Bordetella pertussis* and related species. J. Bact. *74:*133–136.
49. Evans, D. G. 1943. Further experiments on the effects produced by extracts of *H. pertussis* on the blood sugar of rabbits. J. Path. Bact. *55:*269–274.
50. Evans, D. G. 1947. The failure of whooping-cough and adult sera to neutralise *pertussis* toxin. J. Path. Bact., *59:*341–342.
51. Evans, D. G., and F. T. Perkins. 1955. Tests for agglutinin production by pertussis protective antigen, SPA. J. Path. Bact. *69:*329–331.
52. Feldman, R. A., and J. F. Schwartz. 1968. Possible association between cytomegalovirus infection and infantile spasms. Lancet *2:*180–181.
53. Felton, H. M., and E. W. Flosdorf. 1946. Detection of susceptibility to whooping cough. I. Institutional experiences with pertussis agglutinogen as skin test reagent. J. Pediat. *29:*677–686.
54. Felton, H. M., and W. F. Verwey. 1955. The epidemiological evaluation of a non-cellular pertussis antigen. Pediatrics *16:*637–651.
55. Felton, H. M., and C. Y. Willard. 1944. The current status of prophylaxis by *Haemophilus pertussis vaccine.* J.A.M.A. *126:*294–299.
56. Fishel, C. W., A. Szentivanyi, and D. W. Talmage. 1962. Sensitization and desensitization of mice to histamine and serotonin by neurohumors. J. Immun. *89:*8–18.
57. Fishel, C. W., A. Szentivanyi, and D. W. Talmage. 1964. Adrenergic factors in *Bordetella pertussis*-induced histamine and serotonin hypersensitivity of mice. *In:* Landy, M., and Braun, W. (eds.). Bacterial Endotoxins. Institute of Microbiology, Rutgers, The State University, New Brunswick, N.J., pp. 474–481.
58. Fleming, D. S., L. Greenberg, and E. M. Beith. 1948. The use of combined antigens in the immunization of infants. Canad. Med. Assoc. J. *59:*101–105.

59. Flosdorf, E. W., H. M. Felton, A. Bondi, Jr., and A. C. McGuinness. 1943. Intradermal test for susceptibility to and immunization against whooping cough using agglutinogen from Phase I *H. pertussis*. Amer. J. Med. Sci. *206:*421–425.

60. Flosdorf, E. W., and A. C. Kimball. 1940. Separation of the Phase I agglutinogen of *H. pertussis* from toxic components. J. Immun. *39:*475–494.

61. Gardner, R., H. Bohner, and M. Pittman. Reactivity of germ-free and conventionl mice to pertussis vaccine. *In:* Proceedings of the Tenth International Congress of the Permanent Section of Microbiological Standardization, Prague, Czechoslovakia, Sept. 19–23, 1967 (*in press*).

62. Gardner, R. A., and M. Pittman. 1965. Relative stability of pertussis vaccine preserved with Merthiolate, benzethonium chloride, or the parabens. Appl. Microbiol. *13:*564–569.

63. Gordon, J. E., and R. I. Hood. 1951. Whooping cough and its epidemiological anomalies. Amer. J. Med. Sci. *222:*333–361.

64. Gray, D. F. 1946. Some factors influencing the virulence of *Hemophilus pertussis* Phase I. Aust. J. Exp. Biol. Med. Sci. *24:*301–311.

65. Gruenewald, R., E. G. Allen, S. Levine, and E. J. Wenk. 1961. Studies on mechanism of ascites produced by pertussis vaccine. Proc. Soc. Exp. Biol. Med. *108:*109–111.

66. Haire, M., D. S. Dane, and G. Dick. 1967. Reactions to combined vaccines containing killed *Bordetella pertussis*. The Medical Officer *117:*55–58.

67. Hazen, L. N., G. G. Jackson, Chang Shi-Man, E. H. Place, and M. Finland. 1951. Antibiotic treatment of pertussis. J. Pediat. *39:*1–16.

68. Holt, L. B., V. Spasojevic, J. M. Dolby, and A. F. B. Standfast 1961. Immunity in mice to an intracerebral challenge of *Bordetella pertussis*. J. Hyg. *59:*373–378.

69. Hornibrook, J. W. 1939. Cultivation of Phase I *H. pertussis* in a semi-synthetic liquid medium. Public Health Rep. *54:*1847–1851.

70. Hornibrook, J. W., and J. J. Ashburn. 1939. A study of experimental pertussis in the young rat. Public Health Rep. *54:*439–444.

71. Iida, T., N. Kusano, A. Yamamoto, and M. Konosu. 1966. An immunofluorescence study of the action of antibody in experimental intracerebral infection of mice with *Bordetella pertussis*. J. Path. Bact. *92:*359–367.

72. Iida, T., N. Kusano, A. Yamamoto, and H. Shiga. 1962. Studies on experimental infection with *Bordetella pertussis*. Bacteriological and pathological studies on the mode of infection in mouse brain. Jap. J. Exp. Med. *32:*471–494.

73. Ipsen, J., and H. E. Bowen. 1955. Effects of routine immunization of children with triple vaccine (diphtheria-tetanus-pertussis). Amer. J. Public Health, *45:*312–318.

74. Ishida, S. 1968. Characterization of the body weight-decreasing toxicities in mice by the lymphocytosis-promoting factor and the heat-labile toxin of *B. pertussis* and endotoxin. Jap. J. Med. Sci. Biol. *21:*115–135.

75. Jaffe, V. R. 1955. Incidence of pertussis in vaccinated and unvaccinated children. J. Pediat. *47:*716–719.

76. Jochims, J. 1928. Ein Beitrag zur Keuchhusten-encephalopathie. Z. Kinderheilk. *45:*326–332.

77. Joó, I., Z. Pusztai, and V. P. Juhász. 1961. Histamine-sensitizing activity of various pertussis vaccines. Z. Immunitätsforsch. *121:*143–158.

78. Kasuga, T., Y. Nakase, K. Ukishima, and K. Takatsu. 1953. Studies on *Haemophilus pertussis*. Part I. Antigen structure of *H. pertussis* and its phases. Kitasato Arch. Exp. Med. *26:*121–133.

79. Katsampes, C. P., A. M. Brooks, and W. L. Bradford. 1942. Toxicity of washings from *H. pertussis* for mice. Proc. Soc. Exp. Biol. Med. *49:*615–618.

80. Kendrick, P., and G. Eldering. 1935. Significance of bacteriological methods in the diagnosis and control of whooping cough. Amer. J. Public Health *25:*147–155.

81. Kendrick, P., and G. Eldering. 1939. A study in active immunization against pertussis. Amer. J. Hyg. (Sect. B) *29:*133–153.

82. Kendrick, P. L., G. Eldering, M. K. Dixon, and J. Misner. 1947. Mouse protection tests in the study of pertussis vaccine: A comparative series using the intracerebral route for challenge. Amer. J. Public Health *37:*803–810.

83. Kendrick, P., G. Eldering, C. Hornbeck, and J. Baker. 1955. A study of the stability of pertussis vaccine under different conditions of storage. Amer. J. Public Health *45:*1131–1137.

84. Kendrick, P., G. Eldering, and M. Thompson. 1946. Reenforcing or "booster" injection of pertussis vaccine in previously immunized children of kindergarten age. Amer. J. Dis. Child. *72:*382–388.

85. Kendrick, P. L., J. J. Miller, and G. M. Lawson. 1935–1936. Tentative methods for the bacteriological diagnosis and control of whooping cough. *In:* Year Book of the American Public Health Association, New York, pp. 200–206.

86. Kendrick, P. L., E. L. Updyke, and G. Eldering. 1949. Comparison of pertussis cultures by mouse protection and virulence tests. Amer. J. Public Health 39:179–184.

87. Kind, L. S. 1953. Inhibition of histamine death in pertussis-inoculated mice by cortisone and Neoantergan. J. Allerg. 24:52–59.

88. Kind, L. S. 1953. The altered reactivity of mice after immunization with *Hemophilus pertussis* vaccine. J. Immun. 70:411–420.

89. Kind, L. S. 1954. Inhibition of histamine death in pertussis-inoculated mice by Dibenzyline, an adrenergic blocking agent. J. Allerg. 25:33–35.

90. Kind, L. S. 1956. Effects of heat on the sensitizing and shocking properties of *Hemophilus pertussis*. J. Immun. 77:115–118.

91. Kind, L. S. 1958. The altered reactivity of mice after inoculation with *Bordetella pertussis* vaccine. Bact. Rev. 22:173–182.

92. Klimovitskaya, V. E., E. A. Baeva, F. L. Leites, and V. M. Bolotovsky. 1967. [A study of reactogenic and allergic properties of vaccines with a pertussis component in experimental conditions and in epidemiological trial.] Zh. Microbiol. No. 1, pp. 145–148.

93. Kurokawa, M., S. Ishida, S. Iwasa, S. Asakawa, and K. Kuratsuka. 1968. Attempts at analysis of toxicity of pertussis vaccine. I. Body weight-decreasing toxicity in mice. Jap. J. Med. Sci. Biol. 21:137–153.

94. Kurokawa, M., S. Iwasa, and S. Ishida. 1965. On a possible new kind of toxic substance produced by *Bordetella pertussis*. Jap. J. Med. Sci. Biol. 18:161–165.

95. Kuwajima, Y., T. Matsui, and M. Kishigami. 1957. The growth-supporting effect of some anion exchange resins for phase I Haemophilus pertussis. Jap. J. Microbiol. 1:375–381.

96. Kuwajima, Y., and M. Niwa. 1964. [Chemical constituents of *Bordetella* bacteria.] Tanpakushitsu Kakusan Koso 9:717–724.

97. Lacey, B. W. 1960. Antigenic modulation of *Bordetella pertussis*. J. Hyg. 58:57–93.

98. Lambert, H. J. 1965. Epidemiology of a small pertussis outbreak in Kent County, Michigan. Public Health Rep. 80:365–369.

99. Landy, M., and W. Braun (eds.). 1964. Bacterial Endotoxins. Institute of Microbiology, Rutgers, The State University, New Brunswick, N.J.

100. Lapin, J. H. 1943. Whooping Cough. Charles C Thomas, Springfield, Ill.

101. Lawson, G. M. 1933. Epidemiology of whooping cough. Amer. J. Dis. Child. 46: 1454–1455.

102. Lee, J. M., and P. K. Olitsky. 1955. Simple method for enhancing development of acute disseminated encephalomyelitis in mice. Proc. Soc. Exp. Biol. Med. 89:263–266.

103. Leslie, P. H., and A. D. Gardner. 1931. The phases of *Hemophilus pertussis*. J. Hyg. 31: 423–434.

104. Levine, S., and R. Gruenewald. 1962. Ascites in the rat produced by pertussis vaccine. Exp. Mol. Pathol. 1:104–112.

105. Levine, S., and E. J. Wenk. 1961. Studies on the mechanism of altered susceptibility to experimental encephalomyelitis. Amer. J. Path. 39:419–441.

106. Levine, S., E. J. Wenk, H. B. Devlin, R. E. Pieroni, and L. Levine. 1966. Hyperacute allergic encephalomyelitis: adjuvant effect of pertussis vaccines and extracts. J. Immun. 97:363–368.

107. Litvak, A. M., H. Gibel, S. E. Rosenthal, and P. Rosenblatt. 1948. Cerebral complications in pertussis. J. Pediat. 32:357–379.

108. Madsen, T. 1925. The bacteriology, diagnosis, prevention and treatment of whooping cough. Boston Med. Surg. J. 192:50–60.

109. Maitland, H. B., and A. Guérault. 1958. Some surface components of *Haemophilus pertussis:* Immunising antigen, histamine-sensitising factor and agglutinogen. J. Path. Bact. 76:257–274.

110. Maitland, H. B., R. Kohn, and A. D. MacDonald. 1955. The histamine-sensitizing property of *Haemophilus pertussis*. J. Hyg. 53:196–211.

111. Manchester Public Health Laboratory. 1965. Whooping-cough in Manchester, 1963–64. Monthly Bull. Minist. Health 24:104–110.

112. Mannerstedt, G. 1934. Pertussis in adults. J. Pediat. 5:596–600.

113. McFarlan, A. M., E. Topley, and M. Fisher. 1945. Trial of whooping-cough vaccine in city and residential nursery groups. Brit. Med. J. 2:205–208.

114. McGuinness, A. C., J. G. Armstrong, and H. M. Felton. 1944. Hyperimmune whooping cough serum. J. Pediat. 24:249–258.

115. Medical Research Council. 1951. The prevention of whooping-cough by vaccination. Brit. Med. J. 1:1463–1471.

116. Medical Research Council. 1953. Treatment of whooping-cough with antibiotics. Lancet 1:1109–1112.

117. Medical Research Council. 1956. Vaccination against whooping-cough: Relation between protection in children and results of laboratory tests. Brit. Med. J. 2:454–462.

118. Medical Research Council. 1956. Poliomyelitis and prophylactic inoculation against diphtheria, whooping-cough and smallpox. Lancet *2:*1223–1231.
119. Medical Research Council. 1959. Vaccination against whooping-cough: Final report. Brit. Med. J. *1:*994–1000.
120. Miller, J. J., Jr., H. K. Faber, M. L. Ryan, R. J. Silverberg, and E. Lew. 1949. Immunization against pertussis during the first four months of life. Pediatrics *4:*468–478.
121. Miller, J. J., Jr., R. J. Silverberg, T. M. Saito, and J. B. Humber. 1943. An agglutinative reaction for *Hemophilus pertussis*. II. Its relation to clinical immunity. J. Pediat. *22:* 644–651.
122. Mishulow, L., L. S. Sharpe, and L. L. Cohen. 1953. Beef-heart charcoal agar for the preparation of pertussis vaccines. Amer. J. Public Health *43:*1466–1472.
123. Morbidity and Mortality Weekly Report. Annual Supplement. Summary 1966. Reported incidence of notifiable diseases in the United States. 1966. *15*(No. 53):4–5.
124. Morbidity and Mortality Weekly Report. 1967. Pertussis—Michigan. *16:*379.
125. Morbidity and Mortality Weekly Report. 1968. Pertussis—Oregon. *17:*6.
126. Morse, S. I., and S. K. Riester. 1967. Studies on the leukocytosis and lymphocytosis induced by *Bordetella pertussis*. II. The effect of pertussis vaccine on the thoracic duct lymph and lymphocytes of mice. J. Exp. Med. *125:*619–628.
127. Mudd, S., H. M. Felton, and J. Smolens. 1948. Responses of human subjects to vaccines in saline-in-mineral oil emulsion. II. *Hemophilus pertussis* vaccines. J. Immun. *58:* 41–47.
128. Muggleton, P. W. 1967. Vaccines against pertussis. Public Health *81:*252–264.
129. Munoz, J. 1963. Symposium on relationship of structure of microorganisms to their immunological properties. I. Immunological and other biological activities of *Bordetella pertussis* antigens. Bact. Rev. *27:*325–340.
130. Munoz, J. 1964. Hypersensitivity reactions induced in mice treated with *Bordetella pertussis. In:* Landy, M., and Braun, W. (eds.). Bacterial Endotoxins. Institute of Microbiology, Rutgers, The State University, New Brunswick, N.J., pp. 460–473.
131. Munoz, J., and R. K. Bergman. 1968. Histamine-sensitizing factors from microbial agents, with special reference to *Bordetella pertussis*. Bact. Rev. *32:*103–126.
132. Munoz, J., and B. M. Hestekin. 1963. Antigens of *Bordetella pertussis*. III. The protective antigen. Proc. Soc. Exp. Biol. Med. *112:*799–805.
133. Munoz, J., and B. M. Hestekin. 1966. Antigens of *Bordetella pertussis*. IV. Effect of heat, Merthiolate, and formaldehyde on histamine-sensitizing factor and protective activity of soluble extracts from *Bordetella pertussis*. J. Bact. *91:*2175–2179.
134. Nagel, J. 1967. Isolation from *Bordetella pertussis* of protective antigen free from toxic activity and histamine sensitizing factor. Nature *214:*96–97.
135. Nelson, R. L. 1939. The neurological complications of whooping cough. A review of the literature with the reports of two cases of pertussis encephalitis. J. Pediat. *14:*39–47.
136. Newman, B., G. Gavis, and S. Weinberg. 1954. Treatment of pertussis with intramuscular oxytetracycline. Antibiot. Chemother. *4:*934–938.
137. Olson, B. H., G. Eldering, and B. Graham. 1964. Stabilization of pertussis vaccine in the presence of benzethonium chloride. J. Bact. *87:*543–546.
138. Ospeck, A. G., and M. E. Roberts. 1944. Pertussis antitoxin: its relationship to protection in actively and passively immunized mice and rabbits. J. Infect. Dis. *74:*22–31.
139. Parfentjev, I. A. 1950. The effect of antihistaminics on mice hypersensitive to *H. pertussis* vaccine. Yale J. Biol. Med. *23:*28–31.
140. Parfentjev, I. A. 1955. Anaphylaxis and histamine shock in mice. Proc. Soc. Exp. Biol. Med. *89:*297–299.
141. Parfentjev, I. A., and M. A. Goodline. 1948. Histamine shock in mice sensitized with *Hemophilus pertussis* vaccine. J. Pharmacol. Exp. Ther. *92:*411–413.
142. Parfentjev, I. A., M. A. Goodline, and M. E. Virion. 1947. A study of sensitivity to *Hemophilus pertussis* in laboratory animals. I. The hypersensitivity of laboratory animals to *Hemophilus pertussis*. J. Bact. *53:*597–601.
143. Parfentjev, I. A., M. A. Goodline, and M. E. Virion. 1947. A study of sensitivity to *Hemophilus pertussis* in laboratory animals. II. *Hemophilus pertussis* allergen and its assay on laboratory animals. J. Bact. *53:*603–611.
144. Parfentjev, I. A., M. A. Goodline, and M. E. Virion. 1947. A study of sensitivity to *Hemophilus pertussis* in laboratory animals. III. The formation of antibodies and the development of sensitivity in laboratory animals injected with *Hemophilus pertussis* antigens. J. Bact. *53:*613–619.
145. Parfentjev, I. A., and W. L. Schleyer. 1949. The influence of histamine on the blood sugar level of normal and sensitized mice. Arch. Biochem. *20:*341–346.
146. Pennell, R. B., and E. H. Thiele. 1951. Studies on the fractionation of *Hemophilus pertussis* extracts. J. Immun. *66:*627–633.

147. Piersma, H. D., F. W. Bingham, A. E. Bolyn, A. H. Brueckner, H. A. Dettwiler, W. W. Frankhouser, D. M. Marshall, and C. Newman. 1962. Recent laboratory experience in the U.S.A. with the pertussis toxicity test. Round Table Conference on Pertussis Immunization, Prague. Vol. 1, pp. 111–118.

148. Pillemer, L., L. Blum, and I. H. Lepow. 1954. Protective antigen of *Haemophilus pertussis*. Lancet *1:*1257–1260.

149. Pittman, M. 1951. Influence of sex of mice on histamine sensitivity and protection against *Hemophilus pertussis*. J. Infect. Dis. *89:*296–299.

150. Pittman, M. 1951. Comparison of the histamine-sensitizing property with the protective activity of pertussis vaccines for mice. J. Infect. Dis. *89:*300–304.

151. Pittman, M. 1951. Sensitivity of mice to histamine during respiratory infection by *Hemophilus pertussis*. Proc. Soc. Exp. Biol. Med. *77:*70–74.

152. Pittman, M. 1952. Influence of preservatives, of heat, and of irradiation on mouse protective activity and detoxification of pertussis vaccine. J. Immun. *69:*201–216.

153. Pittman, M. 1954. Variability of the potency of pertussis vaccine in relation to the number of bacteria. J. Pediat. *45:*57–69.

154. Pittman, M. 1956. Pertussis and pertussis vaccine control. J. Wash. Acad. Sci. *46:*234–243.

155. Pittman, M. 1957. Effect of *Haemophilus pertussis* on immunological and physiological reactions. Fed. Proc. *16:*867–872.

156. Pittman, M. 1958. Variations du pouvoir protecteur des différents vaccins anticoquelucheux: leur rapport avec la protection de l'être humain. Rev. Immun. (Paris) *22:*308–322.

157. Pittman, M. 1962. Instability of pertussis-vaccine component in quadruple antigen vaccine. J.A.M.A. *181:*25–30.

158. Pittman, M. 1962. Some factors which influence potency evaluation of pertussis vaccine. Round Table Conference on Pertussis Immunization, Prague. Vol. 2, pp. 219–234.

159. Pittman, M. 1967. Mouse strain variation in response to pertussis vaccine and tetanus toxoid. International Symposium on Laboratory Animals, London, 1966. *In:* Symp. Series Immunobiol. Standard. Vol. 5. Karger, Basel/New York, pp. 161–166.

160. Pittman, M., and C. B. Cox. 1965. Pertussis vaccine testing for freedom-from-toxicity. Appl. Microbiol. *13:*447–456.

161. Pollock, M. R. 1947. The growth of *H. pertussis* on media without blood. Brit. J. Exp. Path. *28:*295–307.

162. Powell, H. M., C. G. Culbertson, and P. W. Ensminger. 1951. Charcoal agar culture medium for preparing *Hemophilus pertussis* vaccine. Public Health Rep. *66:*346–348.

163. Preston, N. W. 1963. Type-specific immunity against whooping-cough. Brit. Med. J. *2:* 724–726.

164. Preston, N. W. 1965. Effectiveness of pertussis vaccine. Brit. Med. J. *2:*11–13.

165. Preston, N. W. 1966. Potency tests for pertussis vaccines: doubtful value of intracerebral challenge test in mice. J. Path. Bact. *91:*173–179.

166. Preston, N. W., and P. Garrity. 1967. Histamine-sensitizing factor of *Bordetella pertussis* differentiated from immunogens by neutralization and passive protection tests. J. Path. Bact. *93:*483–492.

167. Proom, H. 1947. The immunological aspects of experimental *Haemophilus pertussis* infection. J. Path. Bact. *59:*165–180.

168. Public Health Service Advisory Committee on Immunization Practices. 1966. Diphtheria, tetanus, and pertussis vaccines. Morbidity and Mortality Weekly Report *15:*416–418.

169. Pusztai, Z., and I. Joó. 1967. Influence of nicotinic acid on the antigenic structure of *Bordetella pertussis*. *In:* Ann. Immunologiae Hungaricae. Medicina Verlag, Budapest, pp. 62–67.

170. Pusztai, Z., I. Joó, and I. Kiss. 1960. Some observations on the growth of *Bordetella pertussis* in liquid shaken cultures. Path. Microbiol. *23:*192–200.

171. Regan, J. C., and A. Tolstoouhov. 1936. Relations of acid base equilibrium to the pathogenesis and treatment of whooping cough. New York J. Med. *36:*1075–1087.

172. Report of the Committee on Immunization and Therapeutic Procedures for Acute Infectious Diseases. 1951. American Academy of Pediatrics, Evanston, Ill., pp. 4–6.

173. Report of the Committee on the Control of Infectious Diseases. 1966. American Academy of Pediatrics, Evanston, Ill., p. 93.

174. Roberts, M. E., and A. G. Ospeck. 1944. A pertussis toxin-antitoxin neutralization technique. J. Infect. Dis. *74:*14–21.

175. Rowatt, E. 1955. Amino acid metabolism in the genus *Bordetella*. J. Gen. Microbiol. *13:* 552–560.

176. Rowatt, E. 1957. Some factors affecting the growth of *Bordetella pertussis*. J. Gen. Microbiol. *17:*279–296.

177. Rowley, D. A., J. Chutkow, and C. Attig. 1959. Severe active cutaneous hypersensitivity in the rat produced by *Hemophilus pertussis* vaccine. J. Exp. Med. *110:*751–770.
178. Sako, W. 1947. Studies on pertussis immunization. J. Pediat. *30:*29–40.
179. Sako, W., W. L. Treuting, D. B. Witt, and S. J. Nichamin. 1945. Early immunization against pertussis with alum precipitated vaccine. J.A.M.A. *127:*379–384.
180. Sanyal, R. K. 1960. Histamine sensitivity in children after *Pertussis* infection. Nature *185:*537–538.
181. Sato, Y., and K. Nagase. 1967. Isolation of protective antigen from *Bordetella pertussis*. Biochem. Biophys. Res. Commun. *27:*195–201.
182. Sauer, L. 1933. Immunization with bacillus pertussis vaccine. J.A.M.A. *101:*1449–1451.
183. Sauer, L. 1946. Whooping cough: prevention and treatment. Med. Clin. N. Amer. Jan., pp. 45–59.
184. Sauer, L. W., W. H. Tucker, and E. Markley. 1944. Immunity responses to mixtures of diphtheria toxoid and pertussis vaccine. J.A.M.A. *125:*949–952.
185. Schachter, M. 1953. Le pronostic neuropsychologique des enfants ayant d'une coqueluche précoce non compliquée. Praxis *42:*464–466.
186. Schayer, R. W., and O. H. Ganley. 1961. Relationship of increased histidine decarboxylase activity to *Bordetella pertussis* vaccine sensitization of mice. J. Allerg. *31:*204–213.
187. Schuchardt, L. F., J. Munoz, W. F. Verwey, and J. F. Sagin. 1963. The relationship of agglutinogen to other antigens of *Bordetella pertussis*. J. Immun. 91:107–111.
188. Smolens, J., and S. Mudd. 1943. Agglutinogen of *Hemophilus pertussis*, Phase I, for skin testing. J. Immun. *47:*155–163.
189. Soboleva, V. D. 1947. [The effectiveness of hyperimmune serum with whooping cough.] Zh. Mikrobiol. No. 5, pp. 33–37.
190. Someya, S. 1966. Studies on the prophylactic effect and untoward reactions of pertussis-diphtheria combined vaccine. IV. Comparative investigation on the antibody productivity and temperature increase in infants inoculated with the combined vaccines (PD, PDT) and tetanus toxoid. Bull. Inst. Public Health *15:*57–62.
191. Someya, S. 1967. Studies on the prophylactic effect and untoward reactions of pertussis-diphtheria combined vaccine. V. Relationship between the results from field trials and laboratory tests. Bull. Inst. Public Health *16:*23–32.
192. Sprunt, D. H., and D. S. Martin. 1943. In vivo neutralization of pertussis toxin with pertussis antitoxin. Amer. J. Path. *19:*255–265.
193. Standfast, A. F. B. 1951. The virulence of *Haemophilus pertussis* for mice by the intra-nasal route. J. Gen. Microbiol. *5:*250–267.
194. Standfast, A. F. B. 1951. The Phase I of *Haemophilus pertussis*. J. Gen. Microbiol. *5:*531–545.
195. Standfast, A. F. B. 1958. Some factors influencing the virulence for mice of *Bordetella pertussis* by the intracerebral route. Immunology *1:*123–134.
196. Standfast, A. F. B. 1958. The comparison between field trials and mouse protection tests against intranasal and intracerebral challenge with *Bordetella pertussis*. Immunology *1:*135–143.
197. Standfast, A. F. B., and J. M. Dolby. 1961. A comparison between the intranasal and intra-cerebral infection of mice with *Bordetella pertussis*. J. Hyg. *59:*217–229.
198. Strean, L. P., D. Lapointe, and E. Dechene. 1941. Clinical studies in immunity to pertussis with the use of pertussis skin testing toxin and antiendotoxin. Canad. Med. Assoc. J. *45:*326–332.
199. Stronk, M. G., and M. Pittman. 1955. The influence of pertussis vaccine on histamine sensitivity of rabbits and guinea pigs and on the blood sugar in rabbits and mice. J. Infect. Dis. *96:*152–161.
200. Sutherland, I. W. 1963. The protective activity of components of *Bordetella pertussis* cell walls. Immunology *6:*246–254.
201. Sutherland, I. W., and J. F. Wilkinson. 1961. A new growth medium for virulent *Bordetella pertussis*. J. Path. Bact. *82:*431–438.
202. Verwey, W. F., and E. H. Thiele. 1949. Studies on the antigenicity of toxic extracts of *Hemophilus pertussis*. J. Immun. *61:*27–33.
203. Weihl, C., H. D. Riley, and J. H. Lapin. 1963. Extracted pertussis antigen. Amer. J. Dis. Child. *106:*210–215.
204. Widelock, D., N. F. Martorana, and M. Schaeffer. 1966. The effect of pertussis vaccine on fetal wastage in mice. II: The sparing effect of glucose. Amer. J. Public Health *56:*1588–1591.
205. Wilson, G. S. 1967. The Hazards of Immunization. The University of London, The Athlone Press, London.
206. World Health Organization. 1964. Requirements for Pertussis Vaccine. World Health Organization Tech. Rep. Ser. No. 274, pp. 25–40.

207. Zakharova, M. S. 1958. [Problems of specific prevention of pertussis.] *In:* Zakharova, M. S. (ed.). [Specific Prevention of Pertussis.] Medgiz, Moscow, pp. 3–19.
208. Zakharova, M. S. 1964. [Pressing problems of special prophylaxis of whooping cough.] Vestnik Acad. Med. Sci., pp. 36–43.
209. Zellweger, H. 1959. Pertussis encephalopathy. Arch. Pediat. *76:*381–386.

# Chapter 12

# NEISSERIA AND NEISSERIAL INFECTIONS

NEYLAN A. VEDROS AND GEORGE A. HOTTLE

*School of Public Health, University of California, Berkeley, California*

The Neisseria comprise a genus of aerobic, nonsporulating, nonmotile, oxidase-positive, gram-negative cocci. Besides the two important human pathogens, *Neisseria meningitidis* and *Neisseria gonorrhoeae*, there are approximately 30 other species that reportedly have been found inhabiting human or animal mucosa. Of the numerous biochemical tests available, acid production from sugars is usually employed for initial species identification. The pathogenic members are distinguished by their fermentation of glucose and maltose (*N. meningitidis*) and of glucose only (*N. gonorrhoeae*). Other species ferment various sugars or have variable fermentative capacities. It should be pointed out that sugar fermentation as a criterion for species identification is far from satisfactory. As an example, it is not uncommon to isolate gram-negative, oxidase-positive diplococci from the human nasopharynx which ferment only glucose. These isolates would thus be identified as *N. gonorrhoeae*.[14] Highly specific agglutinin antisera usually suffice to resolve the issue. In addition to the somatic polysaccharide shared by all Neisseria, the gonococci share a number of minor antigenic components with the meningococci. Suitable cross-absorption removes most if not all of the cross-reacting antibodies to meningococci in antigonococcal sera.

Meningococci exhibit much greater variation than the gonococci. This is best demonstrated by their serologic diversity. Table 1 shows the currently accepted sero-group designation as adopted by the International Committee on Bacterial Nomenclature in 1950.[5] Major epidemics prior to World War II were caused by Group A strains, whereas Group B was predominant during interepidemics. Group C strains appeared in the early 1940's and are presently isolated in 10 to 15 per cent of the meningitis cases in the United States. In 1960 an increased number of meningococcal cases began to appear in the United States and Group B strains were the predominant isolate. Since 1964, however, increasing numbers of isolates could not be typed with antisera to

TABLE 1.    *Relationship among the Various Classifications of Meningococci** 

| DOPTER AND PAURON, 1914 | ROCKEFELLER INSTITUTE (WOLLSTEIN, 1914) | GORDON AND MURRAY, 1915 | GRIFFITH AND SCOTT, 1916 | PULLON, 1917 | NICOLLE, DEBAINS, AND JOUAN, 1918 | EVANS, 1920 (TROPINS) | COMMON USE SINCE 1940 | RECOMMENDED BY COMMITTEE 1950 |
|---|---|---|---|---|---|---|---|---|
| Meningococcus | Normal | I | I | C | A | R | I | A |
| | Irregular | III | | A | | | | |
| Parameningococcus α, β, γ | Parameningococcus | II | II | B | B | S | II | B |
| | | IV | II | | B | Z | IV | D |
| | | | | | C | | II alpha | C |
| | | | | | D† | | | |

* From Branham, S. E. 1953. Serological relationships among meningococci. Bacteriol. Rev. 17:175–188.
† Relation of this D to other groups is unknown.

Groups A, B, C, and D. This new serologic group has been tentatively identified as Group E[45] and is closely related to the Type Y recently isolated in Europe.[40]

Further evidence of the variability of meningococci is the appearance of a distinct serologic group and then its complete disappearance. An example of this is the isolation of Group D strains in the 1929 Chicago epidemic and their absence from cases and carriers since.

The subdivision of gonococci into immunological types is less distinct. *In vitro* cultivation of the gonococci results in antigenic alteration and loss of virulence. Four clonal types ($T_1$ to $T_4$) were described in 1963 and a correlation was demonstrated between colonial morphology ($T_1$, $T_2$) and virulence for man. Types $T_1$ and $T_2$ obtained from patients are characterized by their glistening convexity, dark brown to black coloration, and small size (0.5 mm. and 0.4 mm., respectively). Types $T_3$ and $T_4$ (avirulent for man) are characterized by their nearly flat elevation, minimal coloration, and larger size (1.0 to 2.0 mm.). Extended studies have shown that except for colonial morphology and saline-autoagglutinability (virulent $T_1$ and $T_2$ isolates show positive auto-agglutination) no definitive classification of the gonococci is indicated by antigenic analysis, nutritional requirements, or virulence for experimental animals.[24]

## GENETICS

Transformation was first demonstrated in *N. meningitidis* by Alexander and Redman.[2] The DNA was extracted from Group A cells which were known to exhibit iridescent growth on Mueller-Hinton medium and to show capsular swelling. This DNA was added to Group C cells which were negative for these two characteristics. After an appropriate incubation, as few as $10^4$ Group C cells showed both iridescence and capsular swelling.

Further studies on the genetic competence of meningococci became possible with the development by Catlin and Schloer in 1962[8] of a well defined medium which was suitable for transformation. Initially, drug resistance markers were used, but the preparation of auxotrophic mutants by Jyssum and by Lie permitted more complex experiments and genetic mapping. The auxotrophs were prepared by using a combination of ultraviolet light and penicillin. Later studies showed that nitrous acid was the best mutagen and the mutants obtained required one or more amino acids for growth in addition to the defined medium.[27, 28]

In bacterial transformation, competence has been defined as the capacity of bacteria to absorb DNA molecules from their environment and to become genetically transformed.[43] Although the exact nature of competence is unknown, in most species studied it seems to develop only during specific times in the growth cycle. The phenotypic expression of competence in meningococcal cells was found all through the regular growth cycle. The highest transformation frequency was obtained in the early part of the logarithmic growth phase. It was suggested that meningococci, in contrast to other bacterial species, have a degree of competence directly related to their metabolic activity. This was substantiated by kinetic experiments. The rapidity with which meningococcal transformants began to divide after expression was 5 to 10 minutes, as opposed to 1 to 2 hours for pneumococci. Although meningococci are capable of transformation at all stages of the growth cycle, studies in mixed cultures (str-r$^+$ and ery-r$^+$) indicated that maximum transformation occurred late in the growth phase. This is consistent with the studies of Catlin[7] and Lie,[29] who found that extracellular DNA in meningococcal cultures had transforming capability.

Employing 10 strains of meningococci which had transforming capabilities for streptomycin resistance, Jyssum and Lie[23] attempted to transform these cells after broth passage. They observed that the ability to transform (designated as the competent state, cp$^+$) was lost in different strains at rates varying from 0.40 to greater than 99.5. The incompetent cells (cp$^-$) were kept for over two years and in no case did a reversion to competence occur. Attempts to convert cp$^-$ to cp$^+$ by mutagenic agents, by exposure to DNA from cp$^+$ cells, or by animal passage were unsuccessful. In a later study, Jyssum and Jyssum found a mutant that was capable of going from cp$^-$ to cp.$^+$[22] A nutritional auxotroph that had gone from cp$^+$ to cp$^-$ with respect to streptomycin was tested for competence by DNA coding for the amino acid needed for growth. Cells that were cp$^+$ for the amino acid were then tested for their capability of being transformed to streptomycin resistance. This was possible and those cells were considered to have reverted from cp$^-$ to cp$^+$. These cp$^+$ cells were then found to lose their competence at the same rate as other competent cells of the strain. It was suggested that the reason for this reversion was that cp$^+$ cells contain a genetic determinant of the plasmid type. Cells that regain competence but are currently incompetent (cp) have the plasmid in the cytoplasm. Totally incompetent cells have only the cellular DNA.

These hypotheses were studied at the molecular level. The assumption was made that cells in the stationary phase of growth contain a single DNA molecule, while those in the exponential phase of growth are dividing and have parts of their DNA doubled. It was also assumed that the DNA molecule in meningococci begins replication from a given point and that markers closer to this point will be double more often that markers farther away. The relative ratio of transformation of markers in the exponential phase to those in the

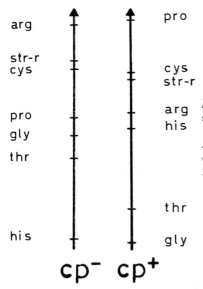

*Figure 1.* Replication charts of the chromosome in a competent (cp⁺) and an incompetent (cp⁻) variant of *Neisseria meningitidis.* (From Jyssum, K. 1965. Polarity of chromosome replication in *Neisseria meningitidis.* J. Bacteriol. *90:*1182–1187.)

stationary phase was compared for six amino acids and streptomycin. Genetic maps were constructed by considering those markers with the highest ratios to be closest to the point of replication and vice versa. Maps for both cp⁺ and cp⁻ are shown in Figure 1.[21] If DNA molecules are circular, then cp⁺ cells begin replication at a point different from cp⁻ cells and in opposite directions. Later studies were made on the transforming activity of the DNA of different densities of cp⁺, cp, and cp⁻ cells. The material was obtained by cesium chloride density gradients and biological activity, determined at various density peaks. Results supported the hypothesis that those cells that can regain competence, but currently are incompetent (cp), contain a cytoplasmic plasmid.

## CARRIER STATE

An important aspect of neisserial diseases has been the carrier state, the condition in which apparently healthy individuals harbor the bacteria. Although the healthy carrier is not unique to neisserial infections, it has been and still is the subject of intense study and controversy, particularly in meningococcal disease.

The literature on studies of meningococcus carriers is voluminous and the reader is referred to the reviews of Murray[38] and of Branham.[4] The meningococcus has a predilection for growing on the mucous membranes of man's oral cavity, but the epidemiology of the conversion of the healthy carrier into a patient with a typical case of cerebrospinal meningitis is unknown. In the past studies have usually been concerned with the nature of meningococcus carried, the length of time it can be isolated from the oral cavity, and environmental factors affecting the carrier rate. Only recently have studies been concerned with man's immunological response to the presence of the bacteria in the oral cavity and the role played by these phenomena in man's natural immunity to meningococcal disease.

Until recently all major epidemics of cerebrospinal meningitis throughout the world were caused by Group A strains of meningococci. Both contact and noncontact carriers harbored Group A strains indistinguishable from those isolated from the meningococcal patient. During World War I, studies in the British Army indicated that an epidemic could be expected if the carrier rate rose to 20 per cent or greater. Adequate "spacing out" of the men in their sleeping quarters apparently controlled the spread of infection. This magic figure of 20 per cent carrier rate as a prelude to an epidemic was shown by later studies to be invalid. Evidence was presented that the biological nature of the meningococcus carried was the important variable which forecast an epidemic rather than the number of carriers.[16, 33] During interepidemic periods in the 1930's, 1940's, and 1950's, 5 to 10 per cent of the population were healthy carriers of Group B meningococci. The numbers of healthy carriers varied and often reached a high figure without occurrence of cases. A similar situation exists today in the United States. Beginning in 1963, an increase in the number of meningococcal cases was noted in several military camps. Whereas Group B strains were usually predominant in interepidemic periods, this sero-group was now present in the majority of carriers and cases. The carrier rate in seasoned troops (past recruit training) reaches as high as 75 to 90 per cent with no cases of meningococcal disease. Whether or not the past epidemic situation with Group A strains will occur in this country remains to be seen.

The changing serological pattern of meningococci carried in the population was not apparent until the Group B strains resistant to sulfadiazine were found to cause disease in 1963.[35] In retrospect, it was recognized that during and soon after World War II it was the Group A strains which were so well controlled by sulfadiazine. The impending change, however, was forecast in 1954 by Love and Finland.[30] These authors observed that among 50 strains isolated from patients or carriers that year there were 6 per cent Group A, 44 per cent Group B, 24 per cent Group C, and 26 per cent untypable. These strains showed a wide range of susceptibility to sulfadiazine. With the changing pattern in isolates, it is no longer possible to terminate the carrier state with sulfadiazine or other drugs. Millar et al.[35] found that 1 million units of penicillin, given daily for four days, was ineffective in eradicating meningococci from the nasopharynx. Similar results were obtained by Leedom et al.,[26] who noted that treatment of contacts of patients with meningococcal disease for four days with penicillin G, phenoxymethyl penicillin, or tetracycline produced no change in the carrier state. Bristow et al.[6] reported that at one naval training center there had been a cyclical increase in meningococcal meningitis since 1960. In 1961 there were nine cases and in 1962 there were 23 cases with one death. By the use of mass prophylaxis with oral sulfadiazine a major epidemic may have been avoided in 1962. In 1963, when meningitis due to Group C appeared, the administration of oral sulfadiazine seemed to prevent further disease for a short time early in the year. About a month later, when Group B infections appeared in recruits, cases continued to appear despite medication. Later, the treatment of all recruits with 1 million units of oral penicillin V daily for four days did not stop the occurrence of cases. Attempts to lower the carrier rates with tetracycline (0.5 gm. twice daily for two days), oxytetracycline (0.5 gm. twice daily for four days), and V-Cillin K (1.2 million units

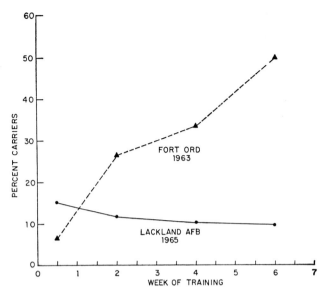

*Figure 2.* A decrease in the percentage of men carrying *N. meningitidis* at Lackland Air Force Base (solid line) during six weeks of basic military training. Broken line shows the usual trend of carrier rates (adapted from Gauld et al.[15]) reported from other military recruit training centers. (From Farrell, D. G., and E. V. Dahl. 1966. Nasopharyngeal carriers of *Neisseria meningitidis*. J.A.M.A. *198*:1189–1192.)

daily for six days) were successful for no more than several days, after which the carrier state reappeared. The epidemic was controlled by stopping the influx of new recruits and by environmental control measures.

The experience of the Air Force, as described by Farrell and Dahl,[11] was different from that reported by Gauld et al.[15] (see Figure 2). Between January 1 and March 31, 1965, 496 men were studied to determine carrier state. It was found that 15.9 per cent were positive on entry and 9.7 per cent were positive at the end of the six week training period; 68.3 per cent of the positive isolations were Group B and 15 per cent of these were resistant to sulfadiazine. There were no cases of meningitis at this base. This experience was in sharp contrast to that at Fort Ord, where carrier rates went from 20 per cent to 80 per cent during eight weeks of basic training. Ninety per cent of the strains isolated from the men were found to be Group B and about 50 per cent of them were resistant to sulfadiazine. Apparently the difference in the carrier rates at the two military bases was due to the character of the strains which occurred in the two populations.

It is generally concluded that there are no drugs currently available which will eliminate the meningococcal carrier state. The role that carriers play in man's natural immunity to meningococcal infection is not well defined. Evidence that the majority of carriers are truly infected was shown by the intracellular growth of the meningococci in the epithelial cells of the nasopharynx.[39] This was further substantiated by the observation that approximately 75 per cent of carriers produce circulating antibodies specific for meningococci. There appeared to be no correlation between the presence of antibodies or degree of antibody rise and the frequency of isolation of the bacteria from the nasopharynx.[46]

Determination of the carrier state with *N. gonorrhoeae* is difficult and obviously not an accurate estimation of the reservoir of infection in the population. In a recent report, however, it was found that a high percentage of females were carrying the organisms but were completely symptomless and not aware that they were infected.[31] This carrier state provided a reservoir which served to perpetuate infection among males. Four different treatment regimens were employed, and it was found that one treatment, which consisted of 2.4 million units of procaine penicillin G in oil followed by another injection of the same amount of aqueous procaine penicillin, resulted in clearing the infection in 89 per cent of the carriers. It was estimated that there were 3.3 per cent treatment failures and 8.4 per cent reinfections after treatment. It was concluded that this treatment regimen was the most efficient of the four tested in preventing reinfection.

## CHEMOTHERAPEUTIC AGENTS

The development of sulfonamide drugs as effective chemotherapeutic agents provided the means for control of meningococcus carriers and patients with this disease during the last 25 years. The appearance of Group B strains as the prime etiological agent in carriers and cases should have forewarned us of impending sulfonamide-resistant isolates. The Group B strains have always shown great variability in their sensitivity to sulfadiazine, an observation that has recently been confirmed.[12] It is interesting to speculate on the reasons for the appearance of these sulfadiazine-resistant strains. As early as 1964, in a study of 100 Marine recruits, it was found that 65 per cent were carrying Group B strains sensitive to $<1.0$ mg. per 100 ml. of sulfadiazine. From the remaining 35 noncarriers *N. perflava* was isolated, which showed resistance to $>10.0$ mg. per 100 ml. of sulfadiazine. Transformation of sulfadiazine resistance from the *N. perflava* to the sensitive meningococci was easily accomplished in the laboratory. The suggestion that this transformation could occur in nature was made in an independent study. An alternative explanation is that sulfadiazine selectively permits the growth of sulfadiazine-resistant strains. Although this theory is logical and attractive, it has not been proved conclusively in limited trials at various military camps. The question of whether all incoming military recruits and case contacts should receive oral sulfonamide prophylaxis is currently being debated. The epidemiology picture is further complicated by the recent appearance of Group A sulfonamide-resistant strains in North Africa.[1] Among 91 strains isolated from the cerebrospinal fluid of hospital cases, 90 per cent grew in the presence of 1 mg. per 100 ml. of sulfadiazine; 49 per cent in 5 mg. per 100 ml.; and 10 per cent in 10 mg. per 100 ml. This is the first report of a severe meningococcal meningitis epidemic in which Group A isolates were found to be sulfonamide-resistant.

The extreme variability of the meningococci and interest in its genetic competence prompted studies in antibiotic sensitivity long before the appearance of sulfonamide-resistant strains. The most complete surveys were carried out by Love and Finland,[30] and more recently by Eickoff and Finland.[10] A

TABLE 2.    *Susceptibility of Meningococci to Antibiotics*

| | 1954 STUDY* | | 1965 STUDY† | |
| Drug | MIC‡ | Range | MIC | Range |
|---|---|---|---|---|
| Penicillin | 0.02 | 0.004–0.2 | 0.06 | 0.01–1.8 |
| Ampicillin | — | — | 0.20 | 0.05–0.4 |
| Erythromycin | 0.2 | 0.04–3.1 | 0.4 | 0.1–1.4 |
| Novobiocin | — | — | 0.3 | 0.02–1.4 |
| Tetracycline | 1.6 | 0.4–6.3 | 0.5 | 0.2–1.5 |
| Oxytetracycline | 1.6 | 0.4–3.1 | — | — |
| Chloramphenicol | 3.1 | 0.8–6.3 | 0.7 | 0.2–1.5 |
| Cephalothin | — | — | 1.0 | 0.4–3.0 |
| Cloxacillin | — | — | 2.0 | 0.4–12.5 |
| Nafcillin | — | — | 5.0 | 0.8–12.5 |
| Carbomycin | 6.3 | 0.8–25.0 | — | — |
| Streptomycin | 6.3 | 1.6–25.0 | 15.0 | 6.3–40.0 |
| Neomycin | 6.3 | 1.6–12.5 | — | — |
| Gentamicin | — | — | 10 | 3.1–20.0 |
| Kanamycin | — | — | 13.0 | 3.1–20.0 |
| Polymyxin B | 50.0 | 25.0–200.0 | >100 | 25.0–>100 |
| Bacitracin | 100.0 | 1.6–200.0 | 30 | 12.5–100 |
| Vancomycin | — | — | >100 | 50–>100 |
| Sulfadiazine | 1.6 | 0.4–200.0 | 0.16 | 0.04–>40 |

* These strains included 3 GrA, 22 GrB, 12 GrC, and 13 untypables.[30]
† These strains included 55 GrB and 1 GrC. They were isolated December, 1963, to May, 1964.[10]
‡ Minimal inhibitory concentration.

TABLE 3.    *Newer Antibiotics Effective Against* Neisseria meningitidis

| ANTIBIOTIC | MIC* μg./ml. | REMARKS | REFERENCE |
|---|---|---|---|
| Cephaloglycin | 1.25 | Unstable. Only 12 hr. incubation valid | 48 |
| Cephaloridine | 1.25 | Stable | 48 |
| Nalidixic Acid | 5.0 | All of 167 strains | 13 |
| Hydroxynalidixic acid | 0.5 | All of 27 strains | 13 |
| Spectinomycin | 20–25.0 | 19 of 27 strains | 32 |

* Determined on agar medium of the Mueller-Hinton type; MIC = minimal inhibitory concentration.

summary of these results is shown in Table 2. These data show no appreciable difference in the strains isolated at the two time periods. Searches have been made for other antibiotics with the hope that active nontoxic drugs would be found for use in those cases in which strains resistant to sulfadiazine or penicillin are encountered or in which hypersensitivity of the patient to the drug is a factor.[13] McCarthy et al.[34] studied the susceptibility of eight types of penicillin on *N. meningitidis* and *N. gonorrhoeae* and found that, with the exception of penicillin G, phenylmercaptomethyl penicillin was the most active. It had a mean minimal inhibitory concentration of 5.3 times that of benzyl penicillin (penicillin G). Since both these penicillins are sensitive to penicillinase, they would not be effective for mixed infections in which one of the bacteria was resistant. Penicillins of the phenoxymethyl and phenoxyethyl series and dimethoxyphenyl penicillin, which are insensitive to penicillinase, were only slightly less active than the phenylmercaptomethyl penicillin. Other antibiotics which were found inhibitory to *N. meningitidis* are shown in Table 3.

Ivler et al.,[20] working with 70 strains isolated from cases of meningococcic meningitis, showed that the strains resistant to 10 mg. per ml. of sulfadiazine elaborated 2.5 times as much PABA as sensitive strains during 24 hour incubation.

In the laboratory, resistance to streptomycin and penicillin has been developed in *N. meningitidis* and *N. gonorrhoeae*.[36, 37] Resistance to streptomycin was very much easier to develop than resistance to penicillin. Since penicillin continues to be the mainstay in the treatment of both types of infection, this work can serve to warn us that penicillin resistance of both Neisseria species is possible and may develop at any time when the disease is seen.

In a study of changes in sensitivity of gonococci to penicillin, it was pointed out that whereas in 1955 practically all strains were susceptible to 0.03 $\mu$g. per ml. of penicillin G, by 1962 in some areas of the United States 60 per cent of the routine isolations required from 0.06 to 0.36 $\mu$g per ml. to suppress growth. This led Thayer and Axnick[42] to define arbitrarily a resistant strain as one which will grow in 0.06 $\mu$g. per ml. or higher concentration of penicillin. The susceptibilities of 52 gonococcal isolates to 10 penicillins are shown

TABLE 4. *Susceptibilities of 52 Gonococcal Strains to Ten Penicillins*

| | MINIMAL INHIBITORY CONCENTRATION $\mu$g./ml. | |
| --- | --- | --- |
| | *Median* | *Range* |
| Penicillin G | 0.18 | 0.003–0.39 |
| Ampicillin | 0.15 | 0.009–0.62 |
| Penicillin O | 0.37 | 0.005–1.48 |
| Phenoxymethyl penicillin | 1.25 | 0.049–6.54 |
| Phenoxyethyl penicillin | 1.25 | 0.037–10.0 |
| Synnematin B | 1.29 | 0.16 –3.22 |
| Dimethoxyphenyl penicillin | 2.50 | 0.18 –10.0 |
| Oxacillin (P-12) | 5.0 | 0.075–20.0 |
| Nafcillin (Wy-3277) | 5.0 | 0.15 –40.0 |
| SKF 12141-Z | 10.0 | 0.037–40.0 |

TABLE 5. *Susceptibility of Neisseria gonorrhoeae* to Antibiotics*

| ANTIBIOTIC | MIC[†] $\mu$g./ml. | MIC RANGE $\mu$g./ml. |
| --- | --- | --- |
| Penicillin | 0.24 | 0.003 to 1.0 |
| Cephalothin (Keflin) | 2.0 | 0.1 to 24.0 |
| Cephaloridine | 10.0 | 0.32 to 16.0 |
| Nalidixic acid | 1.0 | 0.5 to 1.0 |
| Hydroxynalidixic acid | 1.5 | 0.5 to 2.5 |
| Gentamicin | 4.0 | 1.5 to 6.0 |
| Vancomycin | 40.0 | 10 to 40 |
| Colistimethate | Not done | 20[‡] |

* Forty-nine strains isolated from cases which were not cured by penicillin.
† Minimal inhibitory concentration, midpoint value on the susceptibility curve of the 49 strains.
‡ Fewer than half the strains were inhibited at this level.

in Table 4. Of the drugs examined, penicillin G and ampicillin were more active than the others. Penicillin O was almost as effective, but it had a wider range of inhibition. There was no evidence that any of the other penicillins were any more active than penicillin G against resistant strains of gonococci.

Martin et al.[32a] studied 49 strains of *N. gonorrhoeae* from penicillin treatment failures. These strains showed susceptibilities to eight antimicrobial agents as listed in Table 5. Studies of this nature are important because of the three factors concerning present treatment of gonorrhea:

1. Some patients are hypersensitive to penicillin.

2. The drug should be injectable in a single dose because of the factor of patient reliability.

3. The effectiveness of penicillin in treatment of these infections has been seriously reduced by emergence of resistant strains of gonococci.

In a comparison of the susceptibilities of penicillin-sensitive and penicillin-resistant strains of gonococci, Martin et al.[32] reported the following results:

| Antibiotic | 21 Penicillin-Sensitive Strains | | 53 Penicillin-Resistant Strains | |
| --- | --- | --- | --- | --- |
| | MIC* | MIC† RANGE | MIC | MIC RANGE |
| Penicillin G | 0.015 | 0.003–0.03 | 0.23 | 0.06–0.91 |
| Spectinomycin | 10.5 | 10–12.5 | 11.7 | 10–12.5 |
| Lincomycin | 18.5 | 10–30.0 | 30.5 | 15–40.0 |

* In units per ml. or μg. per ml.; midpoint of MIC (minimal inhibitory concentration) curve for the series of strains.

† Extremes in units per ml. or μg. per ml. in MIC curve for the series of strains.

These data illustrate the difference in *in vitro* sensitivity to penicillin of strains which are classed as sensitive and as resistant. This slight difference may explain why increases in treatment dosages brought about cures when doses of lesser magnitude did not.

Thayer and Martin[41] utilized the resistance of *N. meningitidis* and *N. gonorrhoeae* to certain antibiotics for preparation of a selective medium for isolation of the bacteria from human tissues. With a chocolate agar containing, per milliliter, 3 units vancomycin, 7.5 μg. colistimethate, and 12.5 units nystatin, a medium has been prepared which permits rapid isolation and identification of both species of Neisseria.

## PATHOGENESIS

Meningococci are strict parasites of man and gain entry into the human body via the nasopharynx. The organisms may be isolated from the nasopharynx, tonsils, anterior superior nares, and sputum in that order of decreasing frequency. The mechanisms of initial implantation and growth on the oral cavity mucous membranes are unknown, but are most probably influenced by the various known bactericidal substances present in saliva.[47] Occasionally, a local inflammatory reaction occurs and a mild pharyngitis with catarrh may be a predisposing factor to movement of the meningococcus across the mucous membrane into the vascular system. There is apparently no relationship between the incidence of upper respiratory viral infections and either carrier or case rate.

Once the microorganisms enter the blood, bacteremia develops in those rare, susceptible individuals who become patients of this disease. The person who is susceptible may be the one whose phagocytes cannot handle the invading microorganisms at this crucial period. Since cases of meningococcal disease are rare when compared to the number of carriers, the very high immunity that man has to infection may be related not only to the antiphagocytic antibody, but also to the potent bactericidal antibody previously described for this microorganism.[19] There have been approximately 3000 cases per year of meningococcal meningitis in the United States for the last few years. This low incidence of disease has precluded any definitive studies on the incubation period of meningococcal disease in the infected carrier and on the subclinical immunogenic stimulus for protective antibody in the infected carrier.

The clinical symptoms of meningococcemia are acute sepsis, fever, chills, malaise, and prostration. The typical rash appears early in the disease and consists of petechial or maculopapular lesions (up to 15 mm. in size) which involve the skin and mucous membranes. The petechiae may progress to actual necrosis or in mild cases may disappear within a few days. The bacteria can readily be isolated from the petechiae by inoculation into prewarmed blood-broth. Bacteremia plays a major role in the case mortality of this disease, as shown in a study of 300 fatal cases in which it was noted that meningococcemia with or without adrenal hemorrhage accounted for over half the cases.[9] Chronic meningococcemia is rare, but has been described in approximately 150 cases.[3] The clinical picture consisted of episodes of severe fever and chills, petechical rashes of two to three days' duration, and arthralgia or true arthritis. A consistent finding was headache and loss of weight, usually associated with anorexia.

Once the bacteria are distributed throughout the body, metastatic lesions may appear in various sites such as the joints, ears, lungs, adrenal glands, and, most important of all, the central nervous system. Invasion of the central nervous system is marked by inflammation and irritation of the meninges. Experimental evidence is lacking as to the mechanism in which microorganisms reach the meninges via the blood.[18] The symptoms associated with meningitis are muscular spasms, stiff neck, positive Kernig and Brudzinski signs, and convulsions and bulging of the fontanelles in infants.

The role of endotoxin in the pathology of both gonococcal and meningococcal disease is still unresolved. The hemorrhagic manifestations common to this disease suggest the Shwartzman phenomenon. The "Waterhouse-Friderichsen syndrome" has been implicated in meningococcal disease and is characterized by widespread vascular dysfunction, causing shock by the pooling of peripheral blood. Studies with meningococcal endotoxin in rabbits and experimental meningitis in rabbits, guinea pigs, and monkeys suggest the importance of this toxin in the pathogenesis of this disease, but do not rule out other toxic materials described with this organism.

TABLE 6.   *Antimeningococcus Vaccination in Africa to the South of the Sahara**

| | | | VACCINE PREPARATION | | |
| YEAR | PLACE | *Type Org.* | *Treatment* | *Dosage* | RESULTS |
|---|---|---|---|---|---|
| 1915 | Sudan | Unknown | Unknown | Unknown | Unknown |
| 1930 | Sudan | 5 GRP IV | Heat-phenol | $5 \times 10^8$ | No evidence |
| 1931 | Sudan | 9 GRP B | Heat autolysis | $2 \times 10^9$ | Questionable |
| 1934 | Congo | 25 GRP A | Heat-phenol | $6 \times 10^8$ | Questionable |
| 1936–40 | AEF† | 8 GRP A | Heat | $5 \times 10^9$ | Very good |
| 1937 | Niger | 5 GRP A | Autolysed | $5 \times 10^8$ | Good |
| 1938 | AOF‡ | 5 GRP A | Autolysed | $5 \times 10^8$ | Questionable |
| 1940–42 | Cameroun | 8 GRP A | Heat | $5 \times 10^9$ | Questionable |
| 1946 | AOF | 8 GRP A | Heat | $5 \times 10^9$ | Questionable |
| 1946–47 | AEF | 8 GRP A | Heat | $5 \times 10^9$ | Questionable |
| 1950 | Chad | 8 GRP A | Heat | $5 \times 10^9$ | Questionable |

* Data from Lapeyssonnie, L. 1963. La méningite cérébro-spinale en Afrique. Bull. WHO (Suppl.) *28*:1–843.
   † French Equatorial Africa.
   ‡ French West Africa.

The degree of immunity following meningococcal infection is not known. Although they are rare, there are well documented cases of multiple attacks of meningitis in the same person.[44] The antibody response in patients is typical. The peak complement-fixing antibody titer is reached in two to three weeks and then declines. In one case, an individual suffered two episodes of meningitis. A Group B strain was isolated in each episode, but the nature of the antibody response indicated a subtle antigenic difference between the two otherwise indistinguishable isolates.[46]

Gonorrhea is characterized by its sudden onset following an incubation period of from one to 30 days (mean, three to five days). Symptoms include frequent, urgent, and painful urination, with profuse mucopurulent discharge. The organisms penetrate the stratified columnar cells of the male urethra and reach the subepithelial connective tissue in 72 to 96 hours. Leukocytes, mast cells, and lymphocytes accumulate in the region of Littre's glands and ducts and the lacunae of Morgagni. These cells, plus serum, form the yellow discharge characteristic for the disease. In the female, the cervical glands, Skene's glands, and Bartholin's glands are the sites of primary infection. The gonococci are also responsible for ophthalmia neonatorum and vulvovaginitis in the newborn and prepubescent female, respectively.

## PREVENTION

Effective control of clinical cases of meningococcal infection with sulfonamide compounds was clearly demonstrated during World War II. Although more deaths were due to meningococcal disease than to any other infectious agent,[9] widespread chemoprophylaxis probably prevented a much graver situation. Because of the appearance of sulfadiazine-resistant strains, the ineffectiveness of gamma globulin and other drugs, and the limited success of environmental control, serious attempts are being made to develop a suitable vaccine. Although data are scanty, numerous vaccine trials in Africa over the last 30 years have been unsuccessful (Table 6).[25] Greenberg and Cooper[17] have recently prepared a lysed cell vaccine composed of numerous strains indigenous to Africa. It is hoped that field trials with this preparation will be successful.

# References

1. Alexander, C. E., W. R. Sanborn, G. Cherriere, W. H. Crocker, Jr., P. E. Ewald, and C. R. Kay. 1968. Sulfadiazine-resistant group A *Neisseria meningitidis*. Science *161:* 1019.
2. Alexander, H. E., and W. Redman. 1953. Transformation of type specificity of meningococci. Change in heritable type induced by type-specific extracts containing desoxyribonucleic acid. J. Exp. Med. *97:*797–806.
3. Bloom, D. S. 1965. Chronic meningococcemia. Calif. Med. *103:*87–90.
4. Branham, S. E. 1940. The meningococcus (*Neisseria intracellularis*). Bacteriol. Rev. *4:*59–96.
5. Branham, S. E. 1953. Serological relationships among meningococci. Bacteriol. Rev. *17:*175–188.
6. Bristow, W. M., P. F. D. Van Peenen, and R. Volk. 1965. Epidemic meningitis in naval recruits. Am. J. Public Health *55:*1039–1045.
7. Catlin, B. W. 1960. Interspecific transformation of *Neisseria* by culture slime containing deoxyribonucleate. Science *131:*608–610.
8. Catlin, B. W., and G. M. Schloer. 1962. A defined agar medium for genetic transformation of *Neisseria meningitidis*. J. Bacteriol. *83:*470–474.
9. Daniels, W. B. 1950. Cause of death in meningococcic infection. Am. J. Med., *8:*468–473.
10. Eickoff, T. C., and M. Finland. 1965. Changing susceptibility of meningococci to antimicrobial agents. New Eng. J. Med. *272:*395–398.
11. Farrell, D. G., and E. V. Dahl. 1966. Nasopharyngeal carriers of *Neisseria meningitidis*. J.A.M.A. *198:*1189–1192.
12. Feldman, H. A. 1966. Meningococcal disease, 1965. J.A.M.A. *196:*391–393.
13. Feldman, H. A., and C. Melnyk. 1965. *In vitro* susceptibility of sulfonamide-resistant meningococci to nalidixic and hydroxynalidixic acids. Antimicrobial Agents and Chemotherapy—1964, pp. 440–443.
14. Fiumara, N. J., H. M. Wise, and M. Mony. 1967. Gonorrheal pharyngitis. New Eng. J. Med. *276:*1248–1250.
15. Gauld, J. R., R. E. Nitz, D. H. Hunter, J. H. Rust, and R. L. Gauld. 1965. Epidemiology of meningococcal meningitis at Fort Ord. Am. J. Epidemiol. *82:*56–72.
16. Glover, J. A. 1918. "Spacing out" in prevention of military epidemics of cerebro-spinal fever. Brit. Med. J. *11:*509–512.
17. Greenberg, L., and M. Y. Cooper. 1965. A somatic antigen vaccine for the prevention of meningococcal cerebrospinal meningitis. Bull. WHO *33:*21–36.
18. Harter, D. H., and R. G. Petersdorf. 1960. A consideration of the pathogenesis of bacterial meningitis: Review of experimental and clinical studies. Yale J. Biol. Med. *32:*280–309.
19. Heist, G. D., S. Solis-Cohen, and M. Solis-Cohen. 1922. A study of the virulence of meningococci for man and of human susceptibility to meningococcic infection. J. Immunol. *7:*1–33.
20. Ivler, D., J. M. Leedom, L. D. Thrupp, P. F. Wehrle, B. Portnoy, and A. W. Mathies, Jr. 1965. Naturally occurring sulfadiazine-resistant meningococci. Antimicrobial Agents and Chemotherapy—1964, pp. 444–450.
21. Jyssum, K. 1965. Polarity of chromosome replication in *Neisseria meningitidis*. J. Bacteriol. *90:*1182–1187.
22. Jyssum, K., and S. Jyssum. 1965. Variation in density and transformation potential in deoxyribonucleic acid from *Neisseria meningitidis*. J. Bacteriol. *90:*1513–1519.
23. Jyssum, K., and S. Lie. 1965. Genetic factors determining competence in transformation of *Neisseria meningitidis*. I. A permanent loss of competence. Acta Pathol. Microbiol. Scand. *63:*306–316.
24. Kellogg, D. S., Jr., I. R. Cohen, L. C. Norins, A. L. Schroeter, and G. Reising. 1968. *Neisseria gonorrhoeae*. II. Colonial variation and pathogenicity during 35 months *in vitro*. J. Bacteriol. *96:*596–605.

25. Lapeyssonnie, L. 1963. La méningite cérébro-spinale en Afrique. Bull. WHO (Suppl.) 28:1–843.

26. Leedom, J. M., D. Ivler, A. M. Mathies, Jr., L. D. Thrupp, J. C. Fremont, P. F. Wehrle, and B. Portnoy. 1967. The problem of sulfadiazine-resistant meningococci. Antimicrobial Agents and Chemotherapy—1966, pp. 281–292.

27. Lie, S. 1965. On the effect of penicillin in the production of auxotrophic mutants of *Neisseria meningitidis*. Acta Pathol. Microbiol. Scand. 63:609–614.

28. Lie, S. 1965. Production of recombinants in mixed cultures of *Neisseria meningitidis*. Acta Pathol. Microbiol. Scand. 64:130–139.

29. Lie, S. 1965. Studies on the phenotypic expression of competence in *Neisseria meningitidis*. Acta Pathol. Microbiol. Scand. 64:119–129.

30. Love, B. D., Jr., and M. Finland. 1954. *In vitro* susceptibility of meningococci to eleven antibiotics and sulfadiazine. Am. J. Med. Sci. 228:534–539.

31. Lucas, J. B., E. V. Price, J. D. Thayer, and A. Schroeter. 1967. Gonorrhea in the female, diagnosis and treatment. New Eng. J. Med. 276:1454–1459.

32. Martin, J. E., Jr., S. B. Samuels, W. L. Peacock, Jr., and J. D. Thayer. 1965. *Neisseria gonorrhoeae* and *Neisseria meningitidis* sensitivity to spectinomycin, lincomycin, and penicillin G. Antimicrobial Agents and Chemotherapy—1964, pp. 437–439.

32a. Martin, J. E., Jr., J. D. Thayer, S. B. Samuels, and J. B. Lucas. 1966. *In vitro* antimicrobial susceptibility of *Neisseria gonorrhoeae* from penicillin treatment failures. Antimicrobial Agents and Chemotherapy—1965, pp. 366–368.

33. Maxcy, K. F. 1937. The relationship of meningococcus carriers to the incidence of cerebrospinal fever. Am. J. Med. Sci. 193:438–445.

34. McCarthy, C. G., G. Wallmark, and M. Finland. 1961. *In vitro* activity of various penicillins. Am. J. Med. Sci. 241:143–159.

35. Millar, J. W., E. E. Siess, H. A. Feldman, C. Silverman, and P. Frank. 1963. *In vivo* and *in vitro* resistance to sulfadiazine in strains of *Neisseria meningitidis*. J.A.M.A. 186:139–141.

36. Miller, C. P., and M. Bohnhoff. 1947. Studies on the action of penicillin. VI. Further observations on the development of penicillin resistance by meningococcus *in vitro*. J. Infect. Dis. 81:147–156.

37. Mills, F. 1949. The exponential development of penicillin resistance by *Neisseria*. J. Infect. Dis. 85:1–4.

38. Murray, E. G. D. 1929. The Meningococcus. H. M. Stationary Office, London, England.

39. Sanborn, W. R., and N. A. Vedros. 1966. Possibilities of application of complement fixation, indirect hemagglutination, and fluorescent antibody tests to epidemiology of meningococcal infection. Health Lab. Sci. 3:111–117.

40. Slaterus, K. W., C. Ruys, and I. G. Sieberg. 1963. Types of meningococci isolated from carriers and patients in nonepidemic period in the Netherlands. Antonie van Leeuwenhoek J. Microbiol. Serol. 29:265–271.

41. Thayer, J. D., and J. E. Martin. 1966. Improved medium selective for cultivation of *N. gonorrhoeae* and *N. meningitidis*. U. S. Public Health Repts. 81:559–562.

42. Thayer, J. D., and N. W. Axnick. 1964. Susceptibility of gonococci to ten penicillins. Antimicrobial Agents and Chemotherapy—1963, pp. 427–429.

43. Tomasz, A., and R. D. Hotchkiss. 1964. Regulation of the transformability of pneumococcal cultures by macromolecular cell products. Proc. Nat. Acad. Sci. U.S. 51:480–487.

44. Van Peenen, P. F. D. 1965. Second attacks of meningococcal meningitis. Calif. Med. 103:132–134.

45. Vedros, N. A., J. Ng, and G. Culver, 1968. A new serological group (E) of *Neisseria meningitidis*. J. Bacteriol. 95:1300–1304.

46. Vedros, N. A., D. H. Hunter, and J. H. Rust. 1966. Studies on immunity in meningococcal meningitis. Military Med. 131:1413–1417.

47. Vedros, N. A., P. J. Robinson, and R. A. Gutekunst. 1966. Isolation and characterization of a bacterial inhibitor from human throat washings. Proc. Soc. Exp. Biol. Med. 122:249–253.

48. Wick, W. E., and W. S. Boniece. 1965. *In vitro* and *in vivo* laboratory evaluation of cephaloglycin and cephaloridine. Appl. Microbiol. 13:248–253.

# Chapter 13

# CHOLERA

ABRAM S. BENENSON

*The Jefferson Medical College of*
*Philadelphia, Philadelphia, Pennsylvania*

Cholera is one of the most catastrophic of the diseases to which the human is subject. An individual in perfect health is stricken and can be dead within as few as four hours. "To see individuals well in the morning & buried before night, retiring apparently well & dead in the morning is something which is appalling to the boldest heart."[66] It is dramatic when an individual suddenly develops diarrhea so profuse that he literally pours forth his body fluids until be becomes unconscious and dies; but when this happens to an appreciable proportion of the population almost simultaneously, it is not surprising that the uneducated should consider this a divine manifestation, undoubtedly in retribution for the sins of the profane. The heavy devastations wrought by the disease among the intemperate, among the prostitutes, and among the poor lent credence to this belief. Indeed the Governor of New York in 1832 stated, "An infinitely wise and just God has seen fit to employ pestilence as one means of scourging the human race for their sins, and it seems to be an appropriate one for the sins of uncleanliness and intemperance."[67] When reputable citizens and clergymen themselves came down with the disease, it was assumed that there were vices hidden from man but clear to God, for which just punishment was being exacted.

Six times cholera has emerged from its heartland in Bengal, spreading over the western world in pandemic waves lingering for five to 20 years. It crossed the Atlantic, causing epidemic disease in the United States in 1832 to 1835, 1848 to 1850, 1854, 1865 to 1867, and 1873.[60, 64] Each pandemic left behind overfilled cemeteries and decimated families. No other disease could, with such startling rapidity, wreak the havoc of cholera.

> Cholera first appeared at Newburn on the 4th of January, 1832, and, more severely, on the 10th. Then on the 15th there was another of the sudden outbursts so typical of the disease, fifty people—almost one in ten of the whole population—being attacked between nightfall and noon next day. By the end of the epidemic on the 2nd February 274 cases had

occurred—one person in every two in the population—and there had been sixty-five deaths, nearly one person in every eight; a rate of mortality paralleled nowhere else and one that was not to be explained till many years later.[48]

Little wonder that the word "cholera" became, among some social groups, one of the more terrible of curse words!

During the twentieth century the cholera situation has been much more favorable. The sixth pandemic lingered in Eastern Europe and Russia until 1923, but on the whole the disease remained in its normal locus in the delta of the Ganges and Brahmaputra. In 1947, a sharp outbreak occurred in Egypt. In 1958 and 1959, an outbreak in Bangkok led to the establishment of the SEATO-Cholera Research program which set up a research laboratory, first in Bangkok and then, when cholera disappeared from Thailand, in Dacca, East Pakistan. International interest in cholera was developed, and the World Health Organization became actively involved. Funds became available for research, resulting in the mounting of several investigational programs by Thai, Pakistani, Indian, Philippine, Japanese, British, Australian, and American investigators.

A localized focus of cholera had been known for many years on the island of Celebes in the East Indies; here the disease was caused by an organism whose biological characteristics were in some respects different (it is polymyxin resistant, resistant to Mukerjee phage IV, chicken cell agglutinating, and hemolytic) from those of the classical *Vibrio cholerae* traditionally associated with the epidemic disease. This was the so-called El Tor strain, which, although not considered of epidemic potential, spread out of this area in 1961 to invade Hong Kong, the Philippine Islands, Taiwan, Korea, South Viet Nam, and Thailand; in 1964, it extended into India and displaced the classical organism; it spread across West Pakistan, Afghanistan, and Iran in 1965, and into Iraq and the adjacent areas of Russia in 1966. This has been called the seventh pandemic. In 1967, however, instead of spreading, the incidence of cholera was reduced, the borders constricted. In 1968, a low number of cases have been reported, disease occurring principally in Pakistan and in India, with very few cases reported from Nepal, Thailand, Cambodia, Viet Nam, Malaysia, Singapore, and the Philippines. The disease in West Pakistan this time has been caused by the classical biotype of *V. cholerae*.

The popular reaction to the seventh pandemic was in sharp contrast to that to earlier waves. Its geographical progress was watched with concern but no panic. The scientists working with the disease had achieved such success and confidence in the management of the clinical disease that it could be discussed and described as an "experiment of nature."[25] However, serious logistical problems remain in providing the necessary materials and, more important, in conveying to the practitioners the proper techniques. Because of this, concern was often extreme among responsible officials of some developing countries, and restrictive (and ineffectual) measures were sometimes taken which had serious impact on the economy of the country.

But, as an experiment of nature, cholera continues to provide most fascinating and enigmatic interrelations between host and parasite.

# WHAT IS CHOLERA?

First, just what is "cholera"? Purists and some dictionaries would define it as a severe dehydrating diarrhea.[54] The cases were differentiated into epidemic or "Asiatic cholera" and the sporadic "cholera nostras." In 1883 Koch demonstrated the association of *V. cholerae* with cases of Asiatic cholera, and since then many have defined "cholera" as a severe diarrhea caused by *V. cholerae*.[15] A problem arises in deciding when a diarrhea is "severe"; some consider as "cholera" any clinical diarrhea associated with *V. cholerae*, and some report as cholera any infection with this organism, symptomatic or not, since it might have serious implications.

After the vibrio was identified as the etiological agent, cases of dehydrating diarrhea which occurred in "cholera" countries were always assumed to be caused by this organism. When bacteriological cultures were made, usually only in research laboratories, the causative vibrio was recovered in only 50 to 80 per cent of cholera cases. In Delhi during the outbreak in 1965 to 1966, *V. cholerae* was isolated from only 22.9 per cent of patients admitted to the Infectious Disease Hospital as suspected cholera cases.[59] Extensive bacteriological, serological, and epidemiological studies carried out in the Dacca laboratory,[48] and confirmed in Calcutta,[9] have shown that severe dehydrating diarrhea frequently occurs in the absence of vibrios. These cases differ in several ways from those that are associated with vibrios. Cases associated with *V. cholerae* usually occurred as focal outbreaks, not infrequently with several members of the family stricken within a very few days of each other. In the Dacca area the incidence was greatest among children and the epidemic peak occurred in December and January. Cases without vibrios, "nonvibrio cholera," on the other hand, occurred as isolated cases and no association of cases with each other could be established. These patients were predominantly adult (over 12 years of age), and epidemic peaks occurred in March and April. Clinically, the two diseases are usually indistinguishable on admission of the patients; hemoconcentration is as severe whether vibrios are present or not. Only after therapy is initiated does the difference become clear; the patient whose disease is associated with vibrios may continue to purge for five or six days, whereas when vibrios are absent, purging stops in a day or two after rehydration. When the stool is red-brown or pinkish in color, *V. cholerae* are most unlikely to be present. As yet, no bacterium or virus has been associated with this clinical state, even though resemblances to staphylococcal enterotoxin poisoning are noted; nonvibrio cholera is lethal, and grouping of cases with a common food item has not been seen. This might be the "cholera nostras" of the last century, a disease no longer seen in well developed areas, but constituting a greater total problem than the vibrio as a cause of disease, except in epidemic cholera years. In addition, noncholera vibrios have been shown to be capable of producing severe dehydrating diarrhea resembling cholera.[52] Thus, factors evoking the physiological changes which result in the clinical syndrome of severe dehydrating diarrhea are not restricted to *V. cholerae*.

After 85 years of study of the *V. cholerae* we still do not know how disease is produced. Since the days of John Snow and William Budd, it has been generally accepted that an organism must be ingested, and that infection ensues.

This infection causes a diarrhea so intense that a patient may pass as much as 50 per cent of his body weight per rectum in a 24 hour period and, over the course of his illness, require the infusion of several times his body weight to match the output of rice water stools. These stools are rich in bicarbonate (45 mEq./l.) and potassium ion (15 mEq./l.).[75] Vomiting often occurs, intensifying the condition. Purging continues until the patient goes into shock; 60 per cent or more die if not treated.

## WHAT CAUSES THE FLUID LOSS?

Vibrios are found within the lumen of the intestinal tract, from one end to the other; they lie close to but do not penetrate the mucosa.[41] They are present in the same density in the upper as in the lower gastrointestinal tract. But the presence of vibrios in the upper and lower reaches of the gut, with no symptoms, and the ability to produce disease with cell-free material in several animal models, argue against fluid loss as a direct effect of the presence of bacteria. The search naturally turns to the question of toxins. The heat-stable nondialyzable O-antigen (lipopolysaccharide) does not elicit fluid accumulation in any test system.[43] Huber and Phillips demonstrated that the cholera stool and culture filtrates of cholera vibrios contained a heat-stable dialyzable factor which prevented the active transport of sodium ions across short-circuited frog skin, i.e., inhibition of the sodium pump.[62] On a theoretical basis, if sodium is not absorbed it will draw fluid into the lumen to maintain isotonicity. This factor would offer a rational explanation for fluid loss.

However, Finkelstein isolated a nondialyzable heat-labile factor (choleragen) which produces severe diarrhea when placed in the small intestine of rabbits less than 16 days of age in which the sodium pump inhibiting factor was ineffective.[17] The choleragen elaborated by an El Tor Ogawa vibrio is serologically identical to that produced *in vitro* by a classical Inaba vibrio.[18] Benyajati[7] reported that choleragen caused severe diarrhea in a human volunteer to whom it was administered, and it also produced fluid outpouring in the dog.[10] Burrows and his coworkers have shown, using the infant rabbit and isolated ileal loops in the adult rabbit, that a thermolabile nondialyzable culture filtrate material produced diarrhea or ballooning of the loop, while the sodium pump inhibitory toxin did not produce fluid accumulation.[43] Craig[13] demonstrated the presence in cholera stool and culture filtrates of a factor which produces capillary permeability 24 hours after injection into guinea pig or rabbit skin; a similar permeability of the mucosal capillaries could result in increased plasma-to-lumen flow and the diarrhea could then be explained by increased exsorption rather than decreased insorption. It has not been possible to physically separate the skin permeability factor from the loop or infant rabbit factor, suggesting that these may be different methods of measuring one toxin. However, some preparations with a high skin activity have proved to be relatively poor in diarrhea-producing effect in the dog.

The demonstration in some organisms of "adherence factors"[3, 42] which enable the vibrios to adhere to red cells or mucosal cells offers an explanation for the heavy concentration of vibrios seen close to the mucosal surface. This propinquity may be a critical factor in developing disease, since the mucosal cell would then be exposed to the highest concentrations of the effective "toxin." This hypothesis finds support in Freter's finding[19] that small amounts of intraluminal anti-O serum prevent fluid accumulations without interfering with vibrio multiplication during the first four hour period; but the vibrios are predominantly free in the lumen of the intestine, whereas with normal serum they are concentrated on the mucosal surface.

The extrapolation from the animal model to the human is always fraught with hazard. At the moment the evidence would clearly incriminate the heat-labile nondialyzable toxin elaborated by the vibrio as the factor responsible for diarrhea production.

# WHAT IS THE MECHANISM OF FLUID PRODUCTION?

Even when the responsible bacterial factor is defined, this does not explain the mechanism of excess fluid production. Because of the denuded epithelia usually seen on autopsy of cholera patients, the fluid loss had been ascribed, since the days of Virchow, to an exposed submucosa; i.e., the intestine wept like burned skin. However, in 1959, Gangarosa, using the Crosby capsule to obtain biopsies from the living cholera patient, showed with his coworkers that the mucosa was intact, with only some edema and increased cellularity.[21] The protein content of the rice-water stool is very low;[62] Gordon[24] showed by the intravenous injection of $^{131}$I-tagged polyvinyl pyrrolidone that there was no increased leakage into the lumen of the gut, indicating that the mucosal barrier was intact. Thus the integrity of the mucosal barrier was established both anatomically and functionally.

Greenough has postulated that the excess fluid may arise from excess outpouring of fluid into the duodenum because of hypersecretion of secretin or secretin-like hormones.[29] Gordon has pointed out the effectiveness of gastrin and of secretin in increasing intestinal fluid, and the resemblance of the cholera diarrhea to that seen with noninsulin-secreting islet cell tumors of the pancreas.[25] Studies of changes in intestinal absorption[46] and of mucosal enzyme levels (adenosine triphosphatase)[38] have shown a decrease in activities as great in simple gastroenteritis as in cholera, and the degree of impairment did not correlate with the severity of diarrhea.

Pathophysiological studies are underway in several laboratories which promise to clarify this issue in the near future. In general, these suggest that there clearly is an increased plasma-to-lumen flow and relatively little fall, if any, in the lumen-to-plasma flow; i.e., the sodium pump inhibition plays little if any part in the phenomenon. Of great potential importance is the observation that glucose increases the movement of sodium from the lumen to plasma, carrying with it sufficient water to offer a method to control the diarrhea of the cholera patient.[50]

# EXTRAINTESTINAL PARTICIPATION IN DEVELOPMENT OF DISEASE

In the development of disease, however, in contrast with infection, more than the intestinal mucosa itself may be affected directly by the bacteria or its products or be involved. As indicated earlier, pancreatic and hepatic hypersecretion has been postulated as an important source of fluid production. The characteristic rice water stool of the cholera patient in the first few days of purging is devoid of bile pigment; later, still during purging, bile pigment is present. This has led to the assumption that the bile duct might be obstructed mechanically, either by edema or by spasm of the sphincter. However, patency of the ducts during this "acholic" period has been demonstrated by the recovery of a large fraction of intravenously injected sulfobromophthalein dye from the rice water stool.[11] Greig in 1913 reported the recovery of vibrios, usually in pure culture, from 30 per cent of 271 gallbladders removed from fatal cholera cases; the gallbladders were examined with great care to assure no surface contamination.[32] He noted "round the biliary passages and also between the columns of liver cells there is a well marked round-celled infiltration similar to that observed in the wall of the gallbladder";[34] we have also observed a mononuclear cell infiltration in the portal areas of fatal cholera cases.[14] Pollitzer[65] cites the controversy between those who claimed that the bile is infected by retrograde invasion up the biliary tree and those who felt that a transient bacteremia, perhaps restricted to the portal circulation, provides the route for infecting the liver. In our monkey studies,[37] vibrios were recovered from liver or bile of 43 per cent of monkeys who were sacrificed, with bacteriological samples taken while the animals were anesthetized, and in 39 per cent of monkeys who died naturally, indicating that, at least in this animal species, infection was not the consequence of an agonal or postmortem invasion. The liver parenchyma of 20 monkeys was cultured either at autopsy or by needle biopsy; *V. cholerae* were recovered from five, all within eight days of challenge. In four of these monkeys the bile duct had been ligated one to four weeks before challenge to prevent retrograde infection of the biliary tract; although not all monkeys developed deep jaundice, assurance that ligation had been complete, it is unlikely that the vibrios would have ascended the bile ducts in all these animals. Gangarosa et al.[23] reported the recovery of vibrios from a liver biopsy from a convalescent cholera patient. Despite the failure of careful studies to demonstrate penetration of the mucosa by vibrios,[16, 41] these observations suggest that a transient bacteremic phase, restricted to the portal circulation, may be involved in the development of clinical disease, and this direct insult to the liver may participate in inciting the characteristic outpouring of fluid. Even if it is not contributory to the disease, this phenomenon has great importance in the natural history of the disease.

# MANAGEMENT OF THE CLINICAL CASE

While we may not understand precisely what is responsible for the excessive outpouring of fluid in cholera and how this is effected, we have learned how to manage the clinical case. This disease is unique in that we are able to correct the systemic changes easily and rapidly; in this, as in very few other conditions, the physician can see the magic of his ministrations. A moribund, unconscious, pulseless patient at the door of death will, within the space of an hour, be sitting up in bed, fully conscious, alert, comfortable, and happy. Other than the continuing pouring of fluid into the lumen of his gastrointestinal tract, the patient enjoys good health (if one ignores the flow of diarrheal fluid out and intravenous replacement in).

Cholera has been treated unsuccessfully by a wide variety of drugs and procedures; success has been achieved by the rationale and methods recommended in 1831 by O'Shaughnessy, who was 22 years old at the time. He noted that the blood had lost a large proportion of its water and of its "neutral saline ingredients," and "of the free alkali contained in healthy serum, not a particle is present in some cholera cases and barely a trace in others."[57] For treatment, he proposed "first, to restore the blood to its natural water content; secondly, to restore its deficient saline matters."[58] To accomplish this, one could "inject into the veins a tepid water holding a solute of the normal salts of the blood." Latta actually performed intravenous injections in 1832. Unfortunately this mode of therapy was discarded with the other 101 recommended but useless treatments of the day, to be rediscovered in the early twentieth century by British workers in India and American workers in the Philippines.

Working in Egypt in 1947 and in Bangkok in 1958 and 1959, Phillips and his United States Navy coinvestigators quantitatively defined the extent of the changes in total fluids and electrolytes and demonstrated that the life of the cholera patient was saved by correcting these deficiencies.[63] Isotonic saline could replace the fluid loss and bring the patient out of shock, and the acidosis could be corrected with 500 ml. of 2 per cent sodium bicarbonate for each 4 liters of saline. After initial rehydration, homeostasis was maintained by infusing these solutions at a rate to match the measured stool volume; potassium deficiency was made up by mouth or by adding potassium chloride to the fluid after initial rehydration was completed.

This regimen worked excellently in Thailand, the Philippines, and Viet Nam, but physicians in Pakistan and India claimed that it would cause pulmonary edema in their patients. When the Pakistan-SEATO Cholera Research Laboratory began operations in Dacca, East Pakistan, this assertion was found to be correct. Severely dehydrated cholera patients sometimes were admitted in shock with râles in their lung bases; other times they would develop evidence of pulmonary edema after rehydration with saline was initiated. Was this evidence of vibrio toxins? Empirically, however, it was observed that the administration of alkali caused the signs of pulmonary edema to disappear. As a consequence, the therapy was modified so that correction of acidosis was carried out concurrently with rehydration, by using a single solution which incorporated the essential electrolytes in the concentrations present in the rice-water stool. A solution containing 5 grams of sodium chloride, 4 grams of sodium bicarbonate, and 1 gram of potassium chloride per liter provided 135 mEq./l. $Na^+$, 47.6 mEq./l. $HCO_3^-$, and 13.5 mEq./l. $K^+$ and 98.5 mEq./l. $Cl^-$, a close match to the cholera stool which contains 140 mEq./l. $Na^+$, 45 mEq./l. $HCO_3^-$, and 15 mEq./l. $K^+$ and 100 mEq./l. $Cl^-$.[30] When profound hyperventilation and râles were present, treatment was often started with infusion of isotonic sodium bicarbonate solution (12 grams/l.).[28]

When antibiotics became available they were tried in the treatment of cholera but had little if any effect in reducing the case fatality rate, even though the vibrios were sensitive to the drug, because the fluid and electrolyte aberrations were not corrected. However, the patient with severe cholera whose water and electrolyte levels have been corrected and are maintained at normal levels may continue to purge large volumes of stool containing $10^8$ to $10^9$ vibrios per milliter for five to six days. Since there is a relation between the volume of diarrhea and the number of vibrios passed per hour,[40] it would be logical then that an antibiotic which eliminates these vibrios would terminate the diarrhea. Studies in Dacca[28] and in Calcutta[8] have proved this to be true, and have established that antibiotic therapy is an important accessory to the rehydration therapy of cholera, shortening the period of intensive patient care. While an antibiotic can eliminate the etiological organism, it cannot correct the lethal shock and acidosis. Death from cholera is a secondary phenomenon; it is not the direct action of the organism or its products, but the resulting fluid and electrolyte disturbances which kill the patient.

With treatment directed from the first against the acidosis as well as the dehydration (largely with the 5-4-1 solution, the volume of fluid determined by clinical observation and measurement of stool volume), cholera has become an innocuous disease, and, when these measures are supplemented by tetracycline administration, easy to manage. Thus, among 769 consecutive cases treated in the hospital of the Pakistan-SEATO Cholera Laboratory in Dacca, there were only five deaths, a case fatality rate of 0.65 per cent; the case fatality rate (0.61 per cent) of children under ten years of age (including 268 children under five) was comparable to that of adults (see Table 1). In a rural hospital in the Matlab Bazar area with only rudimentary facilities, the case fatality rate was 0.81 per cent; the rate for those under ten was 0.75 per cent.[47]

These results were in sharp contrast to those obtained elsewhere with children; the essential difference in therapy was the inclusion of alkali in the initial rehydrating solution. While it might have been preferable to use hypotonic saline solutions for the rehydration of children,[35] these children, once rehydration was adequate to restore renal function, have been able to adjust physiologically. Fluids and water by mouth were permitted *ad lib*. In the light of this favorable experience, there is no justification for complicating the already tenuous logistics by specifying two multiple solutions, one for adults and a second for children.

TABLE 1.   *Mortality in Cholera Cases Treated by Pakistan-SEATO Cholera Research Laboratory Personnel**

| AGE GROUP | DACCA HOSPITAL | | | MATLAB TREATMENT CENTER | | |
|---|---|---|---|---|---|---|
| | *Cases* | *Deaths* | *C.F.R.*† | *Cases* | *Deaths* | *C.F.R.*† |
| 0–10 | 327 | 2 | 0.61% | 268 | 2 | 0.75% |
| >10 | 442 | 3 | 0.68% | 228 | 2 | 0.88% |
| Total | 769 | 5 | 0.65% | 496 | 4 | 0.81% |

* From Lindenbaum et al. 1966. Cholera in Children. Lancet *7*:1066–1068.
† Case fatality rate.

## STUDIES ON ACIDOSIS

The clinical evidence of pulmonary hypertension observed on admission of some cholera patients, and the complete disappearance of systemic abnormalities when normal fluid and electrolyte levels are restored, argued against any systemic "toxic" effect of cholera, and suggested that cholera might offer a relatively pure model for the study of acidosis, shedding light on the pathophysiology of clinical cholera. Acidosis is not an uncommon problem as a complication of diabetes and nephritis, and several research groups had been concerned with its effect on hemodynamics. To explore these questions, a team under Dr. Réjane Harvey came from the Cardiopulmonary Laboratories of the Columbia Medical Division of Bellevue Hospital, New York, to Dacca, where careful studies were performed on 23 hypotensive patients. These studies[36] showed that acidosis was associated with a redistribution of blood from the peripheral to the central circulation, probably by a peripheral vasoconstriction and a reduction of venous reservoirs. This provides an explanation for the sometimes perplexing paradox of the pulseless patient who continues to be clear mentally and able to carry on surprising degrees of activity and locomotion. This also explains the engorgement of the pulmonary bed, since added fluid disproportionately increases the central blood pool and the heart is literally overloaded. When this added fluid is isotonic saline, a bad situation is aggravated since purging continues to withdraw bicarbonate ion, and the blood pH could fall progressively to levels as low as 7.0, approximating lethal ranges.[27] However, when the rehydrating fluid contains base, as practiced in Dacca and by the Johns Hopkins group working at Calcutta, the blood pH rapidly returns toward normal and the correction of acidosis results in a more even distribution of the circulating blood volume, eliminating overload of the central circulation.

## HOST-PARASITE SYMBIOSIS

If it becomes infected, the biliary tract provides a safe haven for vibrios, permitting their persistence and constituting the reservoir of the disease. Persistent infection has been demonstrated for at least four years in a convalescent patient in the Philippines,[2] who exhibits the paradox of negative stools but positive duodenal aspirates. In Iran, a similar phenomenon was observed in eight of 38 convalescent patients; a saline purge was positive for vibrios but rectal swabs were consistently free of vibrios.[22] In Calcutta, 43 convalescent cholera patients were studied during convalescence or after recovery; vibrios were isolated from two whose routine stool cultures were negative.[74] In Dacca, the phenomenon of vibrio isolation from the bile or small intestine while the rectum or colon was free of vibrios was seen not infrequently in monkeys,[37] but was observed in only one patient. Her daily rectal swabs were positive for classical Inaba *V. cholerae* for eight days, and then became negative. Cholera vibrios were grown from a gastric aspirate taken on the nineteenth day after onset of diarrhea, and the rectal swabs were positive from the twenty-first to twenty-fourth days, again from the thirty-first to thirty-seventh days, and on the forty-first and forty-second days. A duodenal aspirate on the forty-second day was negative—cholecystokinin was not used. On the forty-fourth day after onset of illness, the patient decided that enough studies had been done and departed.

The greater frequency of this finding among Philippine, Iranian, and Calcutta cases has been attributed to the differences in the infecting organism, since these cases were caused by the El Tor biotype while the classical organism has been the cause of cholera in Dacca. However, it seems more logical to consider the carrier state in cholera analogous to that in typhoid fever; i.e., it is established more frequently when the acute disease occurs in one who has some preexisting inflammation or scarring in the gallbladder; it is more frequent the older the typhoid patient.[1] Serological surveys[53] indicate that the initial vibrio infection in the Dacca area occurs in children and, when adult disease occurs, it usually does so in one who already has a basic immunity. On the other hand, in the Philippines and in Iran, nonendemic areas, adults were experiencing their initial infections; there is reason to believe that the level of endemicity in Calcutta is not as high as in the Dacca area. One can postulate that immunity from prior exposure prevents invasion of the biliary tract (an argument for a portal bacteremia); therefore, in hyperendemic areas, this bacteremia occurs only in children whose biliary tracts are still clean. On the other hand, where a broad base of immunity does not exist, the likelihood of cholelithiasis or chronic disease at the time of initial vibrio infection is great (the two positive cases reported by Wallace were in patients 72 and 65 years old; our Dacca case was in a 50 year old housewife), so that if invasion by vibrios occurs, the gallbladder offers a nutritious sheltered locus where the organisms can survive through interepidemic periods. The environment in the cecum and colon is inimical to the survival of the vibrios, possibly because of the high fatty acid content, so that they are killed in transit and the stools are negative. However, a rapid intestinal flow due to enteric infection or dietary indiscretions may cause emergence of viable vibrios capable of initiating a chain of infection which can culminate in an outbreak of disease.

It must be noted that while the carrier state provides a reservoir for the survival of *V. cholerae*, it is relatively ineffective for the transmission of disease. The patient who passes liter after liter of fluid containing $10^9$ vibrios per milliliter is, by many orders of magnitude, a better contaminator of food, water, and fomites, than the person whose formed stool may contain $10^3$ to $10^5$ vibrios per gram. The assumption that the carrier does not transmit disease, however, is untenable.[33, 76]

## INFECTION OR DISEASE?

One of the more fascinating aspects of cholera is the fact that infection with *V. cholerae*, as with other organisms, does not necessarily result in clinical disease. Approximately 20 per cent of the household contacts of cholera patients were found by rectal swabbing to be infected,[56] but less than half of these developed diarrheal disease. In approximately half of these patients the disease produced was a simple diarrhea which did not particularly inconvenience the patient, and recovery occurred without hospitalization and without treatment. Despite the absence or paucity of symptoms, these individuals develop antibody responses comparable to those seen after fullblown disease, indicating that these are truly infections.[5] Prospective studies by MacCormack et al. suggest that there may be 100 to 1000 infections for every case of clinical cholera.[26]

Variations in clinical response can be attributed to differences in: (1) the "virulence" of the organism; (2) host factors (other than immunity); (3) the dose of organisms ingested; (4) the metabolic state of the organisms or their substrate; and (5) immunity.

## Differences in Virulence of the Organism

Variations in "epidemic potential," in the severity of the diarrhea, or in case fatality rates from year to year, or at the beginning and end of an outbreak, or from place to place, have been frequently noted.[51] These changes have been attributed, at least in part, to changes in the "virulence" of the organism. Thus, the El Tor vibrio has been considered to be of low virulence because the clinical disease due to this strain in the Philippines and Viet Nam was milder than that seen in India and Pakistan where the classical vibrio was the etiological organism; i.e., purging was less in volume and shorter in duration. However, when the El Tor strain invaded India in 1964, and coexisted with the classical strain, it was possible to compare the clinical characteristics of infections with these different biotypes in the same population groups. No significant differences in amount and duration of purging, or in clinical or laboratory findings, could be established.[73] No evidence has yet been presented indicating significant immunological differences between El Tor and classical strains of *V. cholerae*.

## Differences in Host Factors

A more attractive hypothesis would involve variations in host factors, nonspecific as well as specific immunity (which will be discussed later). Variations in susceptibility are evident even when cholera is introduced into a population for the first time. In 1832, Dr. Henry Gaulter investigated 200 cholera cases and could establish contact with a known cholera case in only 26; clearly exposure was to mild or asymptomatic cases in many if not most instances.[49] Perhaps of even more direct import is the difference in the relative mildness of the disease in children as compared to adults in the same outbreak.[6] Marked nutritional, cultural, and ethnic differences exist between the people of the Philippines and Viet Nam on the one hand, and those of India and Pakistan on the other, which offer more likely explanations for the difference in severity of disease than vibrio strain differences.

Cholera has always been recognized as predominantly a disease of the poor. Claims by moralists that cholera is the consequence of alcoholic debauchery or merely of indulgence* are hardly tenable since the disease is hyperendemic in a

---

* Even Snow[71] explained the difference in the progress of the disease in England and Scotland on the basis that the English do not drink unboiled water except in warm weather, while "in Scotland, on the other hand, unboiled water is somewhat freely used at all times to mix with spirits; I am told that when two or three people enter a tavern in Scotland and ask for a gill of whisky, a jug of water and tumbler glasses are brought in with it."

nondrinking Moslem population. This then directs attention to nutritional or other deficiencies as the significant predisposing factor. However, no specific nutritional factor has yet been incriminated. In studies carried out in East Pakistan, there was no evidence of deficiency in thiamine nutrition; Vitamin B-12 levels were normal in almost all patients; most cholera patients had normal sodium folate levels and the frequency of subnormal levels was less than in a group of patients with nonspecific acute diarrheal disease. Serum ascorbic acid levels varied widely, but mean values did not differ significantly from those of patients who did not have cholera or from values of the general population.[68] The epithelial changes noted in biopsies of Thai cholera patients[21] suggested that the malabsorption syndrome might represent the key host factor; subsequent studies showed that this represented the more usual mucosal pattern of the Asiatic,[12, 46, 72] and there was no correlation between cholera and the severity of this condition. American Peace Corps personnel developed the same mucosal pattern.[45] Studies on monkeys were equally noncontributory initially; in approximately 10 per cent of those challenged orally an acute diarrheal state developed; others merely passed vibrios for roughly one week. A diet of vitamin-free casein or of rice and salt did not increase the likelihood that oral challenge would result in a cholera-like disease. Potassium and mineral depletion likewise had no significant effect.

At this point in our studies two laboratory infections occurred in the United States.[69] The first case was one of simple diarrhea from which V. cholerae was recovered. However, the second case must be considered to be clinical cholera. This 42 year old male laboratory technician had been ill for six weeks before he was exposed to vibrios, and he had failed to regain an 18 pound weight loss sustained during his influenza-like illness. Infection in these two individuals was caused by a laboratory strain which had been maintained in the lyophilized state for over six years. On the basis that this strain might be highly "virulent," it was used to challenge monkeys but produced only asymptomatic infections with positive rectal swabs for up to ten days after challenge, despite the administration of doses as large as $3.5 \times 10^{12}$ organisms. To test whether the weight loss noted in the American patient might have a bearing, four monkeys were fed a rice and ascorbic acid diet; after they had lost a significant amount of their body weight they were challenged orally. On the following day one was dead and a second moribund; the third died after 21 days with vibrios in the upper intestinal tract but none at the rectal level; the fourth also died on the twenty-first day, with no clear cause, and no vibrios were recovered. Monkeys that had been maintained on the usual adequate monkey diet were challenged with a comparable dose and showed no sign of illness; they were stool-positive for six to seven days and no vibrios could be isolated on sacrifice on the fifteenth and twenty-seventh days. These results can only be considered suggestive; these studies were exploratory, on inadequate numbers of animals, and not fully controlled; the outbreak of the Pakistani-Indian conflict prevented the performance of the crucial experiment. This experience brought to mind a monkey who had been held in the experimental room without having been challenged, but nevertheless developed a severe vibrio-positive diarrhea and died. At autopsy advanced tuberculosis was found.

These observations lead to a conviction that host factors are of critical importance, and suggest that qualitative protein deficiency, a more likely aberration in a poorly fed population, needs more careful investigation. The case for its importance rests on inference from individual case histories and on extrapolation from results on another animal species, both insecure pillars for scientific fact.

### DIFFERENCES IN THE DOSE OF ORGANISMS INGESTED

An explanation for the high incidence of disease among the poor might be found in the insanitary conditions in which these poorly nourished individuals reside. Inadequacies of water supply and waste disposal facilities greatly increase the likelihood that vibrios will be ingested and that the dose will be large. Volunteer studies with typhoid fever have clearly demonstrated the relationship between the numbers of typhoid bacilli fed to healthy male volunteers and the likelihood that symptoms of disease will appear. Twenty-five per cent of these volunteers developed disease symptoms when $10^5$ organisms were administered; 50 per cent were clinically affected after ingesting $10^7$ organisms. Once illness occurred, the clinical courses were comparable regardless of the infecting dose, but the length of the incubation period did vary inversely with the size of the dose.[39] The final answer in cholera will also depend on volunteer studies. We do know that on many occasions people use vibrio-contaminated water without known clinical disease resulting; in other situations, water is clearly incriminated as the vehicle, if not the source, for infection. Cultural traits, such as the Bengali preference for *panta bhat* (wherein water is added to cooked rice and allowed to stand overnight, constituting an excellent culture medium for any vibrios which might be included), might explain, on a dose basis, the greater frequency and severity of clinical cholera in Bengal as compared to Viet Nam.[4] Unfortunately, field studies involve too many uncontrollable variables to provide the final answer to this question.

### DIFFERENCES IN THE METABOLIC STATE OF THE ORGANISMS OR THEIR SUBSTRATE

Accumulating evidence of the part played by vibrio toxins in the pathogenesis of cholera raises the question whether preformed toxin is necessary to initiate a vicious cycle. As indicated above, toxin alone can produce the characteristic response in the various animal models, and toxin is formed *in vivo*.[13, 62] It is conceivable that clinical disease is initiated by preformed toxin ingested together with the infecting dose of vibrios; further toxin is produced in the toxin-induced fluid. This requires an epidemiological reorientation—water then would play its part by contaminating foods which can serve as a substrate for toxin production; infection from water would result only in an asymptomatic but immunizing infection. More data are needed before this hypothesis can be accepted.

### DIFFERENCES IN IMMUNITY

Finally, while specific immunity has a great impact on the host-organism interrelationship, its mechanism of action is yet to be clearly defined. Controlled field studies[6, 55, 61] have now established that a killed whole-cell antigen can confer relatively good resistance to infection, and that the relative immunity of the population or segments thereof can be estimated by the mean vibriocidal antibody level.[53] Manifestation of this immunity is seen in the lack of age selectivity when cholera first enters a population group,[61] while, in endemic areas, it is predominantly an infection of children.[6, 55] The vaccines used in the field trials have not contained toxin and conferred only antibacterial immunity. Data are not yet available to establish whether this is more than humoral immunity, i.e., the contribution of cellular immunity (delayed hypersensitivity), and whether the immunity is effected by intraintestinal antibodies (coproantibodies). Freter[20] has claimed that parenteral immunization results in only a transient (several weeks) spillover of antibody into the intestinal lumen. The Dacca studies have shown the persistence of increased resistance for at least two years after a single dose of an unusually potent vaccine.[6] It is difficult to accept the hypothesis that the initial parenteral injection sensitized these individuals so that they responded with coproantibody formation from natural exposure to vibrios,[20] while those who did not receive the cholera vaccine neither developed coproantibody nor became infected after the same natural exposure to vibrios and subsequently responded as well as or better than those receiving the relatively degraded parenteral antigens.

While control of diphtheria might be achieved by establishing antibacterial factors, the establishment of antitoxic immunity has permitted effective control of the disease, even though bacterial infection may actually persist in the population.[12] The promise that specific cholera toxins responsible for the disease symptoms will be identified raises the hope that an antitoxic immunity may be feasible. While the picture at the moment is clouded by such findings as the presence of toxin-neutralizing potency in the sera of children with no other evidence of past vibrio infection, and the cholera symptoms appearing in the face of these antibodies,[5] it is possible that antitoxic immunity can be achieved which will be as enduring and as effective as that against the toxins of tetanus and diphtheria, in contrast to the relative immunity lasting only six months which follows the present bacterial vaccines.

Within one life span cholera has evolved from a dreadful cataclysm to an "experiment of nature," providing experienced research workers a model for the study of aberrant electrolyte, fluid, and intestinal physiology. Our adequate understanding of the therapeutic considerations makes the willful challenge of health volunteers completely feasible—actually indicated—to provide the essential understanding of immunity and susceptibility.

The evolution of our knowledge of cholera stands as a tribute to the memory of Dr. Joseph E. Smadel, a virologist and rickettsiologist who became fascinated by the problem of cholera and, as chairman of the NIH Cholera Advisory Committee, instigated the programs whose fruition we can report. We can best echo his words at the Cholera Conference in Dacca, in 1960, marking the opening of the laboratory: "These things have been accomplished only because many people, professional and lay, were convinced that the control and eventual eradication of cholera are worthy objectives and not beyond the reach of man."[70]

# *References*

1. Armijo, R., Pizzi, A., and Lobos, H. 1967. Prevalence of Typhoid Carriers after Treatment with Chloramphenicol. Bol. Ofic. Sanit. Panamer. *52:*295–302.
2. Azurin, J. C., Kobari, K., Barua, D., Alvero, M., Gomez, C. Z., Dizon, J. J., Nakano, E., Suplido, R., and Ledesma, L. 1967. A Long-term Carrier of Cholera: Cholera Dolores. Bull. WHO *37:*745–749.
3. Bales, G. L., and Lankford, C. E. 1961. An Adherence Factor of *Vibrio cholerae.* Bact. Proc. *60:*118.
4. Benenson, A. S., Ahmad, S. Z., and Oseasohn, R. O. 1965. Person-to-Person Transmission of Cholera. Proc. of the Cholera Research Symposium, January 24–29, 1965. pp. 332–336. Honolulu, Hawaii. Bethesda, Maryland. U.S. Department of Health, Education, and Welfare, Public Health Service.
5. Benenson, A. S., Saad, A., and Mosley, W. H. 1968. Serological Studies in Cholera. 2. The Vibriocidal Antibody Response of Cholera Patients Determined by a Microtechnique. Bull. WHO *38:*277–285.
6. Benenson, A. S., Mosley, W. H., Fahimuddin, M., and Oseasohn, R. O. 1968. Cholera Vaccine Field Trials in East Pakistan. 2. Effectiveness in the Field. Bull. WHO *38:*359–372.
7. Benyajati, C. 1966. Experimental Cholera in Humans. Brit. Med. J. *1:*140–142.
8. Carpenter, C. C. J., Sack, R. B., Mitra, P. P., and Mondal, A. 1964. Tetracycline Therapy in Cholera. Bull. Calcutta Sch. Trop. Med. *12:*30–32.
9. Carpenter, C. C. J., Barua, S. R., Sack, R. B., Wallace, C. K., Mitra, P. P., Khanra, S. R., Werner, T. S., Duffy, T. E., and Oleinick, A. 1966. Clinical Studies in Asiatic Cholera. V. Shock-producing Acute Diarrheal Disease in Calcutta: A Clinical and Biochemical Comparison of Cholera with Severe Non-cholera Diarrhea, 1963–1964. Bull. Johns Hopkins Hosp. *118:*230–242.
10. Carpenter, C. C. J., Sack, R. B., Feeley, J. C., and Steenberg, R. W. 1968. Site and Characteristics of Electrolyte Loss and Effect of Intraluminal Glucose in Experimental Canine Cholera. J. Clin. Invest. *47:*1210–1220.
11. Cole, J. R., and Greenough, W. B., III. 1965. Patent Bile Ducts at the Time of Colorless "Rice-water" Stool in Cholera. Lancet *2:*972–973.
12. Craig, J. P. 1962. Diphtheria: Prevalence of Inapparent Infection in a Nonepidemic Period. Amer. J. Public Health *52:*1444–1452.
13. Craig, J. P. 1965. A Permeability Factor (Toxin) Found in Cholera Stools and Culture Filtrates and its Neutralization by Convalescent Cholera Sera. Nature *207:*614–616.
14. Dammin, G. J., Benenson, A. S., Feldman, D., Formal, S. B., Goldstein, H. B., Merrill, T. G., and Sprinz, H. 1965. Clinical and Histopathologic Correlations in Acute Diarrheal Disease. Proc. of the Cholera Research Symposium, January 24–29, 1965. pp. 205–210. Honolulu, Hawaii. Bethesda, Maryland. U.S. Department of Health, Education, and Welfare, Public Health Service.
15. Dorland's Illustrated Medical Dictionary. 1957. 23rd Ed. p. 272. W. B. Saunders Co. Philadelphia.
16. Dutt, A. R. 1967. Distribution of *Vibrio cholerae* in the Intestine. Indian J. Med. Res. *55:* 314–317.
17. Finkelstein, R. A., Norris, H. T., and Dutta, N. K. 1964. Pathogenesis of Experimental Cholera in Infant Rabbits. 1. Observations on the Intraintestinal Infection and Experimental Cholera Produced with Cell-Free Products. J. Infect. Dis. *114:*203–216.
18. Finkelstein, R. A., Sobocinski, P. Z., Atthasampunna, P., and Charunmethee, P. 1966. Pathogenesis of Experimental Cholera: Identification of Choleragen (Procholeragen A) by Disc Immunoelectrophoresis and its Differentiation from Cholera Mucinase. J. Immun. *97:*25–33.
19. Freter, R. 1964. Comparison of Immune Mechanisms in Various Experimental Models of Cholera. Bull. WHO *31:*825–834.

20. Freter, R. 1965. Coproantibody and Oral Vaccines. Proc. of the Cholera Research Symposium, January 24–29, 1965. pp. 222–228. Honolulu, Hawaii. Bethesda, Maryland. U. S. Department of Health, Education, and Welfare, Public Health Service.

21. Gangarosa, E. J., Beisel, W. R., Benyajati, C., Sprinz, H., and Piyaratn, P. 1960. The Nature of the Gastrointestinal Lesion in Asiatic Cholera and its Relation to Pathogenesis: A Biopsy Study. Amer. J. Trop. Med. *9:*125–135.

22. Gangarosa, E. J., Saghari, H., Emile, J., and Siadat, H. 1966. Detection of *Vibrio cholerae* Biotype *El Tor* by Purging. Bull. WHO *34:*363–369.

23. Gangarosa, E. J., Sanati, A., Saghari, H., and Feeley, J. C. 1967. Multiple Serotypes of Vibrio Cholerae Isolated from a Case of Cholera. Lancet *1:*646–648.

24. Gordon, R. S., Jr. 1960. The Failure of Asiatic Cholera to Give Rise to "Exudative Enteropathy." SEATO Conference on Cholera. Dec. 5–8, 1960. pp. 54–57.

25. Gordon, R. S., Jr. 1965. Cholera as an Experiment of Nature. Proc. of the Cholera Research Symposium, January 24–29, 1965. pp. 293–295. Honolulu, Hawaii. Bethesda, Maryland. U.S. Department of Health, Education, and Welfare, Public Health Service.

26. Gordon, R. S., Jr. 1968. Summary of United States-Japan Cholera Symposium. Gastroenterology *54:*471–475.

27. Greenough, W. B., III, Gordon, R. S., Jr., Rosenberg, I. S., Davies, B. I., and Benenson, A. S. 1964. Tetracycline in the Treatment of Cholera. Lancet *1:*355–357.

28. Greenough, W. B., III. 1965. Pancreatic and Hepatic Hypersecretion in Cholera. Lancet *2:* 991–994.

29. Greenough, W. B., III. 1965. Cholera. Method of Pakistan-SEATO Cholera Research Laboratory. *In* Current Therapy, edited by H. F. Conn, pp. 7–9. W. B. Saunders Co. Philadelphia.

30. Greenough, W. B., III. 1966. *In* Cholera. Combined Clinical Staff Conference at the National Institutes of Health. Ann. Intern. Med. *64:*1332–1338.

31. Greenough, W. B., III, 1967. The Relevance of Cholera to American Medicine. Milit. Med. *132:*596–601.

32. Greig, E. D. W. 1913. An Investigation on the Occurrence of the Cholera Vibrio in the Biliary Passages. Indian J. Med. Res. *1:*44–58.

33. Greig, E. D. W. 1913. An Investigation of an Epidemic of Cholera Caused by a "Carrier." Indian J. Med. Res. *1:*59–63.

34. Greig, E. D. W. 1914. Lesions of the Gallbladder and Biliary Passages in Cholera: A Bacteriological, Histological and Experimental Study. Indian J. Med. Res. *2:*28–45.

35. Griffith, L. S. C., Fresh, J. W., Watten, R.H., and Villaroman, M. P. 1967. Electrolyte Replacement in Pediatric Cholera. Lancet *1:*1197–1199.

36. Harvey, R. M., Enson, Y., Lewis, M. L., Greenough, W. B., III, Ally, K. M., and Panno, R. A. 1968. Hemodynamic Studies on Cholera—Effects of Hypovolemia and Acidosis. Circulation *37:*709–728.

37. Hassan, S. I., Greenough, W. B., III, Gordon, R. S., Jr., and Benenson, A. S. 1965. The Rhesus Monkey as an Experimental Cholera Model. Proc. of the Cholera Research Symposium, January 24–29, 1965. pp. 276–278. Honolulu, Hawaii. Bethesda, Maryland. U. S. Department of Health, Education, and Welfare, Public Health Service.

38. Hirschhorn, N., and Rosenberg, I. H. 1968. Sodium-Potassium-Stimulated Adenosine Triphosphatase of Small Intestine in Man: Studies in Cholera and Other Diarrheal Diseases. J. Lab. Clin. Med. *71:*28–39.

39. Hornick, R. B., Woodward, T. E., McCrumb, F. R., Snyder, M. J., Dawkins, A. T., Bulkeley, J. T., de la Macorra, F., and Corozza, F. A. 1967. Typhoid Fever Vaccine—Yes or No? Med. Clin. N. Amer. *51:*617–623.

40. Huber, G. S. 1965. The Significance of the Number of Vibrios Seen in Rice-water Stools. Proc. of the Cholera Research Symposium, January 24–29, 1965. pp. 41–44. Honolulu, Hawaii. Bethesda, Maryland. U.S. Department of Health, Education, and Welfare, Public Health Service.

41. La Brec, E. H., Sprinz, H., Schneider, H., and Formal, S. B. 1965. Localization of Vibrios in Experimental Cholera: A Fluorescent Antibody Study in Guinea Pigs. Proc. of the Cholera Research Symposium, January 24–29, 1965. pp. 272–275. Honolulu, Hawaii. Bethesda, Maryland. U.S. Department of Health, Education, and Welfare, Public Health Service.

42. Lankford, C. E., and Legsomburana, U. 1965. Virulence Factors of Choleragenic Vibrios. Proc. of the Cholera Research Symposium, January 24–29, 1965. pp. 109–119. Honolulu, Hawaii. Bethesda, Maryland. U.S. Department of Health, Education, and Welfare, Public Health Service.

43. Leitch, G. J., Burrows, W., and Stolle, L. C. 1967. Experimental Cholera in the Rabbit Intestinal Loop: Fluid Accumulation and Sodium Pump Inhibition. J. Infect. Dis. *117:* 197–202.

44. Lindenbaum, J., Greenough, W. B., III, Benenson, A. S., Oseasohn, R., Rizvi, S., and Saad, A. 1965. Non-vibrio cholera. Lancet *1*:1081–1083.

45. Lindenbaum, J., Kent, T. H., and Sprinz, H. 1966. Malabsorption and Jejunitis in American Peace Corps Volunteers in Pakistan. Ann. Intern. Med. *65*:1201–1209.

46. Lindenbaum, J., Alam, A. K. M. J., and Kent, T. H. 1966. Subclinical Small-Intestinal Disease in East Pakistan. Brit. Med. J. *2*:1616–1619.

47. Lindenbaum, J., Gordon, R. S., Hirschhorn, N., Akbar, R., Greenough, W. B., III, and Islam, M. R. 1966. Cholera in Children. Lancet *1*:1066–1068.

48. Longmate, N. 1966. King Cholera. The Biography of a Disease. p. 49. Hamish Hamilton Ltd. London.

49. Longmate, N. *Op. cit.* p. 106.

50. Love, A. H. G. 1965. The Effect of Glucose on Cation Transport. Proc. of the Cholera Research Symposium, January 24–29, 1965. pp. 144–147. Honolulu, Hawaii. Bethesda, Maryland. U. S. Department of Health, Education, and Welfare, Public Health Service.

51. McGrew, R. E. 1965. Russia and the Cholera 1823–1832. pp. 47, 52, 98. Univ. of Wisconsin Press. Madison and Milwaukee.

52. McIntyre, O. R., Feeley, J. C., Greenough, W. B., III, Benenson, A. S., Hassan, S. I., and Saad, A. 1965. Diarrhea Caused by Non-Cholera Vibrios. Amer. J. Trop. Med. *14*:412–418.

53. Mosley, W. H., Benenson, A. S., and Baruï, A. 1968. A Serological Survey for Cholera Antibodies in the Cholera Vaccine Field Trial Population in Rural East Pakistan. 2. A Comparison of Antibody Titers in Immunized and Control Populations and the Relationship of Antibody Titer to Cholera Case Rate. Bull. WHO *38*:335–346.

54. Onions, C. T. Editor. 1955. The Oxford Universal Dictionary. p. 306. Oxford University Press. London.

55. Oseasohn, R. O., Benenson, A. S., and Fahimuddin, M. 1965. Cholera Vaccine Field Trial in Rural East Pakistan (First Year of Observation). Lancet *1*:450–453.

56. Oseasohn, R., Ahmad, S., Islam, M. A., and Rahman, A. S. M. M. 1966. Clinical and Bacteriological Findings Among Families of Cholera Patients. Lancet *1*:340–342.

57. O'Shaughnessy, W. B. 1831. Letter to the Editor. Lancet *1*:490. Cited by Peterson, M. L. 1968. Physician as a Scholar: Changing Roles in the Twentieth Century. Pharos *31*: 43–46.

58. O'Shaughnessy, W. B. 1832. Report on the Chemical Pathology of the Malignant Cholera. Highley. London. Cited by Peterson, M. L. 1968. Physician as a Scholar: Changing Roles in the Twentieth Century. Pharos *31*:44.

59. Pal, S. C., Murti, D. K., Misra, G. V. S., Chuttani, C. S., Pandit, C. G., and Shrivastav, J. B. 1967. Bacteriological Investigations of Cholera Epidemics in Gurgaon District and in Delhi during 1965–66. Indian J. Med. Res. *55*:810–814.

60. Peters, J. C., and McClellan, E. 1875. A History of the Travels of Asiatic Cholera. *In* The Cholera Epidemic of 1873 in the United States. pp. 515–695. Government Printing Office. Washington.

61. Philippines Cholera Committee. 1965. A Controlled Field Trial of the Effectiveness of Cholera and Cholera El Tor Vaccines in the Philippines. Bull. WHO *32*:603–625.

62. Phillips, R. A. 1963. The Patho-physiology of Cholera. Bull. WHO *28*:297–305.

63. Phillips, R. A. 1967. Twenty Years of Cholera Research. J.A.M.A. *202*:610–614.

64. Pollitzer, R. 1959. Cholera. World Health Organization Monograph Series No. 43. pp. 11–95. World Health Organization. Geneva.

65. Pollitzer, R. *Op. cit.* pp. 476–480.

66. Rosenberg, C. E. 1962. The Cholera Years. The United States in 1832, 1849, and 1866. p. 3. University of Chicago Press. Chicago.

67. Rosenberg, C. E. *Op. cit.* p. 41.

68. Rosenberg, I. H., Greenough, W. B., III, Lindenbaum, J., and Gordon, R. S., Jr. 1966. Nutritional Studies in Cholera. Influence of Nutritional Status on Susceptibility to Infection. Amer. J. Clin. Nutr. *19*:384–389.

69. Sheehy, T. W., Sprinz, H., Augerson, W. S., and Formal, S. B. 1966. Laboratory *Vibrio cholerae* Infection in the United States. J.A.M.A. *197*:321–326.

70. Smadel, J. E. 1960. Review of the SEATO-Cholera Research Programme. SEATO Conference on Cholera. Dec. 5–8, 1960. p. 10. Dacca, East Pakistan.

71. Snow, J. 1855. On the Mode of Communication of Cholera. John Churchill, London. (Republished as Snow on Cholera. 1965. p. 117. Hafner Publishing Co. New York.)

72. Sprinz, H., Sribhibhadh, R., Gangarosa, E. J., Benyajati, C., Kundel, D., and Halstead, S. 1962. Biopsy of Small Bowel of Thai People. With Special Reference to Recovery from Asiatic Cholera and to an Intestinal Malabsorption Syndrome. Amer. J. Clin. Path. *38*:43–51.

73. Wallace, C. K., Carpenter, C. C. J., Mitra, P. P., Sack, R. B., Khanra, S. R., Werner, A. S., Duffy, T. P., Oleinick, A., and Lewis, G. W. 1966. Classical and El Tor Cholera: A Clinical Comparison. Brit. Med. J. 2:447–449.
74. Wallace, C. K., Anderson, P. N., Lewis, G. W., Segre, G. V., Pierce, N. F., Brown, T. C., Sanyal, S. N., and Waldman, R. H. 1967. Probable Gallbladder Infection in Convalescent Cholera Patients. Lancet 1:865–868.
75. Watten, R. H., Morgan, F. M., Yachai-Na-Songkhla, Vanikiati, B., and Phillips, R. A. 1959. Water and Electrolyte Studies in Cholera. J. Clin. Invest. 38:1879–1889.
76. Yen, C. H. 1964. A Recent Study of Cholera with Reference to an Outbreak in Taiwan in 1962. Bull. WHO 30:811–825.

# Chapter 14

# EPIDEMIOLOGICAL AND IMMUNOLOGICAL OBSERVATIONS IN TYPHOID OF MAN AND ANTHROPOIDS AND IN EXPERIMENTAL SALMONELLOSIS OF LABORATORY ANIMALS

A. L. OLITZKI

*Department of Bacteriology,*
*Hebrew University-Hadassah Medical School,*
*Jerusalem, Israel*

*Salmonella typhi* and the paratyphoid bacteria are the few species among hundreds of *Salmonella* serotypes which have become specifically adapted to parasitism in man. No other species of living beings is known to become infected by them under natural conditions of life, but only under the conditions of experimental laboratory infections. It seems, therefore, that the association of *S. typhi* and man is the latest step of a long evolution, but it cannot be predicted whether it is the final one. If we accept the evolutionary concept, each species represents another step of evolution: *S. typhimurium* attacks man and various species of mammalia and birds, *S. abortus* horses and related species, *S. pullorum* and *S. gallinarum* poultry. We are unable to predict the further evolution of a species like *S. typhimurium*, whether it will continue to remain multipathogenic, or whether descendants of it will become monopathogenic for a single species of mammalia or birds. Even

303

among the anthropospecific pathogens there exist different degrees of adaptation to parasitism in man. Typhoid fever, the disease caused specifically by *S. typhi*, can be a result of ingestion of small quantities of bacteria; paratyphoid fevers, the diseases caused by *S. paratyphi A, B,* and *C,* do not result unless large numbers of bacteria are ingested. Therefore, typhoid outbreaks often are water-borne; paratyphoid outbreaks rarely are.

The association between *S. typhi* and man is an ancient one. In the interest of species survival the host has acquired capabilities for adaptation and defense which are able to damage the cellular integrity of the invader and to terminate its viability in any stage of its invasion. The saprophytic microorganisms of the gastrointestinal tract are the natural allies of man and may act by production of physicochemical conditions unfavorable to the multiplication of the invader, as demonstrated by Bergeim et al.[11] and Freter;[48, 49] by production of bactericidal substances such as peroxides, as shown by Berger[12, 13] and Dold;[28] by production of bacteriocins, as demonstrated by Agarwal[1] and Vassiliadis et al.;[148] or by production of DNA modifying the characteristics of the invader, as demonstrated by Vizir and Chebotar'ova.[149]

Antigenic similarity between nonpathogenic intestinal bacteria and the pathogen effects an early development of antibodies acting on the somatic antigens of the invader, as shown by Kauffmann and Moeller[73] and Rouchdi,[124] and a readiness for immediate response to the antigenic stimulus exerted by it, as described by Gulbrandsen.[63] *S. typhi* has to pass the acid medium of the stomach, enter into the intestines, multiply there, pass through the intestinal mucosa into the Peyer's patches, the mesenteric glands, and the thoracic duct, and invade the blood before the initial clinical symptoms of the disease become apparent. At almost every step of this long road *S. typhi* is exposed to bactericidal substances produced by the host or its natural allies, the microorganisms of the digestive tract. After the invasion of the blood and the big organs, liver and spleen, *S. typhi* is exposed to the bactericidal effect of the antibody-complement system, as explained by Felix,[37] Felix and Olitzki,[41] and Lubinski;[94] the opsonic effect of specific antibodies, as shown by Bhatnagar[15] and Jenkin and Rowley;[70] and engulfment by phagocytes and intracellular devitalization and disintegration, as detailed by Olitzki et al.[110] Nonspecific products of white cells, as described by Gershon,[54] Gershon and Olitzki,[55] and Olitzki and Gershon,[105, 105a] complete the antibacterial effects of the specific immunity reactions demonstrated by Felix.[37] However, these defense mechanisms are not equally active in all body organs. Liver extracts have been found to exert an inhibiting effect on bactericidal serum action and phagocytosis *in vitro*, as demonstrated by Gershon[54] and Olitzki et al.,[107, 110] and on intra- and extracellular lysis *in vivo*, according to Olitzki et al.[107, 112, 116] Crude liver extracts, sodium taurocholate, and glycogen act as powerful infection-promoting substances, enabling intraperitoneal infection of mice with *S. typhi* by small inocula of approximately 20 microorganisms, as demonstrated by Olitzki and Godinger[107] and Olitzki and Kaplan.[112] The long persistence of *S. typhi* in the liver and the bile ducts may be correlated with their relatively low environmental bactericidal potency and the presence of the aforementioned infection-promoting substances. The main toxic product, the endotoxin, is stored in specific organs, as shown by the works of Braude et al.;[20-22] it is detoxicated by different mechanisms, as reported by Landy et al.,[90] Rutenberg et al.,[126] Trapani et al.,[138] and Wiznitzer et al.,[159] and its split products are excreted with the urine, according to Herring et al.[64]

In spite of these adverse conditions, *S. typhi* may gain access to the gall-bladder, the kidneys, or the skin, persist there for years, and finally gain egress through the urine, the feces, and the pus of skin abscesses.

*S. typhi* is not an "obligate parasite." Its capability to utilize ammonium and simple organic compounds as sources of nitrogen, as proved by Oren,[117] and carbohydrates and organic acids as sources of energy, as employed by Olitzki et al.,[113, 114] outside the human body, enables it to continue its existence outside the human body, to survive, and even to multiply.

In spite of the high typhoid morbidity—up to 130 cases per 100,000 —which still exists in many countries, the present situation is not hopeless, and the fact that there exist today 13 countries—Australia, Canada, Denmark, Iceland, Ireland, Japan, Luxembourg, Netherlands, Norway, Philippines, Sweden, Taiwan, and the United States, with a total population of 396 million —which were able to lower the typhoid morbidity below the level of 1 per 100,000 proves that by adequate cooperation between the authorities responsible for preventive and curative medicine, a final eradication of typhoid is a practical possibility within the foreseeable future, at least in countries that have reached morbidity levels lower than 1 per 100,000.[35]

An immense literature has accumulated concerning the mode of action of endotoxins of gram-negative microorganisms, e.g., their effects on the metabolism, white blood cells, body temperature, and sensitivity to epinephrine. For the study of the clinical symptoms of typhoid fever the problem exists whether all these immediate and acute effects observed in experimental animals after injections of endotoxin are analogous or identical with those observed in typhoid patients, or, in other words, whether the clinical symptoms of typhoid are the result of a chronic endotoxin intoxication, or whether other mechanisms are involved in their appearance.

Greisman et al.[58] studied the effects of endotoxin in man. In human volunteers 0.5 $\mu$g. of *S. typhi* endotoxin produced headache, chills, fever, myalgia, malaise, abdominal discomfort, and anorexia. When the same subjects were subsequently infected by viable *S. typhi*, they stated that during the overt typhoid infection their symptoms were remarkably similar to those induced by purified endotoxin. During the early phase of the disease the O-antigen of *S. typhi* was detected in patients' sera by the aid of the precipitin test. The endotoxin is not neutralized by antibodies and appearance of O-antibodies does not lead immediately to a clinical remission.

In their experiments on human volunteers Greisman et al.[58] determined the fever reaction following intravenous injection of endotoxin prior to oral infection with *S. typhi* and during the convalescence. These experiments indicated the development of tolerance during the convalescence. Furthermore, the vascular reactivity of volunteers to intravenous norepinephrine infusions was observed during the preinfection period, during overt disease, and during convalescence. The observations indicated the appearance of hyperreactivity of the vascular system to norepinephrine during typhoid fever which persists

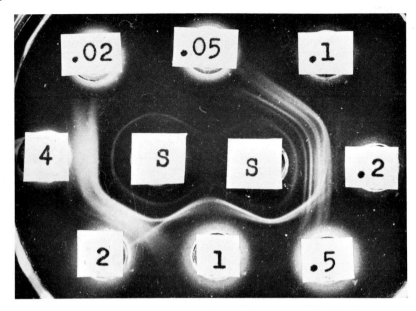

*Figure 1.* $S$ = Immune serum (*Salmonella typhi*, strain O901). In the periphery are graded quantities of *Salmonella hofit*, ranging from 4.0 to 0.02 mg.

into convalescence and subsides by the second to third week after defervescence.

The question arises whether in addition to the O-antigen other toxic substances are able to determine the clinical course of typhoid. *In vivo* experiments did not reveal toxic effects of the H- and Vi-antigen. On the other hand Gershon and Olitzki[56] demonstrated the cytopathogenic effect of Vi-antigen on murine monocytes and Ehrlich ascites tumor cells. These changes were qualitatively different from those exerted by endotoxin, and appeared much earlier. The primary changes were observed on the periphery of the plasma, progressing to the central part of the cell and ending with the destruction of the cell nuclei.

There was no evidence that the plasma antigens described by Olitzki and Godinger[106] exerted any toxic effect. These antigens proved to be completely different from the surface antigens of the Kauffman-White scheme. They are shared by microorganisms which have no common H-, O-, or capsular antigens. Figure 1 shows the reaction of the sonic extract of *S. hofit* (antigenic formula 39:i:1, 5) with $S$ *typhi*, strain O901 immune serum (antigenic formula of *S. typhi:* 9, 12:d:−).

The common antigen described by Kunin et al.[86] was found to be nontoxic. Kessel et al.[75] ascribed some residual toxicity to contamination with O-antigen.

The DNA-conjugated antigens isolated by Boros and Olitzki[18] were not toxic. Summarizing all these results, it seems that the O-antigen of *S. typhi* is its dominating toxic constituent, while the effects of other cell constituents are of minor importance.

Typhoid fever is an interaction between man and a specifically anthropotropic parasite that is seeking survival and egress for temporary existence outside the human body.

There is not an intermediate host, and the obligation of the hygienist is to minimize the probability of survival outside the human body, whereas the obligation of the physician is to minimize the probability of its survival in the host's body and egress from it.

Early hospitalization of patients, and treatment of symptomless excreters and temporary and chronic carriers by antibiotics and (in cases of ineffectiveness of antibiotics) by cholecystectomy, with or without drainage of the common bile duct and irrigation with antibiotics as shown by Erlik and Reitler,[36] should terminate the infectious process and the egress of the pathogens.

Urinary carriers present less of a problem. The urine can be sterilized by antibacterial agents permanently. Each convalescent patient has to be followed up for the disappearance of Vi-agglutinins. Their persistence in a convalescent three or six months after an attack of enteric fever is indicative of the continued presence of *S. typhi*. Such persons should be regarded as potential chronic carriers until the Vi-agglutinins have disappeared or until repeated cultural tests of urine, feces, and bile over a period of three months have proved consistently negative.

The relatively long survival time of *S. typhi* in water, milk, ice cream, cheese, butter, fluid, dried and frozen egg products, and meat and meat products is known; details were reported by Floyd et al.[43, 44] and Olitzki and Grossowicz.[111] Its survival can be terminated by pasteurization or by cooking if the taste and quality of the product is not spoiled or altered by these processes. Shellfish, mainly oysters, constitute a serious problem. In the typhoid cases ascribed to this source there is a case fatality of 25 per cent, as shown by Wilson and Miles.[157] With the exception of this latter source of infection, which seems to be out of control, pasteurization, cooking, and bacteriological control of the subjects handling the food and exclusion of bacillary carriers from any work connected with food preparation or distribution have been effective means in reducing the morbidity; proper sewage disposal and purified water supply and control are the basic sanitary instruments for prevention of typhoid and other enteric infections. The protection of food from contamination by flies by covers or netting and the prevention of multiplication of bacteria in food by cooking or refrigeration are basic requirements of a sanitary food supply by the producer, the dealer, and, finally, the consumer in his own household.

Water may be contaminated by sewage, and food may also be contaminated by water, e.g., canned food, when the cans are cooled by contaminated water. These facts show that pure water and sanitary facilities have to be supplied not only to permanent human residences, but also to camping places, sea beaches, and lakes which attract visitors, sometimes in masses.

The use of phage typing as reported by Batty Shaw and Mackay,[10] Bradley et al.,[19] Craigie and Felix,[24] Craigie and Yen,[25] and Marmion et al.;[96] of biochemical typing as stated by Olitzki et al.;[114] or of phage typing combined with biotyping as shown by Olitzki et al.[114] has elucidated the sources of several epidemics. But this has been done post factum, after the outbreak has occurred, as pointed out in the works of Batty Shaw and Mackay,[10] Bradley et al.,[19] and Marmion et al.[96]

The tracing back of an epidemic to a central source after its outbreak may provide additional experience to the epidemiologist for analogous epidemiological situations in the future. It also may prevent false conclusions concerning the source of the outbreak built up only on the base of circumstantial data, as pointed out by Olitzki et al.[114]

The sewer swab technique enables the hygienist to follow the contamination of the sewage with enteric pathogens back from the main sewer to tributary sewers and finally to the drains of the individual house in which the carrier is living.

All this knowledge which has been accumulated should be effective enough to enable mankind to eradicate *S. typhi* from the surface of the earth. In spite of all this knowledge, the majority of mankind is still living in areas where typhoid is endemic and typhoid morbidity rises periodically to epidemic proportions. It seems, therefore, that the main work to be done today is not so much to accumulate more knowledge or more refined methods of bacteriological diagnosis and typing, but rather an educational work: to bring this knowledge in an adequate and understandable form to all nations of the world. This can be done in the frame of the World Health Organization (WHO), but it can be effectual only with full understanding and cooperation of the local governmental authorities. On one hand, excellent work has been done in vaccination campaigns in which local authorities and representatives of WHO together have planned and organized the performance of the campaign, the determination of the potencies of the vaccines simultaneously in laboratories located in different countries, and the evaluation of the results for further work, as shown by Cvjetanovic and Uemura,[27] Cvjetanovic,[26] Kheifets,[76] Kheifets et al.,[77] and different national and international typhoid commissions[118, 118a, 143, 160, 161] and institutions.[151, 152]

On the other hand, it is still impossible today to obtain information on typhoid morbidity and mortality from a group of countries with a population of over 1500 million owing to the incompleteness or complete lack of information provided by them. Therefore, the main problem at the present seems to be how to let a maximum number of human beings enjoy the benefits of the knowledge of prevention and therapy of typhoid which has accumulated and which the populations of great and developed nations are enjoying today. But, even when the epidemiologist and the physician have done their best according to the present state of our knowledge, there remains still the problem of the education of the individual. Without an adequate health education of the population from the very beginning of childhood, the best work of the sanitary engineer, the epidemiologist, the physician, and the research worker may be annihilated. A person who does not carefully wash his hands after defecation and before starting his meals endangers his family as soon as he becomes a patient or a carrier. A well educated individual, even if he becomes a carrier, will understand his situation and behave himself accordingly.

The research done on nonspecific factors in host resistance has proved that besides sanitation, health education, and adequate therapy of patients and carriers, there exist genetic and environmental factors which determine the resistance of the individual to typhoid infection. In laboratory animals the selection of resistant animal strains has been successful, as seen by the experiments of Webster;[153-155] in human populations selected breeding is impossible. However, our knowledge of the influence of enviromental conditions has expanded. It is clear that an unbalanced diet, mainly lack of animal protein and vitamins, interferes with full development of the humoral and cellular defense mechanisms, according to the experiments of Guggenheim and Buechler,[61, 62] Kligler et al.,[80, 81] and Lassen.[91–93] On the other hand, there are certain forms of hypernutrition, mainly exaggerated protein intake, which lower the resistance, as reported by Smith and Chubb.[134] Certain proteins such as liquid egg white lower the acidity of the gastric content, Arnold,[3, 4] McDaniels,[97] and Nedzel and Arnold[99] have found. The achievement of an adequately balanced nutrition for all men, victory in the fight against undernourishment and hunger, would enhance resistance to typhoid and probably to other bacillary infections.

The influence of climate has been proved by the works of Arnold and Brody,[5] Fisher,[42] Kligler,[78] and Kligler and Olitzki,[82, 83] and it is clear that an extremely high effective temperature lowers gastric acidity and resistance to typhoid. Typhoid does not appear immediately with the appearance of the warm season like dysentery does. In some countries it reaches its peak by the end of the summer (Tables 1, 2, and 3). That means that the resist-

TABLE 1.  *The Seasonal Incidence of Enteric Fevers in Different Countries. Countries with the Peak of Incidence from May to August or with Almost the Same Level of Incidence from May to December (Ratio Maximal Incidence/Minimal Incidence Higher than 1.30)**

| | | | CASES REPORTED | | | RATIO |
| CONTINENT | PERIOD | STATE | *January to April* | *May to August* | *September to December* | MAXIMUM/ MINIMUM |
|---|---|---|---|---|---|---|
| Africa | 1964–1965 | Egypt | 5066 | *19340* | 10836 | 3.81 |
| | 1964–1965 | Ethiopia | 399 | *605* | 360 | 1.68 |
| | 1964–1965 | Kenya | 173 | *257* | 149 | 1.67 |
| America | 1964–1965 | Canada | 79 | *123* | 114 | 1.55 |
| | 1964–1965 | United States | 182 | *361* | *363* | 1.99 |
| | 1964 | Mexico | 2116 | *3319* | 2725 | 1.57 |
| | 1964–1965 | Jamaica | 110 | *156* | 90 | 1.73 |
| | 1964–1965 | Venezuela | 231 | *413* | 355 | 1.79 |
| | 1964–1965 | El Salvadore | 724 | *1036* | 650 | 1.59 |
| Asia | 1964 | Iran | 6519 | *11805* | *11371* | 1.81 |
| | 1964–1965 | Philippines | 110 | *126* | 76 | 1.66 |
| Europe | 1964–1965 | England & Wales | 108 | *938* | 304 | 8.65 |
| | 1964–1965 | Scotland | 22 | *468* | 210 | 9.55 |
| | 1964–1965 | France | 840 | *1482* | *1480* | 1.76 |
| | 1964–1965 | Germany (East & West) | 968 | *2285* | 1532 | 2.36 |
| | 1964–1965 | Hungary | 230 | *398* | 397 | 1.73 |
| | 1964–1965 | Yugoslavia | 1985 | *3458* | 3301 | 1.74 |
| | 1964–1965 | Italy | 5911 | *9663* | 8820 | 1.64 |
| | 1964–1965 | Spain | 2837 | *5107* | 3547 | 1.80 |
| | 1964–1965 | Sweden (all cases of sal- monellosis) | 402 | 1336 | 624 | 3.32 |

* Data from Epidemiological and Vital Statistics Report.[35]

TABLE 2.    *The Seasonal Incidence of Enteric Fever in Different Countries.*
*Countries Where the Peak of the Incidence is in the Autumn*
*(September to December)\**

| CONTINENT | PERIOD | COUNTRY | January to April | May to August | September to December | RATIO MAXIMUM/ MINIMUM |
|---|---|---|---|---|---|---|
| | | | CASES REPORTED | | | |
| Asia | 1964–1965 | Japan | 540 | 632 | 713 | 1.32 |
| | 1964–1965 | Turkey | 1945 | 2483 | 3509 | 1.80 |
| Europe | 1964–1965 | Ireland (North & South) | 14 | 14 | 21 | 1.50 |
| | 1964–1965 | Denmark & Norway | 8 | 23 | 47 | 5.86 |
| | 1964–1965 | Finland | 80 | 102 | 142 | 1.78 |
| | 1964–1965 | Poland | 806 | 994 | 1101 | 1.37 |

* Data from Epidemiological and Vital Statistics Report.[35]

TABLE 3.    *Countries of the Southern Hemisphere with Highest Prevalence of*
*Enteric Fevers from January to April (Hot Seasonal)\**

| CONTINENT | PERIOD | STATE | January to April | May to August | September to December | RATIO MAXIMUM/ MINIMUM |
|---|---|---|---|---|---|---|
| | | | CASES REPORTED | | | |
| Africa | 1964 | South Africa | 1366 | 1012 | 864 | 1.58 |
| | 1964 | Madagascar | 221 | 154 | 134 | 1.65 |
| America | 1964–1965 | Argentine | 810 | 461 | 644 | 1.76 |
| | 1964–1965 | Chile | 4537 | 2373 | 2349 | 1.93 |
| | 1964 | Ecuador | 903 | 843 | 435 | 2.07 |
| | 1964–1965 | Guiana | 261 | 219 | 132 | 1.98 |
| Oceania | 1964–1965 | Australia | 27 | 12 | 26 | 2.92 |
| | 1964–1965 | New Zealand | 38 | 13 | 21 | 1.81 |

* Data from Epidemiological and Vital Statistics Report.[35]

TABLE 4.    *Sudden Changes in the Usual Seasonal Incidence of Enteric Fever in*
*Different Areas by the Appearance of Winter and Summer Epidemics\**

| CONTINENT | STATE | PERIOD | January to April | May to August | September to December | RATIO MAXIMUM/ MINIMUM |
|---|---|---|---|---|---|---|
| | | | CASES REPORTED | | | |
| America | Haiti | 1964 | 258 | 92 | 93 | 2.80 |
| | | 1965 | 64 | 105 | 78 | 1.64 |
| Europe | Czechoslovakia | 1964 | 757 | 290 | 240 | 3.16 |
| | | 1965 | 145 | 156 | 220 | 1.52 |
| | England | 1963 | 197 | 302 | 163 | 1.85 |
| | | 1964 | 51 | 179 | 141 | 3.50 |
| | | 1965 | 66 | 759 | 163 | 11.50 |
| | Scotland | 1963 | 173 | 53 | 10 | 17.30 |
| | | 1964 | 2 | 376 | 193 | 188.00 |
| | | 1965 | 20 | 92 | 17 | 5.40 |

* Data from Epidemiological and Vital Statistics Report.[35]

ance becomes lowered not by a short exposure to an extremely high temperature, but merely by an accumulation of the heat stress during the whole summer. The epidemiological observations were paralleled by the results of animal experiments made by Kligler and Olitzki.[82, 83] If that is true, then protection of man against extremely high effective temperatures is not luxury, but a preventive measure to maintain his natural resistance; adequate ventilation and air-conditioning, construction and planning of towns and individual houses according to the climatic conditions, suitable clothing and, mainly, protecting industrial and agricultural workers against exposure to extremely high temperatures are called for. The adverse effect of sun radiation on resistance has been proved by Kligler and Olitzki[84] and Robertson.[122] This fact demands another attitude to the exposure of the whole body to sun radiation, as is the custom on beaches and in recreation places. Extremely low temperatures lower resistance, too, according to Kligler and Olitzki,[83] Previte and Berry;[119] winter epidemics have been reported (Table 4).[35] It has not yet been studied whether inadequate housing, heating, and clothing of the population were associated with these outbreaks. It is worthwhile to note that in certain equatorial countries no significant differences in typhoid prevalence were observed between the various seasons of the year (cf. Table 5).

The intensive studies of the effects of endotoxin have found their practical application in therapy. The observations of Berry et al.[14] Melby et al.,[98] and Robinson and Smith[123] that adrenalectomy lowers the resistance to endotoxin and that cortisone enhances resistance and inhibits the appearance of endotoxic symptoms have led to an application in therapy of typhoid. Cortisone combined with chemotherapy, mainly chloramphenicol, is a powerful therapeutic regimen which effects an immediate disappearance of the toxic symptoms of the disease, as shown by Kass and Finland,[72] Smadel et al.,[132] and Wisseman et al.[158]

The bacteria of the gastrointestinal tract are the natural allies of man against invasion of pathogens. We know that their destruction by antibiotics is disastrous for man and animals, as demonstrated by Bohnhoff et al.,[17] Formal et al.,[47] Freter,[48–50] Friedman and Halbert,[51] Smith,[133] and Welch

TABLE 5.   *Countries with Almost Equal Incidence of Enteric Fevers during All Seasons of the Year. Ratio Maximum/Minimum Less than 1.3\**

| CONTINENT | PERIOD | STATE | CASES REPORTED | | | RATIO MAXIMUM/ MINIMUM |
|---|---|---|---|---|---|---|
| | | | January to April | May to August | September to December | |
| Africa | 1964–1965 | Congo (Democratic Republic) | 516 | 555 | 442 | 1.25 |
| | 1964–1965 | Sudan | 498 | 549 | 567 | 1.14 |
| America | 1964–1965 | Honduras | 602 | 558 | 600 | 1.08 |
| | 1964 | Peru | 2074 | 2187 | 1759 | 1.24 |
| Asia | 1964–1965 | Ceylon | 873 | 1136 | 1130 | 1.29 |
| | 1964 | Indonesia | 1209 | 1245 | 1182 | 1.06 |

* Data from Epidemiological and Vital Statistics Report.[35]

et al.[156] Only few attempts have been made to colonize in the intestines antagonists to enteric pathogens, e.g., bacteriocin producers, lysogenic strains able to free bacteriophages deleterious for the invader, or free bacteriophages. Since virulence may be changed by genetic processes, recombinations, transformations, and transductions should be tried to fight disease not only by destroying the pathogen, but by changing its pathogenicity. The existence of nonvirulent strains of S. typhi which produce in man a disease with symptoms which in many respects are modifications of its classic symptoms, as reported by Bradley et al.,[19] shows that nature has done this experiment successfully.

There are several modes of action of the normal intestinal flora. So long as gram-negative bacteria are present, they maintain a marked sensitivity of the host to bacterial endotoxin which seems to be essential for resistance to gram-negative infections, as demonstrated by Dubos and Schaedler.[29–32] In so far as nonspecific antigens common with those of the pathogens are in existence, the intestinal bacteria may maintain a high degree of resistance which is rather an immunization process than a nonspecific rise of host's resistance, according to Gulbrandsen.[63] This mechanism can be eliminated by treatment with antibiotics. The production of antibiotics by intestinal bacteria of man has been investigated; the antibiotics seem to be active against shigellae, vibrios, and corynebacteria, but those active against S. typhi seem to be rare, as in the findings of Robbins et al.[121] Furthermore, an antibiotic produced by Escherichia coli acted markedly on a Shigella strain when both microorganisms were given intraperitoneally, whereas after oral administration of both strains no bactericidal effect of the antibiotic on the shigellae was noted by Friedman and Halbert.[51] Since salmonellae are able to produce bacteriocins by themselves, as stated by Agarwal[1] and Vassiliades et al.,[148] there exists the possibility that in the course of infections with these strains, the pathogens exert deleterious effects on the saprophytic intestinal bacteria. Besides the bacteriocins, simple chemical compounds have been found to inhibit bacterial growth in the intestines, e.g., $H_2S$, according to the experiments of Bergeim et al.;[11] volatile fatty acids, according to Bergeim;[11] peroxides; low pH, as shown by Arnold;[3, 4] and the anaerobic conditions which enhance the competition between bacterial species for fermentable carbohydrate sources, as shown experimentally by Freter.[48–50] The role of the lactobacilli as inhibitors of intestinal infections has been emphasized by Dubos and Schaedler[31, 32] and Schaedler and Dubos.[130, 131]

The mouse has been the main laboratory animal for studies on typhoid immunity. Experimental respiratory infections of mice with salmonellae were studied by Oren[117] who showed that the respective $ID_{50}$ for S. typhi, strains Ty2, H901, 0901, Ty1, S. paratyphi B, S. paratyphi C, and S. typhimurium, were: $3.8 \times 10^3$, $5.85 \times 10^4$, $5.85 \times 10^5$, $2.48 \times 10^6$, $3.56 \times 10^2$, $5.53 \times 10^2$, and $8.3 \times 10^1$.

Oren[117] also observed that three consecutive inhalations of strain Ty2 protected mice against a challenge of $10^6$ virulent microorganisms suspended in mucin with typhoid and paratyphoid strains.

Oral infections of mice were carried out by Wassermann and Sommerfeld[150] and Oerskov and Moltke.[102] The authors reported that S. typhi and S. paratyphi B appeared in different organs but there was a steady retrogression of the infection.

The intraperitoneal infection with bacteria suspended in saline was introduced by Grinnel[59] for potency tests in white mice.

Felix[38] emphasized that $10^8$ bacteria equal to $LD_{100}$ have to be inoculated by this route three weeks after the vaccine and 48 hours after the protective serum. Felix and Anderson[39] determined that an alcoholized vaccine is stable enough and keeps its potency more than 10 years in order to serve as standard vaccine.

Landy[87] used the intraperitoneal challenge and found that three immunizing doses of Vi-antigen given subcutaneously, intraperitoneally, and intravenously exerted the same immunizing effect independently of the route of injection. However, there are variations in the results obtained by different authors which seem to depend mainly on the number of immunizing injections and the interval between the last vaccine inoculation and the challenge. The intraperitoneal challenge with the aid of mucin was introduced by Nungester et al.[100] Other pathogenicity-enhancing substances such as fibril cellulose, levans, and dextrans of bacterial origin were introduced by Olitzki et al.,[115] purified O-antigens by Tal and Olitzki,[136] and zymosan by the Polish Typhoid Committee.[118]

The intracerebral challenge was described by Landy et al.[88] and the protecting effect of Vi-antigen against the intracerebral challenge was observed by the same authors.[89]

Chimpanzees were introduced as experimental animals for typhoid research by Gruenbaum.[60] After the animals were fed typhoid bacilli there appeared fever, enteritis, malaise, enlarged Peyer's patches, and positive blood cultures and Widal reactions. These results were confirmed by Edsall et al.,[33] who concluded that typhoid of chimpanzees resembles the mild form of human typhoid seen in childhood. The pathological findings were indistinguishable from those seen in mild typhoid in man. Immunization studies of Gaines et al.[53] showed that in chimpanzees only typhoid induced by large doses of typhoid bacilli conferred immunity to a like number of organisms, while typhoid induced by small numbers of S. typhi was unable to protect against larger numbers of the same strain. These observations are similar to those made by Marmion et al.[96] in man. They observed in two consecutive outbreaks, occurring in the same community within five months, 11 instances of second infection. Gaines et al.[52] proved in chimpanzees the effectiveness of an acetone-killed and dried vaccine and a heat-killed and phenolized vaccine. Both vaccines protected chimpanzees. The O-response was the same and the Vi-antibody titers were low in both instances.

Tully et al.[139] reported that a rough strain devoid of Vi- and O-antigen produced neither fever nor bacteremia in chimpanzees. Strain 0901, devoid of Vi-antigen, produced mild febrile reactions and a few positive blood cultures.

Tully et al.[140] also observed that chimpanzees formerly infected with the rough strain and then rechallenged with the virulent strain $Ty_2$ developed all the symptoms of typhoid. They excluded, therefore, the protection effect of the H-antigen.

Tully et al.[141] exposed two chimpanzees to aerosols of strain $Ty_2$. Evidence of infection, manifested by fever and bacteremia, developed in one of them but not in the other. In both animals the H- and O-titers rose. When both animals were rechallenged five months later by the oral route both presented evidence of immunity to this challenge.

It seems, therefore, that the use of the chimpanzee in immunity studies confirmed the observations made in epidemiological studies[10, 19, 96] and in field trials which were organized in different countries and have already been mentioned.[118, 118a, 143, 160, 161]

The active immunization of laboratory animals and finally of human volunteers has shown that the acetone-killed and dried vaccine is in several experiments superior to other types of vaccines, and Cvjetanovic and Uemura[27] have shown that it is stable enough to serve as a reference vaccine. However, there are also reports that other types of vaccine, mainly heated and phenolized vaccines, exhibited high immunizing potency and were able to reduce markedly the typhoid morbidity, as demonstrated by Kheifets,[76] Kheifets et al.,[77] the Polish Typhoid Committee,[118, 118a] and the Yugoslav Typhoid Commission.[160, 161] In all reports published in this matter an important detail is lacking: the serotype of S. typhi prevalent in the endemic area where the vaccination was carried out. It has been reported in the past that in certain areas intermediate VW strains are prevalent, as observed by Felix et al.[40] and Olitzki et al.,[114] which after in vivo passages may become V-types, as observed by Olitzki et al.[114] However, there are reports on W-types as causative agents of epidemics, as shown by Bradley et al.,[19] and from bacillary carriers non-motile O-forms were isolated by Olitzki[104] which were sensitive to agglutination by O-immune sera. It is possible that in areas where heated vaccines were employed successfully, pure O-strains or W-strains were prevalent.

The increase in virulence in vivo, as observed by Olitzki and Godinger[107, 108] and Olitzki and Kaplan,[112] and the high immunogenic potency of acetone vaccines prepared from bacteria grown in vivo shown by Olitzki and Godinger,[108, 109] open new possibilities to increase the potencies of acetone-dried vaccines. Moreover, the observations of Olitzki and Godinger[109] and Olitzki et al.[116] that free Vi-antigen becomes accumulated in vivo, and the successful application of the purified product as immunizing agent or as adjuvant to an acetone-dried bacterial vaccine by Olitzki and Godinger,[109] may open the way to production of vaccines with higher potencies than those existing at the present.

The observation that S. typhi may lose its virulence when becoming auxotrophic opens additional possibilities of employing auxotrophic strains for the preparation of living vaccines, as demonstrated by Bacon et al.,[6-8] Batson et al.,[9] Formal et al.,[46] Herzberg,[65] and Reitman and Iverson.[120]

Many investigations were carried out in order to determine whether typhoid immunity is mainly correlated with antibody production or with an enhanced activity of phagocytes. For these purposes mouse-pathogenic salmonellae, e.g., S. typhimurium or S. enteritidis, were employed. However, it is questionable whether mouse typhoid can serve as an analog for human typhoid. Human typhoid is in the majority of cases a self-limiting process. According to observations Kligler and Bachi[79] made in the preantibiotic era, the case fatality among Jews in Palestine varied between a minimum of 3 per cent observed in 1939 and a maximum of 8.9 per cent observed in 1925.

According to Felix[37] and Olitzki,[103] the initial bacteremia is finally terminated as soon as a sufficient concentration of O-antibodies has been reached in the patient's serum.

Mouse typhoid produced by virulent strains is a highly deleterious disease yielding with relatively small infecting doses a 100 per cent fatality. According to Ushiba et al.[146] the primary clearance of the blood by antibodies is a transitory one and after the breakdown of the reticuloendothelial system a second, and this time fatal bacteremia follows. The results were extremely contradictory. The conclusions drawn by various investigators are as follows:

1. Mice are protected against mouse typhoid by killed vaccines. The appearance of bacteriolytic antibodies is essential for typhoid immunity. The role of IgM antibodies as active bacteriolytic agents in the presence of complement has been emphasized by Herzberg et al.[66] and Kenny and Herzberg.[74]

2. According to Ushiba et al.,[145, 147] mice are protected against mouse typhoid by living vaccines only, never by killed vaccines. The presence of circulating antibodies is irrelevant, as proved by vaccination experiments of Ushiba et al.[145] with attenuated rough strains or by successful vaccination of very young mice, which were still unable to produce antibodies. Typhoid immunity is, therefore, purely an enhancement of cellular activity.

3. According to Ushiba et al.,[144–147] circulating antibodies in mouse typhoid are essential for the primary clearance of the microorganisms from the blood, while the course of the further processes, the limitation or the further extension of the necrotic foci in liver and spleen, is determined solely by the activity of the reticuloendothelial system. The phagocytic activity determines whether the secondary, i.e., the lethal, invasion of the blood will take place or not. Therefore, the survival depends on phagocytic activity only.

Rowley et al.[125] emphasized the importance of the antibodies as opsonizing agents. Free or cell-bound antibodies may be involved as opsonins. The high degree of activity of living vaccines depends, therefore, on the presence of a specific antigen which is present as an active immunizing agent in living bacteria only. Attempts to isolate this active antigen were reported by Jenkin[69] and Jenkin and Rowley.[70, 71] It was also observed that nonmultiplying bacteria do not immunize; an *in vivo* multiplication is necessary, as demonstrated by Ushiba et al.[146] with streptomycin-dependent organisms.

Whether for the enhanced activity of phagocytes a specific immunization with involvement of specific antigens is necessary or not, is questionable. The resistance to mouse typhoid is determined by hereditary constitution of the white cell population, as observed by Oakberg.[101] It is stimulated by immunization with antigenically unrelated salmonellae, as shown by Tanaka et al.[137] and Sato et al.,[129] or by preexisting infections with microorganisms belonging to biologically or antigenically completely unrelated groups, as observed by Elberg et al.,[34] Howard,[67] Howard et al.,[68] and Sato et al.[129]

The significance of the immunization results exerted by transfer of white cells from the immune donor to a nonimmune receiver has been explained by Akiyama,[2] Ushiba et al.,[146] Kobayashi and Ushiba,[85] and Saito et al.[127, 128] as immunity conferred by the transferred phagocytes. A simultaneous transfer of living bacteria or of antigenic particles has also to be taken into account. According to Sterzl and Hrubešova,[135] the immunity is transferred by RNA modified by the presence of the antigen.

Fong et al.[45] induced resistance by transfer of ribosomes and ribosomal RNA. Mackaness and Blanden emphasized the possible role of immunologically committed lymphoid cells which are present in the peripheral blood and in the regional lymph nodes (see Chapter 2), and Turner et al.[142] described the absorption of 19S antibodies by macrophages. According to Mackaness and Blanden, acquired cellular resistance in infected animals is correlated with a faster rate of killing of the infected bacteria and with a higher proportion of macrophages obtained (see Chapter 2).

Blanden, Mackaness, and Collins[16] also emphasized the critical dimension of the bacterial population existing in the host for the development of resistance of mice infected with *S. typhimurium* and challenged with *Listeria monocytogenes*. The resistance depended on the count of salmonellae present in liver and spleen. Variations in resistance were ascribed to inequality of the bacterial population and of the intensity of the antigenic stimulus exerted by it. A similar observation was made by Collins, Mackaness, and Blanden[23] on mice infected with *S. montevideo* and challenged with *S. enteritidis*. Since these organisms were antigenically unrelated also, these differences must be attributed to inequalities in the intensity of the stimulus exerted by microbial populations of different sizes.

The results of metabolic studies of Gershon and Olitzki[57] on white cells derived from normal mice, from mice treated with killed vaccine, and from those infected with living virulent bacteria indicated that there exist basic differences in metabolism caused by infections with living bacteria on the one hand, and by injections of killed bacteria or their isolated antigens on the other hand.

Several metabolic activities of murine phagocytes were more enhanced by living than by acetone-killed *S. typhi*, and the living strain $Ty_2$ was in this respect more active than the nonvirulent strain O901, though more bacteria of the latter were engulfed. Thus the respective oxygen uptakes (control 1.0) after ingestion of $10^{10}$ living $Ty_2$ living O901, acetone-killed $Ty_2$, and acetone-killed 0901 were 4.4, 3.0, 2.4, and 2.6.

The mitochondria of the phagocytes exposed to the same living and acetone-killed bacteria behaved similarly in the presence of succinate. The respective oxygen uptakes (microliters of oxygen per hour per milligram of protein) were 35.1, 22.0, 25.0, and 21.0. The most marked effect was exerted by the living strain $Ty_2$. Phagocytes taken from mice inoculated with the same bacterial antigens showed also striking differences in this succinic dehydrogenase activity (initial value 100): $Ty_2$ produced a biphasic curve— after a two hour decrease to 39, an increase to 230 lasting 20 hours; with living 0901 a half hour decrease was followed by a gradual transient rise to 137. Dead vaccines produced only transient increases not exceeding 155.

The acid phosphatase activity of phagocytes was strongly enhanced by living $Ty_2$ or purified Vi-antigen and less by exposure to living O901 or purified O-antigen. Basic phosphatase was enhanced only by living $Ty_2$. On the other hand, the enhancement effect of O-antigen on esterase activity was greater than that of Vi-antigen.

Summarizing these results, it becomes clear that several enzymatic activities of phagocytes are stimulated by contact with living bacteria, mainly *in vivo* and to a lower extent *in vitro*, and that the antigenic components O and Vi act differently on different enzymatic activities. Therefore the link between these enhanced enzymatic activities and the enhanced intracellular destruction rate should be investigated in the future.

| S. TYPHI EMPLOYED: | PERCENTAGE OF ACTIVE PHAGOCYTES | AVERAGE INGESTED BACTERIA/PMN | O₂ UPTAKE ($\mu$L. $O_2$/HR./$10^7$ PMNS) | ENHANCEMENT OF O₂ UPTAKE (CONTROL = 1.0) |
|---|---|---|---|---|
| Ty₂ living | 46 | 1.4 | 16.2 | 4.4 |
| O901 living | 60 | 2.8 | 11.2 | 3.0 |
| Ty₂ acetone-killed | 30 | 0.5 | 9.0 | 2.4 |
| O901 acetone-killed | 46 | 1.1 | 9.8 | 2.6 |
| None | — | — | 3.8 | 1.0 |

# References

1. Agarwal, S. C. 1964. Colicinogeny in *Salmonella* serotypes in India. Bull. WHO *30:*444–446.
2. Akiyama, T. 1959. Passive transfer of immunity in experimental typhoid by cell suspensions of immunized animals. Jap. J. Bact. *41:*87–93.
3. Arnold, L. 1930. Alterations in the endogenous enteric bacterial flora and microbic permeability of the intestinal wall in relation to the nutritional and meteorological changes. J. Hyg. *29:*82–114.
4. Arnold, L. 1933. The bacterial flora within the stomach and small intestine. The effect of experimental alterations of acid-base balance and of the age of the subject. Amer. J. Med. Sci. *186:*471–479.
5. Arnold, L., and L. Brody. 1927. Influence of "effective temperature" upon bactericidal action of gastro-intestinal tract. Proc. Soc. Exp. Biol. Med. *24:*832–833.
6. Bacon, G. A., T. W. Burrows, and M. Yates. 1950. The effects of biochemical mutation on the virulence of *Bacterium typhosum:* the induction and isolation of mutants. Brit. J. Exp. Path. *31:*703–713.
7. Bacon, G. A., T. W. Burrows, and M. Yates. 1950. The effects of biochemical mutation on the virulence of *Bacterium typhosum:* the virulence of mutants. Brit. J. Exp. Path. *31:*714–724.
8. Bacon, G. A., T. W. Burrows, and M. Yates. 1951. The effects of biochemical mutation on the virulence of *Bacterium typhosum:* the loss of virulence of certain mutants. Brit. J. Exp. Path. *32:*85–96.
9. Batson, H. C., M. Landy, and A. Abrams. 1949. Avirulent isolate of *Salmonella typhosa* 58 (Panama carrier). Public Health Rep. *64:*671–674.
10. Batty Shaw, A., and H. A. F. Mackay. 1951. Double enteric infection (la fièvre typhoïde intriquée). An account of an epidemic. J. Hyg. *49:*299–314.
11. Bergeim, O., A. H. Hanszen, L. Pincussen, and E. Weiss. 1941. Relation of volatile fatty acids and hydrogen sulphide to the intestinal flora. J. Infect. Dis. *69:*155–166.
12. Berger, U. 1952. Zur Frage der antibakteriellen Wirkung des Speichels. Z. Hyg. Infektionskr. *133:*371–397.
13. Berger, U. 1953. Weitere Untersuchungen zur Frage einer antibakteriellen Speichelwirkung. Z. Hyg. Infektionskr. *136:*94–101.
14. Berry, L. J., and D. S. Smythe. 1964. Effects of bacterial endotoxin on metabolism. VII. Enzyme induction and cortisone protection. J. Exp. Med. *120:*721–732.
15. Bhatnagar, S. S. 1935. Phagocytosis of *B. typhosus* in relation to its antigenic structure and to the antibody components of the sensitizing serum. Brit. J. Exp. Path. *16:*375–384.
16. Blanden, R. V., G. B. Mackaness, and F. M. Collins. 1966. Mechanisms of acquired resistance in mouse typhoid. J. Exp. Med. *124:*585–600.
17. Bohnhoff, M., B. L. Drake, and C. P. Miller. 1945. Effect of streptomycin on susceptibility of intestinal tract to experimental *Salmonella* infection. Proc. Soc. Exp. Biol. Med. *86:*132–137.

18. Boros, D. L., and A. L. Olitzki. 1967. The antigenic activity of native and heat-denaturated DNA isolated from *Salmonella typhosa*, strain Ty2. Biochim. Biophys. Acta *138:*532–541.

19. Bradley, W. H., L. W. Evans, and I. Taylor. 1951. A hospital outbreak of typhoid fever. J. Hyg. *49:*324–334.

20. Braude, A. I. 1964. Absorption, distribution, and elimination of endotoxins and their derivates. *In:* Landy, M., and W. Braun (eds.). Bacterial Endotoxins. Rutgers University Press, New Brunswick, N.J., pp. 98–109.

21. Braude, A. L., F. J. Carey, D. Sutherland, and M. Zalesky. 1955. Studies with radioactive endotoxin. II. Correlation of physiologic effects with distribution by rabbits of lethal doses of *E. coli* endotoxin labelled with radioactive sodium chromate. J. Clin. Invest. *34:*858–866.

22. Braude, A. I., M. Zalesky, and H. Douglas. 1958. The mechanism of tolerance to fever. J. Clin. Invest. *37:*880–881.

23. Collins, F. M., G. B. Mackaness, and R. V. Blanden. 1966. Infection-immunity as the basis of resistance to Salmonella infections. J. Exp. Med. *124:*601–619.

24. Craigie, J., and A. Felix. 1947. Typing of typhoid bacilli with Vi-bacteriophage. Suggestions for its standardization. Lancet *1:*823–827.

25. Craigie, J., and C. H. Yen. 1938. The demonstration of types of *B. typhosus* by means of preparation of type II Vi-phage. 2. The stability and epidemiological significance of W-form types of *B. typhosus*. Canad. Public Health J. *29:*484–496.

26. Cvjetanovic, B. B. 1957. Field trial of typhoid vaccines. Amer. J. Public Health *47:*578–581.

27. Cvjetanovic, B., and K. Uemura. 1965. The present status of field and laboratory studies of typhoid and paratyphoid vaccines: with special reference to studies sponsored by the World Health Organization. Bull. WHO *32:*29–36.

28. Dold, H. 1943. Der bakterienantagonistische Anteil an der Keimschaedigenden Wirkung des Speichels (der Mundhoehlenfluessigkeit). Z. Hyg. Infektionskr. *124:*579–596.

29. Dubos, R. J., and W. Schaedler. 1956. Reversible changes in the susceptibility of mice to bacterial infections. I. Changes brought about by injection of pertussis vaccine or of bacterial endotoxin. J. Exp. Med. *104:*53–65.

30. Dubos, R. J., and W. Schaedler. 1958. Effect of dietary proteins and amino-acids on the susceptibility of mice to bacterial infection. J. Exp. Med. *108:*69–81.

31. Dubos, R. J., and W. Schaedler. 1959. Effect of nutrition on the resistance of mice to endotoxin and on the bactericidal power of their tissues. J. Exp. Med. *110:*935–950.

32. Dubos, R. J., and W. Schaedler. 1960. The effect of the intestinal flora on growth rate of mice and on their susceptibility to experimental infection. J. Exp. Med. *111:*407–411.

33. Edsall, G., S. Gaines, M. Landy, W. D. Tigertt, H. Sprinz, R. J. Trapani, A. D. Mandel, and A. S. Benenson. 1960. Studies on infection and immunity in experimental typhoid fever. I. Typhoid fever in chimpanzees orally infected with Salmonella typhosa. J. Exp. Med. *112:*143–166.

34. Elberg, S. S., P. Schneider, and J. Fong. 1957. Cross-immunity between *Brucella melitensis* and *Mycobacterium tuberculosis:* Intracellular behaviour of *Brucella melitensis* in monocytes from vaccinated animals. J. Exp. Med. *106:*545–554.

35. Epidemiological and Vital Statistics Report. 1965. Typhoid and paratyphoid fevers. *18:* 290–297; 1966. Typhoid and paratyphoid fevers. *19:*2–9, 336–343. World Health Organization, Geneva.

36. Erlik, D., and R. Reitler. 1960. Intrahepatic typhoid infection as cause of the carrier state. Lancet *1:*1216–1218.

37. Felix, A. 1924. The qualitative receptor analysis in its application to typhoid fever. J. Immun. *9:*115–192.

38. Felix, A. 1951. The preparation, testing, and standardization of typhoid vaccine. J. Hyg. *49:*268–287.

39. Felix, A., and E. S. Anderson. 1951. The immunizing potency of alcohol-killed and alcohol-preserved typhoid vaccine after storage for ten years. J. Hyg. *49:*288–298.

40. Felix, A., K. S. Krikorian, and R. Reitler. 1935. The occurrence of typhoid bacilli containing Vi-antigen in cases of typhoid fever and of Vi-antibody in their sera. J. Hyg. *35:*421–427.

41. Felix, A., and A. L. Olitzki. 1926. The qualitative receptor analysis. II. Bactericidal serum action and qualitative receptor analysis. J. Immun. *11:*31–80.

42. Fisher, I. L. 1937. Magensaeure und infektioese Darmerkrankungen. Folia Clin. Orient. *1:*284–293.

43. Floyd, T. M., J. R. Baranski, and M. El-Ganani. 1953. Recovery of human enteric pathogens on meat from butcher shops in Cairo, Egypt. J. Infect. Dis. *92:*224–227.

44. Floyd, T. M., and C. M. Blakemore. 1954. Isolation of human enteric pathogens from ready-to-eat meats from butcher shops in Cairo, Egypt. J. Infect. Dis. *94*:30–33.
45. Fong, J., D. Chen, and S. S. Elberg. 1961. Studies of tubercle bacillus-histiocyte relationship. VI. Induction of cellular resistance by ribosomes and ribosomal RNA. J. Exp. Med. *118*:371–386.
46. Formal, S. B., L. S. Baron, and W. Spilman. 1954. Studies on the virulence of a naturally occurring mutant of *Salmonella typhosa*. J. Bact. *68*:117–121.
47. Formal, S. B., G. Dammin, H. Sprinz, D. Kundel, H. Schneider, R. E. Horowitz, and M. Forbes. 1961. Experimental Shigella infections. V. Studies in germ free animals. J. Bact. *82*:284–287.
48. Freter, R. 1956. Experimental enteric Shigella and Vibrio infections in mice and guinea pigs. J. Exp. Med. *104*:411–418.
49. Freter, R. 1956. Copro-antibodies and bacterial antagonism as protective factors in experimental enteric cholera. J. Exp. Med. *104*:419–426.
50. Freter, R. 1962. *In vivo* and *in vitro* antagonism of intestinal bacteria against *Shigella flexneri*. J. Infect. Dis. *110*:38–64.
51. Friedman, D. R., and S. P. Halbert. 1960. Mixed bacterial infections in relation to antibiotic activities. IV. Shigella-Escherichia coli infections. J. Immun. *84*:11–19.
52. Gaines, S., M. Landy, A. D. Mandel, R. J. Trapani, and A. S. Benenson. 1961. Studies on infection and immunity in experimental typhoid fever. III. Effect of prophylactic immunization. J. Exp. Med. *114*:327–342.
53. Gaines, S., J. G. Tully, and W. D. Tigertt. 1960. Studies on infection and immunity in experimental typhoid fever. II. Susceptibility of recovered animals to reexposure. J. Exp. Med. *112*:1023–1036.
54. Gershon, Z. 1965. The effect of different media on viability, metabolism and phagocytic activity of white cells. Production of a bactericidal substance in the course of phagocytosis *in vitro*. Path. Microbiol. *28*:332–356.
55. Gershon, Z., and A. L. Olitzki. 1965. Monocytin, a protecting substance produced by murine monocytes. Proc. Soc. Exp. Biol. Med. *119*:32–36.
56. Gershon, Z., and A. L. Olitzki. 1966. The demonstration of the toxicity of Vi-antigen on cell cultures and suspensions. Arch. Roum. Path. Exp. Microbiol. *25*:475–482.
57. Gershon, Z., and A. L. Olitzki. 1967. The influence of *S. typhi* cells and their O and Vi-antigens, on the metabolism of murine phagocytes. Boll. Ist. Sieroter. Milan. *46*:490–504.
58. Greisman, S. E., T. E. Woodward, R. B. Hornick, and M. J. Snyder. 1961. Role of endotoxin in typhoid fever. Bull. N.Y. Acad. Med. *37*:493–498.
59. Grinnel, F. B. 1932. A study of the dissociation of the Rawlins strain of Bacterium typhosum with special reference to its use in the production of antityphoid vaccine. J. Exp. Med. *56*:907–918.
60. Gruenbaum, A. S. 1904. Some experiments on enterica, scarlet fever, and measles in the chimpanzee. Brit. Med. J. *1*:817–819.
61. Guggenheim, K., and E. Buechler. 1946. Nutrition and resistance to infection. Bactericidal properties and phagocytic activity of peritoneal fluids in rats in various states of deficiency. J. Immun. *54*:349–356.
62. Guggenheim, K., and E. Buechler. 1948. Nutrition and resistance to infection. The effect of quantitative and qualitative protein deficiency on the bactericidal properties and the phagocytic activity of the peritoneal fluid of rats. J. Immun. *58*:133–139.
63. Gulbrandsen, L. F. 1935. Invasion of the body tissues by orally ingested bacteria and the defence mechanism of the gastro-intestinal tract. Amer. J. Hyg. *22*:257–273.
64. Herring, W. B., J. C. Herion, R. I. Walker, and J. G. Palmer. 1963. Distribution and clearance of circulating endotoxin. J. Clin. Invest. *42*:79–87.
65. Herzberg, M. 1962. Living organisms as immunizing agents against experimental salmonellosis in mice. I. Virulence of auxotrophic mutants. J. Infect. Dis. *111*:192–203.
66. Herzberg, M., K. Kenny, and J. B. Robbins. 1966. Non-absorbable rabbit anti-*Salmonella typhimurium* antibody as detected by the complement-mediated bactericidal reaction. J. Bact. *91*:1548–1555.
67. Howard, J. G. 1961. Resistance to infection with *Salmonella paratyphi C* in mice parasitized with a relatively avirulent strain of *Salmonella typhimurium*. Nature *191*: 87–88.
68. Howard, J. G., G. Biozzi, B. Halperin, C. Stiffel, and D. Mouton. 1959. The effect of *Mycobacterium tuberculosis* (B.C.G.) infection on the resistance of mice to bacterial endotoxin and *Salmonella enteritidis* infection. Brit. J. Exp. Path. *40*:281–290.
69. Jenkin, C. R. 1962. An antigenic basis for virulence in strains of *Salmonella typhimurium*. J. Exp. Med. *115*:731–743.
70. Jenkin, C. R., and D. Rowley. 1963. Basis for immunity to typhoid in mice and the question of "cellular immunity." Bact. Rev. *27*:391–404.

71. Jenkin, C. R., and D. Rowley. 1965. Partial purification of the protective antigen of *Salmonella typhimurium* and its distribution amongst various strains of bacteria. Aust. J. Exp. Biol. Med. Sci. *43*:65.

72. Kass, E. H., and M. Finland. 1950. Effect of ACTH on induced fever. New Eng. J. Med. *243*:693–696.

73. Kauffmann, F., and E. Moeller. 1940. A new type of *Salmonella* (*S. ballerup*) with Vi-antigen. J. Hyg. *40*:246–791.

74. Kenny, K., and M. Herzberg. 1967. Early antibody response in mice to either infection or immunization with *Salmonella typhimurium*. J. Bact. *93*:773–778.

75. Kessel, R. W. I., E. Neter, and W. Braun. 1966. Biological activities of the common antigen of Enterobacteriaceae. J. Bact. *91*:465–466.

76. Kheifets, L. B. 1965. Results of the study of typhoid vaccines in four controlled field trials in the U.S.S.R. Bull. WHO *32*:1–14.

77. Kheifets, L. B., V. Salmin, M. Z. Leitman, M. L. Kuz'minova, A. V. Vasil'eva, I. P. Gal'perin, A. M. Slavina, L. D. Zhdanova, O. G. Pletneva, E. Yu. Varsanova, G. M. Ginzburg, N. G. Glayzer, and E. Yu. Mel'nik. 1965. Comparative evaluation of typhoid vaccines prepared by various methods. Fed. Proc. [Transl. Suppl.] *24*:27–30.

78. Kligler, I. J. 1930. Epidemiology of typhoid fever. Observations on the spontaneous seasonal recurrence of paratyphoid epidemics among guinea-pigs. J. Hyg. *29*:146–156.

79. Kligler, I. J., and R. Bachi. 1945. Analysis of the endemicity and epidemicity of typhoid fever in Palestine. Acta Med. Orientalia *4*:243–261.

80. Kligler, I. J., and K. Guggenheim. 1945. The influence of *Salmonella typhimurium* infection in rats on vitamin A metabolism. J. Hyg. *44*:56–60.

81. Kligler, I. J., K. Guggenheim, and E. Henig. 1945. Susceptibility of vitamin A-deficient and starved rats and mice to a peroral infection with *Salmonella typhi-murium*. J. Hyg. *44*:61–66.

82. Kligler, I. J., and A. L. Olitzki. 1929. Relation of external environment to course of a *B. enteritidis* infection in mice. Science *70*:45.

83. Kligler, I. J., and A. L. Olitzki. 1931. The relation of temperature and humidity to the course of a *B. enteritidis* infection in white mice. Amer. J. Hyg. *13*:349–361.

84. Kligler, I. J., and A. L. Olitzki. 1935. The influence of solar irradiation on the susceptibility of mice to an infection with *S. enteritidis*. Amer. J. Hyg. *22*:1–10.

85. Kobayashi, R., and D. Ushiba. 1952. Studies on the immunity of the experimental typhoid. I. A review of experiments carried out in our laboratory during the past twenty years. Keio J. Med. *1*:35–47.

86. Kunin, C. M., M. V. Beard, and N. E. Helmagyi. 1962. Evidence of a common hapten associated with endotoxin fractions of *E. coli* and other Enterobacteriacae. Proc. Soc. Exp. Biol. Med. *111*:160–166.

87. Landy, M. 1958. Observations on the immune response of the mouse to Vi-antigen. Bull. Res. Counc. Israel [Exp. Med.] *7*:77–88.

88. Landy, M., S. Gaines, and H. Sprinz. 1957. Studies on intracerebral typhoid infection in mice. I. Characteristics of the infection. Brit. J. Exp. Path. *38*:15–24.

89. Landy, M., S. Gaines, and H. Sprinz. 1957. Studies on the intracerebral typhoid infection in mice. II. Immunologic factors concerned in protection. Brit. J. Exp. Path. *38*:25–34.

90. Landy, M., R. C. Skarnes, F. S. Rosen, E. J. Trapani, and M. J. Shear. 1957. Inactivation of biologically active ("endotoxic") polysaccharides by fresh human serum. Proc. Soc. Exp. Biol. Med. *96*:744–746.

91. Lassen, H. C. A. 1929. Ueber den Infektionsverlauf nach oraler Verabfolgung von Bac. aertrycke (Breslau) bei Maeusen bei B-vitaminfreier Kost. Z. Immunitaetsforsch. *63*:110–115.

92. Lassen, H. C. A. 1930. Vitamin A deficiency and resistance against a specific infection. Preliminary report. J. Hyg. *30*:300–310.

93. Lassen, H. C. A. 1932. Die Bedeutung der Vitamine fuer den Verlauf von Infektionen. Z. Immunitaetsforsch. *73*:221–239.

94. Lubinski, H. 1928. Beitraege zur Rezeptorenanalyse. I. Die serologischen Beziehungen zwischen Typhus- und Gaertner Bazillen. Zbl. Bakt. [Orig.] *106*:200–209.

95. Mackaness, G. B., and R. V. Blanden. 1967. Cellular Immunity. Progr. Allerg. *11*:89–140. (Reprinted as Chapter 2 in this volume.)

96. Marmion, D. E., G. R. E. Naylor, and I. O. Stewart. 1953. Second attacks of typhoid fever. J. Hyg. *51*:260–267.

97. McDaniels, H. E. 1931. Effect of egg white in oral vaccination against pneumococcus. Proc. Soc. Exp. Biol. Med. *28*:587–588.

98. Melby, J. C., R. H. Egdahl, I. C. Bossenmaier, and W. W. Spink. 1959. Suppression by cortisone of increased serum-transaminase induced by endotoxin. Lancet *1*:441–444.

99. Nedzel, A. J., and L. Arnold. 1931. Influence of egg white upon the absorption on bacteria from the intestinal tract. Proc. Soc. Exp. Biol. Med. *28:*358–360.

100. Nungester, W. J., L. F. Jourdanais, and A. A. Wolf. 1936. The effect of mucin on infections by bacteria. J. Infect. Dis. *59:*11–21.

101. Oakberg, E. F. 1946. Constitution of liver and spleen as a physical basis for resistance to mouse typhoid. J. Infect. Dis. *78:*79–98.

102. Oerskov, J., and O. Moltke. 1928. Studien ueber den Infektionsmechanismus bei verschiedenen Paratyphus—Infektionen an weissen Maeusen. Z. Immunitaetsforsch. *59:*357–405.

103. Olitzki, A. L. 1928. Die Beziehungen zwischen dem Auftreten stabilotropen Agglutinins im Blute von Typhuskranken und dem klinischen Verlaufe des Typhus. Zbl. Bakt. [Orig.] *106:*247–259.

104. Olitzki, A. L. 1928. Die H- and O-Form des Bac. typhosus und ihr Vorkommen bei Erkrankten und Bazillentraegern. Z. Immunitaetsforsch. *55:*445–450.

105. Olitzki, A. L., and Z. Gershon. 1965. Splenocytin, a protective and curative product of murine spleen cells. Communications, Natl. Congr. Med. Microbiol., Bucharest, p. 217–218.

105a. Olitzki, A. L., and Z. Gershon. 1965. Splenocytin, a protective and curative product of murine spleen cells. Path. Microbiol. *28:*704–712.

106. Olitzki, A. L., and D. Godinger. 1962. Studies on soluble antigens of the Salmonella genus with the aid of the agar gel precipitation technique. Boll. Ist. Sieroter. Milan. *41:* 362–376.

107. Olitzki, A. L., and D. Godinger. 1963. Comparative studies on *Salmonella typhi* grown *in vivo* and *in vitro*. I. Virulence, toxicity, production of infection-promoting substances and DPN-ase activity. J. Hyg. *61:*1–20.

108. Olitzki, A. L., and D. Godinger. 1963. Comparative studies on *Salmonella typhi* grown *in vivo* and *in vitro*. III. The immunizing potencies of acetone-killed vaccines prepared from *in vivo-* and *in vitro*-grown bacteria and the immunizing potency of substances isolated from the infected organs. J. Hyg. *61:*353–363.

109. Olitzki, A. L., and D. Godinger. 1965. Accumulation of a soluble antigen in the peritoneal fluid of guinea-pigs infected with *Salmonella typhi*. J. Infect. Dis. *115:*303–311.

110. Olitzki, A. L., D. Godinger, and Z. Gershon. 1964. The uptake of *Salmonella typhi* by phagocytes and its intracellular viability. Path. Microbiol. *27:*175–201.

111. Olitzki, A. L., and N. Grossowicz. 1968. Fundamentals of bacteriology and immunity [Hebrew]. Kiryath Sefer Edit. Jerusalem *2:*51–52.

112. Olitzki, A. L., and O. Kaplan. 1963. Comparative studies on *Salmonella typhi* grown *in vivo* and *in vitro*. II. The effect of extracts from normal and infected organs on the bactericidal serum action on strains grown *in vivo* and *in vitro*. J. Hyg. *61:*21–30.

113. Olitzki, A. L., and Z. Olitzki. 1959. The infection-promoting effect of intermediates of the tricarboxylic acid cycle on pathogenic and nonpathogenic *Enterobacteriaceae*. J. Infect. Dis. *104:*5–12.

114. Olitzki, A. L., Z. Olitzki, and M. Shelubsky. 1945. Types of *Eberthella typhosa* in Palestine. Trans. Roy. Soc. Trop. Med. Hyg. *39:*167–174.

115. Olitzki, A. L., M. Shelubsky, and S. Hestrin. 1946. Pathogenizing effects of different carbohydrates on *Eberthella typhosa*. Proc. Soc. Exp. Biol. Med. *63:*491–496.

116. Olitzki, A. L., D. Sulitzeanu, N. Sharon, and I. Gelernter. 1961. The accumulation of toxic substances in the organs of mice infected with *Salmonella typhosa* and its relation to the failure of chloramphenicol treatment in the final stages of the infection. Harefuah *61:*57–60.

117. Oren, R. 1956. Influence of the route of infection on the infectivity of *Salmonella*. Ph.D. thesis. Hebrew University, Jerusalem.

118. Polish Typhoid Committee. 1965. Evaluation of typhoid vaccines in the laboratory and in a controlled field trial in Poland. Preliminary Report. Bull. WHO *32:*15–27.

118a. Polish Typhoid Committee. 1966. Controlled field trials and laboratory studies on the effectiveness of typhoid vaccines in Poland. Bull. WHO *34:*211–222.

119. Previte, J. J., and L. J. Berry. 1962. The effect of environmental temperature on the host-parasite relationship in mice. J. Infect. Dis. *110:*201–209.

120. Reitman, M., and W. I. Iverson. 1953. The immunizing properties of dihydrostreptomycin dependent *Salmonella typhosa*. In: Welch, H., and F. Marti-Ibanez (eds.) Antibiotic Annual, 1953–1954. Procedings of the Symposium on Antibiotics, Washington, D.C. Med. Encycl. Inc., New York, pp. 604–608.

121. Robbins, M. L., A. M. Somer, and L. W. Parr. 1957. Variation in the antibiotic producing bacterial flora of the human intestinal tract. J. Bact. *74:*377–380.

122. Robertson, E. C. 1929. A study of the effect of various agents, chiefly sunlight, upon susceptibility of rachitic rats to infection. Amer. J. Hyg. *9:*75–96.

123. Robinson, H. J., and A. L. Smith. 1953. The effect of adrenal cortical hormones on experimental infection. Ann. N.Y. Acad. Sci. *56:757–764.*

124. Rouchdi, M. 1938. Sur la récherche de l'antigène Vi chez les bactéries. C. R. Soc. Biol. *128:1024–1026.*

125. Rowley, D., K. J. Turner, and C. R. Jenkin. 1964. The basis for immunity to mouse typhoid. 3. Cellbound antibody. Aust. J. Exp. Biol. Med. Sci. *42:237–248.*

126. Rutenberg, S. H., F. B. Schweinburg, and J. Fine. 1960. In vitro detoxification of bacterial endotoxin by macrophages. J. Exp. Med. *112:801–807.*

127. Saito, K., T. Akiyama, M. Nakano, and D. Ushiba. 1960. Interaction between *Salmonella enteritidis* and tissue cultured macrophages derived from immunized animals. Jap. J. Microbiol. *4:395–407.*

128. Saito, K., M. Nakano, T. Akiyama, and D. Ushiba. 1962. Passive transfer of immunity to typhoid by macrophages. J. Bact. *84:500–507.*

129. Sato, I., T. Tanaka, K. Saito, and S. Mitsuhashi. 1962. Cellular basis of immunity. III. Cross immunity of the mouse mononuclear phagocytes immunized with live vaccine of *Salmonella enteritidis* against *S. typhimurium, S. choleraesuis, E. coli* and*Mycobacterium tuberculosis.* Proc. Jap. Acad. *38:133–138.*

130. Schaedler, R. W., and R. J. Dubos. 1956. Reversible changes in the susceptibility of mice to bacterial infections. II. Changes brought about by nutritional disturbances. J. Exp. Med. *104:67–84.*

131. Schaedler, R. W., and R. J. Dubos. 1962. The faecal flora of various strains of mice bearing on their susceptibility to endotoxin. J. Exp. Med. *115:1149–1160.*

132. Smadel, J., H. L. Ley, and F. H. Diercks. 1951. Treatment of typhoid fever. I. Combined therapy with cortisone and chloramphenicol. Ann. Intern. Med. *34:1–9.*

133. Smith, D. T. 1952. The disturbance of the normal bacterial ecology by the administration of antibiotics with the development of new clinical syndromes. Ann. Intern. Med. *37:1135–1141.*

134. Smith, H. W., and L. G. Chubb. 1957. The effect of feeding different levels of protein concentrates on the susceptibility of chickens to *Salmonella gallinarum* infection. J. Comp. Path. Ther. *67:10–20.*

135. Sterzl, J., and M. Hrubešova. 1956. The transfer of antibody formation by means of nucleoprotein fractions to non-immunized recipients. Folia Biol. (Prague) *2:21–27.*

136. Tal, C., and A. L. Olitzki. 1948. The toxic and antigenic properties of fractions prepared from the complete antigen of *Shigella dysenteriae.* J. Immun. *58:337–348.*

137. Tanaka, T., I. Sato, K. Saito, and S. Mitsuhashi. 1962. Cellular basis of immunity. IV. Cross immunity of the mouse mononuclear phagocytes immunized with live vaccine of *S. choleraesuis* and *S. typhimurium* against the infection with *S. enteritidis.* Proc. Jap. Acad. *38:288–291.*

138. Trapani, R. J., V. S. Waravdekar, M. Landy, and M. J. Shear. 1962. In vitro inactivation of endotoxin by an intracellular agent from rabbit liver. J. Infect. Dis. *110:135–142.*

139. Tully, J. G., S. Gaines, and W. D. Tigertt. 1962. Attempts to induce typhoid fever in chimpanzees with non-Vi strains of *Salmonella typhosa.* J. Infect. Dis. *110:47–54.*

140. Tully, J. G., S. Gaines, and W. D. Tigertt. 1963. Studies on infection and immunity in experimental typhoid fever. IV. Role of H-antigen in protection. J. Infect. Dis. *112:118–124.*

141. Tully, J. G., S. Gaines, and W. D. Tigertt. 1963. Studies on infection and immunity in experimental typhoid fever. V. Respiratory challenge on chimpanzees with *Salmonella typhosa.* J. Infect. Dis. *113:131–138.*

142. Turner, K. J., C. R. Jenkin, and D. Rowley. 1964. The basis for immunity to mouse typhoid. 2. Antibody formation during the carrier state. Aust. J. Exp. Biol. Med. Sci. *42:229–236.*

143. U.K. Department of Technical Co-operation, Typhoid Panel. 1964. A controlled field trial of acetone-dried and inactivated, and heat-phenol-inactivated typhoid vaccines in British Guiana. Bull. WHO *30:631–634.*

144. Ushiba, D., R. Iwahata, K. Saito, T. Akiyama, and M. Yoshioka. 1954. Studies on the immunity of experimental typhoid. III. A comparative study of active and passive immunization against the infection of mice with *Salmonella enteritidis.* Keio J. Med. *3:73–78.*

145. Ushiba, D., K. Saito, T. Akiyama, M. Nakano, T. Sugiyama, and S. Shirono. 1959. Studies on experimental typhoid: bacterial multiplication and host cell response after infection with *Salmonella enteritidis* in mice immunized with live and killed vaccines. Jap. J. Microbiol. *3:231–242.*

146. Ushiba, D., K. Saito, T. Akiyama, and T. Sugiyama. 1959. Studies on infection and immunity in experimental typhoid viewed from the host cell-parasite relationship. *In:* Mechanisms of Infection and Immunity of Cytopathogenic Bacteria (Symposium of

the 11th Kanto Branch Meeting of the Japan Bacteriological Association). Yamamoto Book Store, Tokyo, pp. 81–101.

147. Ushiba, D., M. Yoshioka, R. Iwahata, and R. Yamagata. 1953. Studies on the immunity of experimental typhoid. II. Effects of the immunization with killed vaccines on *Salmonella enteritidis* infection of mice. Keio J. Med. *2:*75–90.

148. Vassiliadas, P., J. Papavassiliou, A. Glaudot, and P. Sartiaux. 1960. Production de colicines chez les salmonella (étude sur 410 souches). Ann. Inst. Pasteur *99:*926–929.

149. Vizir, P. E., and M. Yu. Chebotar'ova. 1963. Changes in capacity of typhoid bacteria for tryptophan synthesis by assimilation of DNA. Fed. Proc. [Transl. Suppl.] *22:* 1022–1024.

150. von Wassermann, A., and P. Sommerfeld. 1915. Experimentelle Untersuchungen ueber die Wirksamkeit der Typhus und Choleraschutzimpfung. Med. Klin. *11:*1307–1309.

151. Walter Reed Army Institute of Research, Division of Immunology. 1963. Preparation of dried acetone-inactivated and heat-phenol-inactivated typhoid vaccines. Bull. WHO *30:*635–646.

152. Walter Reed Army Institute of Research and International Laboratory for Biological Standards, Statens Serum Institute. 1964. Physical and chemical studies of two dried inactivated typhoid vaccines (Vaccines K and L). Bull. WHO *30:*647–652.

153. Webster, L. T. 1923. Microbic virulence and host susceptibility in parathyroid enteritidis infection of white mice. III. The immunity of a surviving population. J. Exp. Med. *39:*129–135.

154. Webster, L. T. 1924. Microbic virulence and host susceptibility in paratyphoid-enteritidis infection of white mice. IV. The effect of selective breeding on host resistance. J. Exp. Med. *39:*879–886.

155. Webster, L. T. 1933. Inherited and acquired factors in resistance to infection; development of resistant and susceptible lines of mice through selective breeding. J. Exp. Med. *57:* 793–817.

156. Welch, H., C. W. Price, and W. A. Randall. 1946. Increase in fatality rate of *E. typhosa* for white mice by streptomycin. J. Amer. Pharm. Assoc. *35:*155–158.

157. Wilson, G. S., and A. A. Miles (eds.) 1964. Topley and Wilson's Principles of Bacteriology and Immunity. 5th ed. Edward Arnold (Publishers) Ltd., London, pp. 1833–1875.

158. Wisseman, C. L., P. Y. Paterson, J. E. Smadel, F. H. Diercks, and H. L. Ley. 1954. Studies on cortisone and antibiotics for prompt control of typhoid fever and scrub typhus. J. Clin. Invest. *33:*246–275.

159. Wiznitzer, T., N. Better, W. Rachlin, A. Atkins, E. D. Frank, and J. Fine. 1960. In vivo detoxification of endotoxin by the reticulo-endothelial system. J. Exp. Med. *112:*1157–1171.

160. Yugoslav Typhoid Commission. 1957. Field and laboratory studies with typhoid vaccines. Bull. WHO *10:*897–910.

161. Yugoslav Typhoid Commission. 1964. A controlled field trial of the effectiveness of acetone-dried and inactivated and heat-phenol-inactivated typhoid vaccines in Yugoslavia. Bull. WHO *30:*623–630.

162. Zeckwer, I. T., and H. Goodell. 1925. Blood sugar studies. I. Rapid alterations in the blood sugar level of rabbits as result of intravenous injections of killed bacteria of various types. J. Exp. Med. *42:*43–56.

# Chapter 15

# MICROBIAL AND HOST FACTORS IN THE PATHOGENESIS OF BRUCELLOSIS

NORMAN B. McCULLOUGH

*Professor of Microbiology and Public Health and
Professor of Medicine, Michigan State University,
East Lansing, Michigan*

Brucellosis is an acute and chronic infectious disease of domestic animals transmissible to man. Its origin is lost in antiquity. Hughes[58] in his classical monograph relates a disease pattern described by Hippocrates as compatible with brucellosis. References to epidemic abortion in domestic animals and concurrent febrile disease in man date back to the third century B.C.[30] Other historical references of more recent vintage are cited by Hughes.[58] Whether any of these instances really denote the existence of brucellosis is, of course, not known. However, shortly after the modern recognition of the disease, it was found to be present in many areas of the world. We may be reasonably certain that the association of organisms of the genus *Brucella* with disease in domestic animals and man is of long duration.

The verifiable history of the disease commences on the Isle of Malta in 1859 with the detailed clinical descriptions of human illness by Marston,[69] who adequately differentiated this disorder from the enteric and other fevers of man. The microbial cause of the disease was established by Bruce in 1887[16] by the isolation of the bacteria from the spleens of patients dying of Mediterranean fever (Malta fever, undulant fever). He described the organism as a micrococcus and named it *Micrococcus melitensis*. Zammit,[103] in 1905, found that the goats of the Isle of Malta were infected and established the role of the goat reservoir in the genesis of the disease in man. The goat is the chief host of *Brucella melitensis* and the infection is found throughout the world wherever the goat plays an important economic role. *B. melitensis* also infects sheep, particularly milking sheep, throughout its range.

The second member of the genus to be recognized (*B. abortus*) was isolated by Bang[3] in 1897 from the abortion products of cows. He described the organism as a bacillus and its relationship to the "Micrococcus melitensis" of Bruce was not recognized until the classical studies of Alice Evans[27] were published in 1918. Shortly afterward, in 1920, the genus *Brucella* was established to accommodate these closely related organisms.[74] The chief host of *B. abortus* is the bovine and the disease is present in all parts of the world.

The third member, *B. suis*, was isolated in 1914 by Traum[100] from the fetuses of aborting sows. Huddleson later differentiated this organism from *B. abortus*.[52] The hog is the chief host of *B. suis*. The infection is common in North America, in parts of South America, and in Europe. It has been reported in Japan and elsewhere.

These three organisms cause very similar disease states in their respective chief hosts, characterized by abortion of pregnant females, very low mortality, relatively low grade or clinically nonapparent infection, localization, and chronicity. We may speculate that through long association with domestic animals genetic or adaptive changes have occurred tending toward a more perfect state of parasitism. All three species are pathogenic for man, who appears less well able to tolerate the infection than do the chief hosts. Although on a statistical basis minor distinctions in the clinical course of brucellosis in man may be made on the basis of the infecting species, such distinction is not possible in the individual case. The nature of brucellosis in animals and man will be considered in greater detail later in this chapter.

In addition to causing similar diseases these organisms exhibit such similar characteristics that they have long presented problems in identification and speciation. The criteria for distinguishing between them are primarily quantitative, so that no single test is adequate for species identification, but rather a battery of tests is necessary. Further, minor variations in characteristics occur within a given species. Often such stable variant strains may be the only, or the principal, representative of that species within a particular geographic area. To accommodate this situation, biotypes have been established within each species.[62, 94] We now recognize nine biotypes of *B. abortus*, four of *B. suis*, and three of *B. melitensis*.

More recently three newly recognized species have joined the genus *Brucella*. *B. neotomae* was isolated from the wood rat (*Neotoma lepida*) of our western states by Stoenner and Lackman[99] in 1957. It is antigenically similar to the previously mentioned organisms, but differs metabolically, in colonial morphology, and in differential infectivity for mice and guinea pigs. It is not known to infect man or domestic animals, although experimental infection has been produced in swine.[4] *B. ovis* was described by Buddle[17] in 1956 and is the causative agent of ram epididymitis. It is antigenically distinct from the smooth forms of the classical *Brucella* species but shares deeper cell antigens of these organisms.[24] The basic nature of the disease produced in sheep and laboratory animals is similar to that of the other brucelloses. In 1966 Carmichael[18, 19] isolated a brucella-like organism from an aborting beagle bitch, which is now recognized as *B. canis*, the causative agent of infectious canine abortion. It also lacks the smooth antigens of the classical *Brucella* species and so far is not known to infect other domestic animals or man.

In this discussion, the terms "classical species" or "principal species" will be used to refer to *B. abortus*, *B. suis*, and *B. melitensis*. The term brucellosis, unqualified, refers to disease produced by one of these species.

## CHARACTERISTICS OF BRUCELLA

A knowledge of the properties and biology of *Brucella* organisms is essential to an understanding of the disease produced and of host responses to the infection.

The *Brucella*[5] are small, aerobic, coccobacillary, gram-negative rods, non-motile, nonspore forming. Appropriate staining reveals a capsule in smooth cultures. Gelatin is not liquefied. Litmus milk is turned alkaline slowly. Carbohydrates are utilized, but in complex media there is usually little discernible fermentative action; acid is produced in simple synthetic media. An increased carbon dioxide tension is required (*B. abortus*) or stimulatory. Thiamine, nicotinic acid (or nicotinamide), and biotin are required by most strains and pantothenic acid is stimulatory. With the addition of these vitamins *Brucella* will grow in simple, chemically defined media containing ammonium sulfate as the nitrogen source, other inorganic salts, and a single organic source of carbon.[70] Glutamic acid (and some other amino acids) can also serve as the sole nitrogen source.[34, 70, 73] No toxins are produced. Catalase and urease are produced. The organisms do not release an abundance of potent cell-damaging enzymes. Theoretically, this array of properties should well serve these organisms for intracellular life, allowing derivation of required nutrients and nutrilites from the cytoplasmic environment, yet minimizing the potential for rapid destruction of either the parasite or the host cell.

The characteristics used in distinguishing the various species and biotypes of *Brucella* are given in Table 1.

As can be seen, the differences between species, and between biotypes within species, are quite minimal, yet significant differences in virulence and in host preference exist.

To test this seeming homogeneity among the classical members of the genus, and to clarify the taxonomic positions of *B. ovis* and *B. canis*, Hoyer and McCullough[49] undertook deoxyribonucleic acid (DNA) homology studies. In reciprocal DNA-agar competition reactions the polynucleotide sequences of the DNAs of type 1 of each of the classical species, *B. abortus*, *B. suis*, and *B. melitensis*, were found to be similar. These reactions did not distinguish between the species. The DNA from *B. neotomae* was as effective a competitor as that from any of the principal species, whereas the DNA from *B. ovis* was less effective. In further studies,[50] using the membrane filter technique and reciprocal competition reactions among the DNAs of *B. suis*, *B. canis*, and *B. ovis*, these investigators reported that the polynucleotide sequences of *B. canis* DNA were similar to those of *B. suis* (and by inference the other classical species) and that *B. canis* should therefore be included in the genus *Brucella*. The DNA of *B. ovis* was a less effective competitor in the *B. suis* and *B. canis* homologous systems than either of the others, but in reciprocal experiments

TABLE 1.  *Differential Characters of the Species and Their Biotypes of the Genus Brucella*

| Species | Bio-type | $CO_2$ req. | $H_2S$* prod. | Thionin a | b | c | Basic Fuchsin b | c | Agglut. sera a | m | Lysis by phage TB | Glutamic Acid | Orni-thine | Ribose | Ly-sine | Most common host reservoir |
|---|---|---|---|---|---|---|---|---|---|---|---|---|---|---|---|---|
| B. meli-tensis | 1 | − | − | − | + | + | + | + | − | + | − | + | − | − | − | Sheep and goats |
|  | 2 | − | − | − | + | + | + | + | + | − | − | + | − | − | − | Sheep and goats |
|  | 3 | − | − | − | + | + | + | + | + | + | − | + | − | − | − | Sheep and goats |
| B. abortus | 1 | +(−)§ | + | − | − | − | + | + | + | − | + | + | − | + | − | Cattle |
|  | 2 | + | + | − | − | − | − | − | + | − | + | + | − | + | − | Cattle |
|  | 3 | +(−) | + | + | + | + | + | + | + | − | + | + | − | + | − | Cattle |
|  | 4 | +(−) | + | − | − | − | + | + | − | + | + | + | − | + | − | Cattle |
|  | 5 | − | − | − | + | + | + | + | − | + | + | + | − | + | − | Cattle |
|  | 6 | − | − or + | − | + | + | + | + | + | − | + | + | − | + | − | Cattle |
|  | 7 | − | − or + | − | + | + | + | + | + | + | + | + | − | + | − | Cattle |
|  | 8 | + | − | − | + | + | + | + | − | + | + | + | − | + | − | Cattle |
|  | 9 | − or + | + | − | + | + | + | + | − | + | + | + | − | + | − | Cattle |
| B. suis | 1 | − | ++ | + | + | + | − | − | + | − | − | −(+) | + | + | + | Swine |
|  | 2 | − | − | − | + | + | − | − | + | − | − | + | + | + | + | Hares and swine |
|  | 3 | − | − | + | + | + | + | + | + | − | − | + | + | + | + | Swine |
|  | 4 | − | − | + | + | + | + | + | + | + | − | + | + | + | + | Reindeer |
| B. neoto-mae | 1 | − | + | − | − | + | − | − | + | − | − | + | − | +or − | − | Desert wood rat |
| B. ovis | 1 | + | − | + | + | + | + | + | − | − | − | + | − | − | − | Sheep |
| B. canis | 1 | − | − | + | + | + | − | − | − | − | − | − | + | + | + | Dogs |

* A trace, or inconsistent production of small amounts, is regarded as negative.
† The following graded concentrations of dyes (obtainable from National Aniline Division, Allied Chemical & Dye Co., New York) are used: a = 1/25,000,   b = 1/50,000,   c = 1/100,000.
‡ Only four substrates for species differentiation are given in the table. It is recommended that 12 substrates be used.[62]
§ Usually positive; negative varieties occur.

the DNAs of *B. suis* and *B. canis* competed equally with that of *B. ovis*. *B. ovis* appears to be a deletion mutant lacking a small portion of the polynucleotide sequences present in the other members of the genus.

Thus, the *Brucella* comprise a very closely related group of organisms as regards DNA homology. This extensive conservation of DNA polynucleotide sequences is remarkable in view of the fact that members of the genus are worldwide in distribution and have been reported in a wide range of animal hosts. It is suggested that the restrictive nature of the intracellular environment may be a factor in minimizing variation among the members of the genus.

# CHARACTERISTICS OF BRUCELLA ASSOCIATED WITH VIRULENCE

## S ⟶ R VARIATION

The phenomenon of S → R variation is commonplace in bacteriology. However, in interpreting experimental work on *Brucella* such variation assumes unusual significance. The first major contribution in this area was made by

Henry.[45] Using oblique reflected light, he described smooth (S), intermediate (I), rough (R), mucoid brown (RB), and smooth-rough (S[R]) colonial types. Full virulence resided only in the S type, the R, RB, and S[R] being avirulent, and the I of reduced virulence. Huddleson,[56] in exhaustive studies, extended these observations, describing additional colonial types for each species and their pathogenic and antigenic qualities. Remarkably, he never noted reversion of a non-S type to an S type. The author, likewise, in studying hundreds of strains of *Brucella*, many of them over a span of years, has never observed reversion, either spontaneous or induced, *in vitro* or *in vivo*, of a non-S type to a virulent S type. In cloned cultures, once virulence has been lost it has not been regained. Non-S types usually outgrow the S type in culture. Unless meticulous attention is given to this point, cultures suitable at the start of an experiment may become unsuitable before the studies are finished. A great deal of the past work on the pathogenicity and immunology of *Brucella* is difficult to evaluate because smooth, fully virulent cultures were not used. Unfortunately, this fault is not confined to the distant past. While most workers distinguish rough and mucoid forms with ease, few employ rigid criteria for defining the S type and distinguishing it from intermediate (SI) types. Unless virulence titrations are presented it is often impossible to be certain that pure S-type cultures were employed.

Intermediate colonial-type cultures have reduced virulence, often considerably reduced. However, the intermediates (SI$_1$) most closely resembling the S type are still fully antigenic when used as antigen for the agglutination test. Cultures further dissociated have changed in antigenicity. Thus, for preparation of agglutinating antigen, S or SI$_1$ types must be used. Two relatively stable SI$_1$ cultures are in wide use: *B. abortus*, strain 19, used for production of live vaccine for immunization of cattle, and *B. abortus*, strain 1119, the standard strain for production of antigen for the agglutination test. These are both of markedly reduced virulence for guinea pigs, requiring from 500,000 to 1 million cells to produce limited infection. The infective dose of many intermediate strains is in the range of several hundred or several thousand cells. When long term random inbred guinea pigs from the National Institutes of Health colony are employed, 10 or fewer S-type cells of the three classical species regularly infect (ID$_{50}$). Such consistent results cannot be obtained with nonstandard animals; however, the ID$_{50}$ still should be small.

The biochemical (or genetic) mechanisms producing the changes represented in the S $\rightarrow$ R dissociation are unknown. Environmental factors *in vitro* have been explored.[12, 86] Low oxygen tension[38] and accumulation of D-alanine[37] have been implicated as factors promoting the suppression of S cells. There appears to be a loss of surface antigens with modification of surface properties. Virulence is not completely lost in a single step, but is reduced. The change from S to SI$_1$, a minimal change, is accompanied by a significant loss of virulence without detectable antigenic change. A knowledge of the biochemical mechanisms operative at this point of the S $\rightarrow$ R change would probably help to explain why this organism is a pathogen.

As a rule *Brucella* isolates recovered from an infected animal or man are of the S type, although I, R, and mucoid types have occasionally been recovered from tissues of naturally infected animals.[56]

A serum factor has been identified in animals susceptible to brucellosis which, when present in culture media, favors the maintenance of the S type by suppressing the growth of rough and mucoid types.[8-11, 13, 21, 22] This activity was not found in sera from vaccinated or infected animals. Thus, whether it plays a role *in vivo* is questionable.

Despite the emphasis on correlation of virulence with the S types of the classical *Brucella* species, *B. ovis* and *B. canis*, which lack the antigens present in smooth virulent cultures of these species, are pathogenic! However, the apparent limited host ranges of these species may be a reflection of the absence of S antigens.

Huddleson and Stahl[53] studied the catalase activity of a range of cultures of determined virulence and found that high catalase activity was correlated with a high degree of virulence. This finding has been adequately confirmed. Within each species, strains exhibiting high catalase activity are also of a high degree of virulence. Comparisons cannot be made between species as their ranges of catalase activity differ considerably. Within a strain it also holds true. As dissociation progresses there is a decrease of both virulence and catalase activity. The biochemical advantage afforded has not been identified, but one may speculate that since the *Brucella* are strict aerobes, catalase may not only protect the organism against peroxide, but perhaps aid in maintaining an appropriate intracellular oxygen tension in the vicinity of the parasite.

The rate of oxidation of glutamic acid has been shown to be inversely related to virulence in *B. abortus* and *B. suis*.[102] In this instance it appears that the permeability of the bacterial cell to glutamic acid is the rate-limiting factor. It has been proposed that a lower rate of glutamate uptake and oxidation might favor prolongation of the host-parasite relationship by sparing both the bacterial and host cell from rapid depletion of this amino acid. However, an easily rationalized link to virulence is not evident.

In addition to the items mentioned there have been a number of other studies directed toward discovery of metabolic attributes of virulence in *Brucella*. The results either have been negative or have little bearing on current concepts. A recent review is available.[102]

INTRACELLULAR LOCALIZATION OF BRUCELLA

*Brucella* is primarily an intracellular parasite. The tissue of predilection is the reticuloendothelial system and in particular the mononuclear phagocytic cells of this system. However, intracellular growth occurs in many other cell types. The first convincing report of the intracellular nature of the infection was made by Theobald Smith.[89] He described the localization of the organism within the epithelial cells of the bovine fetal membrane. Later, Goodpasture and Anderson[38] infected the developing chick embryo and noted that the organism entered and multiplied within the ectodermal epithelial cells as well as within monocytes in the exudate surrounding necrotic foci. Meyer[75] described the intracellular occurrence of *B. suis* in the epithelial cells of the renal tubules of man. The intracellular localization and growth of *Brucella* has since been confirmed by many investigators. Even in the blood, unless there is overwhelming infection, the bacteria are present within leukocytes.[7]

To be sure, after cell destruction and the formation of micro or gross abscesses, or in fulminating infection, extracellular growth also occurs, but the intracellular aspects largely determine the nature and course of the disease.

As discussed in another section, study of the ability of *Brucella* to multiply within mononuclear phagocytes maintained in tissue culture has shed much light on the nature of virulence. Virulent strains have this ability, while avirulent strains do not.

### OTHER MICROBIAL FACTORS

Two other attributes of *Brucella* cells are of concern to us. Tissue hypersensitivity to *Brucella* antigen is a prime characteristic of *Brucella* infections. This is predominantly of the delayed or tuberculin type of hypersensitivity. Dead organisms or fractions thereof rarely produce sensitization (dermal hypersensitivity). Actual multiplication of the organisms within the host (intracellularly?) appears necessary. In the author's laboratory, live, virulent, streptomycin-dependent organisms, unable to multiply, given by repeated injections, failed to engender dermal hypersensitivity in guinea pigs. Many preparations, from whole killed cells to purified fractions, have been used to elicit an intradermal test response. The nucleoprotein fraction[54] is best known. Other protein and lipoprotein fractions of varying degrees of purity elicit the response. A carbohydrate fraction permits detection of immediate reactions associated with specific precipitins in the serum.[6]

Smooth and intermediate types of *Brucella* cells contain a potent endotoxin of the Boivin type.[54] Preparations made from the classical species are of equal toxicity[91] and those made from strains of reduced virulence (*B. abortus*, strain 19) are just as toxic as those from virulent smooth strains. As dissociation progresses, the endotoxin is lost and rough strains are devoid of this material. Neither the ability to sensitize the host nor the endotoxin content appears to be determinant of virulence, although once infection occurs, they both play important roles in the host response.

# HOST REACTIONS

### HUMORAL IMMUNITY

The host responds to *Brucella* infections by elaborating the usual array of antibody activity which can be demonstrated as bactericidins, agglutinins, opsonins, precipitins, and complement-fixing antibody.

Immunization of animals with killed cells stimulates antibody production, but produces little, or insignificant, immunity to challenge with virulent strains. The multiplication of organisms within the host seems essential for induction of serviceable immunity. *B. abortus*, strain 19, an intermediate colonial type of markedly reduced virulence, has been used for many years for calfhood vaccination. It produces a mild limited infection and a serviceable, but far from solid, immunity. It will not protect goats against *B. melitensis*, or swine against *B. suis* infection. In Russia, it is in use for human immunization. The protection afforded appears minimal, requiring annual revaccination. The pathogenicity of this strain for man, together with its limited effectiveness, has precluded its widespread use for human immunization. Elberg[26] developed a strain of *B. melitensis*, a revert from a streptomycin-dependent strain, which is similarly useful in immunization of goats.

There are numerous reports, such as those of Smith et al.[88] and Keppie et al.,[63] of the effectiveness of soluble antigens, chemical fractions, and cell wall preparations in inducing demonstrable immunity in laboratory animals. One should not become too enthusiastic about such reports, even from a theoretical standpoint, until a nonliving preparation is shown to produce serviceable immunity in one of the chief hosts against its preferentially infecting species of *Brucella*.

The molecular types of antibody appearing in brucellosis have been studied most extensively in cattle. In conformity with the pattern expressed in other diseases, macroglobulins (19S, IgM) appear early after infection or vaccination, followed shortly by the appearance of 7S (IgG) antibody which ultimately becomes dominant and may entirely replace the IgM class.[83, 85]

After vaccination with *B. abortus*, strain 19, the 19S component predominated throughout a three month period of study.[84] In some relatively recent cases of naturally infected cattle, IgG has been reported, as well as IgM singly, and IgM and IgA together. In some long standing cases only IgG antibody was exhibited. Agglutinins and complement-fixing activity were present in both the IgM and IgG classes, while the IgA species did not fix complement.[83] A similar distribution of agglutinins and complement-fixing antibody in brucellosis has been reported for human sera.[46]

The prozone phenomenon in the agglutination test occuring in the sera of patients with chronic brucellosis may be partially due to "blocking" antibody.[39] The concept of "blocking" antibody as incomplete antibody able to unite with antigen but not promote agglutination has received a great deal of attention. Adequate coverage of this concept in the *Brucella* antigen-antibody system, as well as in other systems, can be found in the publications of Hall and Manion,[41] Zinneman et al.,[104] and Glenshur et al.[35] Huddleson,[57] working with bovine sera, found that sera could be made to "block" by treatment with ion exchange resins; they could be reactivated by addition of appropriate cations (calcium was more efficient than sodium), or by digestion with trypsin. These changes were accompanied by changes in electrophoretic mobility. The "blocking" phenomenon was ascribed to reversible complexing of normal antibody with a nonantibody globulin.

Precipitins have been reported in association with chronic disease with abscess formation; they are usually absent in acute infections.[36]

The bactericidal activity of serum or plasma is of interest.[40, 55, 59] Serum or plasma from normal animals and man, in the presence of complement, has significant, nonspecific, killing power against *Brucella*. Such activity is also demonstrable during acute brucellosis. In chronic infections, however, a specific inhibitor appears which prevents the lethal activity of antibody plus complement. When such sera are highly diluted or absorbed with *Brucella* antigen, killing activity becomes demonstrable. Increased bactericidal activity also follows immunization of cattle with *B. abortus*, strain 19. This increase in specific bactericidal antibody as a result of infection or immunization undoubtedly plays some role in immunity. Its role is tempered by the specific and nonspecific clearing mechanisms which remove *Brucella* from the blood, and by the induced specific inhibitor in chronic infection.

Specific antibody acting as opsonin is a factor in promoting phagocytosis by both polymorphonuclear leukocytes and fixed phagocytes. *Brucella* are rapidly cleared from the blood of animals with demonstrable antibody. They are not, however, rapidly killed and once sequestered within cells are protected from further bactericidal action of the blood. Such opsonizing activity probably is a factor in promoting the localization of infection.

### CELLULAR IMMUNITY

The controversy over cellular immunity versus humoral immunity has waxed and waned, and has been continued since the days of Metchnikoff. The concept of cellular immunity as a separate immunological mechanism totally independent of humoral factors has gained adherents in recent years. A significant portion of the evidence for this view derives from studies of the behavior of mononuclear phagocytes derived from *Brucella*-infected animals when again confronted with these organisms. The situation is confused by our lack of understanding of the detailed mechanisms involved in delayed allergy and by technical difficulties in determining the behavior of host cells and of intracellular *Brucella* in *in vitro* experiments. The more pertinent research findings bearing on this concept in brucellosis are discussed.

Phagocytosis of *Brucella* by polymorphonuclear leukocytes, particularly in the presence of immune serum, is easily demonstrated. However, the microorganisms are not quickly killed within these cells; *in vitro* at least, many organisms remain viable for several days and are released when the leukocytes disintegrate. The mononuclear phagocytes, the tissue macrophages and fixed phagocytic cells of the reticuloendothelial system, are mainly responsible for the destruction of *Brucella* in both the normal and the immune animal.

Pullinger,[81] in 1936, demonstrated an increased resistance to infection with *B. abortus* in guinea pigs receiving simultaneous inoculation with virulent tubercle bacilli. He suggested that this resistance was nonspecific and due to the extensive mononuclear cellular reaction provoked by the tubercle bacillus. In later work (1938),[82] using *Listeria monocytogenes* to induce a transient cellular reaction, and giving small inocula of *B. abortus* at various intervals in the same extremity of the animals, he demonstrated a similar but transient increased resistance. Employing appropriate histological studies, this resistance was related to the protective action of macrophages in lymphoid tissue which had been mobilized in response to the injection of *L. monocytogenes*. Since the cellular response was transient, the induced resistance waned after a few days. These studies suggested that mobilized macrophages provided a nonspecific increased resistance to *Brucella* infection. Confirmatory reports[44, 77] have appeared, including *in vitro* studies[25] of the resistance of immune monocytes. In the latter instance a nonspecific (?) immune serum factor was necessary for full expression of monocyte resistance.

With the development of tissue culture techniques, more definitive experiments were conducted on the intracellular growth of *Brucella* and on the role of the macrophage (mononuclear phagocytes) in immunity in brucellosis. Holland and Pickett[47] found that smooth *B. abortus* organisms could multiply in chick embryo fibroblasts while nonsmooth forms failed to do so. Using a tissue culture system that allowed mononuclear cells to survive *in vitro* for several days, Pomales-Lebrón and Stinebring[80] studied the ability of smooth *B. abortus* organisms to multiply in peritoneal mononuclear cells removed from normal guinea pigs and those from guinea pigs that had been infected with a virulent strain of *B. abortus* 16 months previously (immune cells). Streptomycin in the culture fluid prevented the growth of extracellular forms but did not inhibit intracellular growth. They found that in cells from normal animals *B. abortus* multiplied abundantly (as much as 100-fold) but produced no obvious cell toxicity until the cells were filled with organisms. Disruption of cells then occurred. The intracellular growth of *B. abortus* was markedly inhibited in cells taken from immune animals. These results were confirmed and extended by Holland and Pickett.[48] Using cells from rats and mice as well as from guinea pigs, these workers found that smooth cultures of all three species of *Brucella* multiplied extensively in normal monocytes, but growth was markedly inhibited in immune monocytes. The addition of fresh, homologous, *Brucella* antiserum to the culture fluid produced no detectable effect on the growth or survival of *Brucella* organisms in either normal or immune cells. Nonsmooth organisms multiplied slightly in normal monocytes but were greatly restricted in immune cells.

In their experiments the latter investigators attempted to distinguish between the roles of delayed hypersensitivity and cellular immunity. Desensitization of immunized guinea pigs prior to harvest of the monocytes did not diminish the ability of the cells to inhibit intracellular growth. Cells taken from animals immunized with living rough *B. suis*, and which exhibited a delayed skin hypersensitivity to smooth *Brucella* antigen, failed to inhibit intracellular growth of either smooth *Brucella* or of the homologous rough strain. Cells from animals immunized with heat-killed organisms also did not inhibit growth. These animals had high seroagglutination titers but skin tests failed to reveal delayed allergy.

They also attempted to test these results *in vivo*. Groups of mice consisting of untreated controls, passively immunized animals, mice immunized with heat-killed *Brucella*, and mice actively immunized with live virulent *B. abortus* were given challenge doses of smooth *B. suis*, mucoid *B. suis*, and *B. abortus*, strain 19. Extracellular growth was controlled by streptomycin treatment (no resistant cultures were recovered). Survival of the challenge strains in the spleens of the mice was determined by quantitative spleen culture 15 days after inoculation. The mice previously immunized with virulent *Brucella* apparently rid their spleens of all three challenge strains whereas the other groups did not differ from the controls.

An interesting observation was made that the intracellular growth of *Brucella* was not inhibited in all cells from immune animals, although it was in most of them. This may partially explain the continued existence of infection in chronic brucellosis. In similar studies[14] it was found that R cells rapidly destroyed the normal monocytes which ingested them even though they did not multiply therein. *B. abortus*, strain 19, failed to multiply in the cells and disintegrated rapidly intracellularly.

Braun et al.[15] also reported that immunization of guinea pigs with killed *B. abortus* failed to confer upon monocytes the ability to prevent intracellular growth of virulent *Brucella*. However, the rate of multiplication was somewhat less than in cells removed from normal animals.

A pertinent observation throughout these experiments (if observed at the proper time intervals) was the evidence of cytotoxicity in immune monocytes upon exposure to *Brucella* antigen. This is suggestive that specific delayed hypersensitivity played a role in some or all of these experiments.

These studies emphasize the role played by the mononuclear phagocytes in immunity in brucellosis. They do not, however, settle the question of "cellular immunity" entirely divorced from humoral factors.[61] The specific cytotoxicity of *Brucella* antigen for cells from immune animals suggests that cell-bound antibody is involved. Further, the presence of antibody-forming cells in the monocyte preparations cannot be excluded. In the author's laboratory, in preparations of seemingly pure monocytes derived from the peritoneal cavity of guinea pigs immunized against egg albumin, antibody production has been demonstrated regularly for periods of two weeks, and occasionally for as long as six weeks. The presence of a few antibody-forming cells could conceivably affect the behavior of the monocyte preparations toward *Brucella*. The presence of streptomycin in the maintenance medium cannot be ignored. Although it does not inhibit the growth of *Brucella* in normal cells, it may well do so in damaged cells, and injury and death of immune monocytes has been a prominent feature in most of these experiments.

We may conclude that correlation of the amount of circulating antibody, and of specific dermal hypersensitivity, with the "cellular immunity" exhibited by monocytes from infected animals, has been reasonably denied. However, hypersensitivity at the cell level, and the presence of cell-bound antibody, or small amounts of free antibody, have not been excluded. Indeed, delayed hypersensitivity of the reacting mononuclear phagocytes appears to be an integral part of cellular immunity. Further, in the systems tested, once developed, cellular immunity seems nonspecific, the cells being as active against heterologous bacteria as against the *Brucella*.

## Effect of Intracellular Growth on Brucella

The question naturally arose of the possible effect on *Brucella* of continued intracellular residence. Stinebring and Kessel[96] cultured *B. abortus* in guinea pig mononuclear phagocytes for 27 continuous passages (terminated by contamination), and in rat (naturally resistant) monocytes for 14 passages (minimal growth). The organism showed no change in the characteristics measured. In subsequent work[97] it was found that *Brucella* cells harvested after intracellular residence in normal guinea pig monocytes showed an increased resistance to the effect of bactericidal bovine serum. However, if incubated in growth medium for a few hours (approximately one generation time), the cells returned to normal sensitivity. When cultured in monocytes from guinea pigs infected for from one to 14 weeks, similar increased resistance occurred. However, there was an irregular tendency for organisms harvested from cells taken from animals infected for seven or more weeks to be more sensitive to the bactericidal action of bovine serum than those grown in cells from normal animals or from animals with shorter duration of infection. In further experiments[98] it was shown that intracellularly grown *Brucella* were not only more resistant to the bactericidal action of normal serum, but were phagocytized more readily and had an enhanced ability to survive and multiply within the phagocytes.

## HYPERSENSITIVITY

The role of specific hypersensitivity in the manifestations of brucellosis in man has received considerable attention. Allergic skin reactions in veterinarians following manual removal of a retained placenta in infected cows are well known.[54] Laboratory workers chronically exposed to *Brucella* antigens often become exceedingly sensitive. Following exposure, particularly by the respiratory route, to nonviable *Brucella* antigens, they may exhibit all the symptomatology of an attack of acute brucellosis. The injection of intradermal test material, or other antigenic preparations, into highly sensitive individuals may result not only in a severe necrotizing local reaction, but in a systemic reaction as well. Cases of "chronic brucellosis" due to *Brucella* allergy have been encountered, and symptoms have ceased when exposure was interrupted. Particularly distressing reactions have developed after accidental injection of *B. abortus*, strain 19, vaccine into hypersensitive individuals.[72]

Spink[93] has emphasized the role of specific allergy in human brucellosis. In four patients accidentally infected with *B. abortus*, strain 19, in whom the incubation periods were definitely known, he observed very short incubation periods in two, who were known to be allergic prior to exposure. The other two did not react to the intradermal test upon admission. He has postulated that, in man, the onset of symptoms may be determined by the development of a state of hypersensitivity.

Although our knowledge on this point is grossly inadequate, hypersensitivity does not appear to play as prominent a role in infected domestic animals as it does in man.

Delayed hypersensitivity to *Brucella* antigens usually develops after one or more weeks of infection. The usual method of demonstrating specific hypersensitivity is to determine the cutaneous reactivity following the intradermal injection of *Brucella* antigen. Brucellergen, a nucleoprotein fraction, is widely used, as are whole killed cell suspensions. The nucleoprotein fraction is well standardized and yields more specific and easier read reactions. The response is entirely similar to that evoked by tuberculin in sensitized subjects.

In recent years attention has been directed toward detecting cellular hypersensitivity by direct confrontation of tissue cells with antigen. A number of interesting observations have been made.

Heilman et al.[42] studied the response of cells in spleen explants from normal and *Brucella* infected guinea pigs maintained in plasma clots and exposed to killed *B. suis* cells. The antigen markedly inhibited the migration of cells from the explants derived from infected animals and there was concurrent evidence of cytoplasmic damage. The macrophages were affected to a greater degree than leukocytes and fibroblasts, but degenerative changes were noted in all these cells. Specific antiserum reduced the toxic effects. In later studies[43] this group of investigators obtained similar results using nucleoprotein fractions (brucellergens) instead of whole *Brucella* cells. The brucellergens of all three principal species specifically retarded cell migration of sensitized cells and produced cytotoxic damage. The macrophage was the most sensitive cell. The reaction was specific and was not prevented by the presence of specific immune serum. Stinebring et al.[95] confirmed the cytotoxic effect of *Brucella* extracts on splenic cells from infected guinea pigs and reported a lack of correlation between tissue sensitivity and dermal sensitivity. Carpenter et al.[20] developed a cytometric assay employing trypsinized spleen cells in tissue culture and a quantitative procedure. They reported that cells from infected animals exposed to *Brucella* antigens evidenced no changes for the first six hours; but after 24 to 48 hours over 80 per cent of the macrophages became detached from the wall of the culture tube and underwent rapid cytolysis.

Darlington and Scherago[23] studied the effect of brucellergen on leukocytes obtained from the "buffy coat" of guinea pig blood. The leukocytes were maintained in plasma clots. Brucellergen (in the strength used) had no effect on leukocytes from normal animals but retarded the migration of cells from animals previously infected with *B. abortus*. The guinea pigs developed positive reactions to the intradermal test with brucellergen one week after infection. However, leukocyte sensitivity did not appear until the fourth week and waned after the eighth week although the intradermal test remained positive.

Delayed hypersensitivity to *Brucella* antigens, then, is a generalized phenomenon with several types of tissue cells partaking in the reaction. One would expect differing degrees of hypersensitivity in different cells and tissues. It is not surprising that there is not strict correlation with the results of the relatively gross intradermal reaction. The marked damage incurred by sensitized cells in the presence of specific antigen is to be noted. It undoubtedly has a bearing on the pathology and symptomatology of brucellosis.

## ENDOTOXIN

The importance of endotoxin in infections due to gram-negative bacteria is well known, although the mechanism of action is unclear.[66] Spink[92] and associates have emphasized the role of endotoxin in human brucellosis. Its action appears entirely comparable to that of other endotoxins. One microgram of *Brucella* endotoxin administered intravenously to a patient with brucellosis caused a rise in temperature to 105°F., severe frontal headache, photophobia, myalgia, and arthralgia. The relative roles of endotoxin and hypersensitivity are difficult to evaluate, if indeed they are mechanistically separable. In any event, we must accord endotoxin a very significant role in the symptomatology of brucellosis.

All serious students of human brucellosis have noted the severe impact of the disease on the nervous system, central and autonomic, functional and affective. The probable role of endotoxin in the genesis of these disorders has been emphasized.[92] One possibility that has not received attention is the possible production of ammonium ion through the action of bacterial urease and a consequent toxic effect on the nervous system. Local inflammatory lesions are known to occur, on occasion, throughout the central nervous system, and there may be a meningoencephalitis during the acute stage of the disease. Evidence of organic brain disease in chronic brucellosis has been presented.[2]

Some confusion has existed concerning the activity of *Brucella* endotoxin since many laboratory animals not previously exposed to *Brucella* antigen do not react as they do to other endotoxins. Lately it has become clear that prior exposure to the organism or its endotoxin is a prerequisite for eliciting the reactions. Studies of the reactivity of cells maintained *in vitro* have considerably clarified the events that follow reexposure of cells to endotoxin.

Cytotoxicity of *Brucella* endotoxin for macrophages depends upon prior sensitization.[65] Cells from infected animals show toxic changes; those from normal animals do not. Cytotoxicity was prevented by prior treatment of immune cells with goat antiguinea pig globulin, suggesting that specific cell-bound antibody plays an essential role in the cytotoxic reaction to endotoxin. Immunization with killed organisms failed to sensitize the cells to endotoxin. Administration of *Brucella* endotoxin together with Freund's adjuvant induced the usual responses to endotoxin upon subsequent dosage (depression of water intake, increase in hemolysin-producing cells in the spleen, enhancement of antibody formation, delayed hypersensitivity).[33]

The protein component of endotoxin appears necessary to induction of reactivity to subsequent exposure.[31, 32]

At the present time it is impossible to deny specific cellular hypersensitivity a role in the effects of *Brucella* endotoxin. In fact, it appears to be an essential part of the mechanism of the reaction. This does not imply that endotoxin does not have some effects not dependent upon cellular hypersensitivity.

### The Granuloma

Although the tissue changes in brucellosis offer aspects in common with those in other infectious diseases, the basic and characteristic reactions are provided by the mononuclear phagocytes and lead to formation of granulomas. The granulomatous nature of brucellosis was first recognized by Fabyan[28] in 1912 in experimentally infected guinea pigs and confirmed by Jaffé.[60] Löffler and Albertini[67] described granulomas in human material and later Albertini and Leberherr[1] reviewed the pathology of brucellosis in detail. Further confirmatory reports have appeared for man[71, 79, 90] and a variety of laboratory animals (monkeys,[51] mice,[29] dogs,[68] rats, and rabbits[76]).

The details of the formation and evolution of the hepatic granuloma following infection with *B. abortus* have been reported by Braude.[7] Employing the mouse for the early stages (six days) and the guinea pig for later stages (up to one year), he followed closely the events occurring in the blood and liver tissue. Presumably this model reflects the development of similar lesions in other tissues.

Following intraperitoneal injection of a massive dose of virulent *Brucella,* the organisms appeared in the blood in 90 minutes. Many of them were within polymorphonuclear leukocytes. After 24 hours, extracellular forms were rarely seen in the blood. Circulating leukocytes and mononuclear cells containing *Brucella* were readily demonstrated for five days. In the liver, after three hours, increasing numbers of parasitized leukocytes were seen in the sinusoids, and later the sinusoids were packed with leukocytes, often in focal aggregations. Some of these groups included one or more Kupffer's cells which also contained organisms. At 24 hours the number of leukocytes was reduced, many of them apparently phagocytized by Kupffer's cells, which now appeared in focal aggregations and contained enormous numbers of *Brucella.* Up to 72 hours the parasitized Kupffer's cells were present in small groups. By 120 hours the cellular aggregates had increased in size and had the typical appearance of granulomas. Two types were seen: one composed almost entirely of epithelioid cells, presumably originating from collections of Kupffer's cells, and the other a mixture of epithelioid cells and polymorphonuclear leukocytes, traced to the original aggregates of polymorphonuclears and Kupffer's cells in the sinusoids. Later the small granulomas fused to form larger lesions, some with central hyaline necrosis. *Brucella* organisms were sparse in these lesions. As the tissue reaction subsided the cellular elements became reduced in numbers and by the end of a year no residuals remained.

In an attempt to determine the role of hypersensitivity in the development of the granulomas, infected guinea pigs were given weekly injections of killed *B. abortus* to render them anergic as judged by the results of the intradermal reaction to brucellergen. This did not affect the development of granulomas. However, the intradermal reaction does not necessarily reflect the hypersensitivity status of the cells involved in the reaction.[95] This evidence cannot be accepted as denying a role for cellular hypersensitivity in the formation of the granuloma.

The details of abscess formation have not been fully clarified. However, it takes but a bit of imagination to envisage the development of an abscess from these same focal collections of parasitized polymorphonuclear leukocytes and mononuclear phagocytes which give rise to the granuloma.

## LOCALIZATION

The sequence of events described by Braude[7] in formation of the hepatic granuloma, together with the propensity of *Brucella* for growth within mononuclear phagocytes, aided by the blood-clearing effect of opsonizing antibody, and potentiated by the reaction of sensitized tissues to *Brucella* antigen, should adequately explain the localization of *Brucella* and the development of localized lesions. Pregnant susceptible animals perhaps provide a special case.

In the chief hosts of the principal species of *Brucella,* during the initial stages of infection, localization in the placenta and fetal products leading to abortion is a prominent feature of brucellosis. Following the observation that erythritol is a stimulant to the growth of *Brucella* organisms, Smith and co-workers[78, 87, 101] demonstrated the presence of erythritol in the bovine placenta and postulated that it played a role in this selective localization. In an extended study,[64] they found that erythritol was also present in the placenta of the sheep, goat, and hog, which are susceptible to brucellar placentitis, and absent in the placenta of humans, rabbit, guinea pig, and rat, which rarely develop this complication. In addition, erythritol was found to be present in the seminal vesicles and testicles of the bull, ram, goat, and boar, tissues similarly prone to the localization of *Brucella* infection.

Although a potentiating role of erythritol in the development of placentitis seems rational from the results of these studies, other factors should not be dismissed. It should be noted that placental localization and abortion is a prominent feature of *B. canis* infection of dogs (at least of the beagle). Whether the placenta of this species contains erythritol is not known. However, *B. canis* has been found not to be stimulated by, or to oxidize, erythritol. Similarly, *B. ovis* in sheep adheres to the characteristic localization of the classical species, yet does not oxidize erythritol, which is present in the placenta of this animal.

## A SPECULATIVE MODEL

Through synthesis of clinical observations and the results of basic studies, we can arrive at a fair understanding of the pathogenesis of brucellosis. A partially speculative model is presented.

Although the *Brucella* are quite resistant to environmental factors and may remain alive outside the host for weeks or months, the most important means of transfer is by direct contact with an infected animal, or its tissues, or with secretions and excretions recently parted from the host. The usual portal of entry is through mucous membranes. In some species the skin may be an important entry route. In exposure by aerosols, or through ingestion of food, entry is mainly through the mucous membranes of the oropharynx and upper respiratory tract. The conjunctivae provide an efficient route of entry.

In susceptible animals, once the bacteria pass the primary barrier, they enter the lymphatics and are transported to the regional lymph nodes, often within polymorphonuclear leukocytes. If entry is by implantation, the initial local cellular response is an accumulation of polymorphonuclear leukocytes which ingest the organisms. If the dosage is massive, a local mononuclear cell response follows. The polymorphonuclear leukocytes are ineffective against the organisms which may actually multiply within them. The bacteria, mostly intracellular, reach the regional lymph nodes. Here the primary contest occurs, the outcome of which determines whether progressive infection develops.

Whether the organisms are transported free or within phagocytes, in the regional lymph nodes multiplication occurs within the fixed and sequestered mononuclear phagocytes. If the organisms are not disposed of and multiply significantly, death of some host cells occurs, with the release of bacteria, and also of nucleoproteins and other cell contents, which stimulates an intense local mononuclear cell proliferation and activation. The bacteria, after growth within cells, are more resistant to the bactericidal action of normal blood, are more readily phagocytized, and are well adapted to an intracellular existence. The destruction of some bacteria and the release of antigenic material activates the antibody-forming mechanism. Specific hypersensitivity of the mononuclear phagocytes develops. Whether this occurs directly or by transfer from sensitized lymphocytes is not known. Later, generalized hypersensitivity develops as a result of migration of cells and dissemination of the stimulus.

From the observed rates of dissemination of *Brucella* throughout the body, the outcome of the contest in the regional lymph nodes is probably determined primarily by the effectiveness of nonspecific mechanisms. If these are unable to dispose of the bacteria, they are transported via the lymphatics and the blood, mainly within polymorphonuclear leukocytes and circulating mononuclear phagocytes.

The details of sequestration of parasitized cells in the liver sinusoids have been presented. Presumably similar events occur in other sites throughout the reticuloendothelial system. The time lapse before dissemination, and the amount of antigenic material released to the circulation during the regional phase of infection, probably determine whether humoral factors and specific hypersensitivity play any role during this period of dissemination and localization. If antibodies are present, their opsonic action would promote phagocytosis. With development of specific hypersensitivity the intensity of the local inflammatory response is increased, with more destruction of both tissue cells and infecting bacteria. At some stage after generalized dissemination, the release of significant amounts of endotoxin, together with other products of inflammation, locally and to the general circulation, provides a strong stimulus to the further generalized development of humoral and cellular immune responses, and ushers in the manifestations of systemic disease. The amount of endotoxin released and the degree of cellular hypersensitivity present are largely responsible for the magnitude of the response.

If the infection progresses beyond the initial stages of generalized dissemination, release of bacteria from necrotic cells occurs, outstripping the phagocytic cell response, and the extracellular multiplication of *Brucella* becomes a prominent feature. Here, specific humoral factors may play a significant role in limiting the infection. Many organisms are exposed to the direct bactericidal action of the blood and body fluids. The opsonic activity of specific antibody promotes phagocytosis and its action may continue intracellularly and contribute to the effectiveness of the nonspecifically acting macrophage. Hypersensitivity of the tissues adds its localizing action. Granulomas have developed, and when nonsuppurating granulomas do not contain the infection, abscesses may form, or extensive tissue invasion and necrosis may occur. Functional derangement due to localized lesions, the effect of endotoxin on sensitized tissues, and the action of other products of inflammation produces clinical disease.

It should be remembered that the intracellular growth of *Brucella* is not confined to the macrophage, but occurs in a variety of cells of ectodermal and mesodermal origin. These cells presumably lack the defensive capabilities of the macrophage. The author has observed gross numbers of intracellular *Brucella* organisms in hepatic parenchymal cells from surgical specimens of human liver.

As the humoral and cellular immune mechanisms bring the infection under control, perhaps aided by the development of endotoxin tolerance, and by partial desensitization of tissues due to an excess of antigen, a predominantly intracellular phase returns. After termination of the infection a relative immunity is present.

If infection is not completely eliminated, an uneasy equilibrium between intracellularly multiplying *Brucella* and the forces of humoral and cellular immunity may result in chronic and relapsing disease. A more likely explanation, in most cases, is that discrete foci of infection persist which are relatively inaccessible to the humoral and cellular defenses. These may be micro and gross abscesses, walled off granulomatous lesions, or foci in cysts and glandular follicles, bone marrow, and so forth which continuously or intermittently release organisms, endotoxin, and other products to the general circulation. Latent infection and long incubation periods in brucellosis may well be due to a balance between the well adapted intracellular organisms and the nonspecific host defenses.

## THE CHALLENGE

Many gaps remain in our understanding of the *Brucella*-host interaction. The basic questions remain unanswered. What properties of the organism allow it to multiply within the cells of the major defense system of the host? An understanding of these properties might partly explain why the organism is a pathogen. Does it produce protective, toxic, or antigenic material intracellularly that is absent, or present only in small amounts, in cultures grown *in vitro?* How does the organism damage and kill a parasitized cell? How does a mononuclear phagocyte destroy the organism? What are the exact details whereby a specifically sensitized cell is damaged and killed by the organism or its antigens? What is "cellular immunity"? These are but a few of the questions that can be asked. The answers might be applicable to many other systems, or point the way to unravel the similarities and differences.

Among the intracellular parasitic bacteria the *Brucella*, by virtue of technical ease of handling and lack of antigenic relationship with other groups of bacteria, are the organisms of choice for investigation of the details of intracellular parasitism, hypersensitivity, endotoxin action, and basic cellular immune responses. An array of species and biotypes, differing in slight degree, is available for study of the factors responsible for host preferences. The techniques of modern molecular genetics offer intriguing possibilities for further application to this group of organisms. In spite of past advances in our knowledge, the genus *Brucella* presents a fertile field for study of a wide variety of basic problems.

# References

1. von Albertini, A., and W. Lieberherr. 1937. Beiträge zur pathologischen Anatomie der Febris undulans Bang. Frankfurt Ztschr. Pathol. *51*:69–97.
2. Apter, N. S., W. C. Halstead, C. W. Eisele, and N. B. McCullough. 1948. Impaired cerebral functions in chronic brucellosis. Am. J. Psychiatry *105*:361–366.
3. Bang, B. 1897. Die Aetiologie des seuchenhaften (infectiosen) Verwerfens. Ztschr. f. Tiermed. *1*:241–278.
4. Beal, G. A., R. E. Lewis, N. B. McCullough, and R. M. Claflin. 1959. Experimental infection of swine with *Brucella neotomae.* Am. J. Vet. Res. *20*:872–875.
5. Bergey's Manual of Determinative Bacteriology, 7th Ed. 1957. p. 404–406. Williams & Wilkins Co., Baltimore.
6. Braude, A. I. 1948. Dermal hypersensitivity in human brucellosis. Staff Meet. Bull. Univ. of Minnesota Hosp. *19*:254–266.
7. Braude, A. I. 1951. Studies in the pathology and pathogenesis of experimental brucellosis. II. The formation of the hepatic granuloma and its evolution. J. Infect. Diseases *89*: 87–94.
8. Braun, W. 1946. Dissociation in *Brucella abortus:* A demonstration of the role of inherent and environmental factors in bacterial variation. J. Bacteriol. *51*:327–349.
9. Braun, W. 1946. The effect of serum upon dissociation in *Brucella abortus:* A demonstration of the role of selective environments in bacterial variation. J. Bacteriol. *52*:243–249.
10. Braun, W. 1949. Studies on bacterial variation and selective environments. I. The nature of the selective serum factor affecting the variation of *Brucella abortus.* J. Bacteriol. *58*:291–297.
11. Braun, W. 1949. Studies on bacterial variation and selective environments. II. The effects of sera from *Brucella*-infected animals and from normal animals of different species upon the variation of *Brucella abortus.* J. Bacteriol. *58*:299–305.
12. Braun, W. 1950. Variation in the genus *Brucella*, p. 26–36. *In* Brucellosis, A Symposium. Am. Assoc. Adv. Sci., Washington, D. C.
13. Braun, W. 1953. Bacterial Genetics, p. 238. W. B. Saunders Co., Philadelphia.
14. Braun, W., A. Pomales-Lebrón, and W. R. Stinebring. 1958. Interactions between mononuclear phagocytes and *Brucella abortus* strains of different virulence. Proc. Soc. Exptl. Biol. Med. *97*:393–397.
15. Braun, W., R. W. I. Kessel, and A. Pomales-Lebrón. 1962. Failure of vaccination with killed brucellae to modify monocyte-bacterium interactions. Proc. Soc. Exptl. Biol. Med. *109*: 875–878.
16. Bruce, D. 1887. Note on the discovery of a micro-organism in Malta fever. Practitioner *39*:161–170.
17. Buddle, M. B. 1956. Studies on *Brucella ovis* (N. Sp.). A cause of genital disease of sheep in New Zealand and Australia. J. Hyg. *54*:351–364.
18. Carmichael, L. E. 1966. Abortions in 200 beagles. J. Am. Vet. Med. Assoc. *149*:1126.
19. Carmichael, L. E., and D. W. Bruner. 1968. Characteristics of a newly recognized species of *Brucella* responsible for infectious canine abortions. Cornell Vet. *58*:579–592.
20. Carpenter, C. M., M. Fukuda, and C. L. Heiskell. 1962. Cytometric assay of toxicity of *Brucella* antigens for sensitized and nonsensitized cells from the guinea pig. J. Exptl. Med. *115*:613–621.
21. Cole, L. J., and W. Braun. 1950. Studies on the chemical nature of a normal plasma factor which suppresses variation of *Brucella abortus.* J. Immunol. *64*:111–122.
22. Cole, L. J. 1950. Purification of the bovine γ-globulin factor which suppresses variation in *Brucella abortus.* J. Immunol. *65*:485–490.
23. Darlington, R. W., and M. Scherago. 1960. The *in vitro* sensitivity to brucellergen of leucocytes from guinea pigs experimentally infected with *Brucella abortus.* J. Infect. Diseases *106*:106–110.
24. Diaz, R., L. M. Jones, and J. B. Wilson. 1968. Antigenic relationship of the Gram-negative organism causing canine abortion to smooth and rough brucellae. J. Bacteriol. *95*: 618–624.
25. Elberg, S. S., P. Schneider, and J. Fong. 1957. Cross-immunity between *Brucella melitensis* and *Mycobacterium tuberculosis:* Intracellular behavior of *Brucella melitensis* in monocytes from vaccinated animals. J. Exptl. Med. *106*:545–554.
26. Elberg, S., and W. K. Faunce. 1957. Immunization against *Brucella* infection. VI. Immunity conferred on goats by a non-dependent mutant from a streptomycin-dependent mutant strain of *Brucella melitensis.* J. Bacteriol. *73*:211–217.
27. Evans, A. C. 1918. Further studies on *Bacterium abortus* and related bacteria. II. A com-

parison of *Bacterium abortus* with *Bacterium bronchisepticus* and with the organism which causes Malta fever. J. Infect. Diseases *22*:581–593.

28. Fabyan, M. 1912. A contribution to the pathogenesis of B. abortus, Bang. II. J. Med. Res. *26*:441–487.

29. Feldman, W. H., and C. Olson. 1935. The pathogenicity of *Brucella abortus* for white mice. J. Infect. Diseases *57*:212–222.

30. Fleming, G. 1871. Animal Plagues, p. 548. Chapman and Hall, London.

31. Freedman, H. H., E. A. Fox, and B. S. Schwartz. 1967. Antibody formation at various times after previous treatment of mice with endotoxins. Proc. Soc. Exptl. Biol. Med. *125*:583–587.

32. Freedman, H. H., E. A. Fox, R. S. Willis, and B. S. Schwartz. 1967. Role of protein component of endotoxin in modification of host reactivity. Proc. Soc. Exptl. Biol. Med. *125*:1316–1320.

33. Freedman, H. H., A. E. Fox, R. S. Miller, and B. S. Schwartz. 1968. Induced sensitization of normal laboratory animals to *Brucella abortus* endotoxin. J. Bacteriol. *95*:286–290.

34. Gerhardt, P., and J. B. Wilson. 1948. The nutrition of brucellae: Growth in simple chemically defined media. J. Bacteriol. *56*:17–24.

35. Glenshur, H., H. H. Zinneman, and W. H. Hall. 1961. Significance of the blocking antibody in experimental brucellosis. J. Immunol. *86*:421–426.

36. Glenshur, H., U. S. Seal, H. H. Zinneman, and W. H. Hall. 1962. Serum precipitins in human and experimental brucellosis. J. Lab. Clin. Med. *59*:220–230.

37. Goodlow, R. J., L. A. Mika, and W. Braun. 1950. The effect of metabolites upon growth and variation of *Brucella abortus*. J. Bacteriol. *60*:291–300.

38. Goodpasture, E. W., and K. Anderson. 1937. The problem of infection as presented by bacterial invasion of the chorio-allantoic membrane of chick embryos. Am. J. Pathol. *13*:149–174.

39. Griffitts, J. J. 1947. Agglutination and an agglutinin-"blocking" property in serums from known cases of brucellosis. U. S. Pub. Health Ser., Public Health Rep. *62*:865–875.

40. Hall, W. H. 1950. The bactericidal action of human blood against *Brucella* and its specific inhibition, p. 87–93. *In* Third Inter-American Congress on Brucellosis, Pan American San. Bur., Washington, D. C.

41. Hall, W. H., and R. E. Manion. 1953. Comparison of the Coombs test with other methods for *Brucella* agglutinins in human serum. J. Clin. Invest. *32*:96–106.

42. Heilman, D. H., D. H. Howard, and C. M. Carpenter. 1958. Tissue culture studies of bacterial allergy in experimental brucellosis. I. The effect of *Brucella suis* whole antigen on cultures of spleen from normal and *Brucella*-infected guinea pigs. J. Exptl. Med. *107*:319–332.

43. Heilman, D. H., E. Rice, D. H. Howard, H. E. Weimer, and C. M. Carpenter. 1960. Tissue culture studies of bacterial allergy in experimental brucellosis. II. The cytotoxicity of nucleoprotein fractions of brucellae. J. Immunol. *85*:258–267.

44. Henderson, D. W., M. C. Lancaster, L. Parkman, and S. Peacock. 1956. The influence of a pre-existing respiratory infection on the course of another superimposed by the respiratory route. Brit. J. Exptl. Pathol. *37*:597–611.

45. Henry, B. S. 1933. Dissociation in the genus *Brucella*. J. Infect. Diseases *52*:374–402.

46. Heremans, J. F., J. P. Vaerman, and C. Vaerman. 1963. Studies on the immune globulins of human serum. II. A study of the distribution of anti-*Brucella* and anti-diphtheria antibody activities among γss-, γIM- and γIA-globulin fractions. J. Immunol. *91*:11–17.

47. Holland, J. J., and M. J. Pickett. 1956. Intracellular behavior of *Brucella* variants in chick embryo cells in tissue culture. Proc. Soc. Exptl. Biol. Med. *93*:476–479.

48. Holland, J. J., and M. J. Pickett. 1958. A cellular basis of immunity in experimental *Brucella* infection. J. Exptl. Med. *108*:343–360.

49. Hoyer, B. H., and N. B. McCullough. 1968. Polynucleotide homologies of *Brucella* deoxyribonucleic acids. J. Bacteriol. *95*:444–448.

50. Hoyer, B. H., and N. B. McCullough. 1968. Homologies of deoxyribonucleic acids from *Brucella ovis*, canine abortion organisms and other *Brucella* species. J. Bacteriol. *96*:1783–1790.

51. Huddleson, I. F., and E. T. Hallman. 1929. The pathogenicity of the species of the genus *Brucella* for monkeys. J. Infect. Diseases *45*:293–303.

52. Huddleson, I. F. 1931. Differentiation of the species of the genus *Brucella*. Am. J. Pub. Health *21*:491–498.

53. Huddleson, I. F., and W. H. Stahl. 1943. Catalase activity of the species of *Brucella* as a criterion of virulence, p. 57–63. *In* Studies in Brucellosis II, Michigan Agr. Exper. Sta., Tech. Bull. No. 182.

54. Huddleson, I. F. 1943. Brucellosis in Man and Animals. The Commonwealth Fund, New York.

55. Huddleson, I. F., E. E. Wood, A. R. Cressman, and G. R. Bennett. 1945. The bactericidal action of bovine blood for *Brucella* and its possible significance. J. Bacteriol. *50:*261–277.

56. Huddleson, I. F. 1952. The dissociation pattern in the species of the genus *Brucella*, p. 7–63. *In* Studies in Brucellosis III, Michigan Agr. Exper. Sta., Mem. No. 6.

57. Huddleson, I. F. 1964. Studies of the nature and activity of blocked agglutinins in *Brucella* antiserums. Am. J. Vet. Res. *25:*315–324.

58. Hughes, M. L. 1897. Mediterranean, Malta, or Undulant Fever. Macmillan and Co., Ltd., London.

59. Irwin, M. R., and D. T. Berman. 1950. Bactericidal tests in brucellosis, p. 85–97. *In* Brucellosis, A Symposium. Am. Assoc. Adv. Sci., Washington, D. C.

60. Jaffé, R. H. 1922. Über die experimentelle Infektion des Meerschweinchens mit dem Bac. melitensis (Bruce) und dem Bac. abortus (Bang). Arch. pathol. Anat. *238:*119–134.

61. Jenkins, C. R., and D. Rowley. 1963. Basis for immunity to typhoid in mice and the question of "cellular immunity." Bacteriol. Rev. *27:*391–404.

62. Jones, L. M. 1967. Report to the international committee on nomenclature of bacteria by the subcommittee on taxonomy of brucellae. Minutes of meeting, July 1966. Intern. J. System. Bacteriol. *17:*371–375.

63. Keppie, J., K. Witt, and H. Smith. 1963. Cross immunization of guinea pigs with products of *Brucella abortus, melitensis* and *suis*. Brit. J. Exptl. Pathol. *44:*84–87.

64. Keppie, J., A. E. Williams, K. Witt, and H. Smith. 1965. The role of erythritol in the tissue localization of the brucellae. Brit. J. Exptl. Pathol. *46:*104–108.

65. Kessel, R. W. I., W. Braun, and O. J. Plescia. 1966. Endotoxin cytotoxicity: Role of cell-associated antibody. Proc. Soc. Exptl. Biol. Med. *121:*449–452.

66. Landy, M., and W. Braun. (ed.). 1964. Bacterial Endotoxin. Rutgers Univ. Press, New Brunswick, N. J.

67. Löffler, W., and A. von Albertini. 1930. Pathologisch-anatomische Befunden bei sogennanten Febris undulans des Menschen. Krankheitsforchung *8:*1–16.

68. Margolis, G., W. D. Forbus, and G. P. Kerby. 1945. The reaction of the reticuloendothelial system in experimental brucellosis in dogs. Am. J. Pathol. *21:*753–768.

69. Marston, J. A. 1861. Report on Fever (Malta). (Great Britain) Army Med. Rept. 3, p. 486–521.

70. McCullough, N. B., and L. A. Dick. 1943. Growth of *Brucella* in a simple chemically defined medium. Proc. Soc. Exptl. Biol. Med. *52:*310–311.

71. McCullough, N. B., and C. W. Eisele. 1951. *Brucella* hepatitis leading to cirrhosis of the liver. Arch. Internal Med. *88:*793–802.

72. McCullough, N. B. 1963. Medical care following accidental injection of *Brucella abortus,* strain 19, in man. J. Am. Vet. Med. Assoc. *143:*617–618.

73. McCullough, W. G., R. C. Mills, E. J. Herbst, W. G. Roessler, and C. R. Brewer. 1947. Studies on the nutritional requirements of *Brucella suis*. J. Bacteriol. *53:*5–15.

74. Meyer, K. F., and E. B. Shaw. 1920. A comparison of the morphologic, cultural and bio-chemical characteristics of *B. abortus* and *B. melitensis*. Studies on the genus *Brucella* nov. gen. I. J. Infect. Diseases *27:*173–184.

75. Meyer, K. F. 1943. Observations on the pathogenesis of undulant fever, p. 439–459. *In* Essays in Biology in Honor of Herbert M. Evans. Univ. of California Press, Berkeley, Calif.

76. Nyka, W. 1948. Estudio histobacteriológica de los lesiones producidas por brucela en animales y hombres, p. 675. *In* Primera Reunión Interamericana de la Brucelosis. Hosp. Gen., Mexico, D. F.

77. Nyka, W. 1956. Enhancement of resistance to tuberculosis in mice experimentally infected with *Brucella abortus*. Am. Rev. Tuberc. Pul. Diseases *73:*251–265.

78. Pearce, J. H., A. E. Williams, P. W. Harris-Smith, R. B. FitzGeorge, and H. Smith. 1962. The chemical basis of the virulence of *Brucella abortus*. II. Erythritol, a constituent of bovine fetal fluids which stimulates the growth of *Br. abortus* in bovine phagocytes. Brit. J. Exptl. Pathol. *43:*31–37.

79. Pedro Pons, A., R. Bacardi Noguera, and R. Alvarez Zamora. 1945. Hídago melitocócico: Estudio histopatológica des mismo, mediante la punción biópsica aspiradora. Med. Clin. *5:*15–20.

80. Pomales-Lebrón, A., and W. R. Stinebring. 1957. Intracellular multiplication of *Brucella abortus* in normal and immune mononuclear phagocytes. Proc. Soc. Exptl. Biol. Med. *94:*78–82.

81. Pullinger, E. J. 1936. The influence of tuberculosis upon the development of *Brucella abortus* infection. J. Hyg. *36:*456–466.

82. Pullinger, E. J. 1938. Induced tissue resistance to *Brucella abortus* infection. J. Pathol. Bacteriol. *47*:413–422.

83. Rice, C. E., J. Tailyour, and D. Cochrane. 1966. Ultracentrifugal studies of sera from cattle vaccinated or naturally infected with *Brucella abortus*. Canadian J. Comp. Med. Vet. Sci. *30*:270–278.

84. Rose, J. E., and M. H. Roepke. 1964. Physicochemical studies on post-vaccinal *Brucella* agglutinins in bovine serum. Am. J. Vet. Res. *25*:325–328.

85. Rose, J. E., G. Lambert, and M. H. Roepke. 1964. Ultracentrifugation and heat-inactivation studies on seroagglutinins of pregnant heifers artificially infected with virulent *Brucella abortus*. Am. J. Vet. Res. *25*:329–332.

86. Sanders, E., and I. F. Huddleson. 1956. The influence of environmental conditions on the growth and dissociation of *Brucella abortus*. Am. J. Vet. Res. *17*:324–330.

87. Smith, H., A. E. Williams, J. H. Pearce, J. Keppie, P. W. Harris-Smith, R. B. FitzGeorge, and K. Witt. 1962. Foetal erythritol: A cause of the localization of *Brucella abortus* in bovine contagious abortion. Nature *193*:47–49.

88. Smith, H., J. Keppie, J. H. Pearce, and K. Witt. 1962. The chemical basis of the virulence of *Brucella abortus*. IV. Immunogenic products from *Brucella abortus* grown *in vivo* and *in vitro*. Brit. J. Exptl. Pathol. *43*:538–548.

89. Smith, T. 1919. A characteristic localization of *Bacillus abortus* in the bovine fetal membranes. J. Exptl. Med. *29*:451–456.

90. Spink, W. W., F. W. Hoffbauer, W. W. Walker, and R. A. Green. 1949. Histopathology of the liver in human brucellosis. J. Lab. Clin. Med. *34*:40–58.

91. Spink, W. W., and D. Anderson. 1954. Experimental studies on the significance of endotoxin in the pathogenesis of brucellosis. J. Clin. Invest. *33*:540–548.

92. Spink, W. W. 1956. The Nature of Brucellosis. Univ. of Minnesota Press, Minneapolis.

93. Spink, W. W. 1957. The significance of bacterial hypersensitivity in human brucellosis: Studies on infection due to strain 19 *Brucella abortus*. Ann. Internal Med. *47*:861–874.

94. Stableforth, A. W., and L. M. Jones. 1963. Report of the subcommittee on taxonomy of the genus *Brucella*. Speciation in the genus *Brucella*. Intern. Bull. Bacteriol. Nomen. Taxon. *13*:145–158.

95. Stinebring, W. R., J. A. Flick, and A. Pomales-Lebrón. 1958. Lack of correlation between skin test and "tissue" sensitivities in guinea pigs infected with *Brucella abortus*. Proc. Soc. Exptl. Biol. Med. *97*:21–23.

96. Stinebring, W. R., and R. Kessel. 1959. Continuous growth of *Brucella abortus* in mononuclear phagocytes of rats and guinea pigs. Proc. Soc. Exptl. Biol. Med. *101*:412–415.

97. Stinebring, W. R., W. Braun, and A. Pomales-Lebrón. 1960. Modified serum resistance of bacteria following intracellular residence. Ann. N. Y. Acad. Sci. *88*:1230–1236.

98. Stinebring, W. R. 1962. Characteristics of intracellularly grown *Brucella abortus*. J. Infect. Diseases *111*:17–24.

99. Stoenner, H. G., and D. B. Lackman. 1957. A new species of *Brucella* isolated from the desert wood rat, *Neotoma lepida*, Thomas. Am. J. Vet. Res. *18*:947–951.

100. Traum, J. 1914. Annual Report of the Chief, Bureau of Animal Industry, U. S. Dept. of Agr. p. 30.

101. Williams, A. E., J. Keppie, and H. Smith. 1962. The chemical basis of the virulence of *Brucella abortus*. III. Foetal erythritol a cause of the localization of *Brucella abortus* in pregnant cows. Brit. J. Exptl. Path. *43*:530–537.

102. Wilson, J. B., and B. L. Dasinger. 1960. Biochemical properties of virulent and avirulent strains of brucellae. Ann. N. Y. Acad. Sci. *88*:1155–1166.

103. Zammit, T. 1905. A preliminary note on the examination of the blood of goats suffering from Mediterranean fever, p. 83. *In* Reports of the Commission on Mediterranean Fever, Part 3. Harrison and Sons, London.

104. Zinneman, H. H., H. Glenshur, and W. H. Hall. 1959. The nature of blocking antibodies in human brucellosis. J. Immunol. *83*:206–212.

# Chapter 16

# SYPHILIS AND THE TREPONEMATOSES

THOMAS B. TURNER

*School of Medicine, Johns Hopkins University, Baltimore, Maryland*

Treponemal microorganisms form but one tiny segment of the biological forces involved in life and health and death. Even in the realm of infectious disease, one might regard them as constituting only a minor problem in comparison with the vast disease potential of the viruses, rickettsias, and other bacteria. Yet from the study of even this small fragment one may fashion a biological model that provides a framework about which one's knowledge, concepts, and hypotheses of the interaction between man and his parasites can be built.

In another context, too, one of the treponemal diseases, syphilis, since its dramatic appearance on the stage of Western civilization as the great pox some 500 years ago, has been so surrounded by historical and sociological overtones that it has acquired a cultural significance beyond that of most diseases. While new facts concerning the history of syphilis are unlikely to emerge, changing biological concepts may lead to new interpretations of old historical observations.

To most mature students of the infectious diseases the survival capabilities of human pathogens are impressive. Since the emergence of vaccines and the advent of the antibiotic drugs, man has triumphed in many battles against his parasites, but there is a lingering sense that maybe the war has yet to be won. So with syphilis and the other treponematoses; even the preeminent position of penicillin as the ultimate in therapeutic agents is being challenged, proof that it is too early to relegate to the category of useless knowledge a better understanding of the basic interrelationship between host and parasite in these diseases.

It is not feasible in this chapter to give supporting data for many of the statements made and conclusions drawn, but guidance will be given in the bibliography to those who wish to pursue some aspect of the overall problem. Much of the basic information on which this chapter rests will be found in the monograph entitled *Biology of the Treponematoses* by Turner and Hollander,[69] which also contains a list of references to data published by the authors, their colleagues, and others. Two other recent publications, one by Willcox and Guthe[74] and the other by Guthe and Idsøe,[30] contain extensive bibliographic material which will be used without repetition here. The references at the end of this chapter will be limited to more recently published work and to a few papers reporting work that provides special substance to the questions discussed in the text.

## THE PROBLEM OF CLASSIFICATION

As a simple working classification of the spirochetes pathogenic for man, three large groups may be recognized: the *Treponema*, the etiological agents of syphilis and syphilis-like disease, together designated the treponematoses; the *Leptospira*, which give rise to Weil's disease and related clinical syndromes; and the *Borrelia*, the etiological agents in the relapsing fever group of diseases. It is worth noting that each of these large groups of spiral microorganisms has distinctive morphological features, specific antigenic qualities, and a characteristic disease picture in man and animals.

There are other spiral microorganisms that are of interest to the biologist and taxonomist, but which appear to be of no medical importance and consequently have not been extensively studied. A few of these appear to be free-living species but the vast majority exist only in intimate contact with an animal host. Some may cause disease in lower forms of life, but most are members of the indigenous microflora of the animal in which they reside, and as such may even play a role in host survival. An example of the latter is the spirochete(s) that comprises the sex ratio factor in species of *Drosophila*; the presence of this microorganism in maternal insects seems to inhibit the production of male progeny.[57]

The spirochetes that are nonpathogenic for mammals vary greatly in size and shape. Some are morphologically similar to the pathogens and are classified in the same genera. Examples of these can be found among the common inhabitants of the mouth and lower bowel. There are, in addition, many other distinctly smaller or larger spirochetes which are not well classified at the present time. It is hoped that eventually the role of these microorganisms in the scheme of things will be better delineated.

The genus *Spirillum*, which, as its name suggests, may have a spiral form, is found in various mammalian species and may produce disease in man (e.g., one form of rat-bite fever). However, spirilla are not classified among the spirochetes, for unlike the latter they possess a rigid cell wall and polar flagella. These bacteria are closely related to the vibrios and as such are basically comma or S shaped. Confusion with spirochetes occurs primarily when these organisms undergo chaining.

Each of the three large groups of spirochetes referred to above contains both species that are pathogenic for man or animals and species that are not. Like most other groups of microorganisms they do not exhibit a high degree of host specificity in terms of their pathogenicity, and the *Treponema, Leptospira,* and *Borrelia* pathogenic for man also have some degree of pathogenicity for a wide variety of animal species. Indeed, as a generalization, infectious agents that are highly pathogenic for one animal usually have some degree of pathogenicity for other hosts including man, and the spectrum in this regard is broader than is generally recognized. *Mycobacterium leprae* and the virus of infectious hepatitis appear to be among the exceptions to this generalization.

For some reason not easy to fathom, the spirochetes and especially the *Treponema* have acquired in medical and microbiological circles an aura of mystery beyond that of most microorganisms. Partly responsible perhaps has been the inability to cultivate pathogenic treponemes on artificial media, thus making their study quite difficult. Moreover, relatively few investigators have given serious attention to the treponematoses in recent years, a situation which may have stemmed from the notion that arsphenamine drugs, and more recently penicillin, provide effective control measures against the spread of these diseases, a rather dubious assumption, as will be seen later.

Because of lack of definitive data, the question of classification of the spirochetes will not be pursued in detail. Suffice it to say that simple morphological characterization serves a utilitarian purpose in that it identifies the major disease-producing group of spirochetes. Within the *Treponema* group further differentiation at present rests largely on the type of disease from which the strain was isolated and on the infectious picture produced in laboratory animals. For further details concerning this problem see *Biology of the Treponematoses.*[69]

It is probable that progress in this area will come through the application of modern techniques of electron microscopy, cytochemistry, and immunochemistry. A committee sponsored by the World Health Organization is now addressing itself to the whole problem of the classification of the spirochetes.

As already pointed out, the spirochetes which give rise to the three major groups of disease, the treponematoses, the leptospiroses, and the relapsing fevers, have few characteristics in common except their spiral form, and even this is distinctively different for each group. The point would scarcely warrant reiteration were it not for the persistent fantasy that continues here and there in contemporary literature that assumes relationships which have not in fact been demonstrated, and which lead to unsupportable conclusions concerning diagnosis and treatment of these diseases in man. Even the ontological thesis proposed by Cockburn,[10] that all spirochetes are descended from a common stem, while attractive, has indeed little fact to support it.

Recognizing that new information may lead to different conclusions, it will serve a useful purpose for the present to keep firmly in mind that these large groups of spirochetal diseases, the treponematoses, the leptospiroses, and the relapsing fevers, seem to have no closer relationship to one another than any one of them has, say, to streptococcal infections. Added to the wealth of bacteriological, immunological, clinical, and epidemiological data bearing on this point is now the evidence from the different reactions of these three groups of spirochetes to the complex spectrum of the antibiotic drugs.


## THE ENIGMA OF CULTIVATION

Despite the great forward movement in medical microbiology in the latter part of the nineteenth century, made possible by the cultivation of many bacteria on artificial media, and the equally great nascent period of the nineteen thirties and forties which led to the cultivation of viruses and rickettsia in fertile eggs and tissue culture, successful cultivation of *T. pallidum* and related pathogenic treponemes has still not been accomplished in a reproducible manner. Apparent success has been reported, promising leads produced, closely related spirochetes tantalizingly cultivated, yet ability to grow disease-producing treponemes *in vitro* eludes us. A valuable bibliography is given by Willcox and Guthe.[74]

Noguchi in 1911 reported the cultivation of *T. pallidum* on artificial media; the validity of his observations is still debated and his claims have not been substantiated. He and others have indeed grown spirochetes which at times bear a close resemblance morphologically to *T. pallidum*, but the cultivated organisms do not invoke infections in laboratory animals, nor do large quantities of the microorganisms evoke an immune response to virulent treponemes in laboratory animals.

The extensive studies on these cultivable strains, which appear to be identical with spirochetes commonly found as saprophytes in the mouth and bowel in man and animals and at times in other locations, have certainly not been without value. It has been shown that the strains flourish in an atmosphere of reduced oxygen tension, that they require for their growth some factor thus far found only in mammalian serum, and that their requirements for minerals, vitamins, and other nutritional factors are complex. Moreover, these cultivable spirochetes have certain antigenic components in common with virulent *T. pallidum*, and the ability to produce large quantities of the material has been useful in the area of serological tests for syphilis. It is assumed that what is learned about the nutritional and other environmental factors affecting the growth of these spirochetes and about their antigenic composition will contribute to a better understanding of disease-producing treponemes, but this assumption thus far contains a larger degree of intelligent hope than of demonstrated relevance.

A number of investigators have approached the problem of cultivation of virulent *T. pallidum* and related treponemes from another direction through the study of factors which promote *survival* of treponemes *in vitro*. Despite the failure to observe actual multiplication, these studies have yielded important by-products.

Thus, Nelson and Steinman[51] showed that *T. pallidum* can be maintained in a motile and virulent state *in vitro* for upwards of 11 days, and the conditions necessary for such survival were further defined by Steinman and Eagle and by Weber.[74] In all these studies with pathogenic treponemes, the experience gained in growing nonvirulent saprophytic spirochetes was very valuable. Two practical applications have been made of the knowledge arising from this work. Most important is the treponemal immobilization test devised by Nelson and Mayer.[52] This test, which will be considered more at length later on, constitutes a major advance in the serological diagnosis of the treponematoses. Also, the ability to maintain virulent treponemes in a viable state *in vitro* for several days has permitted *in vitro* studies of the effectiveness of antibiotics and other spirochetocidal substances, in a preliminary if not a definitive fashion.[19]

So there is on the one hand the ability to isolate and perpetuate *in vitro* many strains of saprophytic spirochetes which have some relationship both morphologically and antigenically to *T. pallidum*. The best known of these strains is the Reiter spirochete,[74] although other strains isolated by different workers, including Noguchi, are available in various laboratories.

On the other hand, flowing likewise from assiduous application of bacteriological knowledge in this area, we have the ability to maintain virulent *T. pallidum* and related treponemes in a viable state *in vitro* for several days, a technique which permits their study in a variety of highly useful ways.

But remaining is this enigma of the cultivation of the causative agent of syphilis and other treponemal diseases. Why has this lonely bastion not fallen to the tremendous scientific advances both before and after *T. pallidum* was discovered? Has it been due to some uniquely complex biological property of the treponeme? Possibly, but one suspects that this property that seems so elusive now, once known will be explainable by already familiar phenomena. Is it due to lack of effort on the part of well qualified scientists? Certainly many able investigators have tried and failed. Could it be that through sheer lack of numbers the chance is more remote of some one among them having a brilliant flash of insight that might illuminate the problem? It is perhaps idle to speculate on these intangibles. Yet the successful cultivation of *T. pallidum* must remain as a major scientific objective. The accomplishment of this objective would in all probability open avenues of approach to the treponematoses that one can hardly foresee today. Like an unscaled mountain peak it stands as a living challenge to each generation so long as it remains unconquered.

While the subject of growth and survival of treponemes is being discussed, mention should be made of the observations of the author[67] in the nineteen thirties that *T. pallidum* would survive for long periods when frozen at the temperature of dry ice (approximately $-76°C.$). It was known at the time that certain viruses could be preserved by freezing and desiccation. Although treponemes would not withstand desiccation, it was observed that they seemed to be relatively undamaged by freezing alone, and thus began the era of deep freezes for the storage of infectious agents. *T. pallidum* has been repeatedly shown to be virulent for rabbits after periods of 10 to 15 years. Suspension in a diluent of 10 per cent glycerin further minimizes damage (Hollander and Nell, 1954). More recently the use of liquid nitrogen at a temperature of $-130°C.$ or below has been shown by Guthe[29] to be simpler and more efficient as a freezing and storage medium for sera, and the method has been applied to the preservation of treponemes by Dr. Paul Hardy in our laboratory and by Dr. A. Vaisman, Institut Alfred Fournier, Paris.

## SELECTED ASPECTS OF PATHOGENESIS

It is the interaction of man with a variety of infectious agents, and the effect of the internal and external environment on both host and parasite, that form the essence of this book and therefore of this chapter on syphilis and related diseases. Directed ultimately to the question are indeed most of the studies on the treponematoses, whether they utilize the techniques of molecular biology or clinical observation, immunochemistry, or epidemiology. But it will be useful in approaching the overall problem to view the host-parasite relationship in a somewhat narrower context, recognizing that from questions raised by the disease in man will likely come the stimulus for further exploration in the clinic and in the laboratory in an effort to illuminate some of the puzzling aspects of these questions.

The slowly evolving course of syphilis in man has been well known since the early sixteenth century: the incubation period of several weeks following infection, the primary lesion with its satellite lymph node enlargement, the generalized or secondary phase, and the tertiary stage of destructive lesions. A parasyphilitic or quaternary stage, as reflected by the development of aortitis, tabes dorsalis, or general paresis, had been fairly well established through clinicoepidemiological observations by the last quarter of the nineteenth century. Only the concept of the latent stage, at least in its present-day biological relationship, was a product of the rapid succession of important discoveries during the first decade of the present century.

Study of the disease in laboratory animals and in man by more sophisticated clinical methods has certainly enlarged our understanding of the biological "succession of the seasons" in syphilis, but the importance of these studies lies less in their details than in the larger conceptual relationship derived from the composite picture they paint. For viewing the total picture of syphilis, and, in a comparative sense, of the other treponematoses, the biological model that can be projected today differs in many rather vital respects from that which would have been conjured up a few decades ago. It is these aspects of the pathogenesis of syphilis to which the next few sections will be devoted. The general course of some of the other treponematoses, such as yaws and pinta, or the natural treponemal infection of rabbits, is well known and will be dealt with here in only a comparative sense.

### ONE DISEASE OR MANY?

For centuries clinical and epidemiological observers have distinguished syphilis and yaws in man as distinct disease entities. Other syndromes which had certain distinguishing features were also recognized and given separate names, such as pinta, bejel, and a host of other names which gained only local currency.

With discovery of the causative treponeme, development of serological tests, and introduction of new therapeutic agents it became obvious that all of these "diseases" had many features in common, to the extent that it seemed reasonable and useful to blanket them under the more inclusive term, treponematoses. But this device is merely a convenience and does not necessarily gainsay the utility of distinguishing different members of the group if indeed they are sufficiently different to warrant it. This latter statement really begs the question, which after all quickly becomes a philosophical one around the question of when in fact may two diseases be said to be different.

A substantial portion of the monograph by Turner and Hollander[69] was devoted not to debating the issue but to presenting data from which the reader could make his own judgments. The basic materials of that study were five strains of treponemes isolated from syphilis patients, supplemented by 14 other strains, from as many syphilis patients; seven strains of treponemes from yaws patients, supplemented by less complete studies on two others; three strains isolated from bejel patients; two from patients with nonvenereally transmitted endemic syphilis; two strains from patients with a treponemal disease called dichuchwa from Bechuanaland; and one strain from a rabbit with naturally occurring *T. cuniculi* infection.

One of the questions asked in our laboratory was a long but essentially simple one: Do strains of treponemes from patients with these various syndromes, when inoculated into animals (mainly rabbits and hamsters) which are being maintained under the same environmental conditions, induce as a group a disease picture which has distinguishing characteristics? The answer to be derived from a mass of accumulated data is: Yes, they do differ as a group, especially the syphilis and the yaws strains.

Reduced to its simplest terms, the yaws strains gave rise to a type of orchitis which was rarely encountered with syphilis strains. Also, the yaws strains usually induced a skin lesion at the site of inoculation in hamsters whereas the syphilis strains failed to do so in all but a small minority of instances, although treponemes could be found in the local lymph nodes in most. Strains from the other syndromes tended to conform more to the yaws pattern than to the syphilis pattern. The one cuniculi strain studied induced a response in the rabbits testes different from either syphilis or yaws, but conformed to the syphilis pattern in hamsters.

It can be stated, therefore, not only that there are recognizable differences between syphilis and yaws in man but that the infecting organism of each disease when perpetuated in laboratory animals under essentially the same environmental conditions produces distinguishing features. It seems reasonable to conclude that these differences reside basically in the treponeme itself.

Armed with these facts, the clinician, the epidemiologist, the microbiologist, or the health administrator may do whatever he finds most useful or most congenial to his personal philosophy of disease. If he wishes to emphasize the similarities, which are abundant, he can use the inclusive term, treponematosis; or, wishing to accentuate the differences for whatever reason, he has ample scientific basis for using the older names.

No convincing evidence is available concerning the factors in the treponeme responsible for these differences. It has been suggested on the basis of simple laboratory observations[69] that the ability of a particular strain of treponeme to produce a mucoid material may play some role in the phenomenon, but this is largely speculative, and the difference may lie in genetic characteristics of a different nature.

## Is T. Pallidum Significantly Modified by Animal Passage?

Experimentalists are not ordinarily deluded into believing that a laboratory animal model of a disease is a faithful reflection of the same infection in man; perhaps the closer the animal to man in the evolutionary scale, e.g., the chimpanzee, the more nearly may it mirror the disease in man. Yet in the study of certain aspects of the host-parasite interaction, it is possible to isolate a particular phenomenon, subject it to repeated testing even in the lower laboratory animals, and thereby justify some degree of extrapolation of the data in terms of the disease in man.

But another haunting question often arises, particularly in the case of strains of organisms long since separated from their natural host, man, to wit: Has the strain been modified by perpetuation in its new host to the extent that experimental results may not be validly transferred from the laboratory model to the natural disease?

In syphilis, there is reassuring evidence on this point from two sources. Much of the experimental work with syphilis has been carried out with the well known Nichols strain of T. pallidum which was isolated by Nichols and Hough in 1912[74] and has been carried in laboratory animals, mainly rabbits, ever since. It so happens, however, that at intervals during this time laboratory accidents have occurred which resulted in the infection of laboratory workers with this strain, and documented instances have been reported in 1913, 1914, 1924, 1952, 1954, 1965, and 1966, the latter by Chacko[6] in whose paper a complete bibliography will be found. Moreover, in 1953 Magnuson and his associates[45] carried out a series of studies in which human volunteers were infected with the Nichols strain.

The sum of all these observations has been that the Nichols strain of T. pallidum remains fully virulent for man and, to the extent observed, the character of the infection in man has not been appreciably altered by prolonged animal passage.

From another direction comes evidence of a different kind. Following discovery of T. pallidum in 1905 investigators have from time to time attempted to establish the infection in laboratory animals, and in the aggregate several hundred isolations have been recorded in the literature. The author and associates, for example, have had occasion to attempt to transfer strains of treponemes from man to laboratory animals over a period of many years. The purposes of these isolations were simply to obtain strains of treponemes from various sources for comparative studies; altogether in excess of 40 strains have been isolated by me or under my immediate supervision. Both from the literature and from my own experience, I am impressed with the comparative ease of establishing infection in rabbits or hamsters from material taken directly from man. In the case of rabbits, in which my experience has been largest, intratesticular inoculation of known treponeme-containing material is followed in the vast majority of instances by the development of an orchitis which in its essential features differs in no way from the one observed on subsequent passages. In other words, the rabbit (and with reservations based on less experience, the hamster too) from the very first is a congenial host for strains of treponemes which have been in their natural host, man, for millennia. Detailed data on the isolation of these strains have been presented elsewhere in another connection.[70]

### NUMBER OF T. PALLIDUM REQUIRED TO INFECT

The earlier studies by Morgan and Vyronis[74] and Magnuson, Eagle, and Fleischman[74] indicated that infection in rabbits could be established with very small numbers of treponemes, so small indeed that with the techniques employed it seemed possible that infection might have been established with one treponeme. Later Magnuson et al.[45] determined the smallest number of organisms of the Nichols strain of *T. pallidum* required to infect 50 per cent of rabbits (the so-called $ID_{50}$ dose) to be 23, with the $ID_{50}$ of the same inoculum for man to be 57. These figures are obviously of the same order of magnitude and indicate the high infectivity for both man and rabbits of treponemes obtained from fresh lesions of rabbits. One can only speculate about the relative infectivity of treponemes from the disease in man but the results of attempted transfers from man to animals suggest that here too only a few organisms are required to infect.[70]

Indeed, little is known about the infecting capabilities of bacteria in general. Whether in an inoculum of, say, 100 organisms all are equally infective and have a concerted effect in establishing infection, or whether in fact only a small proportion of the total number are capable of infecting a new host has not been determined for most species. In syphilis at least it appears that in certain types of material virtually all treponemes have infective capacity. It may be that the role of mucoid material as discussed below is significant in favoring the parasite over the host.

### EVENTS CONCOMITANT WITH THE INCUBATION PERIOD

It is often written that *T. pallidum* cannot penetrate the intact skin, and doubtless this elemental body defense does present a formidable barrier. But such knowledge is of little comfort in view of the frequency of minuscule breaks in the skin and the active motility of treponemes. It is know from experiments in rabbits that virulent *T. pallidum* placed on presumably normal mucous membrane surfaces frequently find their way to the deeper layers of the dermis, beyond the reach of a local treponemicidal material, within 4 hours. Moreover, it seems likely that intact mucous membrane can be breached by *T. pallidum*, but again minute breaks in the membrane may provide the entrance. The point, however, is of little practical importance, except to note that inflamed and injured areas of the skin or mucous membrane present a particularly favorable environment for implantation and multiplication of the treponeme.[8]

The incubation period in syphilis is usually defined as that interval of time elapsing between implantation or inoculation of the organism and appearance of a lesion at that site, this primary lesion being historically labelled "chancre." Both the concept and the clinical observations are valid and useful, but as in other diseases this incubation period is one of considerable biological activity.

For example, a number of different kinds of studies have indicated that *T. pallidum* multiplies in the rabbit at a rate approximating one generation about every 33 hours.[69] Expected, therefore, would be a shortening of the incubation period by about 4 days for each tenfold increase in the number of organisms inoculated, and this in fact can be observed experimentally within fairly narrow limits. Assuming that a certain critical mass of treponemes is required to induce a clinically recognizable lesion, it can be postulated that starting with a single treponeme the longest incubation period should be in the order of 60 days, assuming a straight line logarithm multiplication. While observable incubation periods exceed this figure in some instances, the fact is that in the vast majority of instances most incubation periods in both animals and man are considerably shorter than 60 days. At the other end of the scale, when $10^7$ organisms are injected intradermally in the rabbit, a specific lesion usually develops within 48 to 72 hours. It should be noted that the experiments of Hollander et al.[33] showed that the mere presence of a few treponemes over a long period of time did not lead to the induction of a clinically recognizable lesion. While the foregoing observations were made principally with the Nichols strain, our experience with other strains of *T. pallidum* suggest that this same general pattern obtains. Incubation periods with *T. pertenue* and *T. cuniculi* tend to be longer, but whether this is a reflection of a slower rate of division or of a lesser degree of tissue reaction to the same number of treponemes is not known, although the latter situation seems to be the more likely one.

These studies in rabbits clearly indicate that the duration of the incubation period is primarily a function of the number of *T. pallidum* injected; if inoculation is intradermal, the lesion is easily observed and the incubation period is more accurately determined than when inoculation is at some other less visible site, such as into the testis.

Concomitant with the multiplication of treponemes at the site of inoculation, tissue changes are invoked and these changes, which can be detected in the rabbit within 48 to 72 hours after injection of a small inoculum (500 *T. pallidum*), have the characteristic earmarks of syphilis—lymphocytic infiltration, cuffing of small vessels, and early presence of mucoid material. In other words, although gross tissue changes in the form of a primary lesion may not be recognized for days or weeks, these are but the culmination of progressive tissue changes at the microscopic level which begin during the earliest days of the infection (Rich et al., 1933; Ferris and Turner, 1937; Turner and Hollander, 1957[69]).

One other event of practical import is that from the earliest hours after implantation of *T. pallidum* some treponemes make their way beyond the immediate site of implantation, quickly reach the local lymph nodes and blood, and establish what is in effect a generalized infection. It is probably the active motility of *T. pallidum* which endows it with the capacity to move in tissues, for at times one sees in infected fresh tissue organisms with the most active motility, the spiral form elongating to virtually a straight line as it moves snake-like through the tissues.

Experimentally, *T. pallidum* has been found beyond the local site within minutes after injection, but to what extent the injection itself might force treponemes into lymph and vascular channels is a question. Suffice it to say that even when this factor does not enter the picture, treponemes still move beyond the local site within hours, so that almost from the very beginning syphilis is irrevocably disseminated.[74]

While many of the observations and conclusions just mentioned have been derived from animal experiments, it seems likely that these same events occur in much the same pattern in the natural infection of man. It has been clearly established, as indicated earlier, that *T. pallidum* from patients with early syphilis usually suffer no significant decline in their biological activity when first transferred to a rabbit host, and it seems reasonable to conclude that another nonimmune human host would provide a no less favorable medium. Thus it seems safe to assume that the incubation period in man is largely a product of the number of *T. pallodum* implanted, with associated mild trauma playing some role in providing a favorable local environment. Likewise, therapeutic excision of primary lesions in man, as frequently performed during the last century, revealed that generalized syphilis was not thereby prevented.[7] The frequent failure of local prophylaxis when applied several hours after exposure and the few recognized instances in which syphilis was transmitted by transfusion during the incubation period also indicate that in man syphilis does not long remain a local infection.

## FACTORS INFLUENCING THE SECONDARY OR GENERALIZED STAGE OF SYPHILIS

From the local site of inoculation, treponemes move through lymph channels and eventually through the blood to be widely disseminated throughout the patient's body. While the most common secondary lesions are those of the skin and mucous membrane, clinically recognizable lesions have been observed in almost every structure of the body—lymph nodes, liver, spleen, kidneys, heart, bones, joints, larynx, ocular structures, meninges, and brain. Treponemes have been demonstrated in most of these tissues as well as in various body fluids, e.g., blood, milk, tears, and ostensibly normal cerebrospinal fluid. Recovery of treponemes from most of these same organs can readily be accomplished in the experimental disease in monkeys, rabbits, mice, and other rodents.

Factors that influence the location of generalized lesions in man cannot be defined with any degree of accuracy. Perhaps chance distribution of treponemes may be one; perhaps local tissue temperature is important, for it is known that *T. pallidum* multiplies more readily at a temperature slightly below normal internal body temperature (see below); and doubtless there are other factors of which we are largely ignorant at this time.

In general, skin lesions of the secondary stage tend to be individually smaller than the primary lesion, a phenomenon that can be attributed to the progressive development of immunity.

It seems likely that symptoms such as malaise, low grade fever, arthralgia, and headache arise from direct action of *T. pallidum* on relevant tissues. No evidence of the production of an exotoxin by *T. pallidum* has been adduced; the symptoms mentioned above may be ascribed either to the action of a mild endotoxin or to tissue changes induced by the organism. For, as indicated earlier, one characteristic of the secondary stage of syphilis is the constant presence, often in large numbers, of *T. pallidum* in all lesions, and in many tissues and body fluids in which no gross changes can be recognized.

## What Makes One Strain of Treponeme More Virulent than Another?

Virulence is not easy to define or to measure. The term will be used here to indicate the extent of disease produced by a given number of treponemes of one strain in comparison with that of another. Within this general context it can be observed that certain strains of *T. pallidum* are more virulent than others. Among the many strains the author has worked with, several stand out as being constantly more virulent than most.

For example, among five strains carried through successive rabbit passages for many years in Chesney's laboratory and which were observed personally by me, three (the Nichols and Truffi strains and Strain F) were highly virulent in the sense that they produced extensive lesions upon intracutaneous or intratesticular inoculation, and invoked lesions in the uninoculated testis in a high proportion of animals; huge necrotic lesions involving the scrotum were often observed.

On the other hand, two other strains (Strain C and Strain H) consistently induced a much less extensive local lesion, and metastatic lesions were less frequent and less extensive when they occurred. Likewise, in the many strains isolated by my associates or myself and carried for a number of passages in rabbits these same differential characteristics were noted. The Chicago strain, for example, from the first animal passage has been more virulent in this sense than most of the others isolated, and an occasional strain has been consistently less virulent. It might be added that yaws strains virtually without exception show less tissue change by either intratesticular or intracutaneous inoculation than even the least virulent syphilis strains.

That recognizable differences in virulence of strains occur, therefore, seems well established; the unanswered question is, what factors appear to determine this difference? We have been able to identify only one factor, which if not the cause of the difference is at least fairly consistently identified with it. This is the amount of mucoid material developing in the initial lesion. We have discussed the nature and significance of this material elsewhere.[69] Suffice it to say here that it appears to be hyaluronic acid or some closely related material since it is hydrolyzed by hyaluronidase, and there is further evidence, as yet inconclusive, that this mucoid material is the forerunner of the extremely indurated tissue so characteristic of the typical "hard chancre" in man and of the older initial lesions in rabbits. It is postulated that a sulfating of the hyaluronic acid occurs, to produce chondroitin sulfate, which has been identified in excessive amounts in these indurated lesions.

A further piece of this incompleted puzzle is the fact that injection of cortisone early in the course of experimental syphilis in the rabbit leads to an excessive production of mucoid material, together with a tremendous proliferation of treponemes in the lesion.[69] It is postulated that this hyaluronic acid-like material is produced by the treponeme, rather than by the tissue in response to the treponeme. It has been also suggested that the mucoid substance is in the nature of capsular material. It is known that the action of specific antibody *in vitro* is hastened when hyaluronidase and lysozyme are used,[74] suggesting again that some surface substance that inhibits the action of antibody is thereby removed from the treponeme.

One is enabled therefore to build a hypothesis, however shaky, that the more mucoid material produced by the treponemes of a particular strain, the more virulent the strain, although it must be conceded that the mucoid material could merely accompany virulence and not be an essential part of it.

The presence of this mucoid substance probably serves also to provide an environment more favorable to the treponeme, in that movement is easier, antibody is less accessible to it, and the normal cellular defenses of the tissues are obstructed. Parenthetically, while no clear role has been assigned to phagocytic cells in the defense against treponemal infections, it is too early to assume that their role in treponemal infections is negligible.

## LATE SYPHILIS

Once immunity is well established, treponemes, while present in many tissues, are less abundant and as a rule lesions tend to be smaller. The disease may be clinically asymptomatic for years, a stage referred to as latent syphilis, although such a designation merely indicates the absence of readily detectable signs and symptoms of the disease, and much biological activity may be going on at the microscopic level. For example, Frazier et al.[21] have shown that during the course of latent syphilis in the rabbit treponemes may be shed into the blood at intervals, indicating that *T. pallidum* which are known to be present in various organs must not simply be lying dormant in some microscopic focus. The interesting problem of latency will be referred to later.

## THE GUMMA

A striking feature of syphilis in man, which has no well defined counterpart in experimental syphilis in the rabbit, is the gumma of late syphilis. This is a combined hypertrophic and destructive lesion most frequently involving the skin but which may occur in almost any tissue or organ, especially bone, muscle, liver, and testes. It is characterized histologically by massive infiltration of lymphocytes and endothelial cells, cuffing of arterioles to the point of obliteration, with accompanying tissue death, and paucity of treponemes since they are rarely found by staining, darkfield examination, or infectivity tests. Gummata heal rapidly with antisyphilitic treatment. They may also occur in yaws.

Evidence related to the pathogenesis of the gumma is meagre. Treponemes can usually be found by diligent search, which together with prompt response of the lesion to specific therapy suggests strongly that the gumma develops in direct response to the action of treponemes. As an aside, the prompt response of the gumma to iodides has never been convincingly explained. The proliferative nature of the lesion, which is out of proportion to the number of treponemes, suggests that an element of hypersensitivity is operative, but again evidence on the point is meagre. Suggestive are the observations by the author[66] and by Magnuson et al.[45] that reinoculation of syphilis patients, especially those with late syphilis, with either *T. pertenue* or *T. pallidum* resulted in the development of a proliferative and destructive skin lesion, devoid of detectable treponemes, at the point of inoculation. The observations of Csonka,[69] who used killed *T. pallidum* for intradermal injection, point to the same conclusions.

### Effects of Environmental Temperature

It is firmly established that *T. pallidum in vivo* is sensitive to temperature changes. From observation of the experimental disease in rabbits, it is clear that the treponeme produces lesions more readily in areas where the dermal and subdermal temperature is 35 to 36°C. than in areas approximating "normal" body temperature of the rabbit, which is 37 to 39°C. This phenomenon may be one explanation for the development of extensive orchitis following direct inoculation and for the frequent occurrence of generalized lesions on the extremities, tail, and areas from which fur has been removed. Details of these observations are given elsewhere.[69]

To a limited extent similar temperature effect can be noted in the natural disease of man, although here doubtless the situation is more complex and correlations are more difficult to establish. While the phenomenon may be used to explain the common occurrence of lesions of the extremities and other dermal areas, it can scarcely be evoked to explain the occurrence of perineal condylomata and mucous membrane lesions of the mouth and genital tract, and there is much mystery concerning factors that determine the location of lesions in man.

On the other end of the scale *T. pallidum* is known to be adversely affected in both man and experimental animals by temperatures a few degrees above normal body temperature; hence the physiological basis of hyperthermia in the treatment of syphilis.[3] Little information is available on the mechanism of this temperature effect. It is not known whether the effect is directly upon the treponeme through perhaps some alteration in enzyme activity, or whether some change in activity of tissue components, such as the wandering cells, is the important element.

Regardless of the mechanism of the effect of environmental temperature, among the practical conclusions to be drawn from the observations are, first, that in investigations of the experimental disease environmental temperature can be a significant variable and should be controlled, and, second, since at cool temperatures the treponeme is at an advantage vis-à-vis the host, infectivity tests should always be made in experimental animals maintained at moderately cool temperatures (15 to 18°C.).

In line with the common observations that the experimental disease in rabbits tends to be substantially milder at warm than at cool environmental temperatures, one is led to speculate upon this effect in man if maintained over many generations. Might the observed differences between yaws and syphilis in man be accounted for simply by the long continued effects of environmental temperature? One can only speculate on the question, yet that such an effect might have occurred seems a reasonable supposition. In as yet unpublished experiments by the author and his associates, the Chicago strain of *T. pallidum*, a notably virulent one, was maintained in parallel series of animal passages, one maintained at approximately 15°C., and the other at approximately 30°C. While the disease picture in the warm-room animals was consistently milder than its cold-room counterpart, after 9 years the former substrain when inoculated in rabbits maintained at cool temperatures behaved just as did the cold-room substrain; in other words, there seemed to be no reversion to the yaws type. Reversions in the opposite direction have been noted[69] and will be referred to later.

### HORMONES

The effect of the corticosteroids on the course of experimental syphilis has been reviewed above as well as elsewhere.[69] Suffice it to say that these hormones have a profound effect, with results similar to those observed in many other infectious diseases.

Sex-related hormones also have a significant effect on the experimental disease, as shown by Magnuson, Rosenau, and Greenberg,[44] among others, although it seems fair to say that these hormones have never been tested under the optimal experimental conditions that are available today. In general, administration of female hormones tends to make the disease milder, and male hormones, more severe.

## CHANGING CONCEPTS OF IMMUNITY IN SYPHILIS

Since the discovery of *T. pallidum* in 1905, concepts of immunity in syphilis have undergone three fairly clear-cut stages, each successively current for about two decades. Even before that eventful period, however, it had been firmly established on the basis of autoinoculation and reinoculation experiments in man, as well as from epidemiological observations, that an individual with syphilis was largely free from the risk of a second full-blown attack, and various "laws," such as Colles' and Profeta's, having to do with the immunity to syphilis of mother and father and child under various circumstances, had already been promulgated.[7]

When Ehrlich developed the arsephenamines for the treatment of syphilis in 1910,[30] the experimental syphilologist was handed a tool which few of his confreres working with other infectious agents possessed, namely, a means whereby the infection could presumably be completely eliminated in both man and animals. Thus for the first time the experimentalist and indeed the clinician could study a given host in which syphilitic infection, once present, could with reasonable certainty be assumed to have been eliminated. While this basic assumption has now been challenged, even as to the therapeutic efficacy of penicillin, it is too early to discard all the important studies that were predicated on the notion that the infection had been eliminated.

To oversimplify, the earlier experiments, principally those of the German investigators, showed that reinoculation in both man and animals with untreated disease usually failed to produce a lesion, whereas following curative treatment a second inoculation was often successful. From these observations came the concept of *Infektion-Immunität:* if syphilitic infection remains the host is immune, whereas if it is eliminated the host is susceptible to a second infection. Exceptions to this general rule were noted but were explained away by assuming that the first infection had in fact not been eliminated by therapy.

Chesney, assisted by various colleagues, conducted a series of long and carefully conceived experiments in rabbits,[7] and developed from these the first evidence of the relatively slow buildup of immunity in syphilis. This phenomenon, until then not fully appreciated, underlay some of the erroneous interpretation of the earlier workers. Chesney showed, for example, that in rabbits reinfection immunity increased progressively during the initial three months of infection, and if curative therapy was initiated at various times in this period the animals could be left with varying degrees of resistance.

Once immunity was fully developed it persisted in the absence of infection for a long time and usually to the end of the animal's life. Again, discussion revolved around the question of whether or not the first infection had in fact been eliminated by the arsenical drugs, but the weight of evidence indicated that it had.

From these studies, which were widely confirmed, came the concept of *Echte-Immunität* ("true immunity"), as opposed to *Infektion-Immunität.* In other words, once the host tissue had been adequately exposed to the antigenic stimulus of the treponeme, the immune reaction persisted after elimination of the original stimulus. It is rather curious in retrospect how little impact this debate seems to have had on the concept of immunity in general, for it seems to have been accepted that Chesney's concept merely brought the situation in syphilis in line with that in other infections; even in the prepenicillin era it was assumed that in many diseases immunity persisted long after the antigenic stimulus was no longer present. This certainly seems to be the case in respect to some of the toxins, notably tetanus, and while it is assumed that the well demonstrated long lasting immunity in some of the virus diseases persists for years after the virus is no longer present, the absence of the infectious agent in these instances is often difficult to prove beyond a reasonable doubt.

It should be noted that Chesney fully perceived the quantitative nature of immunity in syphilis, as well as its slow development. In some instances immunity is of very high degree, in which the host is solidly resistant not only to the induction of new lesions but to establishment of asymptomatic infection as well, whereas in other instances it is of a lower order of effectiveness.

Another important concept promulgated during the fourth and fifth decades of this century was that immunity in syphilis was a "tissue immunity," as opposed to a "humoral immunity," since no evidence of the presence of circulating antibodies could be adduced; it early became clear that the presence of antibodies active in the Wassermann test and related reactions did not correlate with the presence of immunity, a subject which will be referred to later.

The term tissue immunity has always been rather loosely applied and has been subject to various interpretations. Used in its original sense, it usually meant simply that the animal or human subject was refractory to inoculation of an infectious agent in the absence of demonstrable circulating antibody. The term cellular resistance, a more precise one, is now in current use but a good deal of confusion persists. This whole subject has recently been reviewed by Mackaness and by Good (Chapters 2 to 4) and will not be pursued in detail here. These authors point out that the term cellular immunity has been used to connote what appears at first to be two different phenomena.

In the one, the host's mononuclear phagocytes show increased destructive capacity for ingested organisms, a form of immunity which can be transferred with cells but not with serum. The evidence indicates that small amounts of antibody are present on these wandering macrophagic cells, whether through actually being produced by the cell or through adherence to the cell after being produced at some other site. The situation is further complicated by the observations of Mackaness and his associates that cells initially stimulated by *Mycobacterium tuberculosis* also acquired enhanced capacity to inactivate intracellularly apparently unrelated organisms such as the listeria, brucellae, and salmonellae. In other words, this type of cellular immunity is evoked by an ostensibly specific immunological reaction, but may be nonspecific in its antimicrobial effects.

The second meaning of the term cellular immunity has been applied to the rejection phenomenon in transplanted tissue. Mackaness and Blanden, however, suggest that the two phenomena may be more closely related immunologically than might appear on the surface, and their review is concerned to a considerable extent with that aspect of the problem. There seems no doubt, therefore, that antibody in one form or another enters into the mechanism of antitissue immunity. Whether this is through cells acting as passive vectors of antibody, especially by the adherence of antibody to the surface of monocytes and macrophages, or whether through circulating lymphocytes which actually manufacture antibody after proper stimulus, is not certain at this time.

No convincing evidence has been adduced to show that treponemes are actively phagocytized, yet it does seem clear that in the immune animal treponemes are in a sense immobilized or held *in situ* or at least rendered incapable of producing a lesion, and this has been interpreted as a manifestation of tissue immunity in the classic concept of Metchnikoff. For example, the simple but elegant experiment of Reynolds[59] in Chesney's laboratory showed that *T. pallidum* from tissue explants placed in a nonimmune host both multiplied and migrated to the regional lymph node, whereas in the immune host they remained alive but multiplied little if at all and did not migrate. Similar results were also obtained by Waring and Fleming with a slightly different approach.[72]

With the demonstration of "protective antibodies" in syphilis by the author[68] and discovery of the immobilization phenomenon by Nelson and Mayer[52] it became clear that there is indeed a humoral expression of immunity in syphilis, thus bringing the concept of the nature of immunity in syphilis squarely in line with the general concepts of immunity in most infectious processes. Further studies have shown that following elimination of infection a slow waning of resistance probably occurs.

In a sense, then, we know no less and no more about immune mechanisms in the treponematoses than in the majority of other infectious diseases. In retrospect the general immunologist could have profited by being more cognizant of advances being made in the immunology of syphilis and related diseases, less ready to regard them as a thing apart. And clearly, the experimental syphilologist must regard any advance in the understanding of other infectious processes as having probable pertinence to his own studies. These statements would be trite indeed, were not the rather dismal lessons of history to the contrary.

Having seen the gradual emergence of a concept of immunity in syphilis which fits our classic notions of immunity in the general run of infectious diseases, we must now be prepared to have these notions shaken or at least substantially modified. Studies on the "slow-viruses,"[26] on some of the tumor viruses,[37] and on certain species of mycoplasma[20] suggest that mechanisms hitherto only dimly perceived may be operative in a determinative manner.

Whatever the biological attributes and determinants of immunity in syphilis may eventually prove to be, it seems clear that in the untreated infection the delicate balance eventually achieved between host and parasite, a state referred to loosely as latent syphilis, presents one of the most interesting and challenging problems in host-parasite interaction. It is not known what mechanisms permit *T. pallidum* to remain for long periods in a particular host apparently without multiplying, and without producing anything but minor histological evidence of tissue damage, but without loss of inherent virulence, for when transferred to a new host these organisms seem to spring to life with their initial vigor in a manner suggesting that they have been essentially unaltered by this long subjection to the inhibitory environment.

Could it be the simple interplay between antigen and antibody, like foxes and rabbits on an island, the one waxing while the other wanes? If so, what delicate checkmate is so exquisitely sensitive that the organism is on the one hand never eliminated, and on the other not permitted to damage the host. Of course, in the natural disease, while this delicate balance does seem to be present in many, the best evidence is that in a proportion of infected persons the infection is indeed eventually eliminated even in the absence of intervention with drugs (Brunsgaard, Gjestland);[30] and it is well known that, on the other side of the scale, repeated damage to tissues may be produced. The uneasy balance struck in most instances over many years is nevertheless impressive, both clinically and as a biological phenomenon.

If the mechanism of latency in syphilis remains as one of the challenging unknowns in the realm of infectious diseases, accomplishments in terms of new knowledge concerning immune mechanisms in syphilis have none the less been impressive. Indeed, one by one various infectious processes shed their uniqueness as classic phenomena are demonstrated, if one can be permitted such a general term. Protective antibodies have been found in malaria,[11, 12] another world scourge, and recent work with tumor viruses suggests that in some instances antibody may be playing a role in regression of the disease.[37]

It is perhaps presumptuous to suggest that there is necessarily a constant pattern to be found in the reaction of so complex a biological system as that to be found in the higher animals to relatively simple microorganisms that invade them. Yet it is in the nature of man that he seeks unity, perhaps yearns for it, whether as a mystic through God, or as a biologist studying life, or as a physicist trying to delimit the universe; and even these move toward a common point. The more one seeks the whole, the more parts one discovers, yet at rare intervals great synthesizing flashes bring simplicity from complexity. Perhaps it is the race, then, that is important, but a race without a goal is no race at all.

## MORPHOLOGY OF TREPONEMES

The scholarly persistence and technical competence of Schaudinn, who first saw *T. pallidum* under the lightfield microscope, becomes even more impressive as instruments of greater sophistication are applied to the study of these organisms.[74] It should be recalled, too, that it was Karl Landsteiner, in one of his many major contributions to bacteriology and immunology, who developed darkfield microscopy, thus moving the study of treponemal diseases a step further along the road.[40]

Soon after application of the electron microscope to biomedical problems, Mudd and his colleagues[49] first provided an insight into the fine structure of the treponemal group of organisms. Their micrographs, excellent for their period, gave a preview of many of the subsequent findings as instruments and techniques were further refined.

The next few years brought a number of other studies on the ultrastructure of treponemes,[74] but the recent investigations of Pillot and his associates in Paris,[56] Ovčinnikov and his group in Moscow,[55] and Jepsen and associates in Copenhagen[33a] using ultrathin sections have revealed details of morphology hitherto only vaguely sensed. The description that follows will be largely a summary of the findings of these three groups of investigators.

*T. pallidum* may be regarded as a long sinuous spiral cylindrical cell contained within membranes. This cell is about 0.2 micron thick. There is an external envelope, a cytoplasmic membrane, cytoplasmic substance, and bundles of fibrils. The outer envelope is about 70 to 90 Å thick, the outer edge being somewhat more dense than the inner. Lying between this outer envelope and the cytoplasmic membrane are bundles of fibrils which stretch from one end of the treponeme to the other, and wind in helical coils around the cytoplasm. These structures, which are 100 to 200 Å thick, are analogous to the flagella of eubacteria. They arise from the ends of the cell and those originating from different ends overlap along much of the cell length. The free ends of fibrils may extend beyond the distal end of the cell. The tension of the fibrillar

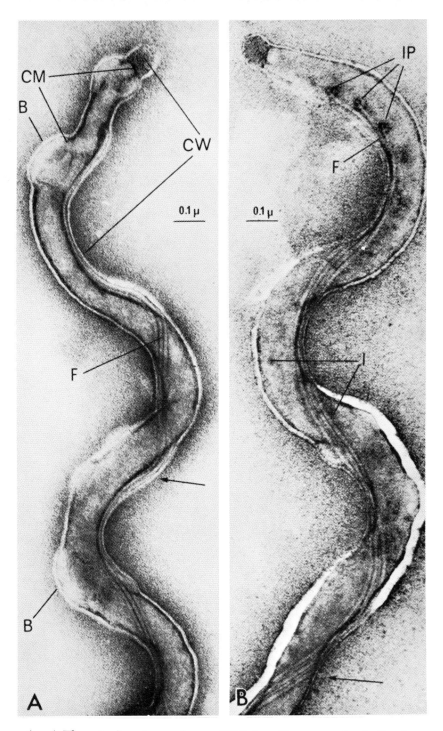

*Figure 1.* *A*, The cytoplasmic membrane (*CM*) is well seen as a borderline between zones 1 and 2 of the organism. Beyond *CM* is cell wall material (*CW*) only. *CW* is seen in close contact with *CM* except in the regions of lower electron density, blebs (*B*), and the part of the cell where the fibrillar bundle (*F*) passes straight along the cytoplasmic body (arrow). Formalin fixation; negative staining; 1 per cent ammonium molybdate. Magnification 90,000 ×.

*B*, The three zones at the tip of the organism are clearly illustrated. Three fibrils (*F*) with insertion points (*IP*) are seen in zone 3, whereas five fibrils are seen more centrally. Two thin fibrils are present (arrow) and dense inclusions (*I*) are seen. Formalin fixation; negative staining; 1 per cent phosphotungstic acid. Magnification 90,000 ×. (From Jepsen et al.: Acta Path. Microbiol. Scand., 1968, in press.)

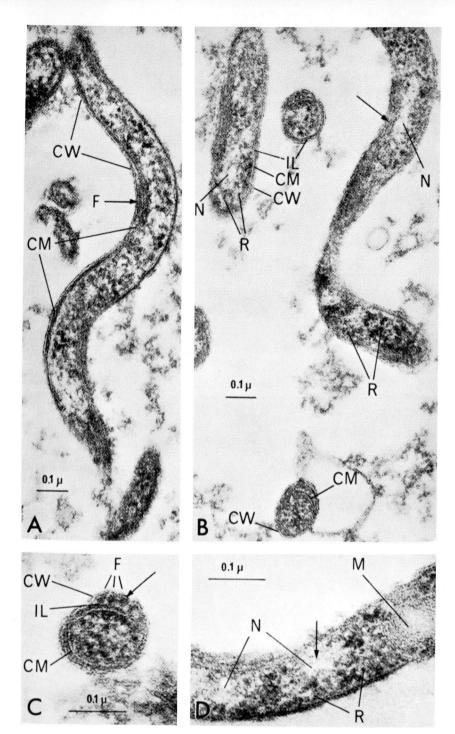

*Figure 2.* *A,* Section showing a sinusoidal piece of an organism. The three-layered cell wall *(CW)* tightly envelops the organism. Fibrils *(F)* are located between *CW* and the cytoplasmic membrane *(CM)* (arrow). Magnification 90,000 ×.

*B,* Section showing pieces of organisms cut at various angles. The cell wall *(CW)* is seen outside the intermediate layer *(IL)* which is adjacent to the outer layer of the cytoplasmic membrane *(CM)*. Ribosomes *(R)* and nuclear regions *(N)* are seen in the interior of the cells. Note double-lined appearance of fibrils (arrow). Magnification 90,000 ×.

*C,* A cross section showing the location of fibrils *(F)* between the three-layered cell wall *(CW)* and the three-layered cytoplasmic membrane *(CM)*. The intermedi-

bundles probably determines the spiral morphology of the treponeme. These fibrils have some of the characteristics of muscle fibrils and it is suggested that the contraction and relaxation of the bundles may account for the movement of the organism.

At each extremity of the treponeme are rather dense bodies resembling the head of a snake and these serve as points of insertion, or origin, for the fibrils. The actual point of insertion of the fibril is slightly raised and round, and denser and larger than the fibril itself. This body, which has been variously termed "basal granule," "blepharoplast," and so forth, lies within the cytoplasmic substance. In early electron microscopic studies of spirochetes the marked fragility of the cell envelope was not appreciated. Rupture of this membrane permitted the fibrils to float free, thus giving the impression of flagella; it is now generally agreed that treponemes have no true flagella.

The cytoplasmic membrane is extremely thin and encloses the cytoplasm in a cylindrical structure which may vary unevenly in mass as does an earthworm as it moves. The cytoplasm contains various dense structures or granules, some spore-like in their appearance, and it is postulated that these may be nucleoid bodies. Ribosomes, considered to be the site of protein synthesis, are distributed rather evenly in the cytoplasm, and mesomeres, intrusions of the cytoplasmic membrane, are recognized. *T. pallidum* appears to lie exclusively outside the host cells, thus confirming older observations.

In general, the structure of pathogenic and cultivable treponemes is similar. In both, evidence of transverse segmentation is noted, and the consensus is that only transverse division occurs.

A treponeme may undergo transverse division in several places along its length, not merely in one place. Division is preceded by shedding of the old fibrils and the formation of new basal granules and fibrils on either side of the site of division. While it is not possible to be sure of the age of a pathogenic treponeme from a human or rabbit lesion, it is noted that in the cultivable treponeme segmentation increases with age of the culture, and some of these segments appear to become independent granular forms developing into the balloon spheres described by Gelperin.[69] It should be noted that Hardy and Nell[69] found the state of the local environment, osmotic pressure, and other factors to be major determinants in the production of these spheres from cultivable treponemes, but it is not known whether such forms occurring in the living host develop from similar stimuli. Ovčinnikov and Delektorsky[55] postulate that granular forms do occur *in vivo* and that they are one of the stages of resistant survival, a conclusion reminiscent of the earlier contention of Levaditi and his colleagues.[74] The development of granular forms *in vitro* is hastened by a variety of adverse environmental conditions including exposure to immune serum and penicillin. It is still probably an open question whether they are solely expressions of degeneration of the microorganisms or constitute an important stage in the life cycle.

---

ate layer (*IL*) is seen to adhere to the outer layer of *CM*. Hollow subfibrils can be distinguished in individual fibrils (arrow). Magnification 160,000 ×.

*D,* A section illustrating the whorled type of mesosome (*M*). Delicate strands (arrow) are present in the nuclear region (*N*). Ribosomes (*R*) are also seen. Magnification 160,000 ×. (From Jepsen et al.: Acta Path. Microbiol. Scand., 1968, in press.)

Thus far there is no firm indication that a capsule of a mucous nature surrounds the treponeme, although some micrographs strongly suggest the presence of such an envelope.

The Russian workers describe in some detail a porous mass in the head structure of the treponeme and feel that this might be a nuclear excretory organ. They believe the possibilty that treponemes possess a sexual mechanism of multiplication cannot be excluded. The published micrographs of Ovčinnikov and Delektorsky[55] and of Jepsen et al.[33a] are superb.

It is in the nature of basic research of this sort that the practical implications are often obscure for a time, but there can be little doubt that the increase in knowledge concerning this group of organisms will eventually be reflected in terms of the problem in man. The stage now seems set for productive approaches to study of the cytochemistry of these organisms.


## ANTIGENIC STRUCTURE OF TREPONEMES

Study of the antigenic structure of pathogenic *T. pallidum* and related treponemes has been handicapped by inability to obtain large quantities of the organisms relatively free of mammalian tissue. By contrast, much work has been done on cultivable spirochetes, particularly the Reiter organism, but it is difficult to translate the one in terms of the other.

In 1949, d'Alessandro and his colleagues[16] isolated from the Reiter organism a protein fraction which was reactive with syphilitic serum, and with various refinements this fraction is still used for some clinical purposes. This antigen reacts not only with sera from patients with syphilis and other treponematoses, but also with immune sera to cultivable treponemes. Thus it is obviously a group antigen, common to a variety of anaerobic spirochetes, and this greatly limits its diagnostic value. From a practical standpoint, this antigen appears to have little advantage over the common cardiolipin antigens.

More recently, attention has turned to the polysaccharide components of cultivable treponemes in the hope that these might provide antigens of greater specificity. The fractions isolated by Nell and Hardy[50] from the Reiter organism appear to be among the more chemically pure ones in that in their preparation little or no protein was present, a statement which could not be made about some of the fractions prepared by others. This polysaccharide fraction was active in the usual *in vitro* tests with specific antisera to the Reiter treponeme, and also with serum from animals immunized with six of eight other strains of cultivable treponemes. It is of particular interest that serum from rabbits infected with the pathogenic Nichols strain of *T. pallidum* was nonreactive with this fraction. It was concluded by Nell and Hardy that reactions obtained by others with a presumed carbohydrate fraction and the serum of syphilitic animals or patients were due to small amounts of protein contaminating the polysaccharide fraction. They further suggest that the carbohydrate fraction may be species-specific.

Christiansen[9] has attempted to isolate polysaccharide fractions from pathogenic treponemes obtained from rabbit testes, and while such fractions have indeed been obtained and shown to be immunologically active, essentially similar fractions have been obtained from normal rabbit testicular extracts. Again, progress in this area will be largely dependent upon access to a much larger treponemal mass with a minimum of other tissue elements, which can probably be achieved only through cultivation of pathogenic treponemes on artificial media.

In summary, therefore, it appears that cultivable treponemes contain a protein antigen which is widely present in pathogenic as well as non-pathogenic treponemes. Relatively pure polysaccharide fractions tend to be more species-specific and seem not to be common to both pathogenic and nonpathogenic varieties. Lipoidal fractions have purportedly been isolated from both cultivable and pathogenic treponemes, but since this material is so widely present in tissues, including serum, the significance of this finding is difficult to assess.

While, on the whole, fractionation studies of the treponemal group of organisms have thus far been disappointing in their practical import, such studies appear to offer the main hope of clarifying the confusing serological picture in these infections. The investigations have succeeded in producing certain basic information concerning the chemical structure of the organism, methods have been tested, and pitfalls have been recognized to the point where rapid progress in the study of the pathogenic treponemes can be anticipated when cultivation *in vitro* is accomplished.

## SEROLOGICAL TESTS IN RELATION TO INFECTION, DISEASE, AND IMMUNITY

In an era in which the laboratory has contributed so much to diagnostic, therapeutic, and preventive medicine, it is but natural that serological tests for syphilis and related diseases have acquired a halo of definitiveness that often seem to obscure biological and clinical complexities rather than shed light upon them. Reflective clinicians and epidemiologists are aware of the pitfalls, yet because so much of the syphilis iceberg remains below the clinical surface serological tests inevitably constitute an indispensable diagnostic aid. The many different serological tests will not be described in detail, but rather an attempt will be made to translate the information they yield in terms of infection, disease, and immunity, insofar as the evidence permits.

Each test in current use is in essence an *in vitro* reaction between a mixture of antigens and a serum which may and often does contain multiple antibodies reactive to one or more of these antigens. Indeed one can only wonder at the high degree of clinical specificity of the tests. While efforts to define the limits of clinical and epidemiological "specificity" and "sensitivity" of the many tests in current use are entirely praiseworthy, they scarcely seek the root of the problem.

Broadly speaking, serological tests for syphilis are of two kinds: in one, cardiolipin, an apparently nonspecific antigen in the biological sense, is used; in the other, the pathogenic treponeme itself or some component of it serves as the antigen. The first group of tests were in use nearly half a century before the second, and serve as a reference point for much of our clinical and epidemiological data.

When, in 1906, Wassermann and his colleagues,[74] applying the principle of complement fixation as demonstrated by Bordet and Gengou,[4] developed the first clinically useful test, it was believed that the antigen was in fact "specific" in that T. pallidum was abundantly present in the fetal liver extracts employed. It was soon demonstrated, however, that organs from nonsyphilitic persons and animals were equally reactive, and the common source of these antigens today is the heart muscle of beef cattle with cholesterol and lecithin added. Later, with the use of the same antigen and the flocculation phenomenon discovered by Michaelis[47] numerous other tests were developed. Among the many tests for syphilis in which cardiolipin antigen is used are the Wassermann, Hinton, Kahn, Eagle, Sachs-Georgi, Chediak, Meinicke, Venereal Disease Research Laboratories (VDRL), Mazzini, and Brewer slide test. It is somewhat ironic that the names of Bordet, Gengou, and Michaelis have been largely lost in this context.

In 1949, Nelson and Mayer[52] in our laboratory developed a test in which virulent T. pallidum was used as the antigen, and in which the observed reaction was based upon direct action of serum on the treponeme as indicated by immobilization of the motile treponeme in the presence of complement. This was clearly a specific reaction in the biological sense. There was accompanying evidence that immobilization reflected death of the organism; in other words, the antibody might be considered as treponemicidal as well as immobilizing in its action, and it is probably the same antibody active in the protection tests referred to earlier.[68]

Mention should be made of another group of serological tests for syphilis, probably related more closely to the second type than to the first, in which the antigen is composed of nonpathogenic cultivable spirochetes or antigenic fractions derived therefrom. The most commonly used antigen of this type is an extract of the Reiter strain of spirochetes. It contains a protein-nucleic acid complex that reacts with syphilitic serum from which the Wassermann antibody has been removed by absorption, but as noted above it is probably a group antigen common to many treponemal species.

At any rate, it was quite clear that the antibody or antibodies active in the TPI test, as the immobilization test came to be known, were different from Wassermann antibody (that active in the so-called standard serological tests for syphilis) since absorption of serum from a syphilitic patient or animal with cardiolipin antigen largely removed the component of the serum active in the standard tests, whereas activity of the serum in the TPI test remained essentially unaltered.

In the category of "specific" antibody tests may also be placed the fluorescent antibody technique, in which pathogenic treponemes are used as the antigen. It has not been definitely determined whether the same or different antibodies are being detected in the TPI and FTA (fluorescent antibody) tests, but it does seem clear that in each it is not primarily the Wassermann antibody that is being measured.

Thus, demonstrably, there are at least two varieties of antibody found in response to syphilitic infection, and doubtless more. It should be noted, parenthetically, that all the known pathogenic treponemes invoke in man and animals essentially these same antibodies which are reactive in the standard serological tests and in tests using *T. pallidum* as antigen. Despite the different character of the antigens employed in the two types of test it would be unwise to regard the one type of test as being more "specific" than the other; both are useful clinically and epidemiologically, and each probably reveals important though different aspects of the host-parasite interaction. It is the joint task of the experimentalist and the clinician to seek interpretations of these tests in terms of the basic biology of the treponemal infections.

### WASSERMANN ANTIBODY

For a laboratory aid that was so quickly accepted clinically and has been of such enormous usefulness over the years, it is dismaying to realize how limited is our knowledge of the underlying biological and immunological import of Wasserman antibody as revealed by the tests made with cardiolipin antigen. The TPI and FTA tests conform to a more familiar immunological pattern, but the Wassermann type of test does not fit into our usual immunological pigeonholes since the antigen is biologically nonspecific, and this lack of basic understanding eventually imposes limitations on its clinical value. Indeed, cardiolipin has been identified in many mammalian tissues and even in some bacteria.[73]

In attempting to reduce the enigma of the Wassermann antibody to its simplest terms, several points should be noted. (1) Wassermann antibody is produced in large quantities in response to all treponemal infections. (2) The amount of antibody tends to be correlated directly and quite immediately with the degree of tissue reaction to the treponeme; it waxes as the number of treponemes and the tissue reaction increase, and wanes as these decline. (3) The quantity of Wassermann antibody bears no direct relation to immunity; the titer of the antibody is often high at a time when resistance to infection is poorly developed, and the titer is often low when resistance is high. (4) Small quantities of Wassermann antibody are present in the serum of many, probably most, normal persons,[41] and in the presence of certain nontreponemal conditions the amount may increase to the point of giving positive results with the standard serological tests. This is especially true during acute infections, some chronic infections such as leprosy and malaria, and those conditions associated with changes in collagen tissue such as lupus erythematosus.

Earlier studies[35] indicated that Wassermann antibody, although usually found in both the IgM (19S, $\beta$2M globulin) and the IgG (7S, $\gamma$ globulin) fractions, was predominantly contained in the former fraction. Further studies by Laurell[41] and Tringali et al.,[65] in which the sera of patients in various stages of the disease were fractionated, showed that in primary and secondary syphilis the Wassermann antibody although present in both fractions was predominantly in the IgM portion; no consistent pattern was found in later stages of the diseases although the predominance of the antibody in the IgM fraction was probably somewhat less as the disease progressed.

Norins and his associates,[54] working with serum from rabbits experimentally infected, found that the initial Wassermann antibody response was entirely in the IgM fraction, this broadened to include antibody in the IgG fraction as the disease progressed, and late in the course of the experimental disease (i.e., after 2 years) the Wassermann antibody was entirely of the IgG type. Tringali et al. have reported similar findings.[65]

These are valuable observations but it is too early to hazard a guess as to their interpretation in clinical terms. In the light of observations to be referred to next, there is a temptation to hypothesize that the production of large macromolecular type of antibody is indicative of an intense antigenic stimulus, perhaps due to or accompanied by intense tissue reaction, but there is as yet little basis to support such a hypothesis. The same type of antibody is usually produced early in the course of artificial immunization and during the early stages of certain other acute infections.[5]

Nevertheless, the data indicate that Wassermann antibody is formed in response to the antigenic stimulus of some component of the treponeme. Such a hypothetical component is clearly shared by many other mammalian tissues including quite obviously the beef heart-cholesterol-lecithin complex, with which the formation of Wassermann antibodies may be induced in the rabbit when combined with a *Schlepper* protein or absorbed on an inert substance such as kaolin. It has also long been suggested that Wassermann antibody is an autoantibody developed in response to some abnormal tissue element formed during the course of treponemal infection; Fredricksson et al. are among the latest proponents of this view.[22] In a biological sense, however, Wassermann antibody is produced almost uniquely, and certainly spectacularly, by the treponeme. Whether this is accomplished directly, as we believe to be the case in viruses, for example, or through some secondary mechanism in which an intermediate antigenic product is postulated has not been finally determined.

On a more pragmatic level, there are many bits and pieces of evidence which in sum suggest that the levels of Wassermann antibody reflect in a rough way activity of syphilitic disease. This has long been observed in the experimental disease in rabbits and has been more recently demonstrated again by Frederiksson et al.[22] and in our own laboratory.[71] Clinical experience too in general supports this view, although there are admittedly many exceptions. For example, most patients who have demonstrable syphilitic lesions of the bones exhibit unusually high Wassermann antibody titers. The same is true of patients with congenital syphilis in which stigmata or active lesions are present.

As noted above, there is no indication that Wassermann antibody plays any role in the immune process.

## TREPONEMAL IMMOBILIZING (TPI) ANTIBODY

In contrast to Wassermann antibody, the antibody active in the TPI test develops more slowly during the course of both natural and experimental disease, often reaches a peak later, and persists at high levels for much longer periods after the disease has become clinically quiescent.[1, 22, 69, 75] Even though this antibody may remain at high titer for many years after the infected patient or experimental animal has received supposedly curative treatment, the titer of the antibody tends to decline slowly in both treated and untreated subjects, and in a small proportion of instances undoubtedly becomes negative.

Because of the technical difficulties of the TPI test fewer quantitative studies have been made with this test than with most of the other tests for syphilis in current use.[53] There is a considerable mass of evidence, however, which indicates that there is a rough correlation between the titer of this antibody and immunity;[69] the pattern of the evolution of resistance to re-infection in experimental syphilis corresponds to the rise in titer of TPI antibody, and the persistence of the one, both before and after treatment, in general parallels that of the other.

Studies by Julian et al.[34] indicate that immobilizing antibodies are contained almost exclusively in the IgG fraction of serum, and this might be expected from the slower formation of this antibody during the course of the natural infection and its much longer persistence in waning infections. However, it should be noted that sulfhydryl compounds are present in the medium employed in the treponeme immobilization test, and most IgM antibodies are very susceptible to *in vitro* exposure to such reagents. In other words, the apparent absence of immobilizing antibody in IgM fractions may be an artefact.

## TREPONEMAL AGGLUTINATION TEST

It was early noted that *T. pallidum* under certain *in vitro* conditions would agglutinate in the presence of syphilitic serum. More recently, using concentration methods, McLeod and her associates and Hardy and Nell went further in defining the conditions which enhance and inhibit agglutination, and in subjecting the test to clinical trials. The latter authors[32] described the "ripening" effect in which agglutinability is enhanced by ageing of the antigen and postulated that this effect was due to the progressive loss of mucoid capsular material. Hardy and Nell also showed that both Wassermann and immobilizing antibodies are active in agglutination. Since in the present state of development the agglutination test appears to have no advantage over the technically more simple FTA test, the former is not being used clinically.

## FLUORESCENT TREPONEMAL ANTIBODY (FTA) TEST

The FTA test was devised by Deacon et al.[17] using principles developed by Coons.[15] Because of the relative simplicity of the test, it is being used extensively in various modified forms for diagnostic and research purposes in treponemal diseases. While the test undoubtedly constitutes a major contribution to the technical armamentarium of the syphilologist, it is well documented that multiple antibodies participate in the FTA test.

In one modification of the FTA test, the FTA-ABS test, serum is first absorbed with material derived from cultivable treponemes, usually the Reiter strain, with a view to removing so-called group antibodies to the protein fraction of those organisms. In the initial studies with this absorption technique a sonicate of Reiter treponemes was used, and such antibodies were probably removed selectively. More recently, however, a newer material used for absorption, the so-called sorbent, has been subjected to certain manipulations which almost certainly denature the bacterial proteins originally present;

while the titers of Wassermann antibody and of FTA antibody are reduced it seems doubtful that the group antibody has in fact been selectively removed.

It remains unclear, therefore, whether the FTA test measures primarily immobilizing antibody or distinctly different antibodies. There are instances in which one is positive and the other is not. On the whole, however, there is a high degree of correlation, as reported by a number of workers,[1, 75, 76] and most studies indicate that the FTA test is somewhat more sensitive in detecting long standing syphilitic infection. There are also instances in which the usual tests for Wassermann antibody are positive, and the FTA and TPI tests are negative, the so-called biologic false positive (BFP) reactors, indicating that it is probably not Wassermann antibody that is active in the FTA test.

On the other hand, Norins et al. found that antibody as measured by the FTA-ABS test appeared simultaneously with Wassermann antibody in the very early days of the experimental infection in rabbits, which is not true of the TPI antibody.

Király et al.[36] and Julian et al.[34] have shown that FTA antibody occurs in the IgA, IgM, and IgG fractions of sera in all stages of syphilis. However, these antibodies tend to be predominantly in the IgA and IgM fractions early in the course of the disease and in the IgG fraction in late and latent syphilis. Moreover, Király and his associates have found that treponemal group antibodies tend to be low early in the course of the infection, and proportionately high late in the infection. These authors make the interesting suggestion that nonpathogenic treponemes of the mouth and bowel may provide a continuing stimulus to the production of these group antibodies even in the absence of *T. pallidum* or related pathogenic organisms. From a practical standpoint the FTA test is becoming among the most widely used clinically.

A word of caution in the use of various immunofluorescence procedures should be given at this point. The phenomenon of tagging antibody-carrying serum with fluorescein as developed by Coons has been a great contribution to immunology. However, in applying the method to various problems associated with treponemal infections, it should be noted that sera from syphilitics contain group antibodies that may react in a seemingly specific manner with spirochetes other than *T. pallidum* and closely related pathogenic treponemes. Moreover, many artefacts are observed to take the fluorescent stain and some of these frequently show deceptively spiral forms. Careful control of the procedure is necessary, especially in situations in which *T. pallidum* is not certainly known to be present, as for example when they are being sought in tissue or various body fluids.

## ANTIBODY TO REITER PROTEIN

As indicated in a preceding section, a lipoprotein fraction has been isolated from cultivable treponemes and this material is being used as antigen in another type of complement fixation test for syphilis. Its assessment has been largely on a clinical basis, and while it seems to detect some instances of old infection in patients, the biological basis for the test is even less clear than for the customary Wassermann tests or the TPI test. The Reiter lipoprotein antigen does seem to detect antibodies to treponemal group antigens since injection of animals with this antigenic fraction(s) evokes the production of antibodies that react widely with antibodies to other cultivable strains and to various pathogenic treponemes as well.

### Antibodies to Carbohydrate Fractions of Treponemes

There is little to add to the comments made in the section entitled Antigenic Structure of Treponemes. Chemically and immunologically pure carbohydrate fractions of cultivable treponemes are obtained with difficulty, but they do appear to be species-specific.[50] It has not been possible for technical reasons to prepare such fractions from pathogenic treponemes; presumably these too would be species-specific, and if so, these antigens would be highly valuable in differential diagnosis were they ever to become available for clinical use.

### Biological and Clinical Interpretations

All this is very confusing, since there is inherent conflict between the clinicians' desire for simplicity in the message conveyed by laboratory tests and the complexity of the basic immunological phenomena which together comprise the tests. It may be that a simple antibody type plays the dominant role in a test such as that based on treponemal immobilization, but there is evidence even here that more than one antibody may participate.

As for the FTA test, this simply reveals proteins (i.e., globulins) attached to the treponeme. Therefore, any antibody of any type that can react with *T. pallidum*, (or with any tissue adhering to *T. pallidum*) will be revealed by the test. Somewhat the same situation might likewise be present in the agglutination phenomenon. The ambiguity of the immunological message conveyed by the Wassermann and similar tests and the Reiter protein complement fixation test has already been commented upon. The remarkable clinical specificity of the immobilization test may be a reflection of its relative inefficiency; for similar reasons the FTA test is probably the least specific of all syphilis serology tests, as well as the most sensitive. Strictly speaking, the terms FTA antibody, Wassermann antibody, and so forth are misnomers, but it is not likely that they will be read out of respectable scientific and clinical literature by this fact.

Clearly, much work remains to be done on the significance of the various serological tests for syphilis in terms of the basic biology of the disease. The major difficulty appears to be in the use of antigenic material which contains many antigens in an immunological sense. While differential absorption of sera with various antigens is a step in the right direction, unfortunately only two antigen preparations are available in sufficient quantities to make absorption techniques practical, cardiolipin and the Reiter protein antigen, and because of the nature of each antigen, we are not much further ahead in a precise immunological sense than before absorption.

By way of summary, it can be stated, however, that Wassermann antibody develops earlier than TPI antibody, tends to reach its height at an earlier stage in the disease, declines as the disease moves to an asymptomatic stage, and eventually may fall below readily detectable levels. The TPI antibody, on the other hand, develops more slowly and persists at easily detectable levels much longer; once it reaches a relatively high titer it is less affected by antisyphilitic treatment, even curative treatment. In most of these respects, FTA antibody tends to follow the TPI antibody patterns. As a means of detecting previous syphilitic infection, the TPI and FTA antibody tests are clearly superior, both in theory and in practice, to the standard serological tests for Wassermann antibody. The skillful clinician and epidemiologist, therefore, will use both types of tests in a manner best calculated to help illuminate the particular situation at hand.

In the light of all the evidence, which is admittedly imcomplete, it is now a supportable opinion that persistent high titer Wassermann antibody represents continued biological activity of pathogenic treponemes, and within reasonable limits is an indication for further antisyphilitic treatment. At the same time, it must be kept in mind that danger to life from *T. pallidum* is not necessarily equated with the number of living treponemes in the body or even the degree of tissue reaction they invoke. More significant is the location of the tissue damage. Quite clearly a small area of damage if located in some vital region, such as at the base of an aortic valve or in certain very limited areas of the brain or spinal cord, might be lethal in its import, yet provide minimal antigenic stimulus, and hence be reflected in little or no antibody rise. In other words, low titer serological tests minimize the likelihood of treponemal pathology, but certainly do not altogether rule it out.

These kinds of clinical interpretations are, of course, but rationalizations based on the basic biology of the disease as it is known to us today; new insights and, in particular, new observations and data may lead to wholly different interpretations.

As mentioned above, small amounts of Wassermann antibody are present in the serum of most normal (i.e., nonsyphilitic) persons. Whether this is due to commensal relationship with oral spirochetes or to other factors is not known, but it is known that this antibody may reach readily detectable amounts in some apparently normal persons or in those with various acute and chronic infections. There is presently no laboratory test capable of differentiating such antibody from that present due to treponemal infection, and diagnosis in these circumstances is entirely dependent upon clinical and epidemiological evidence. However, it should be emphasized that Wassermann antibody is rarely present in high titer (8 units or more in the VDRL test) in the absence of treponemal infection. It is in these cases that the TPI and FTA tests may be particularly helpful. In this same connection, it would be surprising in a biological sense if false positive tests for TPI antibody were not occasionally encountered and indeed rare instances of such occurrences have been reasonably well documented.

As an indication of immunity, clearly the tests that measure primarily Wassermann antibody are of no value. There is a fair body of evidence suggesting that there is reasonably good correlation between the level of TPI antibody and resistance to reinfection, but the data are not extensive and the correlations are approximate at best. Evidence is beginning to accumulate that at least one of the antibodies measured in the FTA test may exhibit the same relationships as the TPI antibody.

Finally, it should be noted that while the bulk of the available data on serological tests in treponemal diseases relates to syphilis in man or animals, the indications are from more fragmentary data that the same relationships apply to yaws, and possibly to other treponemal infections such as pinta and *T. cuniculi* infection of rabbits, although in these latter instances the evidence is meagre.

The observations and speculations given above emphasize the value of quantitative, as opposed to qualitative, tests in syphilis and related diseases. Quantitation of Wassermann antibody is a relatively simple procedure, especially with the VDRL test or the modification devised by Portney, Brewer, and Harris,[74] and as techniques for the FTA tests are refined, it may also be relatively easy to quantitate FTA and similar antibodies, all of which will probably add a new dimension to clinical competence in the treponemal diseases.

Further efforts to obtain chemically pure antigenic fractions and continuing characterization of antibodies in treponemal infections should lead to the acquisition of information of great value from a clinical and epidemiological standpoint.

## ARTIFICIAL IMMUNIZATION IN THE TREPONEMATOSES

Little more success has been achieved in the field of artificial immunization in syphilis and related diseases than in the cultivation of pathogenic treponemes. Yet, the problem seems slightly less elusive in that much has been learned in the last few years about the preparation of antigens in general, methods of immunization, and methods of challenge, all of which might conceivably make some contribution to the problem in the treponematoses.

Many investigators have made immunization attempts with killed pathogenic *T. pallidum*, usually harvested from rabbit's testes, or with cultivable treponemes, all with no success or with results which scarcely fall beyond the bounds of chance. All but the most recent attempts have been summarized elsewhere.[69]

Despite failures, hope is insistent that even with presently available materials, some evidence of artificial immunity may eventually be adduced. From a scientific point of view, the clear demonstration of even a slight degree of artificially induced immunity would be a significant advance, providing a needed stimulus to more intensive study. To this end, it is justifiable and indeed desirable to develop a model system in which each element is designed to give maximum chance of success, regardless of how artificial the model might be, so long as adequate controls are in evidence.

As an example of this point of view, examination of protocols of many of the experiments on artificial immunization reveals that the challenge inoculation was unnecessarily severe, a technique calculated to obscure slight degrees of resistance that might have been present. It is known that syphilitic lesions can be regularly produced by intracutaneous inoculations of the order of 100 to 500 *T. pallidum* organisms at each of several sites on the rabbit's back; yet in some experiments inocula of 1 million or more organisms were used.

The basic problem in experiments using pathogenic *T. pallidum* is probably that insufficient antigenic mass is obtainable from the ordinary testicular infections in rabbits, and this is unlikely to be corrected until these organisms can be grown on artificial media. However, better methods of extraction and concentration of treponemes are now available and the administration of cortisone to the infected rabbit enhances the yield of treponemes, so that it might be possible to garner a richer harvest of antigenic material. Likewise, methods of inactivation useful in preparation of viral antigens might be employed to advantage. Use of potentiating materials also might favor success, although many such substances are toxic for the experimental animal, necessitating the employment of groups of control animals injected with potentiating material alone.

One senses, therefore, that the definitive experiments on immunization, even with the limited materials now available, have not yet been done. Certain new approaches have recently been made, as for example the trial of gamma-irradiated treponemes by Miller,[48] with faintly suggestive results. Likewise, Knox[38] has repeated the experiments of others in which large quantities of cultivable treponemes have been used, again with suggestive but unimpressive results.

Unfortunately, little is known concerning what component of the treponeme is antigenic in the sense of inducing resistance, or indeed whether any portion of the cultivable treponemes has such antigenic capacity at all. Yet, the similar morphology, as lately revealed by electron microscopy, and the known reactivity of certain components of cultivable treponemes with serum from patients with syphilis, strongly suggest that the nonpathogenic varieties may possess minute amounts of resistance-invoking material. Since these organisms can be grown in bulk, it might be worth the effort to prepare large quantities of various recoverable fractions of these organisms for definitive immunization trials.

In dealing with pathogenic *T. pallidum*, sheer quantity is probably a major limiting factor and at present it can be corrected only in part, although there are methods of increasing the yield, as indicated above. Another problem, however, arises in selecting methods of inactivation and preservation that best conserve the antigenic capacity which at best can be present only to a limited degree. Careful attention to the experience with viruses in this regard may be of help. But another favorable factor might be in long spacing of antigenic stimuli, keeping in mind the slow buildup of immunity in the natural infection. Such an enterprise requires not only adequate scientific competence, but a high sense of purpose, stable financing, and a stout heart.

It is probable, too, that the full potential of *T. cuniculi* as an immunizing agent has not been fully explored. It is quite clear that rabbits experimentally infected with this species of treponeme develop substantial resistance to syphilis and yaws.[69] It is known, too, that evanescent disease phenomena can be induced in monkeys with *T. cuniculi*, but little is known concerning its infectivity or pathogenicity for man. Fragmentary reports in the older literature suggest that this organism does not produce a local lesion in man on artificial inoculation[69] but those observations cannot be regarded as definitive. Indeed, I would anticipate that a local lesion and perhaps a generalized infection could be induced in man.

More recently it has been suggested that pinta treponemes, if successfully perpetuated in animals, might be explored as a possible immunizing agent.[39a]

## SHIFTING SANDS IN THERAPY

The development of arsphenamine in 1910—the 606 of Ehrlich—heralded a new day in therapy (or so it was thought); for the first time there was a magic bullet that went to the heart of an infectious agent of man (or so it was thought). As time went on it gradually became clear that only a proportion of the treponeme population was killed with any one dose, and on the basis of clinical results, the treatment period was extended further and further by clinicians, reaching into the second year by the nineteen twenties. Moreover, the arsenical drugs employed had a toxicity index for the treponeme that approached the toxicity level for mammalian cells. When an intensive and shortened treatment scheme was proposed for use among American soldiers during World War II, the issue came to the needle point in one dramatic statement by that critical investigator, Harry Eagle, when he drew the arsenical dose curves in relation to cure and toxicity and then said, "Gentlemen, select your mortality." Happily, the sunshine of penicillin soon broke across the problem, making the hard decision unnecessary.

It will serve no useful purpose at this point to reconsider the vast amount of work that went into studies on the application of the arsenical drugs to the treatment of syphilis, and on their mode of action. It is hoped that they have been relegated to the museum of broken hopes, never to be used again.

But it is with a sense of foreboding that one turns to the consideration of penicillin in the treatment of the treponematoses some 25 years after its introduction. The transcending importance of its role in the therapy of syphilis is beyond debate, but the dimensions of its role may not be all-inclusive. While much of the basic information on the mode of action of penicillin derives from studies on bacteria other than treponemes, the findings are consistent among the various species of bacteria studied and probably apply as well to treponemes. Beginning with the fundamental observations of Gale and his associates,[27] it has been conclusively shown that penicillin is active only on growing bacterial cells. The point of action is the cell wall, and the definitive effect is exerted through prevention of the assimilation of mucopeptides. Penicillin has no action on resting cells. These studies have been further developed by Strominger and associates,[61] among others.

While no direct observations are available on the mode of action of penicillin on treponemes, it seems reasonable to assume that it is similar to that on staphylococci, pneumococci, and other species studied. This is supported by the recent demonstration of muramic acid, a mucopeptide component, in treponemes as well as in other genera of spirochetes.[56]

Indirect evidence suggests that the division time of *T. pallidum in vivo* is relatively long, 33 hours as contrasted to 15 to 20 minutes for pneumococci; moreover it is not known whether all or most of the treponemes are dividing in any given situation. This is especially true in the latent stage of a natural or experimental infection in which it is still to be determined whether or not treponemal cell division is proceeding at all, and if so at what rate.

Viewed in this manner, it might be surprising that there is no higher proportion of clinical failures in the treatment of early syphilis in man, which are now estimated to be of the order of 5 to 8 per cent. The assumption has been that in latent syphilis the results of penicillin therapy were equally good, but when viewed critically there is not much evidence one way or another on this point. That the practical therapeutic results are generally good has been concluded from the fact that few patients subsequently developed disease phenomena, and that in many the titers of Wassermann antibody decline. These conclusions are supported by the apparent sterilizing effect of penicillin in old infections of rabbits as indicated by failure to demonstrate infectivity of lymph nodes in treated animals.

These concepts are now being challenged by observations coming from several directions. Collart and his colleagues in Paris,[13, 14] for example, report the demonstration of treponemes as determined by staining techniques in the lymph nodes of both treated animals and treated patients, and in an occasional instance infectivity of these organisms has apparently been demonstrated. The results of Yobs et al.[77] while not wholly conclusive point in the same direction. Moreover, Smith and his colleagues[60] report finding treponemes in patients in a number of situations, particularly in aqueous humor and in spinal fluid, following what has been considered to be adequate penicillin therapy. In at least one instance treponemes recovered from the aqueous humor of a penicillin-treated patient with evidence of old syphilitic keratitis proved to be infectious for rabbits. Treponemes have likewise been found by Goldman and his associates[28] in aqueous humor from patients with treated syphilis, but no positive infectivity tests have been recorded. Whether or not most of the spirochetes demonstrated are in fact *T. pallidum* is still *sub judice.*

These observations are disturbing to our accepted concepts of the efficacy of penicillin, but in the light of the evidence on the fundamental action of penicillin they should probably not be surprising. McDermott has coined the phrase "microbial persistence"[42] to characterize the persistence of resting forms of bacteria in the face of what is considered to be adequate therapeutic doses of a normally effective drug. This has been shown particularly in tuberculous infections in which *M. tuberculosis* has been found to be dormant for years in lymph nodes of patients who have had large doses of streptomycin and potentiating drugs. Bacterial persistence as used by McDermott is not to be confused with true drug resistance or the production of penicillinase by penicillin-resistant bacteria, such as staphylococci. There is no evidence that treponemes ever produce penicillinase or that penicillin-resistant strains in the classic sense ever develop.

Nevertheless, the recent observations mentioned above, if substantiated by others, do suggest that the manner in which penicillin is used should be reviewed. In America, at least, it is customary to give either a single dose or two doses of a long acting penicillin at 1 or 2 week intervals, on the assumption that all treponemes would be destroyed, an assumption for which there is considerable clinical support. The clinical use of penicillin in aqueous solution has been largely abandoned in the treatment of syphilis because of the transient blood levels attained and the inconvenience of giving multiple injections at intervals of several hours. As shown in the review by Guthe and Idsøe,[30] certain preparations of slow absorption penicillin give more persistent blood levels than others, and in the therapy of syphilis presumably the longer substantial blood levels persist the better. But this conclusion while reasonable is being drawn without much knowledge of the state of the treponeme in the tissues of long standing cases of syphilis. Is it a justifiable assumption that every treponeme is indeed in a growth phase at some time during the 1 or 2 weeks that substantial blood levels of penicillin are present? Would wider spacing of doses of the antibiotic be more likely to blanket every treponeme while it is in its growth phase? While there is no evidence to justify modification of present therapeutic practices, the subject is probably worth exploring experimentally.

Although penicillin is one of the least toxic drugs ever developed, it does have antigenic potentialities, and in a substantial proportion of individuals treated penicillin hypersensitivity develops to the point where further administration of penicillin is dangerous. These hypersensitivity manifestations take the form of either immediate reactions, such as anaphylactic shock, which can be fatal, or immediate development of an urticarial rash, or more delayed reactions with timing and symptoms similar to serum sickness. For many reasons, therefore, it would seem wise to push on with the exploration of the value of other therapeutic agents in the treatment of treponemal infections. The best current information is that there are a number of such antibiotic drugs that are preferable to the old arsenicals for this purpose.[30]

Finally, mention should be made of the Herxheimer phenomenon originally described in relation to the treatment of syphilis with the arsenical drugs. The same phenomenon, which consists essentially of an intensification of tissue reactions in the syphilitic lesions, is observed following penicillin therapy. In practice it is a minor problem, usually amounting only to a transient increase in body temperature[58] although there is the possibility that some vital organ such as the optic nerve might be irreparably damaged.

It has generally been supposed that the reaction is due to the lysis of treponemes with the release of a hypothetical endotoxin. It is my opinion, however, that the Herxheimer reaction is due primarily to an initial and transitory stimulating effect of the drug on the treponeme. Supporting evidence for this point of view stems from the frequent observation of intensified growth of antibiotic-sensitive bacteria on agar in a limited zone about the antibiotic reservoir. If this hypothesis is correct, it is probable that the more rapidly the treponeme is killed, the more transient is this stimulatory phase, and logic suggests that a large initial dose of penicillin would be less likely to evoke a Herxheimer reaction than a small one.

The whole subject of the therapy of syphilis has been recently reviewed by Guthe and Idsøe.[30]

## EPIDEMIOLOGICAL CONSIDERATION— TREPONEMAL RESERVOIRS

It is a well documented historical fact that syphilis came sharply into the consciousness of the medical profession in Europe in the closing years of the fifteenth century. Seemingly arising from a focus in the Iberian Peninsula and southern France, the disease was soon recognized in Italy and Germany, and shortly all over Europe and parts of Asia. Indeed, despite the efforts of a number of scholarly medical historians, it has come generally to be believed that syphilis was first introduced into Europe by several of Columbus' sailors returning from the Caribbean Islands in March, 1493, and then spread from Lisbon within the course of 2 or 3 years to engulf the population of Europe in a great epidemic wave under the appellation of the great pox.

To the epidemiologist and syphilologist the very simplicity of this thesis arouses doubt; perhaps it could have happened that way, but did it? For as each circumstantial item is pursued it becomes evident in the light of modern knowledge that postulation of the seemingly simple thesis of the American origin of syphilis presupposes a concatenation of a remarkably complex series of events which seems considerably less likely to have happened than certain alternatives that will be discussed below.

The scholarly historical investigations of Sudhoff cogently support the thesis that syphilis had been endemic in Europe for many centuries, that there was in fact no epidemic in the ordinary sense of that word at the beginning of the sixteenth century, and that its impact on the intelligentsia of Europe was a product mainly of the wholly new way of life sparked by the invention of printing.[62]

At first printed professional medical works were mainly reproductions of treatises centuries old. Contemporary medical writings did not begin to be printed until the fourteen seventies; for example, the first printed treatise on plague by a living author was published in 1473, despite the fact that plague had ravaged Europe throughout the preceding 100 years. The earliest printed reference to syphilis uncovered by Sudhoff was in the Edict from the Diet of Worms issued on August 7, 1495. Konrad Schelling of Heidelberg, who accompanied Philip, Elector of the Palatinate, to the Diet, was ordered to draw up a regimen against the disease. It is significant that the value of mercury in treatment was already recognized, a remarkable fact if indeed the disease had been introduced into Europe only 2 years before. Actually, by 1495, the disease was already well known along the Rhine by the name of malum francium. Within the next 2 years, printed descriptions of the disease were published by Sebastion Brandt in the form of verse; by Joseph Grünpeck, including the famous woodcut showing shafts of punishment producing sores and rash; by Niccolo Leoniceno, Professor of Medicine at Ferrara, who did not regard it as a new disease; by Caspare Torrella of Valencia; and by Hans Widman of Tübingen. All these authors used some modification of the name malum francium given the disease by Schelling.[63]

The disease was identified in Italy in 1494, in the British Isles in 1497, in India in 1498, in Russia in 1499, and in China in 1505. Its rapid spread during this period has been attributed to the unusual movement of armies and to the increased tempo of maritime commerce. There seems little doubt, therefore, that regardless of just how or when syphilis was introduced into Europe the disease gained unusual prevalence in the early years of the sixteenth century and there is good evidence that along with increased incidence the infection tended to be unusually severe in its clinical course, thus gaining the appellation of the great pox as distinguished from the small pox.

Two points in this connection, however, should be noted. First, even in this century cases that might be legitimately designated as the great pox have been observed here and there in the world, including the United States. In these cases patients usually have extensive pustular lesions during the course of secondary syphilis, with accompanying high fever, bone involvement, and a degree of prostration. Secondly, in each of the two recent world wars, the incidence of syphilis has reached significantly higher proportions than during the intervening periods despite the availability of relatively effective drugs. It seems unnecessary, therefore, to postulate introduction of syphilis anew into any area in order to account for its prominence on the disease scene.

To approach the problem from another point of view, in the light of all that is known about the movements of people between the several continents in pre-Columbian times, it stretches credulity to assume that no case of treponemal infection had been introduced into Europe before 1493. Land traffic between Asia and Europe was doubtless centuries old. Peoples had crossed the land and the ice bridge from Asia to North America, and had gone by sea from South America at least to the Pacific Islands. The Norsemen and perhaps the Celts had been to North America and back, probably many times; the Crusaders had moved in large numbers from northern Europe to the Balkans and then to Asia Minor; the travels of Marco Polo and his kind between southern Europe and the Orient in the fifteenth century are well known; the Sahara Desert had been penetrated in both directions; and explorations along the west coast of tropical Africa with incursions inland had antedated Columbus' voyage by half a century.

Elizabeth Donnan, in *Documents Illustrative of the Slave Trade to America*, states, "Neither slavery or the slave trade was new in 1441—For perhaps five centuries trade routes from central Africa, to east and north, had been kept open, and slaves had been carried through eastern parts to the rest of the world, some of them undoubtedly finding their way to the markets of western Europe."[18] In 1444, Europeans themselves first captured natives on the west coast of Africa and brought them by ship to Lisbon, and within a decade this traffic in human beings had become an acceptable and profitable part of European commerce; by 1460, 700 to 800 West Africans were being carried to Portugal annually; it must be presumed that some of these persons had yaws. Many of the eyewitness accounts of the genesis of the enforced movements of people from one place to another are exceedingly moving human documents.[2]

At any rate, it seems highly likely that not only was syphilis present in Europe in a low level endemic form throughout the fifteenth century but that persons with yaws were repeatedly brought into Europe in that period. Indeed Hackett[31] goes much further and postulates that treponemal infections have been virtually worldwide at least since 7000 B.C., with endemic syphilis having been constantly present in Europe in the centuries preceding Columbus' voyage to America. The seven maps in Hackett's monograph convey his concept of the worldwide distribution of the treponematoses since 15,000 B.C.

Impressive as this mass of circumstantial evidence may be, a new fact of great importance has been introduced into the epidemiological equation. This is the finding by Fribourg-Blanc and his associates[23-25] that subhuman primates in certain parts of Central Africa present serological evidence of treponemal infections and have been shown to harbor pathogenic treponemes. The serological findings have been confirmed by Thivolet et al.[64] and by Kuhn et al.[39] Were these primates infected in retrograde fashion from human beings who in turn had received the disease from Europe by way of America? Or is it more likely that they represent an enduring reservoir of treponemal infection of great antiquity? The latter seems much more probable.

Before proceeding further with this line of reasoning, however, cognizance should be taken of the close biological relationships existing among the various treponemal syndromes as discussed in a preceding section, as well as elsewhere.[69] In addition, there is some evidence of an experimental nature which suggests that at times yaws treponemes acquire the ability, whether through true genetic mutation or some other mechanism, to produce a syphilis-like disease.[69] It is not difficult to imagine that the same may happen in man. If convertibility of the various treponemal species can occur in nature, then it is permissible to view all the various treponemal infections of man and animals as one gigantic epidemiological pool, which expands and contracts in response to varying environmental and social factors, a view which the author has long espoused[69] and which forms the basic thesis of Hackett's monograph.[31]

Parenthetically, it should be observed that the role of *T. cuniculi* infection in rabbits in relationship to this pool has not been determined. Was the rabbit originally infected from man, or vice versa, or were the treponematoses established in these two species from a common source?

But, to revert to pre-Columbian fifteenth century, it seems probable that there were many endemic foci of treponemal infections, in the Caribbean, in tropical Africa, in southern Europe, and doubtless in North and South America and Asia. True, the evidence derived from lesions of bones does not support these hypotheses, but both Hrdlička and Williams have pointed out how unreliable such reported evidence can be.[74]

It may never be possible to reconstruct the events of the fifteenth century more definitively than as suggested above. More to the point is the composite epidemiological picture of our own time. Two world wars and the jet age have foreshortened time and distance. Reservoirs of disease are unlikely for long to remain isolated in the way that they might have in centuries past; reservoirs of infectious diseases of whatever kind and wherever located today constitute a potential and frequently an actual threat to the rest of the world. Treponemal infections are no exceptions despite the shield of penicillin.

It would be desirable, too, not to limit our preoccupation to reservoirs of infection in the human population. We need to know more about natural primate infections, and more about the transmissibility of the rabbit disease to man. Finally, it would seem unlikely indeed that natural treponemal infections are limited among the animal kingdom to only primates and rabbits, and one may confidently predict that other animal reservoirs will be uncovered.

Valuable observations on special aspects of the epidemiology of the treponematoses have been published by Grin,[28a, 28b] by Murray et al.,[49a] by Guthe,[30a] and by Medina.[46a] From these observations it seems that we may be current spectators of changing environments that could lead to substantial modification in the epidemiological pattern of the treponematosis. At least two factors appear to be operating simultaneously to create changed environments: one is the widespread and often marked upgrading of worldwide living conditions, especially in the developing countries; the other is the impact of mass examination and penicillin treatment campaigns sparked by the World Health Organization in many of the developing countries. We may be witnessing, without adequate comprehension or documentation, the rare phenomenon of a disappearing disease, or more likely, substantial modification of well known disease patterns.

## SUMMARY COMMENTS

Reviewing the modern era of research on the treponematoses beginning with discovery of *T. pallidum* in 1905, one finds periods of great scientific ferment and rapid advance in knowledge, followed by intervals in which accretion of knowledge went at a more deliberate pace. The waxing and waning of the psychological tide has been equally impressive. The ebb tide was accentuated by the notion that there was little to learn and little that needed to be learned, and in any case it was all too difficult, the difficulty being compounded by ennui on the part of those who provided the material framework within which research is done.

But on the flood tide, whether bolstered by the needs of war or sparked by an élan of one or more imaginative individuals, this tiny segment of human biology came to life, a few good minds were attracted to the field, the hurdles seemed lower when viewed in the long perspective, and once again the possibility existed that some sleepwalker would stumble onto a new fact of great importance.*

How one views the field at any moment may depend in part on the soundness of his sleep the preceding night, upon his natural buoyancy, and upon his faith in the relentless progress of science, however episodic. But all these reservations notwithstanding, a sober judgment at this writing would

---

* This reference is to the great book on the nature of discovery, *The Sleep Walkers*, by Arthur Koestler.

be that knowledge of the treponematoses has increased apace in the twentieth century, following an upward spiral, if one may be permitted the allusion, to the point where the picture in terms of basic biology is strikingly different from that which could have been outlined in 1905.

We see a group of treponemal microorganisms parasitizing man over millenia of both unrecorded and recorded history. Never able completely to destroy its host, the *Treponema* nevertheless have accounted for untold misery and disability and death. Man, on the other hand, fighting back, has fashioned weapons capable of dealing lethal blows to the parasite, yet has never been quite able completely to conquer it. A precarious balance in nature is struck, and it can even be conjectured that the treponeme is on the run. Yet many ramparts are still occupied, reinforced by poverty and ignorance and the deepest stirrings of the sexual urge.

Even were these ramparts to be enveloped one by one, the Army of the Treponeme would probably fall back to the redoubts of the tropics where life probably began and where the battle of the parasite against man seems a little less unequal. And when in our imagination man is finally freed of this parasitizing burden, one can see still in being, not only the primate reservoir, but perhaps countless other mammalian reservoirs, of which the rabbit may be only one. The phenomenon of the "disappearing disease" should be studied.

But to turn from the cosmic to the community level, it is difficult to assess at this point in time just what is being accomplished with the modern approach to the treponematoses. Clearly, yaws, under the impact of WHO control programs, has been materially reduced in terms of both seriousness and incidence, although continuing surveillance is probably necessary to prevent its gradual return. It seems, too, that there is less syphilis than there use to be, again in terms of both serious disease and attack rate. But it may be a little early to be sure that syphilis has reached or will reach negligible proportions. The haunting thought arises that maybe in some instances the infection has only been driven underground, so to speak, where, deep in the tissues of the host, the treponeme may still have mischief-making proclivities.

This then brings us to the clinical unit of one person and his parasites, for in a sense our knowledge of what happens in the community and in the world is based on this host-parasite interaction, which in turn must be interpreted in terms of cellular events. It is at these latter levels that treponemal infections begin to behave in similar fashion to other infectious processes. As Mudd has aptly said, "Nature has few themes, but many variations on those themes."* Our problem is to identify the themes from the cacophony of often apparently unrelated events. While the contributions flowing from the study of other diseases have been many, it must be recognized that in these diseases, too, as well as in the treponematoses, there are many gaps in knowledge. It is a justifiable prediction that study of the treponematoses by intelligent investigators will contribute to a better understanding not only of these diseases, but of other infectious diseases as well, and indeed this has already been the case.

Alert young scientists will go where the action is, where the pioneering

* Mudd, S. Personal communication.

spirit may find the promise of hopes fulfilled. I have tried to convey in the preceding sections a sense of the many opportunities open to the epidemiologist, the clinician, the bacteriologist, the immunologist, and the experimental pathologist in research on the treponematoses, and through this, on host-parasite relations in general.

To those who have the responsibility for dividing up the always limited resources allocable to the future, it will be the part of wisdom not only to keep alive the existing thread of knowledge of the treponematoses, but in respect of these diseases to keep open the door to the anteroom of the sacred chamber of Discovery, into which so few ever qualify to enter.

# *References*

1. Atwood, W. G., J. L. Miller, G. W. Stout, and L. C. Norins. 1968. The TPI and FTA-ABS tests in treated late syphilis. J.A.M.A. *203:*549–551.
2. deAzurura, G. E. 1896. The Chronicle of the Discovery and Conquest of Guinea. First translated into English by Charles Raymond Beazley and Edgar Prestage. Hakluyt Society, London.
3. Boak, R. A., C. M. Carpenter, and S. L. Warren. 1932. Studies on the physiological effects of fever temperatures. III. The thermal death timer of *Treponema pallidum in vitro* with special reference to fever temperatures. J. Exp. Med. *56:*741–750.
4. Bordet, J., and O. Gengou. 1901. Sur l'existence de substances sensibilisatrices dans la plupart des sérums antimicrobiens. Ann. Inst. Pasteur *15:*289–302.
5. Boyd, W. C. 1966. Fundamentals of Immunology. 4th Ed. Wiley, New York.
6. Chacko, C. W. 1966. Accidental human infection in the laboratory with the Nichols rabbit-adapted virulent *Treponema pallidum.* Bull. WHO *35:*809–810.
7. Chesney, A. M. 1927. Immunity in Syphilis. Williams & Wilkins, Baltimore.
8. Chesney, A. M., T. B. Turner, and C. R. L. Halley. 1928. Studies in experimental syphilis. VIII. On the localization of syphilitic lesions in inflamed areas. Bull. Johns Hopkins Hosp. *42:*319–334.
9. Christiansen, A. H. 1964. Studies on the antigenic structure of *T. pallidum.* 5. Attempts to isolate polysaccharide antigen from Nichols pathogenic strain. Acta Path. Microbiol. Scand. *61:*141–149.
10. Cockburn, T. A. 1961. The origin of the treponematoses. Bull. WHO *24:*221–228.
11. Coggeshall, L. T., and H. W. Kumm. 1937. Demonstration of passive immunity to experimental monkey malaria. J. Exp. Med. *66:*177–190.
12. Cohen, S., I. A. McGregor, and S. Carrington. 1961. Gamma-globulin and acquired immunity to human malaria. Nature *192:*733–737.
13. Collart, P., L. J. Borel, and P. Durel. 1962. Etude de l'action de la penicilline dans la syphilis tardive. Persistance du tréponème pale après traitement. I. La syphilis tardive expérimentale. Ann. Inst. Pasteur *102:*596–615.
14. Collart, P., L. J. Borel, and P. Durel. 1964. Significance of spiral organisms found after treatment, in late human and experimental syphilis. Brit. J. Vener. Dis. *40:*81–89.
15. Coons, A. H. 1954. Labelled antigens and antibodies. Ann. Rev. Microbiol. *8:*333–352.
16. D'Alessandro, G., and L. Dardanoni. 1953. Isolation and purification of protein antigen of the Reiter treponeme; study of its serological reactions. Amer. J. Syph. *37:*137–150.
17. Deacon, W. E., V. H. Falcone, and A. Harris. 1957. A fluorescent antibody test for treponemal antibodies. Proc. Soc. Exp. Biol. Med. *96:*477–480.
18. Donnan, E. 1930. Documents Illustrative of the Slave Trade to America. Publication No. 409, Carnegie Corp. of Washington, Vol. 1, pp. 1441–1700.
19. Eagle, H., R. Fleischman, and A. D. Musselman. 1950. The effective concentrations of penicillin *in vitro* and *in vivo* for streptococci, pneumococci, and *Treponema pallidum.* J. Bact. *59:*625–643.

The author wishes to acknowledge the valuable criticisms and suggestions of his colleague, Dr. Paul H. Hardy.

20. Eaton, M. D. 1965. Pleuropneumonia-like organisms and related forms. Ann. Rev. Microbiol. *19:*379–406.

21. Frazier, C. N., A. Bensel, and C. S. Keuper. 1952. Further observations on the duration of spirochetemia in rabbits with asymptomatic syphilis. Amer. J. Syph. *36:*167–173.

22. Fredriksson, T., B. Hederstedt, and S. Rosengren. 1967. A study on the serology in relation to histopathological findings in *T. pallidum*-infected animals and man. WHO/VDT/RES/67.120.

23. Fribourg-Blanc, A., G. Niel, and H. H. Mollaret. 1963. Note sur quelques aspects immunologiques du cynocéphale africain. Bull. Soc. Path. Exot. *56:*474–485.

24. Fribourg-Blanc, A., G. Niel, and H. H. Mollaret. 1966. Confirmation sérologique et microscopique de la tréponématose du cynocéphale de Guinée. Bull. Soc. Path. Exot. *59:*54–59.

25. Fribourg-Blanc, A., and H. H. Mollaret. 1968. Natural treponematosis in the African monkey: Isolation of a strain of pathogenic treponeme and its adaptation to the hamster. WHO/VDT/RES/68.135.

26. Gajdusek, D. C. 1967. Slow-virus infection of the nervous system. New Eng. J. Med. *276:*392–400.

27. Gale, E. F., and E. S. Taylor. 1947. The assimilation of amino-acids by bacteria. 5. The action of penicillin in preventing the assimilation of glutamic acid by *Staphylococcus aureus*. J. Gen. Microbiol. *1:*314–326.

28. Goldman, J. N., and K. F. Girard. 1967. Intraocular treponemes in treated congenital syphilis. Arch. Ophthal. *78:*47–50.

28a. Grin, E. I. 1953. Epidemiology and control of endemic syphilis. Report of a mass-treatment campaign in Bosnia. World Health Organization, Geneva. Monograph Series No. 11.

28b. Grin, E. I. 1962. Endemic treponematoses. St. Johns Hospital Dermatological Transactions, Summer 1962 (London).

29. Guthe, T. 1966. Epidemiological-serological investigations of yaws. Freezing and transport of sera at −150 to −196°C. in liquid nitrogen. Arch. Immun. Ther. Exp. *14:*689–703.

30. Guthe, T., and O. Idsøe. 1968. Antibiotic treatment of syphilis. *In:* Antibiotic Treatment of Venereal Diseases. A. Luger (Ed.) S. Karger, Basel.

30a. Guthe, T. 1969. Clinical, serological and epidemiological features of framboesia tropica (yaws) and its control in rural communities. Acta Dermato-Venereol. Scand. *49:*343–368.

31. Hackett, C. J. 1963. On the origin of the human treponematoses (pinta, yaws, endemic syphilis and venereal syphilis). Bull. WHO *29:*7–41.

32. Hardy, P. H., and E. E. Nell. 1955. Specific agglutination of *Treponema pallidum* by sera from rabbits and human beings with treponemal infections. J. Exp. Med. *101:*367–382.

33. Hollander, D. H., T. B. Turner, and E. E. Nell. 1952. Effect of long-continued subcurative doses of penicillin during the incubation period of experimental syphilis. Bull. Johns Hopkins Hosp. *90:*105–120.

33a. Jepsen, O. B., K. H. Hougen, and A. Birch-Andersen. 1968. Electron microscopy of *Treponema pallidum* Nichols. Acta Path. Microbiol. Scand. *74:*241–258.

34. Julian, A. J., L. C. Logan, and L. C. Norins. 1969. Early syphilis: immunoglobulins reactive in immunofluorescence and other serologic tests. J. Immunol. *102:*1250–1259.

35. Kabat, E. A., and M. M. Mayer. 1961. Experimental Immunochemistry. Charles C Thomas, Springfield, Ill.

36. Király, K., R. Backhausz, A. Jobbágy, J. Lajos, and L. Kováts. 1967. Fluorescent treponemal antibody test with antihuman immune sera of different specificity. WHO/VDT/RES/67.130.

37. Klein, G. 1966. Tumor antigens. Ann. Rev. Microbiol. *20:*223–252.

38. Knox, J. M., W. G. Dacres, D. H. Short, and J. M. Glicksman. 1967. Research on immunology in syphilis. WHO/VDT/RES 67.128. Paper read at the 25th General Assembly and Technical Conference of the International Union Against Venereal Diseases and the Treponematoses (IUVDT), Munich, August, 1967.

39. Kuhn, U. S. G., W. J. Brown, and V. H. Falcone. 1967. Seroreactivity of non-human primates in treponemal and non-treponemal antigen tests for syphilis. WHO/VDT/RES/68.137.

39a. Kuhn, U. S. G., G. Varela, F. W. Chandler, and G. G. Osuna. 1968. Experimental pinta in the chimpanzee. J.A.M.A. *206:*829.

40. Landsteiner, K., and V. Mucha. 1906. Zur Technik der Spirochaetenuntersuchung. Wien. Klin. Wschr. *19:*1349–1350.

41. Laurell, A. B. 1955. On antibodies separated by paper electrophoresis with special reference to the Wassermann reagins. Acta Path. Microbiol. Scand., Suppl. 103, pp. 1–90.

42. McDermott, W. 1958. Microbial persistence. Yale J. Biol. Med. *30:*257–291. (See also Harvey Lecture Series, 1968.)

43. Mackaness, G. B., and R. V. Blanden. 1967. Cellular immunity. Prog. Allerg. *11:*89–140. (Reprinted as Chapter 2 in this volume.)

44. Magnuson, H. J., B. J. Rosenau, and B. C. Greenberg. 1951. The effects of sex, castration, and testosterone upon the susceptibility of rabbits to experimental syphilis. Amer. J. Syph. *35:*146–163.
45. Magnuson, H. J., E. V. Thomas, S. Olansky, B. I. Kaplan, L. De Mello and J. C. Cutler. 1953. Inoculation of syphilis in human volunteers. Medicine *35:*33–82.
46. Mahoney, J. F., and K. K. Bryant. 1934. The time element in the penetration of the genital mucosa of the rabbit by *Treponema pallidum.* J. Vener. Dis. Inform. *15:*1–5.
46a. Medina, R. 1964. Reactions produced in pinta, yaws or syphilis patients on inoculation with *Treponema pertenue* Castellani 1905. WHO/VDT/RES/63.64.
47. Michaelis, L. 1907. Präcipitinreaktion bei Syphilis. Klin. Wschr. *44:*1477.
48. Miller, J. N. 1964. The appearance and persistence of VDRL, RPCF, and TPI antibody during the course and treatment of experimental syphilis in the rabbit. J. Invest. Derm. *42:*367–371.
49. Mudd, S., K. Polevitzky, and T. F. Anderson. 1943. Bacterial morphology as shown by the electron microscope. V. *Treponema pallidum, T. macrodentium* and *T. microdentium.* J. Bact. *46:*15–24.
49a. Murray, J. F., A. M. Merriweather, M. L. Freedman, and D. J. deVilliers. 1956. Endemic syphilis in the Bakwena Reserve of the Bechuanaland Protectorate. A report on mass examination and treatment. Bull. WHO *15:*975–1039.
50. Nell, E. E., and P. H. Hardy. 1966. Studies on the clinical composition and immunologic properties of a polysaccharide from the Reiter treponeme. Immunochemistry *3:*233–245.
51. Nelson, R. A., and H. G. Steinman. 1948. Factors affecting the survival of *Treponema pallidum in vitro.* Proc. Soc. Exp. Biol. Med. *68:*588.
52. Nelson, R. A., and M. M. Mayer. 1949. Immobilization of *Treponema pallidum in vitro* by antibody produced in syphilitic infection. J. Exp. Med. *89:*369–393.
53. Nielsen, H. Aa. 1957. Investigations on the reproducibility of the quantitative *Treponema pallidum* immobilization test. Acta Path. Microbiol. Scand. *40:*119–135.
54. Norins, L. C., L. C. Logan, and A. J. Julian. 1968. Antibodies in the course of syphilis in rabbits. Unpublished observations.
55. Ovčinnikov, N. M., and V. V. Delektorskij. 1966. Ultrathin sections of *treponema pallidum* in the electron microscope. J. Hyg. Epidem. (Praha) *10:*195.
56. Pillot, J., and A. Ryter. 1965. Structure des spirochètes. 1. Etude des genres *Treponema, Borrelia,* et *Leptospira* au microscope electronique. Ann. Inst. Pasteur *108:*791–804.
57. Poulson, D. F., and B. Sakaguchi. 1961. Nature of "sex-ratio" agent in *Drosophila.* Science *133:*1489–1490.
58. Putkonen, T., O. R. Salo, and K. K. Mustakallio. 1966. The febrile Herxheimer reaction in different phases of primary and secondary syphilis. Brit. J. Vener. Dis. *42:*181–184.
59. Reynolds, F. W. 1941. The fate of *Treponema pallidum* inoculated subcutaneously into immune rabbits. Bull. Johns Hopkins Hosp. *69:*53–60.
60. Smith, J. L., C. W. Israel, J. A. McCrory, and R. E. Harner. 1968. Recovery of *Treponema pallidum* from aqueous humor removed at cataract surgery in man by passive transfer to rabbit testis. Amer. J. Ophth. *65:*242–247.
61. Strominger, J. L., and D. J. Tipper. 1965. Bacterial cell wall synthesis and structure in relation to the mechanism of action of penicillins and other antibacterial agents. Amer. J. Med. *39:*708–721.
62. Sudhoff, K. 1917. The origin of syphilis. Bull. Soc. Med. Hist. *2:*15–23.
63. Sudhoff, K. 1925. The earliest printed literature on syphilis, being the tractates from the years 1495–1498. Adapted by C. Singer. Florence, R. Lier and Co.
64. Thivolet, J., J. Sepetjian, and T. Guerraz. 1968. Examination of 667 sera from monkeys of various origins for treponemal antibodies. WHO/VDT/RES/68.136.
65. Tringali, G., C. Del Carpio, and N. Giammanco. 1966. Sensitivity to 2-mercaptoethanol of reagins in human syphilis, in B. F. P. reactors in "normal rabbits." Riv. Ist. Sieroter. Ital. *41:*291–298.
66. Turner, T. B. 1936. The resistance of yaws and syphilis patients to reinoculation with yaws spirochetes. Amer. J. Hyg. *23:*431–448.
67. Turner, T. B. 1938. The preservation of virulent *T. pallidum* and *T. pertenue* in the frozen state: with a note on the preservation of viruses. J. Exp. Med. *67:*61–78.
68. Turner, T. B. 1939. Protective antibodies in the serum of syphilitic rabbits. J. Exp. Med. *69:*867–890.
69. Turner, T. B., and D. H. Hollander. 1957. Biology of the Treponematoses. World Health Organization Series No. 35, Geneva.
70. Turner, T. B., P. H. Hardy, and B. Newman. 1969. Infectivity tests in syphilis. Brit. J. Vener. Dis. *45:*183–196.
71. Turner, T. B., and B. Newman. Unpublished material.

72. Waring, G. W., Jr., and W. L. Fleming. 1951. The effect of partial immunity on dissemination of infection in experimental syphilis. Amer. J. Syph. *36*:368–375.
73. Whang, H. Y., and E. Neter. 1967. Further studies on the effect of endotoxin on antibody response of the rabbit to common antigen of *enterobacteriaceae*. J. Immun. *98*:948–957.
74. Wilcox, R. R., and T. Guthe. 1956. *Treponema Pallidum*. A Bibliographical Review of the Morphology, Culture, and Survival of *T. Pallidum* and Associated Organisms. World Health Organization, Geneva.
75. Wilkinson, A. E., and C. F. A. Rayner. 1966. Studies on fluorescent treponemal antibody (FTA) test. Brit. J. Vener. Dis. *42*:8–15.
76. Wood, R. M., Y. Inonye, W. Argonza, L. Bradford, R. Jue, Y. Jeong, J. Puffer, and H. L. Bodily. 1967. Comparison of the fluorescent treponemal antibody absorption and *Treponema pallidum* immobilization tests on serums from 1182 diagnostic problem cases. Amer. J. Clin. Path. *47*:521–524.
77. Yobs, A. R., S. Olansky, D. H. Rockwell, and J. W. Clark. 1965. Do treponemes survive adequate treatment of late syphilis? Arch. Derm. *91*:379–389.

# Chapter 17

# THE NATURE OF MYCOPLASMAL INFECTIONS

MONROE D. EATON

*Harvard Medical School, Boston, Massachusetts*

The organism of bovine pleuropneumonia was considered a filterable virus until Nocard and Roux (1898) succeeded in growing it in broth contained in a collodion sac inserted into the peritoneal cavity of a rabbit. From such cultures the disease was reproduced in cattle. Although the organisms did not pass out of the collodion sac (and presumably viruses from the rabbit could not pass in), the emergence of toxic products caused extreme emaciation in the rabbits used as hosts. Later the use of media containing serum enabled Borrel et al. (1910) to study in detail the morphology and other properties of *Mycoplasma mycoides*, which for 25 years remained the sole representative of this group. In 1923 the organism causing agalactia in sheep was isolated and several "pleuropneumonia-like" species were described in the early 1930's by Ledingham, Klieneberger-Nobel, Laidlaw, and others. Elford, using gradocol membranes for filterability measurements, obtained results indicating that the minimum viable units were 125 to 175 m$\mu$ in diameter. Thus the existence of the smallest free-living organisms capable of reproducing themselves without assistance from other forms of life was established.

The similarities of pleuropneumonia-like organisms to bacteria without their cell walls (L forms) were soon brought out by the work of Klieneberger (1935) with *Streptobacillus moniliformis*. In cultures of this organism two colony forms regularly appear: the ordinary streptobacillus colonies containing pleomorphic rods and filaments, and much smaller colonies consisting of large polymorphous bodies and small coccoid elements growing down into the medium. Klieneberger propagated the small colonies in pure culture and, noting their similarity to mycoplasma colonies, believed them to be living in symbiosis with *S. moniliformis*. But Dienes and Smith (1942) were able to cause reversion of pure cultures of the L$_1$ form to the streptobacillus. The possible existence of small colony variants (and possibly filterable forms) of bacteria had been studied by Dienes and several other investigators as early as 1930. Later Dienes and his associates produced L variants from numerous species of bacteria. When the mode of action of lysozyme and penicillin in removing or preventing formation of cell walls was defined it became apparent that L forms were phenotypic variants of bacteria sometimes so stable as to suggest that mutation had occured.

Even now the difference between mycoplasmas and stable L forms is a matter of considerable uncertainty. One point of view is that the former have evolved from the latter; hence the distinction becomes a matter of elapsed time (plus an appropriate selective environment). It is not surprising, therefore, that isolates from infected materials have been termed L forms (e.g., Klieneberger's $L_2$, $L_3$, $L_4$) when they were really mycoplasmas. Also, the use of selective media containing penicillin may result in the emergence of L forms of bacteria which can be identified only by their reversion to the original bacterial form, and such reversion may take a long time. So far attempts to produce reversion of mycoplasmas to bacteria in the laboratory have either given completely negative results or aroused suspicions of contamination and acrimonious controversies. The search for bacterial ancestors of the mycoplasmas must be based on some other approach, as discussed later.

For many years mycoplasmas were of much more concern to veterinarians than they were to those working on human medical problems. Bovine pleuropneumonia was a widespread and frequently fatal disease over large parts of the world and still remains a serious problem in certain regions of Africa, Australia, and Eastern Europe. According to Foster (1934),[*] bovine pleuropneumonia first appeared in Switzerland and Germany in 1713 and in England in 1735. By the end of the eighteenth century it had spread over the entire German Empire, France, and Italy. It was carried from England to Australia in 1858 and about the same time from Holland to South Africa. The United States was affected in 1843 and it was only by the most energetic and rigid government veterinary measures that the disease was finally eradicated. Pleuropneumonia of cattle was first recognized in China in the early twentieth century, but is less common in the Near East and India although pleuropneumonia of goats is widespread in those regions. M. mycoides may not be brought into the United States and several other countries, even for laboratory study.

In addition to infection of cattle by two well defined species (M. mycoides and M. bovigenitalium), mycoplasmal infections have been described in goats, sheep, dogs, swine, rats, mice, chickens, turkeys, and possibly cold blooded animals. Pneumonia and other lesions of the respiratory tract (acute or chronic) are considered the most important forms of such infections, but involvement of the oviducts and uterus, mastitis, arthritis, eye infections, septicemia, pericarditis, peritonitis, enteritis, lymphadenitis, subcutaneous cellulitis, myositis, and infections of the heart valves (endocardium) and central nervous system have been described in various species of animals.

Much of the early work on the association of mycoplasmas, and pos-

---

[*] Quoted by Tang et al. (1935) and Klieneberger-Nobel (1962).

sibly L forms, with human infection was done by Dienes and his associates. Dienes and Edsall (1937) isolated a mycoplasma in pure culture from an abscess of Bartholin's gland, and subsequent studies by Klieneberger-Nobel (1960), Stokes (1955), and others have associated these organisms with the urogenital tract. More recently the T strains, which may be a different genus, have been associated with nongonococcal urethritis. (Shepard, 1956). The agent of primary atypical pneumonia, isolated by the author and his colleagues in 1942 and thought to be a virus, was after 20 years shown to be a mycoplasma by Marmion and Goodburn (1961), who first visualized it in chick embryos, and by Chanock, Hayflick, and Barile (1962), who grew it on artificial medium. These observations emphasized the pathogenicity of mycoplasmas for human beings and stimulated research on the biological characteristics of these organisms and their role in human infectious disease. Of the various well defined species so far isolated from man, only *M. pneumoniae*, *M. hominis* type 1, and the T strains seem to have pathogenic properties. The remaining known species, *M. fermentans*, *M. salivarium*, and *M. orale* (*M. pharyngis*), appear to be saprophytes of quite ubiquitous distribution. Numberous unidentified strains have been isolated from the genitourinary tract and from other human material, as reviewed by Hayflick and Chanock (1965).

A group of mycoplasmas found in sewage, compost, and soil has been designated *M. laidlawii*, types A, B, and C, after Laidlaw (1936), who discovered them. These organisms will grow on simpler media than will the species from animals and human beings, but it is still not clear whether their normal habitat is the intestinal tract or whether such organisms are capable of existing independently of higher animals.

## TAXONOMY AND CLASSIFICATION

Mycoplasmas differ from filterable viruses in four important respects: (1) They contain both DNA and RNA, whereas all viruses are thought to contain either one or the other but not both. (2) They are capable of growing on lifeless media because their physiology closely resembles that of some bacteria. (3) Unlike viruses, the mycoplasmas do not appear to be capable of modifying the metabolic machinery of the host cell so as to use it for their own reproduction. They are not dependent on the host cell for energy metabolites or on host ribosomes for protein synthesis directed by foreign messenger ribonucleic acid as from a virus. (4) Mycoplasmas are enclosed in a triple-layered flexible plasma membrane, whereas viruses have an outer coat consisting of protein molecules arranged in geometrical symmetry. However, some viruses do in addition have an outer membrane, apparently derived from modified host cell material.

The principal difference of mycoplasmas from bacteria is the absence of a cell wall containing muramic acid. This is replaced by a stabilized membrane containing cholesterol, in most of the pathogenic species, or lipids containing phosphatidyl glycerol and phosphatidyl glucose in other species. The passage

TABLE 1. *"Intermediate" Agents and Viruses*

|  | MYCOPLASMAS | CHLAMYDIAE | RICKETTSIAE | VIRUSES |
|---|---|---|---|---|
| DNA and RNA | both | both | both | either |
| Cell wall and sensitivity to penicillin | 0 | + | ? | 0 |
| Filterability | + | + | ± | + |
| Growth on lifeless medium | +* | 0 | 0* | 0 |
| Enzyme activity in particle | + | + | + | 0* |
| Replication | ? fission | ? fission | binary fission | exposed† genes |

* One or more exceptions.
† Uncoating, replication of genetic material, synthesis of coat protein, and reassembly.

of mycoplasmas through filters which retain bacteria probably can be attributed to their plastic outer membrane as well as to their small size. As to nutritional requirements, no clear distinction between mycoplasmas and bacteria seems possible except that less is known about the specific nutritional requirements of the former. Dependence on cholesterol, found in some mycoplasmas, has not been found among bacteria.

It is somewhat more difficult to differentiate mycoplasmas from rickettsiae and chlamydiae (bedsoniae), especially if it is true that some mycoplasmas will not grow on lifeless media. Certain agents causing chronic lung disease in animals are indistinguishable from mycoplasmas in fine structure and tissue localization but have not yet been grown on artificial media (Gay, 1967). They also have the same spectrum of sensitivity to antibiotics and gold salts as mycoplasmas do. Although the growth of most species of mycoplasmas is extracellular or on the surface of cells, they are sometimes seen inside cells and the intracellular microcolonies of *M. pneumoniae* closely resemble those of rickettsiae or the chlamydiae (Eaton et al., 1962). They do, however, differ in staining reactions. Some mycoplasmas are reported to have a definite coccobacilliform morphology and uniform size, thus resembling rickettsiae. Also, *R. quintana*, the organism causing trench fever, has been grown on artificial medium (Vinson, 1961) and it has been known for 20 years that other rickettsiae possess some of the enzymes concerned in energy metabolism.

The chlamydiae are clearly distinguishable from mycoplasmas by their sensitivity to penicillin which has been correlated with the presence of a cell wall like that of bacteria. As with rickettsiae, enzymes of energy metabolism and biosynthesis have been demonstrated. However, obligate cellular parasitism may soon disappear as a fixed characteristic of the chlamydiae since one psittacosis agent has shown limited replication in enucleate cytoplasmic fragments.

Although the several agents just discussed differ from viruses in that they appear to replicate by some form of fission, true binary fission, as occurs in bacteria, remains in doubt for the chlamydiae and mycoplasmas. Most of the latter do not seem to exhibit the orderly binary fission observed with bacteria. Freundt (1958) has maintained that reproduction occurs by the formation of elementary bodies in the mycelial structures often observed in mycoplasma cultures.

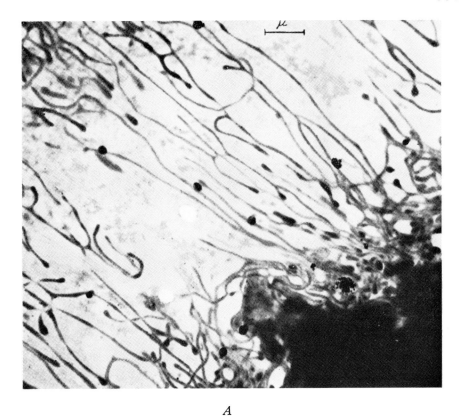

A

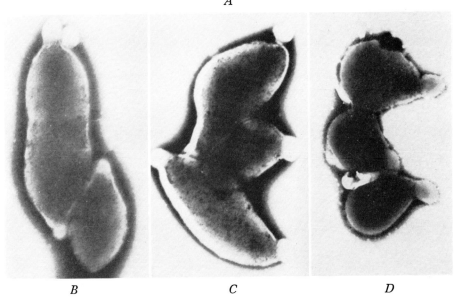

B                          C                          D

*Figure 1.   A, Mycoplasma mycoides.* Electron micrograph of 4 hour colony growing on collodion films floating on serum broth: branching mycelial filaments (×10,300). (From Freundt. 1958. The Mycoplasmataceae. Munksgaard, Copenhagen.) *B, C,* and *D, Mycoplasma gallisepticum.* Electron micrograph of glutaraldehyde-fixed, negatively stained cells, 2 to 4 hour cultures: polar blebs and apparent binary fission (×36,400). (From Morowitz and Maniloff. 1966. J. Bact. *91:*1638–1644.)

TABLE 2.    *Comparison of Some Metabolic Characteristics of* M. pneumoniae
*and Streptococci*

|  | M. PNEUMONIAE | STR. MG | STR. FAECALIS |
|---|---|---|---|
| Catalase | 0 | 0 | 0 |
| Aerobic stimulation (glucose) | + | ND | + |
| α Glycerophosphate → $H_2O_2$ + lactate | + | 0 | + |
| Arginine → Ornithine, $NH_3$, ATP | 0 | +? | + |
| Methylene blue tolerance (%) | 0.02 | 0.005 | 0.1 |

With *M. mycoides* growing on collodion film floating on serum Freundt obtained mycelial filaments extending from the edge of the colony. On the other hand, evidence that *M. gallisepticum* replicates by binary fission has been presented by Morowitz and Maniloff (1966), who used the phospho-tungstic acid negative staining technique and electron microscopy. With *M. laidlawii* the formation of filaments or single coccoid elements depends in part on the kind of fatty acids, especially oleic acid, in the medium (Razin et al., 1966). *M. pneumoniae* forms coccoid elements both *in vitro* (Clyde, 1967) and *in vivo* (Marmion and Goodburn, 1961). However, a recent paper (Bredt, 1968) reports that *M. pneumoniae* forms filments and later grape-like structures when grown on coverslips in broth. T strain colonies are much smaller than those of other mycoplasmas and are composed of coccoid elements. Classification of mycoplasmas into subgroups on the basis of morphology and mode of replication remains uncertain.

Some relatively unique metabolic properties of mycoplasmas may have taxonomic significance not only in classification within the group but also in suggesting evolutionary relationships to bacteria.

For example, *M. pneumoniae* forms hydrogen peroxide under certain conditions. The only bacteria known to form hydrogen peroxide are anaerobes, pneumococci, and some groups of streptococci. Since *M. pneumoniae* grows best

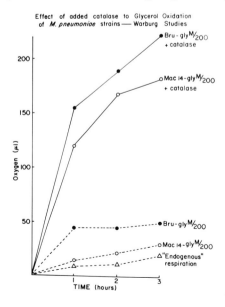

*Figure 2.*    Release by catalase of the hydrogen peroxide inhibition of oxygen uptake in *Mycoplasma pneumoniae* strains Bru and Mac; about $10^9$ organisms suspended in saline with glycerol (gly) as substrate. (From Low, Eaton, and Proctor. 1968. J. Bact. *95*:1425–1430.)

under aerobic conditions it cannot be classed as an anaerobe. The inhibitory effect of hydrogen peroxide on *M. pneumoniae* is relieved by catalase (Low, Eaton, and Proctor, 1968) which is absent or deficient in many strains of mycoplasmas. Rodwell (1967) has reported similar observations for *M. mycoides* (Fig. 2).

The use of biochemical reactions as a basis for taxonomy is fundamental and well known. A comparison of *M. pneumoniae* with two streptococci is shown in Table 2. Streptococcus MG has an antigen in common with *M. pneumoniae*. Catalase, although absent in the organisms listed, is present in other species of mycoplasmas (*M. gallisepticum*) and hence is of taxonomic significance. Although many mycoplasmas grow best at low oxygen tension, *M. pneumoniae* and *M. mycoides* are stimulated in a glucose-containing medium by aeration. *M. pneumoniae*, *M. gallisepticum*, *M. mycoides*, and several other species ferment glucose and this has been used in classification to set them apart from nonfermentative species, as with bacteria. Oxidation of glycerol has not been investigated in detail with mycoplasmas but *M. pneumoniae* apparently uses a pathway common to the group D streptococci and *M. mycoides* in the formation of L-glycerol-3-phosphate, which in the lack of NAD-linked dehydrogenases forms hydrogen peroxide and lactate. Bacteria that do not form peroxide, and probably some species of mycoplasma, ferment glycerol in a different manner.

Another intriguing set of enzymes is that concerned with the utilization of arginine. There are at least two different pathways by which microorganisms may produce ammonia. Many species of mycoplasmas, but not *M. pneumoniae*, use arginine as a source of energy by way of citrulline, carbamyl phosphate, and ATP. The other reaction, by the action of arginase, causes a breakdown of arginine to urea and ornithine without the formation of citrulline and is not known to occur among mycoplasmas.

*M. pneumoniae* is more resistant to methylene blue than most other species of mycoplasmas and this property is shared by group D streptococci. Reduction of tetrazolium salts may prove to be of some value in classifying mycoplasmas (Fabricant and Freundt, 1967) but with some species the reaction is variable, depending upon conditions of growth and the composition of the medium.

Molecular genetic studies of relationships among mycoplasmas, L forms, and bacteria have become useful recently. Base ratio determinations and agar column hybridization of extracted nucleic acids have shown clear relationships among L forms and known bacterial parents. But similar relations between mycoplasmas and hypothetical bacterial ancestors, *M. pneumoniae* and streptococcus MG or *M. hominis* and a diphtheroid D5, have indicated a complete lack of genetic relationship (McGee et al., 1967). It is of interest that *M. pneumoniae* has a base composition quite different from that of most mycoplasmas, suggesting the possibility of a distinct subgroup.

If the presence or absence of constitutive enzymes reflects the existence of corresponding genes, there are innumerable biochemical tests by which genetic homology can be indicated and possible evolutionary relationships indicated. Obviously tests of nucleic acid homology cannot be done with all species of mycoplasmas against all bacteria, but it is hoped that disclosure of unique metabolic properties such as those just discussed will point to those organisms most likely to give positive results in homology measurements.

## GROWTH REQUIREMENTS

Media used for isolation of mycoplasmas are of unknown chemical composition and have been developed empirically. It is doubtful that any medium, even though used successfully for several fastidious species of mycoplasma, would grow all species. The basic constituents are beef heart infusion broth, peptone, and serum or other proteinaceous material, usually in relatively high concentration.

Generally the medium is made selective by the addition of penicillin (1000 units per ml.) and thallium acetate 1:2000 as inhibitors of bacterial growth. In the attempted isolation of mycoplasmas from materials normally free of bacteria, such as blood, bone marrow, or internal organs obtained with aseptic precautions, the omission of penicillin and thallium acetate would be advantageous. Thallium acetate is known to be inhibitory for the T strains of mycoplasma and the possibility that it may prevent growth of other strains should be kept in mind. Penicillin presents the hazard of inducing L form transformations of bacteria, especially when hypertonic media are used. The resulting confusion can be resolved only by serial subcultures in the absence of penicillin to obtain reversion to the parent bacterium. Streptomycin, which has been added routinely with penicillin to eliminate bacteria from materials used in virus isolation, is inhibitory to many species of mycoplasmas, as are numerous other antibiotics and antimycotic agents commonly used in tissue cultures.

With complex media of unknown composition the possibilities of inadvertently including inhibitory substances are considerable. Certain basic media which support growth of some species of mycoplasmas have been found to be inhibitory to other species. Many of the commercial preparations of peptone and agar are inhibitory. Sera of human or animal origin may contain antibodies or other factors capable of preventing or delaying growth, especially when not inactivated at 56°C. Attempts to eliminate these difficulties by isolating the lipoprotein serum fraction required for the growth of many mycoplasmas have been only partially successful because this supplement is unable to support the growth of all species. There may be advantages in using horse serum from which the gamma globulin has been removed.

The successful cultivation of the *M. pneumoniae* and *M. orale* on artificial media resulted from modifications by Hayflick (1965) of the previously available PPLO agar. It appears that the most critical factor was in the preparation of yeast extract. Fresh aqueous extract of baker's yeast was found to be much more effective than other commercial yeast extracts or yeast autolysates then available (Kraybill and Crawford, 1967). Since it is prepared by boiling, the essential nutrients in the yeast extract are heat-stable. On the other hand, heat-labile factors are apparently necessary in the horse serum because heating to 56°C. reduces, but does not abolish, its growth-promoting properties for *M. pneumoniae*.

Although *M. pneumoniae* and *M. mycoides* grow best with mild aeration of the medium, reduced oxygen tension or anaerobiosis may be essential for the growth of T strains and of other species of mycoplasmas, many of which appear to be saprophytic. In atmospheres such as those produced in the candle jar or the Fortner plate (1928) there is increased carbon dioxide as well as reduced oxygen and little is known about the carbon dioxide requirements. Catalase, by decomposing hydrogen peroxide, might increase the aerobic growth of some "anaerobic" strains.

Information about specific nutrients required by mycoplasmas is quite limited. The fermentative strains use glucose aerobically (*M. pneumoniae* and *M. mycoides*) or under anaerobic conditions (*M. fermentans*). Although glucose definitely increases the rate of growth, a precipitous drop in pH to levels of 6.0 to 6.5 may result in rapid loss of viability of the cultures. Lactate, pyruvate, and glycerol can serve as energy sources for some species, and pyruvate also reacts nonenzymatically with hydrogen peroxide to produce acetate, carbon dioxide, and water, thus relieving hydrogen peroxide inhibition.

On the other hand, there are several nonfermenters that cannot utilize glucose at all and must have pentose sugars, either free or as DNA, for biosynthesis of nucleic acids. Arginine can serve as an energy source for species having the dihydrolase enzyme system and in some cases addition of arginine as a supplement has been reported to improve growth.

A few studies on amino acid requirements have revealed marked deficiencies in the ability of mycoplasmas to synthesize these building blocks of proteins. A list of nine amino acids required by *M. hominis* type 2 was published some time ago (Smith, 1955). Rodwell has recently presented evidence that a strain of *M. mycoides* cannot synthesize any of the amino acids. In addition, a requirement for certain amino acids in the form of dipeptides or polypeptides has been indicated. Lack of biosynthetic capabilities apparently also extends to purines, pyrimidines, and other nucleic acid precursors. At least some, if not all, T strains require urea for optimum growth. The metabolic function of this substance is unknown.

The specific requirement of most pathogenic mycoplasmas for cholesterol has been recognized longest and studied in greatest detail. The presence of cholesterol in their membranes differentiates mycoplasmas from bacteria and suggests a resemblance to the plasma membranes of animal cells and some protozoa. The protein fraction of serum which promotes growth contains cholesterol and phospholipid and the protein requirement sometimes is related to binding and detoxifying effects for cholesterol or other lipids. Extraction of the lipids makes the protein inactive. Also, the extracted lipid is inactive unless recombined with protein. The presence of cholesterol in the membrane makes mycoplasmas sensitive to cholesterol reagents such as digitonin and to polyene antibiotics.

## HOST SPECIFICITY AND VIRULENCE

Among the many species of mycoplasmas studied actively by veterinarians over a period of more than 30 years not one has been shown definitely to be infectious for man. Nocard and Roux (1898) reported that material from bovine pleuropneumonia, when injected into horses, sheep, dogs, and pigs, produced no disease. Rabbits, guinea pigs, hamsters, and mice are susceptible. This is quite a different situation from the Bedsonia group in which the only reservoirs for human infections are avian and occasionally mammalian hosts.

In the early studies on the etiology of human primary atypical pneumonia difficulty in crossing species barriers was also encountered. Following leads such as the transmission of yellow fever to the mouse by Theiler, and influenza to the ferret by Smith, Andrews, and Laidlaw, numerous investigators attempted reproduction of atypical pneumonia in many species of animals, some quite exotic, with negative results. Weir and Horsfall (1940), before their apparent success with the mongoose, had tried ferrets, mice, guinea pigs, rabbits, monkeys, voles, hamsters, deer mice, skunks, opossums, and woodchucks. It is not definitely known that the agent which produced lung lesions in the mongoose was indeed *M. pneumoniae;* it could well have been another human virus, and since it was subsequently lost no cross immunity tests could be done with the agent that turned out to be *M. pneumoniae.* In California, this writer's associates concentrated their efforts in rodents as experimental animals, since the George Williams Hooper Foundation at the University of California already had a well developed program for trapping, and kindly made a number of species available. None were significantly susceptible to the primary atypical pneumonia agent. At that time the cotton rat was not unknown in virus research; it had been used for studies on typhus and poliomyelitis. The western cotton rat (*Sigmodon hispidus eremicus*), which is tamer and more easily bred in captivity, was used in preference to the species generally available to laboratory workers (*Sigmodon hispidus hispidus*). In both species pulmonary lesions similar in gross and microscopic pathology to those in human disease developed after intranasal inoculation under ether anesthesia with suspensions of sputum or pulmonary tissue. At the time these studies were in progress, Dr. Harold N. Johnson, investigating an epidemic in Alabama, also obtained lung lesions in cotton rats (see Annual Report of the International Health Division, Rockefeller Foundation, 1942, page 44). When the Syrian hamsters became available for experimental work, animals bred in the California laboratories were found to be as susceptible as cotton rats but other lines seem to be somewhat more resistant to the atypical pneumonia agent. In both cotton rats and hamsters the pulmonary lesions diminished or disappeared on serial passage, indicating that the human material contained a higher concentration of organisms than was present in the lungs of an animal with well developed pulmonary consolidation. This suggests that a toxic factor of *M. pneumoniae* or an enhancing effect of heterologous tissue may participate in the production of pulmonary lesions in cotton rats and hamsters.

In chick embryos variation in growth of the atypical pneumonia agent was encountered but in serial passages up to the eightieth some lots produced pulmonary lesions in cotton rats equal to or greater in extent than those from human material. When *M. pneumoniae* was finally cultured on lifeless medium, small pulmonary lesions were obtained in Western cotton rats with broth cultures of the fifty-eighth passage containing about $10^6$ colony forming units (CFU) per ml. Suspensions of chick embryo tissue were found to contain about $10^7$ CFU per ml. Passage from chick embryo to broth resulted initially in poor growth (about $10^4$ CFU per ml.), and adaptation to artificial medium was necessary.

Most attempts to produce disease in experimental animals with other mycoplasmas of human origin have been fruitless. Freundt (1958) in unpublished experiments did succeed in producing abscesses in rabbits by intratesticular inoculation of human strains; abscesses can also be produced by mixing mycoplasmas with agar or other material before subcutaneous injection. It is, however, not uncommon to obtain mycoplasmas as contaminants in experimental animals inoculated with material from human disease of unknown etiology. Thus *M. neurolyticum* was recovered during studies on toxoplasmosis (Sabin, 1938), in which mice were inoculated intracerebrally, and another mycoplasma, probably *M. pulmonis*, after intranasal inoculation and passage in mice of material from cases of chickenpox (Edward, 1940). During the studies on atypical pneumonia we encountered a contaminant in chick embryos, probably *M. gallisepticum*, which produced extensive pulmonary lesions in cotton rats (van Herick and Eaton, 1945) but was avirulent for hamsters and other rodents. A possible example of contamination from laboratory animals of mycoplasma cultures on cell-free medium may be the organism designated *M. hominis* type 2, which was originally described as a common genital strain in the United States. This species is antigenically indistinguishable from *M. arthriditis*, which is indigenous to rats. Other isolations from human material of mycoplasmas antigenically related to *M. hominis* 2 have recently been reported from Finland by Jansson and Wager (1967). It should be noted that antigenic relationship does not necessarily establish the origin of all strains having the *M. hominis* 2 antigen. There may be antigens in common between rat and human strains.

The fact that most identifiable mycoplasmas can be cultivated on artificial medium would seem to make superfluous the use of chick embryos or tissue cultures. Because of the existence of fastidious strains which will not grow on the presently available lifeless media, and in the absence of convenient laboratory methods of determining virulence, tissue cultures remain valuable. It should be noted that species specificity is demonstrable in tissue cultures. Hence the use of cultures of human tissue for isolation of human pathogens is indicated. With good species matching between host cell and mycoplasmas, cytopathic effects are obtained on the first passage in tissue cultures, as with a mycoplasma from bovine mastitis in calf embryo kidney, or *M. gallisepticum* in chick embryo cultures. Strains of human origin, either pathogenic or sapro-

TABLE 3. Mycoplasma pneumoniae *in Tissue Culture*

| TISSUE | GROWTH | CPE* |
|---|:---:|:---:|
| Chick embryo | | |
| Amnion, CAM | + | O |
| Yolk entoderm | + | O |
| Rh. monkey kidney | + | ± or O |
| Human | | |
| HeLa | ± | O |
| Amnion (WS) | + | + |
| Embryonic lung (E. Davis) | + | + |

* CPE: cytopathic effects.

TABLE 4.    *Pneumonia by Intranasal Inoculation of Chinese Hamsters*

| STRAIN | PASSAGE | INOCULUM CFU*/ML. | PNEUMONIA NUMBER TESTED |
|---|---|---|---|
| Normal chick embryo | | — | 0/9 |
| Mac | CE† 79 | $2 \times 10^7$ | 10/13 |
| Mac | Agar 14 | $4 \times 10^7$ | 0/4 (1 ±) |
| Mac | Agar 125 | $2 \times 10^9$ | 1/3 (1 ±) |
| FH | Agar 67 | $10^8$ | 4/4 |
| FH | Agar 125 | $2 \times 10^8$ | 3/4 (small) |

  * CFU: colony-forming units.
  † CE: chick embryo.

phytic, grew and formed intracytoplasmic inclusions in a tissue culture of human synovial cells (Hayflick and Stinebring, 1960). *M. pneumoniae* will grow in cultures of chick embryo, monkey kidney, human amnion, and human embryonic lung, but it will produce cytopathic effects only in human tissues. In HeLa cells, however, *M. pneumoniae* and other mycoplasmas often grow in the medium or on the cell surface but do not produce cytopathic effects.

In the chick embryo, *M. gallisepticum* and *M. mycoides* produce well defined pathologic changes after amniotic, allantoic, or yolk sac inoculation. Others, such as the T strains (Shepard) and *M. pneumoniae*, grow in considerable abundance but do not produce recognizable pathologic changes. Whittlestone (1967) observed that an apparently saprophytic mycoplasma from pigs with enzootic pneumonia grew readily in chick embryos but the true causative organism, also a mycoplasma, would not grow in chick embryos although it did grow in cultures of swine tissue. It has also been claimed that some mycoplasmas will grow on artificial medium only after yolk sac passage (Barber and Fabricant, 1962). The extensive use of chick embryos in study of avian and other mycoplasmas is open to the risk of contamination by organisms carried by the fowl, but it can be pointed out that viruses passed in chick embryos are usually free of mycoplasmal contaminants which, of course, is not the case with tissue culture passages.

The alteration of mycoplasmas by long passage in cell-free medium is a well known phenomenon. Nocard and Roux suspected that isolates from bovine pleuropneumonia had become attenuated after only 10 to 20 passages in broth sacs in the peritoneal cavity of rabbits, and attenuation of this organism readily occurs both in serum broth and chick embryo passage. On the other hand, *M. pneumoniae* retained its ability to produce pulmonary lesions in cotton rats after about 80 passages in chick embryos. After a comparable number of passages in broth, the growth in chick embryos dropped from $10^7$ to $10^3$ CFU/ml. (Eaton and Low, 1967). A freshly isolated strain of *M. pneumoniae* carried in tissue culture for only two passages produced pneumonia in three of 27 human volunteers and febrile respiratory disease in others (Chanock et al., 1961b), but after passages on cell-free medium illness was produced less frequently (Smith et al., 1967). Evidence for the attenuation of *M. pneumoniae* on artificial medium is supported by experiments in animals. A comparison of egg passage and agar passage strains also indicated a loss of virulence in terms of ability to produce pulmonary lesions in Chinese hamsters, and agar-passed organisms seldom produced gross pneumonic lesions in Syrian hamsters (Dajani, Clyde, and Denny, 1965).

## PATHOLOGY AND PATHOGENESIS

Before it was known that the causative agent of cold agglutinin-positive atypical pneumonia was a mycoplasma, a characteristic pathology of "virus" pneumonia in man and experimental animals was recognized. Nonbacterial pneumonias were seen to have a greater abundance of mononuclear cells than bacterial pneumonias, with interstitial infiltration and mononuclear cuffing of bronchioles and blood vessels. In the few known cases of mycoplasmal pneumonia in man coming to autopsy the gross and microscopic pathologic lesions cannot be differentiated from those of influenza, Q fever, psittacosis, or adenovirus infection (except for the intranuclear inclusions in the latter). The same is true of experimental infection in which the pathologic histology resulting from *M. pneumoniae* cannot be differentiated from that produced by viruses, rickettsiae, or chlamydiae. It should not be inferred, however, that the pathology of nonbacterial pneumonia lacks variety and this is the major source of difficulty in characterizing and differentiating these infections.

Two cases from which the agent later identified as *M. pneumoniae* was transmitted to chick embryos and cotton rats are described by Meiklejohn et al. (1945, and unpublished observations). In one case hospitalized for 6 days before death both lungs were extensively infiltrated with whitish peribronchiolar nodules up to 1 cm. in diameter and confluent nodules up to 4 cm. The pneumonic areas extending from apex to base of both lobes were pink or gray, dry, granular foci of irregular size and shape. The bronchi contained abundant yellowish purulent frothy exudate. The pleural surfaces were smooth and the essential pathological findings were limited to the lungs. Microscopic examination showed almost uniform ulceration of the epithelium in the bronchioles and various combinations of cellular fibrinous or serous exudate in the alveoli. Some alveoli contained patches of polymorphonuclear leukocytes which seemed to be a direct extension from the bronchi. Fibrin in considerable amount was often tightly adherent to alveolar walls and in some areas invasion by young fibroblasts was evident. Many alveoli contained a sparse mononuclear exudate. The epithelial lining of a few bronchi had changed entirely or in part to a stratified squamous type with loss of cilia. Thick collars of round cells around the bronchioles extended into alveolar walls, thickening them markedly.

No bacteria could be seen in the sections of bronchiolar lumens or lung parenchyma, or in impression smears, and cultures remained sterile. Suspensions of the lung tissue inoculated intranasally into cotton rats produced lesions in eight of 27 animals. The agent was carried for over 50 amniotic passages in chick embryos and shown to be antigenically identical with the Mac strain which is still in existence.

The latter strain was isolated from a case more acute and fulminating than the one just described. Death occurred within 2 to 3 days after the onset of illness. Postmortem examination showed almost complete hemorrhagic and edematous consolidation of all lobes without distinct foci. Evidence of acute myocardial involvement was also found (see Rytel, 1964). There was much less cellular reaction in this case, probably because of the overwhelming nature of the infection. Edema fluid and erythrocytes were seen in the alveoli with sparse mononuclear exudate in some areas. There was very little peribronchial, perivascular, or septal infiltration. Although impression smears revealed no bacteria by direct microscopic examination, *Staphylococcus aureus* was cultured from material that had been taken with sterile precautions.

In the experimental pneumonia produced by intranasal inoculation of cotton rats or hamsters with *M. pneumoniae* the extent and character of the pulmonary lesions depends on the number and virulence of the organisms inoculated and also, possibly, on the method of anesthesia. Dajani, Clyde, and Denny (1965), using phenobarbital anesthesia, obtained only minimal pulmonary lesions in Syrian hamsters with inocula up to $10^5$ CFU of a third agar passage following direct isolation on agar. Microscopically the lesions consisted mainly of mononuclear infiltration around bronchi and brochioles with a polymorphonuclear exudate in the lumens. Alveolar thickening and edema were found occasionally. With fluorescein-labeled antibody or special staining techniques small clumps of organisms were found on the surface of the bronchial epithelium and later in deeper layers of the bronchiolar mucosa. There were none in the lung parenchyma. These lesions are probably representative of self-limiting *M. pneumoniae* bronchiolitis as it occurs in man, in which scattered infiltration is often seen by x-ray.

These results in Syrian hamsters are in contrast to the observations of Goodburn and Marmion (1962) and Eaton et al. (1944) with chick embryo passage material and inoculation under ether anesthesia which gave macroscopic lesions of varying extent in over 50 per cent of the hamsters. Lesions in hamsters and cotton rats inoculated with chick embryo material show the changes described in the preceding paragraph with extension to the alveoli. In the consolidated areas there is infiltration of the alveolar walls, mononuclear alveolar exudate, and some polymorphonuclear leukocytes. The alveolar walls contain polyhedral cells with large pale-straining nuclei. Liu (1968) has recently observed that inoculation of *M. pneumoniae* with a pneumococcus in hamsters greatly increases the extent and severity of the pulmonary lesions. On the other hand, streptococcus MG, once thought to have an etiological role in atypical pneumonia, has no synergistic effect with *M. pneumoniae* in cotton rats or hamsters.

In pleuropneumonia of cattle the lymphotropism of *M. mycoides* is quite evident (Adler, 1965). The lung shows a variety of pink, red, and gray lobular consolidation. Invasion of the perivascular lymphatics and extension to the interstitial tissue results in edema of the septa. Compression by accumulated fluids may involve adjacent blood vessels with eventual necrosis. A recent description of experimental caprine pleuropneumonia emphasizes the massive infiltration with lymphocytes in the trachea and bronchial tree and necrosis of the epithelium, with mucous, fibrous, and cellular exudate (Solana and Rivera, 1967). *M. mycoides* also produces perivascular infiltration in the central nervous system, and arthritis resulting from synovitis and necrosis of the joint

A

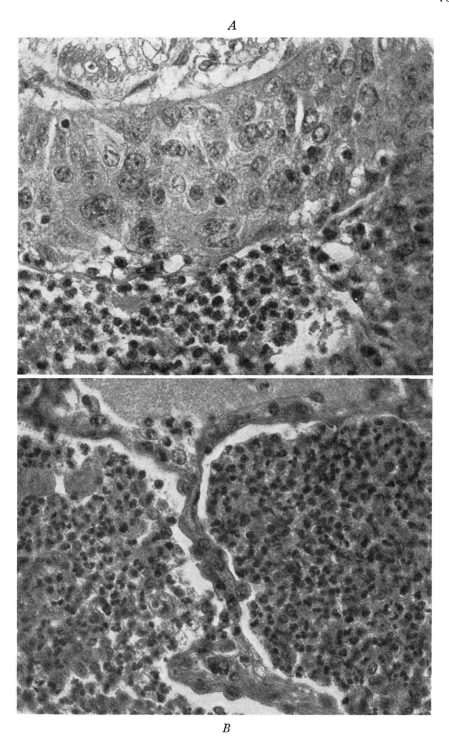

B

*Figure 3.* Sections of lungs from a fatal case of primary atypical pneumonia. Hematoxylin and eosin (×400). *A,* In the alveolar exudate, small mononuclear and polymorphonuclear cells predominate, with occasional macrophages. *B,* Section showing metaplasia of bronchial epithelium. The ciliated columnar epithelium has changed to an irregular stratified squamous type. There is mononuclear infiltration above and to the right; the lumen is below. (From Meiklejohn, Eaton, and van Herick. 1945. J. Clin. Invest. *24:*241–250.)

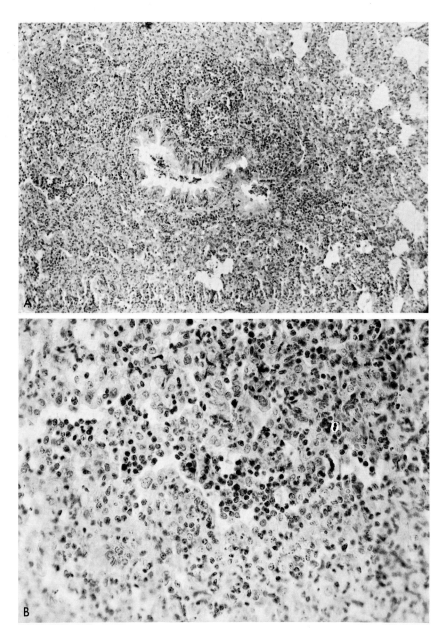

*Figure 4.*    Section of lung from a cotton rat inoculated intranasally with sputum from a patient with primary atypical pneumonia. Animal sacrificed at 10 days. Hematoxylin and phloxine. *A,* Infiltration with lymphocytic cells around blood vessels and bronchioles. Alveolar thickening in various degrees is seen in surrounding areas (×185). *B,* Same showing cellular detail in alveoli. At the center is an alveolar exudate consisting of mononuclear cells and a few polymorphonuclear leukocytes. Alveolar walls contain pathological cells of polyhedral form with large, pale-staining nuclei (×500). (From Eaton, Meiklejohn, and van Herick. 1944. J. Exp. Med. *79:*649–668.)

membrane with lymphocytic infiltration and serous exudate. When *M. mycoides* is inoculated subcutaneously extensive cellulitis results but this property has not been observed in animals inoculated with *M. pneumoniae*, indicating, perhaps, that the latter organism has a tropism limited to the respiratory tract.

In chronic respiratory disease of chickens and turkeys (*M. gallisepticum*) there is involvement of the trachea, air sacs, sinuses, and lungs characterized by formation of lymphoid foci, infiltration with lymphocytes and monocytes, hyperplasia of the epithelium, and granuloma formation (Olesiuk and Van Roekel, 1960).

In contrast to this lymphotropism, in some of the major diseases caused by mycoplasmas abscess formation and sepsis have sometimes been observed in man and animals (Stokes, 1955). *M. hominis* 1 appears to be the most common mycoplasma in abscesses of the genital tract but such cases are relatively rare (Hayflick and Chanock, 1965). This organism also seems able to produce exudative pharyngitis and tonsillitis in experimentally infected human volunteers. Mycoplasmas have been isolated on two occasions from purulent meningitis and abscess of the brain (Paine et al., 1950; Carlson et al., 1951). In animals purulent mastitis and agalactia are common infectious diseases caused by PPLO.

A strain of mycoplasma not previously described but resembling the T strains has been isolated from the chorion, decidua, and amnion of a patient who had a spontaneous abortion (Kundsin et al., 1967). The infected organs showed necrosis of the amniotic membrane and subacute inflammation. Infiltration was mostly polymorphonuclear. Inflammatory exudate, apparently aspirated and swallowed by the fetus, filled the lumens of its bronchi and its stomach without adjacent tissue reaction. There was an unusual sclerosis of placental villi. Subsequently the same strain was isolated from the membranes in three of six spontaneous abortions and from cervical cultures of five of ten women with history of spontaneous abortion.

The affinity of PPLO for serosal membranes is illustrated by a number of animal diseases (Adler, 1965). PPLO other than *M. mycoides* cause fibrino-purulent arthritis in cattle. A septicemic and arthritic disease of goats having similar pathology is apparently transmitted by the respiratory route. There is also meningeal involvement with cellular infiltration of the membranes. This organism is also pathogenic for swine but not for horses, calves, dogs, rabbits, rats, guinea pigs, mice, or avian species. An acute epidemic infectious disease of swine characterized by serofibrinous peritonitis and arthritis has been ascribed to a PPLO. Others have described fibrinous pericarditis, meningitis and other severe serositis often with lymphocytic infiltration associated with *M. hyorhinis* infection of pigs. *M. arthritidis* after intravenous inoculation in mice produces a polymorphonuclear infiltration of the synovial villi accompanied by inflammatory changes in adjacent structures. This is accompanied by proliferation of fibrous tissues, bone, and cartilage. Some of the avian mycoplasmas also cause arthritis. Kerr and Olson (1967) have described chronic vascular lesions produced by experimental infections of chickens with *M. synoviae* or *M. gallisepticum*. Lesions produced in the cardiac arteries and valvular and mural

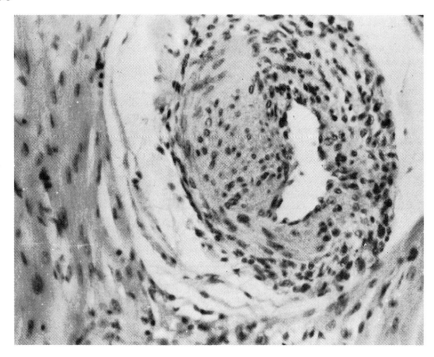

*Figure 5.*   Myocardial artery of chicken infected with *Mycoplasma gallisepticum.* Irregular proliferation of cells of the media with a tendency toward nodule formation (left); lymphocytic and mononuclear cell infiltration with vacuolation of the media (right); 84 days after infection. Hematoxylin and eosin (×312). (From Kerr and Olson. 1967. Ann. N.Y. Acad. Sci. *143:*204–217.)

endocardium were characterized by proliferation of the normal cellular structure as well as generalized reticuloendothelial system proliferation. The disease persisted for as long as 8 months before death.

A good example of the pathology of chronic respiratory infection in mammals is to be found in the disease of mice caused by the agent of mouse catarrh, *M. pulmonis*. Normal-appearing mice carry this mycoplasma in the respiratory and auditory tracts. Some animals develop rhinitis, otitis media, or pneumonia, as evidenced by chattering, torticollis, and labored respiration. Since the pulmonary lesions develop very slowly *M. pulmonis* does not often cause confusion with viruses having a short incubation period, but it may with viruses such as the psittacosis group and that causing enzootic bronchiectasis which also tend to cause chronic infections (Nelson, 1967).

The pulmonary lesions in intranasally infected mice consist of a massive gray focal pneumonia. The bronchi contain abundant leukocytic exudate. There is cuffing of bronchi and blood vessels with lymphocytes and plasma cells and compression or obliteration of the alveoli by accumulated leukocytes and mononuclear cells. The reaction in nasal passages and middle ear is predominantly purulent. Complete resolution of the lesions in experimentally infected mice is rare. Intraperitoneal injection causes infection of the ovaries and oviducts without pneumonia. The organism is also found in the spleen.

## TOXIC PRODUCTS

Although the original experiments of Nocard and Roux with *M. mycoides* suggested the formation in the rabbit peritoneum of a diffusible toxin, others have not been able to demonstrate a clear-cut toxic effect with this organism. There is one report that an extracted lipopolysaccharide gives toxic reactions in rabbits and cattle. Sabin (1941) was the first to show that *M. neurolyticum* from mice produces a true neurotropic exotoxin which is thermolabile, antigenic, and neutralizable. The brain damage associated with the rolling and choreiform reactions to this toxin have recently been studied in more detail by Thomas et al. (1966a). The primary effect after intravenous injection in mice appears to be a permeability reaction in the tissues of the central nervous system so that vital staining of the brain with trypan blue occurs. Depending upon the dose, the toxic reaction begins within 10 to 240 minutes. Microscopic examination shows greatly distended astrocytes, displacement of axons, vacuolization, free extracellular fluid, and myelin degeneration. The toxin has a molecular weight over 200,000 and is digested by trypsin. The 10,000 g sediment from an extract of brain reacts with the toxin so that no effect is produced on intravenous injection of the mixture. The receptor, probably a ganglioside, is heat stable, trypsin resistant, and periodate sensitive.

The neurotoxic properties of *M. gallisepticum* in turkeys are associated with the organisms themselves and not with a soluble endotoxin. Injection of $10^{10}$ to $10^{11}$ organisms causes ataxia, paralysis, rolling, and torticollis after 1 to 9 hours (Thomas et al., 1966b). Polyarteritis and other brain damage was attributed to direct toxic action. However, some multiplication of the injected organisms must be necessary because tetracyclines and, to a lesser extent, gold salts prevent the effect. Intravenous injection of similar suspensions of *M. gallisepticum* in rodents was without effect.

Nonantigenic toxic or potentially toxic products have also been associated with a mycoplasma, presumably *M. gallisepticum* isolated from chick embryos (van Herick and Eaton, 1945). The organism showed only mild pathogenicity in chickens 2 to 10 weeks of age but was quite lethal for chick embryos. Seitz filtrates of the broth cultures or allantoic fluids when inoculated intranasally into cotton rats produced red edematous consolidation of the lungs extending to all lobes with death in 2 to 3 days. Smaller lesions were seen in some of the white rats inoculated intranasally. Other rodents were not susceptible. Intracerebral inoculation had no effect. Animals that recovered from a sublethal dose did not survive reinoculation with a lethal dose. The poison resisted heating to 90°C. for 30 minutes. The relation of this lung poison to the toxic action of suspensions of *M. gallisepticum* described before remains obscure. However, the experiments in turkeys suggested that active metabolism of organisms in contact with susceptible cells produced the damage to cerebral arteries. This might have been mediated through the same substance as the lung poison, which probably also damaged endothelium.

The possible role of peroxides in the hemolytic action and virulence of mycoplasmas has been considered. This idea is somewhat more compelling in the case of mycoplasmas which grow in intimate contact with cell membranes than with bacteria, but it should be remembered that pneumococci and many streptococci, as well as some saprophytic organisms, form hydrogen peroxide. *M. pneumoniae* produces a $\beta$ hemolysin which is present only around actively growing colonies under aerobic conditions and with a dialysate of yeast extract in the medium. The ability of the hemolysin to pass a viscose membrane indicated that it is of low molecular weight, and it is not destroyed by trypsin. Later it was found that catalase prevented formation of the hemolysin (Somerson et al., 1965). Since hydrogen peroxide itself ordinarily forms methemoglobin rather than hemolyzing erthrocytes, some question must be raised as to whether the hemolysin is actually hydrogen peroxide or a product of its action on red cells or constituents of the medium. The nature of the hemolysin is of interest because it may be related to the virulence of *M. pneumoniae* and it has been suggested that cold hemagglutinins found in atypical pneumonia may be antibodies to products resulting from the action of the hemolysin on erythrocytes of the host. Other pathogenic species, including *M. mycoides* and *M. gallisepticum* as well as *M. laidlawii* and some other saprophytes, form hydrogen peroxide and hemolysins (Cole et al., 1968).

It is not inconceivable that mycoplasmas coating cell membranes might cause damage by the formation of other obscure toxic products or by depriving the cell of metabolites such as essential amino acids or nucleoside precursors. The depletion of arginine in tissue cultures contaminated with PPLO is a well known phenomenon. With a strain of mouse ascites lymphoma this depletion of arginine has been related to mycoplasmal toxins which are active *in vitro* but apparently not *in vivo* (Kraemer, 1964). Certain strains, some related to *M. hominis* 1, were lytic for the lymphoma but not for other cell lines. The toxic factor formed on agar, in lysates of the lymphoma, and also in cell cultures resistant to lysis, was able to pass a membrane with pore diameter small enough to retain the mycoplasmas. It is stable at 56°C. for 30 minutes and nondialyzable. Arginine at 2.13 mM. (three times the normal concentration in the tissue culture medium) reverses its inhibitory effect on cell growth. The chemical specificity of this toxin is striking but it is not clear that its effect is actually due to depletion of arginine. Arginine may have some detoxifying effect at higher concentrations. Data on the effect of other amino acids, catalase, keto acids, and other metabolites would be of interest.

With fermentative strains of mycoplasmas which grow in close contact with cell membranes another "toxic" effect might be the local formation of acid. Changes in the cytoplasm adjacent to mycoplasmal growth at the membrane as visualized by electron microscopy have been reported. Whether diffusion of lactic or pyruvic acids into the medium would prevent a damaging drop of pH at the membrane depends on glucose concentration in adjacent fluids and the rate of fermentation, which is often very rapid.


## INTERACTIONS BETWEEN MYCOPLASMAS AND CELLS

Mycoplasmas are sometimes seen in the cytoplasm of cells but strains adapted to artificial medium may become incapable of intracellular growth.

With the possible exception of T strain organisms seen in large mononuclear cells from urethral smears, there is at present no good evidence for the intracellular presence of mycoplasmas in natural infection of man or animals. In tissue cultures of chick embryos various forms of intracellular growth have been described and some evidence for a developmental cycle in the cytoplasm is presented (Hayflick and Stinebring, 1960, Eaton et al., 1962). In Giemsa-stained preparations scattered organisms, small clumps, or microcolonies in various stages of development were seen. Also, electron microscopy of thin sections of cells infected with mycloplasmas has revealed forms resembling PPLO in the cytoplasm, sometimes in vacuoles. The characteristic morphology of *M. gallisepticum,* an oval form with two bleb-like structures, facilitates the identification of intracellular organisms. When these mycoplasmas are mixed with leukocytes phagocytosis and intracellular digestion occurs (Zucker-Franklin et al., 1966). The formation of characteristic osmophilic inclusions was attributed to coalescence of PPLO undergoing digestion in vacuoles with cell lysosomes. Similar osmophilic bodies have been seen by electron microscopy in sections of chick embryo lungs infected with *M. pneumoniae.* The gray lung "virus" and a rat pneumonia agent, which have not been grown in the absence of living cells but resemble mycoplasmas in structure and sensitivity to chemotherapy, form complex cytoplasmic inclusions suggesting an intracellular developmental cycle (Gay, 1967).

The marked tendency of mycoplasmas to interact with cell membranes could lead to their ingestion by varieties of cells that are not thought to have phagocytic abilities. Also there may be species variations among cells but the possible ability of some mycoplasmas to grow in the cytoplasm has not yet been examined critically enough to relate this property to virulence.

Some species of mycoplasmas agglutinate erythrocytes or cause hemadsorption to their colonies. However, this appears to be the exception rather than a general rule. Species that are not known to cause hemagglutination are often found in close association with the surface of cells in tissue culture and some electron microphotographs have even suggested fusion of the membrane of the organism with the cell surface. By use of an orcein staining method (Fogh and Fogh, 1967a) it is possible to count mycoplasmas on cell surfaces. In such measurements the ratio of free to cell-associated mycoplasmas varied from 400:1 to 16:1 at 37°C., but at temperatures of 30° or 24°C. the proportion of free mycoplasmas was higher. *M. pneumoniae* in addition to agglutinating erythrocytes is also capable of adsorbing to its colonies or agglutinating suspended cells from certain established tissue culture lines. In the case of *M. gallisepticum* the receptor on red cells appears to be a compound containing sialic acid. Neuraminidase treatment of turkey red cells prevents agglutination by this organism, and soluble proteins containing sialic acid such as those in egg white or fetal bovine serum inhibit hemagglutination.

Since many tissue cultures used in virus research are contaminated with mycoplasmas the effects on intracellular processes such as viral growth and the production and action of interferon are of interest. Although there is one report of an augmenting effect of mycoplasmas on production of interferon by equine encephalomyelitis viruses, others have been unable to demonstrate that mycoplasmas alone cause interferon production or influence the action of interferon.

It seems advisable therefore to search for other reasons for prevention of virus growth by mycoplasmas such as incipient cytopathic effects or depletion of the medium as in the case of adenovirus which requires arginine for growth (Rouse et al., 1963). A mycoplasma serologically related to *M. orale* suppressed the growth of Rous sarcoma in cultures of human or chick embryo fibroblasts even after its cytopathogenicity had been reduced or eliminated by passage on agar. Growth of influenza virus was not inhibited under similar conditions (Somerson and Cook, 1965).

It has been shown that the characteristics of cell populations in tissue culture may be permanently altered by mycoplasmal contamination and these are irreversible after suppression of the mycoplasmas by antibiotics (Fogh and Fogh, 1967b). This type of change could be attributed either to simple selection by the contamination or to mutations followed by selection. Mitogenesis initiated in lymphocyte cultures by phytohemagglutinin is inhibited by *M. hominis* 1 even when nonviable and also by aqueous extracts of that organism (Morton et al., 1968). The inhibition of mitosis was reversed when the PPLO were removed by changing the medium.

Studies using autoradiograms suggest that PPLO prevent the uptake of tritiated uridine or thymidine into L cells (Nardone et al., 1965). Instead of entering the nucleus or cytoplasm normally, the label remained on the cell surface. We interpret these observations to indicate that the nucleosides were broken down at the cell surface into products not readily taken up by the cell and were perhaps used by the mycoplasmas; this despite the report that "sufficient" label remained in the supernatant fluids to give normal autoradiograms with uncontaminated L cells. Since cell division continued, *de novo* synthesis of DNA was not prevented but this was not measured quantitatively in infected and control cultures. Liberation of acid-soluble products from DNA due to mycoplasmal contamination of HeLa cells or L cells and not attributable to cell destruction has been reported by Randall et al. (1965). Such effects could be most readily explained by intracellular growth of mycoplasmas but the diffusion of mycoplasmal products activating cell nucleases might also be considered.

Fogh and Fogh (1967b) found characteristic chromosome changes in cells of the FL human amnion line after mycoplasmal infection. These consisted in reduction in chromosome number and appearance of new varieties of chromosomes. Observations extending over a period of almost 3 years showed continuous reduction in chromosome numbers from 70 to 76 to ranges between 61 and 66 and a gradual increase in some chromosome aberrations, most notably large telocentric chromosomes. Elimination of the unidentified mycoplasma by Aureomycin treatment of the tissue cultures did not result in an increase in the number of chromosomes or disappearance of the large telocentric forms. Originally the cytopathic effect of the mycoplasma had destroyed most of the cell population and this was followed by outgrowth of cells with changed characteristics, clearly a biological selection. Resistance to mycoplasma and reduction in tumor-producing capacity in the cheek pouch of Syrian hamsters treated with cortisone accompanied a change in culture requirements. Although the original effects in the genetically heterogeneous FL cell line were undoubtedly due to selection, the continued gradual change over a period of years is of interest in suggesting further chromosome alteration by the mycoplasma corresponding to analogous, more rapid effects produced by virus infection. Chromosome damage has also been reported in a human diploid cell strain infected with mycoplasmas (Paton et al., 1965). The relative genetic stability of such diploid cell lines is well known, so that some possibility of a transforming effect of mycoplasmas must be considered.

## SEROLOGY AND IMMUNITY

In general, the various species of mycoplasmas form distinct serological groups with little overlapping. Also, antigenic variation within a species has not yet appeared as frequently as is the case with many bacteria. But recently antigens in common have been discovered in such unrelated species as *M. mycoides* and *M. pneumoniae*. Despite these possible complications serological methods have proved to be the best for identification because biological and biochemical characters often tend to be variable and nondistinctive.

Antisera for typing are usually prepared in rabbits with live, killed, or disrupted organisms. Repeated injections intravenously or by the intramuscular or footpad route, sometimes with Freund's adjuvant, are required. Although antibody responses to many strains of mycoplasma are satisfactory, difficulties are sometimes encountered. Normal rabbits often have low levels of complement-fixing antibodies before immunization but this is rarely the case with precipitating or growth-inhibiting antibodies. The latter, however, may be found in rabbit sera which are not inactivated at 56°C.

Organisms concentrated from broth cultures by centrifugation at high speed may be used to prepare an antigen for agglutination or complement fixation. Merthiolate and formalin have been used as preservatives and in addition boiled antigens are of some interest in connection with recent discoveries regarding the heat-stable antigens of mycoplasmas. The agglutination test was first used extensively by Klieneberger (1938) for the differentiation of species, but difficulties were encountered because of instability of the suspensions and spontaneous flocculation in the absence of antiserum. Also, relatively large amounts of broth culture are required for agglutination as compared with other methods. Recent improvements in this method include use of antiglobulin antibody or specific labeling of the precipitate by the indirect Coons technique.

Of the many serological methods now available the complement fixation test has been in use for the longest time but there are some reasons to doubt the specificity and reliability of this test as applied to mycoplasmas.* Klieneberger-Nobel (1960) used complement fixation in an extensive serological survey of human genital mycoplasmas. It was shown that these strains form a single serological group (*M. hominis* 1). Antibodies were found in 34 per cent of patients from venereal disease clinics and in 2 per cent of blood donors and children. The results were well correlated with rates of isolation of *M. hominis*

---

* The unhappy experiences of the author resulting from the use of tissue infected with *M. pneumoniae* will be detailed later.

from various population groups but others have found less significant differences between diseased and healthy individuals. Although the presence of antibodies suggests infection with *M. hominis* there may be a commensal infection together with bacteria rather than a disease of simple mycoplasmal etiology. Later, in patients with salpingitis, Lemcke and Csonka (1962) were able to show significant changes in antibody titers, in a few cases a rise associated with progress of the disease or a fall following therapy and recovery. In infections with *M. pneumoniae* complement-fixing antibodies are sometimes absent when other serological reactions are positive and the antibody response measured by this method seems more transient than other forms of serological reaction.

The growth inhibition method devised by Edward and Fitzgerald (1954) has undergone many modifications to improve its reliability. Originally based on colony counts on agar plates with and without antiserum, the test recently has employed antiserum on paper discs on seeded agar plates, as in antibiotic sensitivity measurements, or incubation of graded numbers of organism with antiserum followed by subculture on agar. The so-called metabolic inhibition tests are in reality growth inhibition tests except that the indicator is ability to metabolize glucose, urea, or arginine, with formation of acid in the case of glucose metabolism or ammonia in the case of urea or arginine metabolism (Purcell et al., 1967). Rapid growth of the organisms results in a change in color of the phenol red indicator while a marked reduction in the rate of growth by antibody leaves the indicator unchanged. The tests are initiated with a small inoculum and there is no evidence that antibody per se will prevent enzymatic splitting of glucose to acid. Similar considerations probably apply also to the tetrazolium reduction methods.

With *M. pneumoniae* the first demonstration of antibodies in human and animal sera was accomplished by a growth inhibition test in the whole animal (Eaton et al., 1945). Suspensions of infected chick embryo lung were mixed with antiserum and inoculated intranasally into cotton rats or hamsters. The indicator was the appearance of pneumonia. This, of course, was essentially the same procedure as used in neutralization tests for antibodies to influenza virus in the mouse neutralization tests. Analogous methods applied to bacteria are generally less successful although in the useful pneumococcus protection test organism and antiserum were mixed before intraperitoneal injection into mice. With *M. pneumoniae* it was found that "neutralization" was feeble and irregular when the test was performed in chick embryos. In cultures of human tissue cytopathic effects were delayed or sometimes absent but growth of the organisms was not prevented (Eaton et al., 1962). An immune rabbit serum (heated at 56°C. for 20 minutes) that neutralized the atypical pneumonia agent in high titer when tested intranasally in cotton rats was relatively ineffective at a dilution of 1:10 in tissue culture. These difficulties, not ordinarily encountered with neutralization of viruses in tissue culture, could be attributed to a requirement for accessory immunity mechanisms in the case of mycoplasmas, for example, complement, phagocytic cells, and possibly lymphocytes, which are available in the intact animal but absent from chick embryos or tissue cultures. In view of the fact that growth inhibition tests, as measured by metabolism, can be done easily with *M. pneumoniae* it is conceivable that cells in tissue culture may interfere by decomposing the antibody or by protecting the mycoplasma from its action. Although simpler serological methods have now replaced the animal neutralization test, these observations were of interest in revealing the mechanisms of immunity to mycoplasma infectivity and may still be of value with related organisms unable to grow on lifeless media.

The hemagglutination inhibition test with mycoplasmas discovered by van Herick (1945) working in the author's laboratory has been applied extensively in diagnosis and measurements of immunity to avian mycoplasmas. Hemadsorption of guinea pig erythrocytes by the colonies of *M. pneumoniae* on agar is inhibited by immune serum. A hemagglutination inhibition test using erythrocytes suspended in normal horse serum has been described by Feldman and Suhs (1966). Measurement of antibodies to *M. pneumoniae* in man by hemagglutination inhibition correlates well with other methods. There is also an indirect hemagglutination method using antigen-coated, tannic acid-treated red cells.

Liu (1957) first used the immunofluorescence technique of Coons to localize the infection with *M. pneumoniae* in the chick embryo lung, an observation which later facilitated microscopic visualization of the agent by Marmion and Goodburn (1961). Although the use of fluorescein-labeled antibodies has been most extensive with *M. pneumoniae* it is equally applicable with other mycoplasmas to identify agar-grown colonies of various species and to detect mycoplasmal contaminants in tissue culture, and it may eventually prove of value in early diagnosis of mycoplasmal infection. The latter would depend on obtaining cells containing microcolonies or associated mycoplasmas from the respiratory or genital tracts or other locations in suitable form for specific labeling. Sections of infected chick embryo lung were originally used by Liu, Chanock, and others to titrate antibodies to *M. pneumoniae*. A good correlation was obtained with the animal neutralization test.

A comparison of serologic response to *M. pneumoniae* using four different methods—immunofluorescence, complement fixation, indirect hemagglutination, and tetrazolium reduction—has been made by Taylor-Robinson and associates (1966). They characterized the immunofluorescence method as the most effective but it is also the most laborious and technically difficult. Complement fixation using an antigen phenolized and heated to 56°C. for 30 minutes was found to be less sensitive and detected only 85 per cent of *M. pneumoniae* in-

TABLE 5. *Summary of Antibody Responses of Marine Recruits to* M. pneumoniae *Infection as Measured by Immunofluorescence (IMF), Complement Fixation (CF), Indirect Hemagglutination (IHA), and Inhibition of Tetrazolium Reduction (TRI)*\*

| | NUMBER OF PAIRED SERA TESTED | BY ANY TECHNIQUE | IMF | CF | IHA | TRI | BY ALL TECHNIQUES |
|---|---|---|---|---|---|---|---|
| Antibody rise † | 81‡ | 42 | 41 | 36 | 36 | 36 | 31 |
| Mean titers: | | | | | | | |
| Acute | 52 | — | <10 | <4 | 24.5 | 2.2 | — |
| Convalescent | 52 | — | 70 | 28 | 320 | 105 | — |

\* Data from Taylor-Robinson et al., 1966.
† Fourfold or greater.
‡ Febrile respiratory disease and pneumonia, 50; afebrile disease or asymptomatic, 31.

fections diagnosed by other techniques. The indirect hemagglutination test has been suspected of being less specific because relatively high titers of antibodies are found in children and in the acute phase sera of patients with atypical pneumonia. A heterologous immune reaction to other mycoplasmas by indirect hemagglutination may account for detection of antibodies not demonstrated by other tests. The metabolic inhibition test, on the other hand, shows a high degree of both strain and species specificity. Antigenic differences were detected among different isolates of *M. hominis 1* (Purcell et al., 1967). The only metabolic inhibition test available for the T strains of Shepard uses urea as a substrate. Other mycoplasmas are not known to decompose urea to ammonia. A large proportion of adolescents and adults, but not children, were found to have antibodies to one T strain. Titers are generally low and there may be several serological groups.

Heat-labile fractions in normal and immune sera play a part in killing of mycoplasmas. Riggs et al. (1967), working with an unidentified mycoplasma isolated from tissue cultures, found that fresh nonimmune rabbit serum, although inactive by itself, enhanced the killing effect of immune serum which had been heated to 56°C. for 3 hours. The heat-labile factor was removed by reagents which inactivate complement. In addition, human and guinea pig sera had low titers up to 1:40 of natural inhibitory antibody against this strain of mycoplasma. In studies on "neutralization" of *M. pneumoniae* in cultures of human tissue, immune rabbit serum when inactivated had little effect, but delay in the appearance of cytopathic effects and reduction in the number of viable organisms was obtained with untreated serum which had been stored in the frozen state (Eaton et al., 1962). Normal rabbit sera tested in our laboratory also have shown some activity against *M. pneumoniae* in the metabolic inhibition test. Generally, human or animal sera are inactivated at 56°C. before antibodies are titrated in this test and in others that depend on inhibition of growth. Otherwise nonspecific killing may result.

In the titration of antibodies against *M. pneumoniae* by the indirect immunofluorescence technique, with frozen sections of chick embryo lung as antigen, Liu (1961) observed that a heat-labile factor in normal human and guinea pig serum increased the observed antibody titers of convalescent sera. No such enhancement was found with the serum from *M. pneumoniae*-immune rabbits or in similar immunofluorescence reactions with mumps, measles, or influenza virus and human serum. Evidence was presented that the heat-labile factor facilitated combination of *M. pneumoniae* antibody with its antigen but did not affect the combination of the fluorescein-labeled antiglobulin with the human antibody. Similar studies should be done with other PPLO of human origin, such as the genital strains in which low antibody titers are a problem. Additional evidence for participation of heat-labile substances in the combination of mycoplasmal antigens and antibodies is found in an observation with *M. mycoides* polysaccharide antigen which gives a much stronger complement fixation reaction with antibody of bovine origin in the presence of unheated normal bovine serum. In this case the heat-labile factor is probably not complement because this would act in the opposite direction by being present in excess and lowering the observed complement fixation titer.

These observations suggest that heat-labile factors may act by two distinct mechanisms. One is analogous to the classical bactericidal reaction of Bordet as observed with certain gram-negative bacteria. The other, which may involve either a component of complement or some previously unknown heat-labile substance, appears to be characteristic of reactions of human antibody with mycoplasmas but not viruses. In this reaction the accessory factor either facilitates the linkage of antigen and antibody or makes the combination firmer.

The cold agglutinin reaction (Finland et al., 1945) has long been known as a serological peculiarity of atypical pneumonia and some other non-pneumonic diseases. Sera from patients with very high titers give some agglutination of normal human erythrocytes at room temperature and such individuals may partially hemolyze their own erythrocytes, thus developing hemolytic anemia. The cold agglutinin appears to result from an autoimmune response to heterophil antigens possibly involving alteration of cell components by *M. pneumoniae*. Cold agglutinins have not been found in other mycoplasmal infections (except in one case of an infection with *M. hominis 1* in a human volunteer), and experimental animals infected with *M. pneumoniae* do not develop cold agglutinins even when the disease is severe. It may be that the absence of cold agglutinins in experimental infection is related to blood group differences between these animals and man. Schmidt et al. (1965) found that 18 of 25 strains of mycoplasmas when incubated with I-positive human erythrocytes caused inhibition of I antigen reactivity, possibly by splitting off. Also, I antibodies and cold agglutinins are often associated in several diseases, including atypical pneumonia. Therefore in lower animals the absence of a heterophil antigen may account for the failure of cold agglutinins to develop.

The possibility that the cold agglutination is not an autoimmune reaction, but is due to an antigen in common between *M. pneumoniae* and human erythrocytes, has not been excluded. The glycoprotein antigens common to certain bacteria and blood groups ABH(O) are well known, and there is also a close chemical relationship between blood group substances and Forssman antigens. In *M. pneumoniae* there may be an undiscovered weak antigen related to blood group I which stimulates antibodies only in severe infections when a large mass of mycoplasmal antigen is present.

If cold agglutination is indeed a heterophil reaction then it might have been predicted that other heterophil antigens could be activated in primary atypical pneumonia resulting in autoimmune reactions. The author was unaware of this possibility when in 1942 and 1943 an attempt was made to do complement fixation tests using infected hamster lungs. There followed a remarkable series of laboratory events paralleled by the similar independent observations of Thomas et al. (1943).

In acute and convalescent sera, a rise in complement-fixing antibodies was best demonstrated by keeping the test in the refrigerator overnight. Later it was found that the hamster lungs were not actually infected with the atypical pneumonia agent but with an antigenically unrelated virus which had replaced it during serial passages. But with normal hamster lung not all of these paired serum specimens showed a rise in antibodies, suggesting that the antigen involved may be activated by infection with dissimilar agents. Thomas and his associates obtained in 14 of 35 cases of atypical pneumonia an increase in complement-fixing antibodies to suspensions of mouse lung infected with the pneumonia virus of mice, and sera of five of the patients also reacted with dissimilar antigens prepared with viruses of influenza and the psittacosis group.

Shifrine and Gourlay (1965) have reported serological reactions between *M. mycoides* antisera and a galactan from bovine lungs. Also, antigens in common between bacteria and normal tissues are known (Kaplan, 1967, and others). As shown by cross absorption, the antigen involved in nonspecific complement fixation is not the same as the one reacting in cold hemagglutination but it may be activated by a similar process. Supposedly it is more abundant in inflammatory exudates and may occur in one or more of the several kinds of leukocytes. Because of the existence of this reagin the fixation of complement by sera from patients with *M. pneumoniae* infection and any viral antigens grown in tissue may be nonspecific. As a partial control the corresponding normal tissue should always be included in such complement fixation tests.

The serological cross reaction between streptococcus MG and *M. pneumoniae* has now been clearly shown to be due to an antigen in common and is therefore a different category from the heterophil antigen-antibody reactions discussed above. Sera from patients with antistreptococcus MG agglutinins still react at the same titer after absorption with human type O red cells. It is clear then that a third antigen is involved in addition to those for cold hemagglutination and heterophil complement fixation.

Recent studies on the heat-stable antigens of mycoplasmas have revealed that some species possess lipid antigens that are soluble in chloroform-methanol and other organic solvents (Kenny, 1967). Although the lipids by themselves are poor stimulators of antibody formation the lipoproteins of which they are constituents in the whole organism produce high levels of complement-fixing antibody and moderate amounts of growth-inhibitory antibodies. It is apparently one of these lipoprotein antigens which is responsible for cross reactions between streptococcus MG and *M. pneumoniae* as demonstrated by Lemcke, Marmion, and Plackett (1967). Gel diffusion tests indicate that the bacterial and mycoplasmal antigens are partly related rather than identical, and chemical tests suggest the presence of a carbohydrate determinant in the lipid antigen of *M. pneumoniae*. The corresponding component in streptococcus MG seems to be in the cell wall because cross reaction with convalescent sera from atypical pneumonia has been attributed both to a polysaccharide soluble antigen and to a somatic antigen of the decapsulated R variant of the streptococcus (Thomas et al., 1945). Although rabbits immunized with streptococcus MG develop the heterophil antibody they do not do so with *M. pneumoniae* or the L form of streptococcus MG. A possible explanation of these reactions, one way in rabbits and the opposite in human beings, might be found in differences in host response to partial antigens. For example, some pneumococcal polysaccharides are not antigenic in the rabbit but may be in other animals.

Cross reactions between *M. pneumoniae* and *M. mycoides* have also been reported and in this case there may be more than one antigen in common. The lipopolysaccharide antigen discussed earlier which reacts with streptococcus MG antiserum also gives complement fixation with antimycoides bovine convalescent serum. Another fraction of *M. pneumoniae*, extracted by phenol after removal of lipids with chloroform-methanol, gives little reaction with strepto-

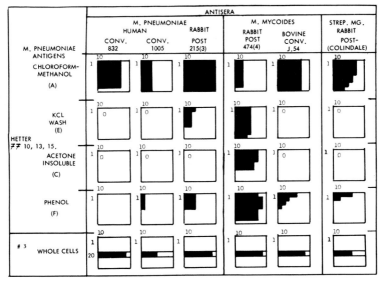

CONV. = CONVALESCENT    POST    POST INOCULATION
PRE - INOCULATION SERA NEGATIVE

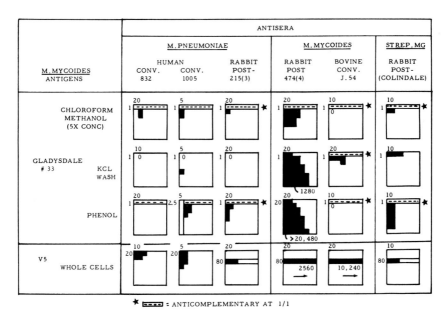

★ ▭ = ANTICOMPLEMENTARY AT 1/1

*Figure 6.* Cross reactions of antisera to *Mycoplasma pneumoniae, M. mycoides,* and streptococcus MG with extracted antigens and whole organisms of the two species of mycoplasma as measured by complement fixation. Each square represents a "chess-board" titration with increasing antigen dilutions downward and serum dilutions across. Whole cells were positive with all antisera, preinoculation sera were negative. The lipid extract (chloroform-methanol) of *M. pneumoniae* shows strong cross reactions, and the phenol extract a smaller cross reaction. Some human convalescent sera give cross reactions with *M. mycoides* antigens. (From Lemcke, Marmion, and Plackett. 1967. Ann. N.Y. Acad. Sci. *143*:691–702; see also Lemcke, R. M., Shaw, E. J., and Marmion, B. P. Aust. J. Exp. Biol. Med. Sci. *43*:761–770, 1965).

coccus MG antiserum but strong reactions with antimycoides rabbit serum. In addition, cross reactions between *M. mycoides* antisera and certain bacteria such as strains of *Escherichia coli, Corynebacterium xerose,* and a streptococcus of Lancefield Group K have been found (Shifrine and Gourlay, 1967). The antigens obtained by aqueous phenol extraction are apparently polysaccharides. In some cases strong precipitin lines of identity were obtained in the agar gel tests; in others, lines were weaker and indicated partial identity. In cattle sensitized to *M. mycoides* several of the bacterial antigens gave immediate allergic skin reactions, and there were reciprocal skin reactions with *M. mycoides* after sensitization with some of the bacterial antigens.

## VACCINES

Immunization against mycoplasmal infection has been studied the longest and most extensively with bovine pleuropneumonia. With live organisms the principle of inoculation by an unusual route to avoid fatal infection, in this case the tip of the tail, has often been applied. Results with killed vaccines have not been promising. Organisms propagated in broth or the yolk sac are commonly used as live attenuated vaccine. These are sometimes lyophilized. Occasionally following vaccination a spreading subcutaneous edema, arthritis, cardiac lesions, small lung lesions, and other complications appear. Piercy (1960) has advocated the inoculation of virulent or near-virulent organisms by the tail-tip route because of the uncertainties of obtaining cultures of the proper degree of attenuation. Encouraging results have been obtained with adjuvants and attenuated cultures.

In avian mycoplasmal infections both vaccination and chemotherapy have been used as methods of control. Some doubts have been expressed about the value of antibody response as a measure of immunity. Killed vaccines were ineffective despite the development of high antibody titers. Attenuated vaccine strains of *M. gallisepticum* have been developed (Luginbuhl et al., 1967) and were inoculated intranasally. Challenge with a virulent strain and attempted isolation of the organisms 7 days later revealed that the virulent strains were not recoverable from vaccinated chicks but were always present in the controls. Treatment of experimentally infected chickens and turkeys with tetracyclines and other antibiotics resulted in lowered mortality and improved growth (Gale et al., 1967). Infection of the eggs and embryos was reduced.

The need for a vaccine against *M. pneumoniae* may be questioned because atypical pneumonia has not been prevalent in the general population in recent years, the disease responds well to broad-spectrum antibiotics, and mortality is low even without chemotherapy. In high-risk populations such as military recruits and college students, the inclusion of *M. pneumoniae* in polyvalent viral vaccines seems justifiable. Chanock and associates (1961a) obtained serologic evidence for *M. pneumoniae* infection in 68 per cent of a group of 238 recruits at a military training center and about half of these developed some form of febrile respiratory disease during the period of observations. The incidence of pneumonia due to mycoplasmal infections of the respiratory tract has been estimated to be as low as 4 per cent in civilian adults, however.

The first studies on experimental immunization with *M. pneumoniae* were done by Eaton and van Herick (1947) in cotton rats and hamsters using chick embryo passage material. It was found that fully virulent material could be inoculated by the intraperitoneal route without the production of pneumonia or other signs of illness. This is quite a different behavior from the highly invasive properties of *M. mycoides*. Formalin did not appear to reduce the antigenicity of the *M. pneumoniae* vaccine, but in any case at least three injections were required to produce solid immunity to intranasal challenge. A close correlation between antibody titer and active immunity could not be demonstrated. Some groups of hamsters receiving intraperitoneal immunization developed pneumonia on intranasal challenge despite the presence of relatively high antibody titers. Immunity in cotton rats lasted for about 3 months, yet some animals had no antibody. Attempts to obtain passive immunization with hyperimmune rabbit strain were not successful. The artificial stimulation of antibodies in rabbits by formalin-inactivated vaccines is related to the number of viable organisms (colony-forming units, CFU) in the suspension before inactivation. Thus broth-grown preparations containing $10^4$ CFU/ml. were barely antigenic, whereas those with $5 \times 10^{10}$ CFU/ml. produced titers of 2000.

In man the presence of growth-inhibitory antibody at titers above a certain level seems closely associated with active immunity to *M. pneumoniae* in both experimental and natural infections. Only one of 10 volunteers who developed antibodies had a febrile illness after challenge with *M. pneumoniae*, but 10 of 13 unvaccinated controls became ill. However, an anomalous effect was observed in volunteers who did not develop antibody following vaccination in that more severe illness appeared than in the control group. This paradoxical enhancement of infection by vaccines of low potency has been found by several investigators. The results of field trials suggest that *M. pneumoniae* vaccine which produces an antibody response in most individuals may be able to reduce by about 50 per cent the incidence of pneumonia caused by this organism in a military population.

The improvement of *M. pneumoniae* vaccines may depend upon the use of highly purified antigens from the organism or the finding of a suitable attenuated strain. Purification of phospholipid antigens has been accomplished and their ability to block growth-inhibiting antibody demonstrated (Sobeslavsky et al., 1966). However, the isolation of a highly antigenic lipoprotein has not yet been accomplished. One may speculate that the immunizing antigen of *M. pneumoniae* is relatively more stable than in other mycoplasmas such as *M. mycoides*.

Strains of *M. pneumoniae* grown on artifical medium show a definite reduction of virulence for man but even after many passages they still produce febrile illness in 5 to 10 per cent of those inoculated by the respiratory route. Whether further attenuation will result in a successful live vaccine or dissociation with loss of essential antigens remains to be seen. Subcutaneous or intradermal inoculation of live attenuated organisms has apparently not yet been tried in man but, in view of the early results with *M. pneumoniae* in experimental animals and present practices in vaccination against *M. mycoides*, experiments on inoculation by the cutaneous route would seem indicated.

# References

Adler, H. E. 1965. Mycoplasms in animals. Advances Vet. Sci. *10:*205–244.

Barber, T. L., and Fabricant, J. 1962. Primary isolation of mycoplasma organisms (PPLO) from mammalian sources. J. Bact. *83:*1268–1273.

Borrel, A., and Dujardin-Beaumetz, E. 1910. Le microbe de la péripneumoniae. Ann. Inst. Pasteur *24:*168–175.

Bredt, W. 1968. Growth morphology of Mycoplasma pneumoniae strain FH on glass surface. Proc. Soc. Exp. Biol. Med. *128:*338–340.

Carlson, H. J., Spector, S., and Douglas, H. G. 1951. Possible role of pleuropneumonia-like organisms in etiology of disease in childhood. Amer. J. Dis. Child. *81:*193.

Chanock, R. M., Hayflick, L., and Barile, M. F. 1962. Growth on artificial medium of an agent associated with atypical pneumonia and its identification as a PPLO. Proc. Nat. Acad. Sci. U.S.A. *48:*41–49.

Chanock, R. M., Mufson, M. A., Bloom, H. H., James, W. D., Fox, H. H., and Kingston, J. R. 1961a. Eaton agent pneumonia. J.A.M.A. *175:*213–220.

Chanock, R. M., Rifkind, D., Krevetz, H. M., Knight, V., and Johnson, K. M. 1961b. Respiratory disease in volunteers infected with Eaton agent: A preliminary report. Proc. Nat. Acad. Sci. U.S.A. *47:*887–890.

Clyde, W., and Kim, K. S. 1967. Biophysical characterization of human mycoplasma species. Ann. N.Y. Acad. Sci. *143,* 425–434.

Cole, B. C., Ward, J. R., and Martin, C. H. 1968. Hemolysin and peroxide activity of mycoplasma species. J. Bact. *95:*2022–2030.

Dajani, A. S., Clyde, W. A., Jr., and Denny, F. W. 1965. Experimental infections with Mycoplasma pneumoniae (Eaton's agent). J. Exp. Med. *121:*1071–1086.

Dienes, L., and Edsall, G. 1937. Observations on the L-organism of Klieneberger. Proc. Soc. Exp. Biol. Med. *36:*740–744.

Dienes, L., and Smith, W. E. 1942. Reproduction of bacteria from the large bodies of Bacteroides funduliformis. Proc. Soc. Exp. Biol. *51:*297–300.

Eaton, M. D., Farnham, A. E., Levinthal, J. D., and Scala, A. R. 1962. Cytopathic effect of the atypical pneumonia organism in cultures of human tissue. J. Bact. *84:*1330–1337.

Eaton, M. D., and Low, I. E. 1967. Propagation of M. pneumoniae and other fastidious strains of mycoplasma. Ann. N.Y. Acad. Sci. *143:*375–383.

Eaton, M. D., Meiklejohn, G., and van Herick, W. 1944. Studies on the etiology of primary atypical pneumonia. A filterable agent transmissible to cotton rats, hamsters, and chick embryos. J. Exp. Med. *79:*649–668.

Eaton, M. D., and van Herick, W. 1947. Experimental immunization with the virus of primary atypical pneumonia. J. Infect. Dis. *81:*116–121.

Eaton, M. D., van Herick, W., and Meiklejohn, G. 1945. Studies on the etiology of primary atypical pneumonia. III. Specific neutralization of the virus by human serum. J. Exp. Med. *82:*329–342.

Edward, D. G. F. 1940. The occurrence in normal mice of pleuropneumonia-like organisms capable of producing pneumonia. J. Path. Bact. *50:*409–418.

Edward, D. G. F. and Fitzgerald, W. A. 1954. Inhibition of the growth of pleuropneumonia-like organisms by antibody. J. Path. Bact. *68:*23–30.

Fabricant, J., and Freundt, E. A. 1967. Importance of extension and standardization of laboratory tests for the identification and classification of mycoplasma. Ann. N.Y. Acad. Sci. *143:*50–58.

Feldman, A. A., and Suhs, R. H. 1966. Serologic epidemiologic studies with M. pneumoniae I. Demonstration of an hemagglutinin and its inhibition by antibody. Amer. J. Epidem. *83:*345–356.

Finland, M., Peterson, O. L., Allen, H. E., Samper, B. A., and Barnes, M. W. 1945. Cold agglutinins. II. Cold isohemagglutinins in primary atypical pneumonia of unknown etiology with a note on the occurrence of hemolytic anemia in these cases. J. Clin. Invest. *24:*458–473.

Fogh, J., and Fogh, H. 1967a. Morphological and quantitative aspects of Mycoplasma-human cell relationship. Proc. Soc. Exp. Biol. Med., *125:*423–430.

Fogh, J., and Fogh, H. 1967b. Irreversibility of major chromosome changes in a Mycoplasma-modified line of FL human amnion cells. Proc. Soc. Exp. Biol. Med. *126:*67–74.

Fortner, J. 1928. Ein einfaches Plattenverfahren zur Zuchtung strenger Anaerobes. Z. Bakt. *108:*155–159.

Foster, J. P. 1934. Some historical notes on contagious pleuropneumonia. J. Amer. Vet. Med. Assoc. *84:*918–925.

Freundt, E. A. 1958. The Mycoplasmataceae. Munksgaard. Copenhagen.

Gale, G. O., Layton, H. W., Shor, A. L., and Kemp, G. A. 1967. Chemotherapy of experimental avian mycoplasma infection. Ann. N.Y. Acad. Sci. *143:*239–255.

Gay, F. W. 1967. Fine structure and location of mycoplasma-like gray lung and rat pneumonia agents in infected mouse lungs. J. Bact. *94*:2048–2061.

Goodburn, G. M., and Marmion, B. P. 1962. A study of the properties of Eaton's primary atypical pneumonia organism. J. Gen. Microbiol. *29*:271–290.

Hayflick, L. 1965. Tissue cultures and mycoplasma. Texas Rep. Biol. Med. *23* (suppl. 1):285–303.

Hayflick, L., and Chanock, R. M. 1965. Mycoplasma species of man. Bact. Rev. *29*:186–221.

Hayflick, L., and Stinebring, W. R. 1960. Intracellular growth of pleuropneumonia-like organisms (PPLO) in tissue culture and in ovo. Ann. N.Y. Acad. Sci. *79*:443–449.

Jansson, E., and Wager, O. 1967. Mycoplasma in collagen diseases and blood dyscrasia. Ann. N.Y. Acad. Sci. *143*:535–543.

Kaplan, M. H. 1967. Multiple nature of the cross-reactive relationship between antigens of group A streptococci and mammalian tissue. *In:* Cross-reacting Antigens and Neoantigens. J. J. Tretin, ed. Williams & Wilkins, Baltimore, pp. 48–60.

Kenny, G. E. 1967. Heat lability and organic solvent solubility of mycoplasma antigens. Ann. N.Y. Acad. Sci. *143*:676–681.

Kerr, K. M., and Olson, N. O. 1967. Cardiac pathology associated with mycoplasmal arthritis in chickens. Ann. N.Y. Acad. Sci. *143*:204–217.

Klieneberger, E. 1935. The natural occurrence of pleuropneumonia-like organisms in apparent symbiosis with Streptobacillus moniliformis. J. Path. Bact. *40*:93–97.

Klieneberger, E. 1938. Pleuropneumonia-like organisms of diverse provenance, some results of an enquiry into methods of differentiation. J. Hyg. (Cambridge) *38*:458–462.

Klieneberger-Nobel, E. 1959. The possible significance of pleuropneumonia-like organisms in human genital infections. Brit. J. Vener. Dis. *35*:20–25.

Klieneberger-Nobel, E. 1960. Pathology and immunology of organisms of the pleuropneumonia group. Ann. N.Y. Acad. Sci. *79*:615–625.

Klieneberger-Nobel, E. 1962. Pleuropneumonia-like Organisms. (PPLO): Mycoplasmataceae. Academic Press, New York.

Kraemer, P. M. 1964. Interaction of mycoplasmas (PPLO) and murine lymphoma cell cultures. Prevention of lysis by arginine. Proc. Soc. Exp. Biol. Med. *115*:206–212.

Kraybill, W. H., and Crawford, Y. E. 1967. Comparison of two agar media for the isolation of mycoplasma from the human oropharynx. Ann. N.Y. Acad. Sci. *143*:401–410.

Kundsin, R. B., Driscoll, S. G., and Ming, P. L. 1967. Strain of mycoplasma associated with human reproductive failure. Science *157*:1573–1574.

Laidlaw, P. P., and Elford, W. J. 1936. A new group of filterable organisms. Proc Roy. Soc. [Biol.] *120*:292–298.

Lemcke, R., and Csonka, G. W. 1962. Antibodies against pleuropneumonia-like organisms in patients with salpingitis. Brit. J. Vener. Dis. *38*:212–217.

Lemcke, R. M., Marmion, B. P., and Plackett, P. 1967. Immunochemical analysis of Mycoplasma pneumoniae. Ann. N.Y. Acad. Sci. *143*:691–702.

Liu, C. 1957. Studies on primary atypical pneumonia. I. Localization, isolation and cultivation of a virus in chick embryos. J. Exp. Med. *106*:455–467.

Liu, C. 1961. Studies on primary atypical pneumonia. III. A factor in normal serum which enhances the reaction between PAP virus and convalescent serum. J. Exp. Med. *113*:111–123.

Liu, C. 1968. In preparation.

Low, I. E., Eaton, M. D., and Proctor, P. 1968. Relation of catalase to substrate utilization by Mycoplasma pneumoniae. J. Bact. *95*:1425–1430.

Luginbuhl, R. E., Tourtellotte, M. E., and Frazier, M. N. 1967. M. gallisepticum: control by immunization. Ann. N.Y. Acad. Sci. *143*:234–238.

Marmion, B. P., and Goodburn, G. M. 1961. Effect of organic gold salts on Eaton's primary atypical pneumonia agent and other observations. Nature *189*:247–248.

McGee, Z. A., Rogul, M., and Wittler, R. G. 1967. Molecular genetic studies of relationships among mycoplasma, L-forms and bacteria. Ann. N.Y. Acad. Sci. *143*:21–30.

Meiklejohn, G., Eaton, M. D., and van Herick, W. 1945. A clinical report on cases of atypical pneumonia caused by a new virus. J. Clin. Invest. *24*:241–250.

Morowitz, H. L., and Maniloff, J. A. 1966. Analysis of the life cycle of Mycoplasma gallisepticum. J. Bact. *91*:1638–1644.

Morton, H. E., Copperman, R., and Lam, G. T. 1968. Some properties of the inhibitor of lymphocyte mitosis derived from mycoplasma. J. Bact. *95*:2418–2419.

Nardone, R. M., Gonzalez, P., and Gaffney, E. V. 1965. Nucleoside incorporation into strain L cells; inhibition by pleuropneumonia-like organisms. Science *149*:1100–1101.

Nelson, J. B. 1967. Pathologic response of Swiss and Princeton mice to M. pulmonis. Ann. N.Y. Acad. Sci. *143*:778–783.

Nocard, E., Roux, E. R., Borrel, A., and Dujardin-Beaumetz, E. 1898. Le microbe de la péripneumoniae. Ann. Inst. Pasteur *12*:240–252.

Olesiuk, O. M., and van Roekel, H. 1960. Pathological and immunological observations concerning avian pleupneumonialike organisms. Ann. N.Y. Acad. Sci. 79:727–740.

Paine, T. F., Murray, R., Perlmutter, I., and Finland, M. 1950. Brain abscess and meningitis associated with a pleuropneumonia-like organism, clinical and bacteriological observations. Ann. Intern. Med. 32:554–562.

Paton, G. R., Jacobs, J. P., and Perkins, F. T. 1965. Chromosome changes in human diploid cell cultures infected with mycoplasma. Nature 207:43–45.

Piercy, S. E. 1960. Observations on the type species Mycoplasma mycoides. Ann. N.Y. Acad. Sci. 79:665–669.

Purcell, R. H., Wong, D., Chanock, R. M., Taylor-Robinson, D., Canchola, J., and Valdesuso, J. 1967. Significance of antibody to mycoplasma as measured by metabolic inhibition techniques. Ann. N.Y. Acad. Sci. 143:664–675.

Randall, C. C., Gafford, L. G., Gentry, G. A. and Lawson, L. A. 1965. Lability of host-cell DNA in growing cell cultures due to mycoplasma. Science 149:1098–1099.

Razin, S., Cosenza, B. J., and Tourtellotte, M. E., 1966. Variations in mycoplasma morphology produced by long chain fatty acids. J. Gen. Microbiol. 42:139–145.

Riggs, S., Sharp, J. T., and Carpenter, R. R. 1967. Factors involved in growth inhibition of mycoplasma by immune serum. Ann. N.Y. Acad. Sci. 143:784–793.

Rodwell, A. W. 1967. The nutrition and metabolism of mycoplasma: progress and problems. Ann. N.Y. Acad. Sci. 143:88–109.

Rouse, H. C., Bonifas, V. H., and Schlesinger, R. W. 1963. Dependence of adenovirus replication on arginine and inhibition of plaque formation by PPLO. Virology 20:357–365.

Rytel, M. W. 1964. Primary atypical pneumonia; current concepts. Amer. J. Med. Sci. 247:84–104.

Sabin, A. B. 1938. Identification of a filterable transmissible neurolytic agent isolated from toxoplasma-infected tissues as a new pleuropneumonia-like microbe. Science 88:575.

Sabin, A. B. 1941. The filterable microorganisms of the pleuropneumonia group Bact. Rev. 5:1–68.

Schmidt, P. J., Barile, M. F., and McGinniss, M. H. 1965. Mycoplasma (Pleuropneumonia-like organisms) and blood group I: associations with neoplastic disease. Nature 205:371–372.

Shepard, M. C. 1956. T-form colonies of pleuropneumonia-like organism. J. Bact. 71:362–369.

Shifrine, M., and Gourlay, R. N. 1965. Serological relationships between galactans from normal bovine lung and M. mycoides. Nature 208:498.

Shifrine, M., and Gourlay, R. N. 1967. Serological relationships between M. mycoides and other bacteria. Ann. N.Y. Acad. Sci. 143:317–324.

Smith, P. F. 1955. Synthetic media for pleuropneumonia-like organisms. Proc. Soc. Exp. Biol. Med. 88:628–631.

Smith, C. B., Chanock, R. M., Friedewald, W. T., and Alford, R. H. 1967. Mycoplasma pneumoniae infections in human volunteers. Ann. N.Y. Acad. Sci. 143:471–483.

Soběslavský, O., Prescott, B., James, W. D., and Chanock, R. M. 1966. Isolation and characterization of fractions of M. pneumoniae. II. Antigenicity and immunogenicity. J. Bact. 91:2126–2138.

Solana, P., and Rivera, E. 1967. Infection of goats in Mexico by Mycoplasma mycoides var. Capri. Ann. N.Y. Acad. Sci. 143:357–363.

Somerson, N. L., and Cook, M. K. 1965. Suppression of Rous sarcoma virus growth in tissue cultures by Mycoplasma orale. J. Bact. 90:534–540.

Somerson, N. L., Purcell, R. H., Taylor-Robinson, D., and Chanock, R. M. 1965. Hemolysin of Mycoplasma pneumoniae. J. Bact. 89:813–818.

Stokes, E. J. 1955. Human infection with pleuropneumonia-like organisms. Lancet 1:276–279.

Tang, F. F., Wei, H., McWhirter, D. L., and Edgar, J. 1935. An investigation of the causal agent of bovine pleuropneumonia. J. Path. Bact. 40:391–399.

Taylor-Robinson, D., Soběslavský, O., Jensen, K. E., Senterfit, L. B., and Chanock, R. M. 1966. Serologic response to M. pneumoniae infection. I. Evaluation of immunofluorescence, complement fixation, indirect hemagglutination and tetrazolium reduction inhibition tests for the diagnosis of infections. Amer. J. Epidem. 83:287–298.

Thomas, L., Aleu, F., Bitensky, M. W., Davidson, M., and Gesner, B. 1966a. Studies of PPLO infection. II. The neurotoxin of M. neurolyticum. J. Exp. Med. 124:1067–1089.

Thomas, L., Curnen, E. C., Mirick, G. S., Ziegler, J. E., and Horsfall, F. L. 1943. Complement fixation with dissimilar antigens in primary atypical pneumonia. Proc. Soc. Exp. Biol. Med. 52:121–125.

Thomas, L., Davidson, M., and McCluskey, R. T. 1966b. Studies on PPLO infection. I. The production of cerebral polyarteritis by Mycoplasma gallisepticum in turkeys. J. Exp. Med. 123:897–912.

Thomas, L., Mirick, G. S., Curnen, E. C., Zeigler, J. E., and Horsfall, F. L. 1945. Studies on primary atypical pneumonia. II. Observations concerning the relationship of a non-hemolytic streptococcus to the disease. J. Clin. Invest. *24:*227–240.

van Herick, W., and Eaton, M. D. 1945. An unidentified pleuropneumonia-like organism isolated during passages in chick embryos. J. Bact. *50:*47–55.

Vinson, J. W., and Fuller, H. S. 1961. Studies on trench fever; propagation of a rickettsia-like organism from a patient's blood. Path. Microbiol. (suppl.) *24:*152–166.

Weir, J. M., and Horsfall, F. L. 1940. Recovery from patients with acute pneumonitis of a virus causing pneumonia in the mongoose. J. Exp. Med. *72:*595–610.

Whittlestone, P. 1967. Mycoplasma in enzootic pneumonia of pigs. Ann. N.Y. Acad. Sci. *143.* 271–380.

Zucker-Franklin, D., Davidson, M., and Thomas, L. 1966. The interaction of mycoplasmas with mammalian cells. I. Hela cells, neutrophils and eosinophils. J. Exp. Med. *124:*521–542.

# INFECTIONS BY VIRUSES

# Chapter 18

# VIRUS INFECTION AND VIRUS DISEASE*

SIR CHRISTOPHER H. ANDREWES

*Honorary Consultant to Common Cold Research*
*Unit, Salisbury, Wiltshire, England*

Many people regard viruses as being invariably malevolent, harmful parasites. A popular book on viruses has the title *The Virus; Life's Enemy.* It is generally known that man and other animals carry in their mouths, throats, and intestinal tracts and on their skin vast numbers of bacteria, and also that the great majority of these are harmless scavengers; some are even beneficent. Fewer people realize that something of the same sort is true about viruses. There are probably many more harmless virus infections than hurtful ones: virus infection and virus disease are by no means the same thing. True, viruses are obligate intracellular parasites; so they cannot play a scavenging role as many bacteria can. They may, however, and commonly do, cause infections, transient or persistent, which give rise to no symptoms at any time.

It was Theobald Smith who first pointed out that the natural tendency of a host-parasite relationship was toward mutual toleration. A too-successful parasite would ensure its own destruction by eliminating all potential hosts or rendering them immune. This is true of viruses as of other parasites. Viruses have therefore tended to become attenuated so that they do not kill all their hosts and so that they spread well enough, yet not too well.

Accordingly, we find everywhere in nature evidence of inapparent virus infections. Wild animals are much more difficult to observe than domesticated ones. Even allowing for this, it seems that virus disease, as opposed to virus infection, is relatively uncommon in the wild. A great deal of disease due to viruses and other parasites is due to man's interference with nature.

We can now consider under a number of headings the many factors concerned in the sad facts that virus infection is not always inapparent and that many viruses cause troublesome diseases among ourselves, our fellow animals,

---

* For a more detailed survey of the ecology of virus-host interaction, the reader is referred to *The Natural History of Viruses,* by Sir Christopher H. Andrewes, W. W. Norton & Company, New York, 1968.

and plants. We cannot deal with the bacteriophages, the viruses attacking bacteria, for we are almost completely ignorant as to what part they play in causing disease of bacteria in nature: we only know them as laboratory pets. Though we deal with various factors in order it must not be forgotten that things are rarely simple and that in the case of many virus diseases several different factors are concerned.

## Virus Disease as Helper of Virus Spread

A great deal of virus disease appears to be accidental, of no benefit to the virus and, obviously, even less helpful to the host. Nevertheless, there are many instances in which the production of some damage to the host is helpful or even necessary to permit spread to fresh hosts. Common cold viruses are helped by causing their victims to sneeze and distribute excessive respiratory secretion in other ways. We shall, however, see later that this is not the whole story. It is likely that the running eyes and noses at the onset of measles similarly help the measles virus to get across from one child to another. We may well imagine that the rash of measles is irrelevant from the virus's point of view; it may occur just because the virus has the power to inflame all sorts of superficial epithelial tissues, the respiratory epithelium being the real target.

It could be supposed that viruses infecting the intestinal tract would be similarly favored by causing diarrhea. Yet the big group of enteroviruses—poliomyelitis, Coxsackie and echoviruses—which do not in general cause diarrhea, seem nevertheless to spread very readily by the fecal-oral route, at least under conditions of poor hygiene. Perhaps if they had needed to cause diarrhea in order to spread, their evolution would have led to that result. There are, of course, virus diseases which do cause diarrhea, virus diarrhea of cattle, transmissible gastroenteritis of swine, and some virus diarrheas of man: as to the agents of the last we are woefully ignorant. We may speculate as to how far the diarrhea is helpful to these agents.

Viruses may be spread wholly from the local lesions which they cause; warts and molluscum contagiosum are examples. Variola can apparently get around either from the respiratory tract or from dried-up crusts. Myxomatosis of rabbits is of interest here. Virus is present in the blood, but never in great quantity; biting insects—mosquitoes or fleas—cannot pick up enough from the blood for effective transmission. Only when they bite the virus-rich raised myxomatous skin lesions do they get their proboscis sufficiently contaminated. So the evolution of the myxoma virus has been directed toward production of a suitable virus-rich skin lesion. It has also tended, as shown by Mykytowycz[7] and by Fenner and Ratcliffe[3] to such a state of attenuation of virus as will permit the infected rabbits to survive for some time and to serve as sources of infections for numerous vectors.

When disease—often encephalitis—is caused by arboviruses, it seems to be quite valueless from the virus's standpoint. One form of vector-borne encephalitis, rabies, is another matter, however. Rabies causes in dogs, foxes, skunks, and other carnivorous vectors a form of encephalitis which causes them to go mad and indulge in promiscuous biting. The virus, which gets into their salivary glands as well as their brains, is thus effectively spread.

An example from the plant world is afforded by yellows of beet. Lesions produced by this virus render it more attractive to aphids, the normal vectors, and infection is thus distributed more widely.[11]

### The Unlucky Few

Many virus infections, for example poliomyelitis, cause in most people only inapparent infections; yet a few unlucky ones suffer serious disease. Poliomyelitis normally remains localized as a harmless infection of the intestinal tract. But probably the balance between virus and host is a delicate one and some abnormal circumstance may upset it, with resulting disease. Paralytic poliomyelitis may occur as a result of tonsillectomy, violent exercise, or injection of some unrelated vaccine; usually it involves the part of the body concerned in the particular stress. Very possibly some similar but undetected circumstance determines the occurrence of paralysis in other unlucky victims. So, too, Japanese encephalitis virus infects thousands of Japanese children, the virus being conveyed from birds by mosquito bite, yet only a small minority of them suffer any harm. Genetic factors may well play a part; people with a particular build have been thought to be unusually poliomyelitis-prone. Certainly there is a vast amount of experimental evidence that genetic factors are important in determining virus susceptibility among mice and farm animals; scrapie in sheep affords a good example.

### Relatively Harmless Virus Disease

Though many host-virus associations seem to end up as wholly inapparent infections, there would seem to be no good reason for elimination by natural selection of diseases so mild as to cause only temporary disability and no deaths. Perhaps we may place in this category some of the minor exanthems which afflict children, and minor respiratory infections such as those caused by some adenoviruses. Why some infections should be inapparent and others remain as mild apparent ones is hard to say. We should not forget, however, that host-virus relations are probably rarely static and that some of these mild illnesses may be on the road to inapparency.

### Incomplete Equilibrium

This brings us to the next point. A virus may be newly introduced, perhaps in ways to be considered in a moment. It may cause disease which will be severe, often fatal, in a wholly susceptible population, and the factors tending toward a more comfortable mutually acceptable equilibrium may not have had time to operate. Myxomatosis again affords an illustration. The virus from South America, when first introduced into Australia, killed over 99 per cent of the rabbits. Now the virus has become attenuated, the rabbits are genetically more resistant, and the disease is killing somewhere between 50 and 90 per cent. Though the most rapid changes in the equilibrium are now over, it is quite likely that we shall end up with a nonfatal local infection such as we see in the natural hosts, the Brazilian *Sylvilagus* rabbits.

### SPREAD TO STRANGE HOSTS

Very important and often serious diseases are caused when a virus spreads to a new host from one with which a harmless equilibrium has long been established. The arboviruses afford many examples, particularly of zoonoses, infections passed to man from some other animal. In most instances of which we are aware, arboviruses exist in nature as harmless infections of vertebrates, carried from one to another by arthropod vectors. In these, too, the infections are inapparent: in fact there are good grounds for believing that the viruses in question were originally parasites of insects. They may be supposed to have used the vertebrate as a means of getting from one insect to another, a contrast to our usual way of looking at the matter.

Some examples are worth more than passing attention. The Eastern and Western equine encephalomyelitis viruses normally circulate among birds, especially water birds, during summer months. In them infection is inapparent; but virus transferred by mosquito bite to horses and to man may cause fatal encephalomyelitis. Such infections are not naturally transmissible in series. Since horses are involved so incidentally there is a tendency nowadays to drop the "equine" from the names of these viruses. It is of interest that disease may be caused by these viruses in a few birds; these are the house (or English) sparrow and the pheasant, neither of them native American species. The fact that these two species were introduced to North America many decades ago shows that inherited resistance has not been acquired in these birds at all rapidly. Overwintering of these viruses may possibly be explained by a basic cycle in small mammals, reptiles, or amphibians from which virus spills over into birds every spring.[1]

Yellow fever was once responsible, along with malaria, for the name "the white man's grave" applied to West Africa. The virus circulates among monkeys, carried by *Aedes africanus* and other mosquitoes. This is jungle yellow fever: superimposed on this cycle is urban yellow fever, which is carried from man to man by *Aedes aegypti*. It is this which kills. Some think there is an undiscovered basic cycle in some other species, spreading intermittently to monkeys. Be that as it may, the African monkeys do not develop overt disease. Nor indeed do most native Africans in scattered villages. Children here may be developing neutralizing antibodies year by year though there is no clinically evident yellow fever to be detected. Here is an example of a virus causing disease, not in a different species, but in a different race of the same species, the white man.

Urban yellow fever and jungle fellow fever occur in South America also. It is likely that the virus was at one time introduced from Africa, for the South American monkeys are not all of them naturally resistant, as are those in Africa. Dead spider monkeys have been found on the forest floor at times shortly preceding the occurrence of outbreaks of yellow fever in man.

There are about 200 arboviruses known, with more turning up every year. Of these something like 50 are known to cause disease in man, and all of these are apparently carried to him by biting insects from some reservoir host. An exception is afforded by yellow fever when the urban cycle involving only man and *Aedes aegypti* is concerned. Dengue viruses may also circulate in populous places in a similar way with the aid of the same mosquito; here, too, the urban cycle is probably superimposed on a jungle cycle involving forest animals. There exist also arthropod-borne diseases of domestic animals, carried to them, we believe, from reservoirs of harmless infection in wild animals: Rift valley fever, African horse sickness, and blue tongue of sheep are examples.

It is not only the arthropod-borne viruses which cause trouble of this kind. The virus of malignant catarrh, a member of the herpesvirus family, causes naturally an inapparent infection in wildebeest or gnu. In the young wildebeest one is persistent viremia for many months.[9] When cattle run on land where these are present, many contract a fatal infection, but how infection spreads is not known. Another herpesvirus, pseudorabies or mad itch, is very fatal to cattle and may afflict them when they are run together with pigs. In pigs the infection may be mild or inapparent but virus is present in their nasal discharges and readily passes to the cattle.[12] In East and South Africa a virus infection can pass from apparently normal wart hogs to pigs, causing high mortality: this is African swine fever. Many more examples of this sort of thing could be quoted.

### INTRODUCTION OF VIRUS INTO A NEW AREA

When an apparently "new" virus disease turns up in an area, it is often difficult to know whether or not there is also a question of transfer from another host species. Two examples can be quoted. In 1959 an epidemic virus disease began in Northern Uganda, spreading rapidly southward and causing disease in 5 million Africans. It was called o'nyong-nyong, which in a local language means twisting up; severe joint pains cause these contortions. It was transmitted by *Anopheles*, a mosquito genus not commonly involved as vectors of arboviruses. It has been suggested that adaptation of a virus from culicine to anopheline mosquitoes may have been associated with a change in pathogenicity for man.

Then in the province of Mysore, in India, an epidemic of a "new" disease occurred especially among forest workers; it was called Kyasanur forest disease. The outbreak in man coincided with finding of dead langur and bonnet monkeys in the forest. It was thought locally that infection was contracted by smelling a dead monkey, but in fact the virus was shown to be transmitted by *Haemaphysalis* ticks. The virus is related to the tick-borne encephalitis viruses of Europe and Asia, but is quite distinct from them; where it came from nobody knows.[14]

Apart from these mysteries, known viruses may cause havoc when spreading to places long free from them: witness the very big outbreaks of yellow fever in the Nuba mountains of the Sudan in 1940 and in Abyssinia from 1959 to 1962. Similarly measles has been unusually severe when introduced after a long period of freedom to the Faeroe Islands (1940) and to Fiji.

### EFFECTS OF CHANGE IN ENVIRONMENT

An apparently new disease may become evident as a result of changes in environment, due to weather or human activity. Such changes may result in a big buildup of virus in a reservoir host in which infection is inapparent. Only then is a spillover into man and other unusual hosts evident. In 1959 the Eastern encephalitis virus became unusually abundant in New Jersey in water birds: in these it was being carried by salt-marsh mosquitoes. A sudden change in the wind brought many of these into inland areas. The virus was introduced there and other mosquitoes began to pick up the virus and carry it over to man and to horses.[4] Heavy rains and floods have elsewhere favored the multiplication of mosquitoes and, as a consequence, of mosquito-borne viruses. It has been suggested that unusual flooding has enabled the Murray Valley virus to spread at times to more southerly parts of Australia from its normal habitat farther north.

Anything man does in a big way, from clearing jungle to draining marshes or irrigating deserts, is likely to alter the balance of nature, harming some species and encouraging others. In the latter event there may be new opportunities for their viruses and other parasites to spread to man.

### ACTIVATION OF LATENT INFECTIONS

A number of viruses are able to exist as persistent latent infections of their hosts. The condition may be found as a sequel to a brief apparent infection, or there may not have been symptoms at any time. We have a clue as to how this comes about through studies of tissue cultures. In these a virus may cause destruction of many cells, but then at times the cultures seem to recover as a result of growth of surviving cells. These may go on growing indefinitely and turning out a certain amount of virus. They also produce some of the antiviral protein, interferon, and these two activities seem to balance out so that cells are no longer destroyed and yet to a limited extent virus can still multiply. It is highly probable that the same thing can go on in the intact animal.

The equilibrium is, however, often unstable both in the tissue culture and in the living animal. Various factors may upset the balance and then disease results. For instance, corticosteroid hormones have a depressing effect on the production of both antibodies and interferon. It is sometimes desirable to give these hormones in order deliberately to suppress the body's immunity mechanism; for instance, in attempting to graft a kidney from a donor who is not genetically identical. When this is done, there may be activation of the latent virus of cytomegalic disease, a member of the herpesvirus family, and the resulting disease may be fatal. More often we only guess how the activation works, but the mechanism may well be similar.

The classical example of activation of a latent infection is afforded by herpes simplex. The "fever blisters" caused by this virus, especially around nostrils and lips, may come as a consequence of a cold in the nose, some feverish illness, or mild allergy: the stimulus is apt to be different among those liable, so-called "habitual herpetikers." The latency usually follows an infection, probably caught as a rule from the mother during infancy. It may at that time present as a widespread stomatitis or the infection may creep in insidiously. There is little doubt that the virus's ability to break forth at intervals is of great survival value to it. If at one time it fails to encounter a susceptible, usually very young, host, then it can keep on trying, time and again, from its successive eruptions of blisters.

The same argument applies in the case of a related virus, that of varicella. This virus, when the chickenpox eruption is over and done with, is apparently able to persist, lying doggo in the central nervous system. Some stimulus in later life activates it in posterior root ganglia and shingles or herpes zoster appears. What the stimulus is we do not know, but as shingles is rather frequent in late life, it may be connected with waning immunity to the varicella-zoster virus. Here again it seems that the virus benefits by getting a chance to start a new chain of infection.[5] A somewhat different method has been adopted by the virus of rubella. This, as is now well known, causes many congenital deformities in babies when the mother has been infected in the first 3 months of pregnancy. These abnormalities do not in themselves help the virus, but they are associated with persistence of virus in the throat of the newborn infants, perhaps for many months. These may infect other infants and also nurses looking after them.

When newly recruited men are brought together in the services for the first time, there are commonly outbreaks of respiratory infections among them. There is evidence that these are not merely a result of unusual opportunities for spreading noxious organisms; it seems that the stresses of a novel, rigidly disciplined life and administration of a whole series of different vaccines may act as stressing factors, converting into an active disease something which might otherwise have been an inapparent infection.[8] We know of the occurrence of infections which are wholly inapparent yet liable to reactivation, largely because of research on laboratory animals. When monkey kidneys began to be used in a big way for tissue culture of polio and other viruses, there began to turn up in those cultures whole series of hitherto unknown viruses. These belong to many families, enteroviruses, adenoviruses, reoviruses, myxoviruses, and herpesviruses. They produce destructive effects under the abnormal conditions of tissue culture, but most of them are not known to cause symptoms in the monkeys: an exception is the B herpesvirus which can cause mouth blistering in macaques.

More important for our present argument are the many diseases which appear in mice and other species when tissues are ground up and used for serial passage to other animals of the same kind. Diseases so produced have often led experimenters astray. The infections thus caused in mice include ectromelia, caused by a member of the poxvirus family, hepatitis, lymphocytic choriomeningitis, encephalomyelitis, diarrhea, and several kinds of pneumonia. Some of these are known to cause sporadic disease in the absence of laboratory manipulations, others are not.

Of special interest are the viruses which cause leukemia or tumors in mice. These when passed serially in the laboratory can be relied upon to cause a high proportion of solid tumors or leukemias in inoculated mice of suitable genetic composition and they are often referred to as oncogenic viruses. It is often forgotten that under natural conditions they are, so far as we know, entirely inapparent infections. The polyoma virus, for instance, is known to be endemic among wild mice, but polyoma-caused tumors among them are not known to occur naturally. Occurrence of spontaneous leukemia due to a virus is only known in inbred stocks of laboratory mice.

Other viruses which are usually inapparent may find conditions very favorable in tumors and may be able to persist there when they would probably have died out in a normal animal. Thus serial passage of tumors or leukemias has led to appearance of fatal hepatitis due to a virus which has been exalted quantitatively or qualitatively as a result of serial passage of the malignant cells which were harboring it.

The viruses which cause in fowls either leukemia or sarcomata such as the well known Rous sarcoma behave in a similar way. There are in many fowls inapparent infections with viruses related to these oncogenic ones. Many fowls without any evidence of malignant disease have, in consequence, antibodies against the Rous sarcoma virus. It is highly probable that the occurrence of many cases of leukemia or sarcoma in certain stocks of fowls is a consequence of inbreeding or the artificial conditions of modern husbandry.

## Upper Respiratory Infections

Some apparently special problems are presented by the minor infections of the human respiratory tract; they are not, however, basically different from others we are considering. Though they are among the commonest infections, there is much that is obscure in their epidemiology. There is, first of all, influenza. At epidemic times there is person to person spread, plain for all to see. There is often, however, no evident increased nasal discharge such as is assumed to be necessary for the spread of colds. We still do not understand where the virus goes between outbreaks, for when an epidemic is over it may be impossible to discover any virus in the lately affected community. True, there may be occasional isolations of virus between epidemics, or serological evidence that the virus is about. Opinions differ as to how far one can account for interepidemic survival of virus in terms of such occurrences. It has been observed that at the end of the winter an epidemic peters out on the fringe of the involved area; and when, 1 or 2 years later, another epidemic spread begins, it may start just in that country in which the previous outbreak had petered out. I myself suspect that virus may keep going in some fashion as a subclinical infection; occasional unusually susceptible people may indicate that the virus is around by suffering from an apparently sporadic attack of flu. Such a hypothetical subclinical spread would seem to be doubtfully effective in immunizing a population.

When we come to the common cold we again have to consider an explanation of its epidemiology in terms of subclinical spread with episodes of obvious "catching" of colds. There is much evidence of how clinically evident colds can be spread; virus is known to come mainly from violently discharged nasal secretions, to pass effectively in medium-sized droplets, and to infect most readily when a landing is made in the nose itself. Yet there is epidemiological evidence that colds may start simultaneously over large areas, often apparently in relation to sudden weather changes; and that such simultaneity cannot easily be explained on a basis of person to person spread.[13] It can readily be argued that a latent infection can be activated by stresses, particularly meteorological ones. Yet this cannot be anything quite like the activation of latent herpes infections, for when a person has a succession of colds they are at times, and probably as a rule, due to different serotypes of rhinoviruses.

I have before now put forward a hypothesis to account for these apparently discrepant findings[2] and I see no reason to change my view. On this notion, rhinoviruses, and probably other upper respiratory pathogens, are constantly being passed from one person to another, obtaining only temporary local lodgment in the nose, neither causing symptoms nor inducing solid immunity. When an appropriate stress is applied, the "temporary lodger" can seize the opportunity to invade wide areas of mucosa; it then causes a clinical cold and the resulting sneezing can spread it to more victims. The activation by stress is of whatever virus happens to be there at the time. In favor of this view is the fact that although rhinoviruses are definitely associated with clinical colds and can cause them experimentally, yet they turn up not infrequently in noses of people who are free from symptoms.

Influenza viruses and rhinoviruses are perhaps special cases: influenza viruses can undergo antigenic changes rather readily and rhinoviruses are of very many serotypes. Other "respiratory" viruses are entities more stable or less diverse. The effects of stresses in activating adenoviruses were considered earlier. In the case of the parainfluenza and respiratory syncytial viruses it is likely that a solid immunity is achieved with difficulty and that, following initial infection in childhood, numerous reinfections can occur, presenting either as colds or being wholly subclinical, yet serving as sources of infection for other people.

### Man-Made Diseases

An outstanding example of an iatrogenic disease, one caused by the physician, is, of course, serum hepatitis. The only known mechanism of spread of any importance is the doctor's syringe which unwittingly transfers the virus from the blood of a carrier. Other means by which the virus is similarly conveyed are less important.

Apart from this, however, man brings trouble upon himself in ways we have discussed earlier. The stresses of multiple vaccinations combine with other factors to cause outbreaks of adenovirus infections in recruits. The gathering together of "pure cultures"—aggregations of a single species—of cattle, sheep, sugar-beet plants, or man himself favors the rapid spread and associated exaltation of virulence which encourage epidemic disease. And finally there are upsets which man causes in the balance of nature when he carries out his large agricultural and other schemes: possible results of these have already been mentioned.

### Unusual Immunological Situation

There seem to be instances in which an animal's immune response, if it is somewhere short of giving complete protection, may actually sensitize, so that illness is worse than in a nonimmunized animal. Mice can thus be sensitized against lymphocytic choriomeningitis virus by giving vaccine subcutaneously.[10]

As a result of immunological tolerance, a virus such as lymphocytic chorio-meningitis may exist in the body yet produce no harmful reaction; the giving of antiserum may then induce a reaction which causes severe symptoms. An effective vaccine against respiratory syncytial virus is hard to produce. If one injects one which is only feebly effective in eliciting antibodies, it may make a child more sensitive than normal to contact with that virus. These are all rather artificial situations; yet they raise the question of whether something similar may not be at the bottom of some natural occurrences. It was suggested many decades ago that some exanthematous rashes were allergic in nature.

### POSSIBLE BENEFICENT VIRUSES

One may finally ask whether virus disease can in the long run be beneficial to the host. Inapparent infection certainly can: the maize hopper *Dalbulus maidis* normally feeds only on maize and a related grass; but when fed on asters already infected with aster yellows virus it not only flourishes but can thrive afterward on other asters and on several other kinds of plants.[6] The virus infection increases its digestive powers!

Bacteria, too, when they carry a bacteriophage in the prophage state are thereby made resistant to other phages.

But overt virus disease is another matter. Caribou and other herbivores are often attacked by wolves. This they doubtless hate; yet they are helped in the long run, for the wolves take the defective or weak ones and thus the stock is improved. It is very doubtful whether parasites such as viruses serve the same end. The predator takes his toll of a few and the survivors are unscathed: the parasite attacks and harms many, simply killing those worst affected. Predation helps to favor the survival of those which are generally fitter—swifter, stronger, more alert: survivors of attack by parasites are on the contrary better than their fellows only because they are specifically resistant to one particular enemy.

We conclude therefore that in the course of evolution, viruses and their hosts are likely to come to terms. One will normally end up with an inapparent infection or with one which is so harmless that natural selection will not wholly eliminate symptoms. Often a lesion of some sort will continue to be found, when its presence is required by the virus for its own perpetuation. Very rarely, however, will this disease be a serious one as rabies is. Were the world static we could hope that in the course of evolution virus diseases would grow less and less troublesome. But the world keeps changing and viruses behave like opportunist creatures, alert to take advantage of change.

## References

1. Altman, R., Goldfield, M., and Sussman, O. (1967). The impact of vector-borne viral diseases in the middle Atlantic States. Med. Clin. N. Amer. *51*:661–671.
2. Andrewes, C. H. (1964). The complex epidemiology of respiratory virus infections. Science, *146*:1274–1277.

3. Fenner, F., and Ratcliffe, F. N. (1965). Myxomatosis. Cambridge University Press.

4. Hayes, R. O., Beadle, L. D., Hess, A. D., Sussman, O., and Bonese, M. J. (1962). Entomological aspects of the Eastern equine encephalomyelitis New Jersey outbreak. Amer. J. Trop. Med., *11:*115–121.

5. Hope-Simpson, R. E. (1965). The nature of herpes zoster: a long-term study and a new hypothesis. Proc. Roy. Soc. Med., *58:*9–20.

6. Maramorosch, K., and Jensen, D. D. (1963). Harmful and beneficial effects of plant viruses in insects. Ann. Rev. Microbiol., *17:*495–530.

7. Mykytowycz, R. (1953). An attenuated strain of the myxoma virus recovered from the field. Nature, *172:*448–449.

8. Pierce, W. C., Stille, W. T., and Miller, L. F. (1963). A preliminary report on the effects of routine inoculations on respiratory illness. Proc. Soc. Exp. Biol. Med., *114:*369–372.

9. Plowright, W., Ferris, W. D., and Scott, G. R. (1960). Blue wildebeest and the aetiological agent of bovine malignant catarrhal fever. Nature, *188:*1167–1169.

10. Seamer, J., Barlow, J., Gledhill, A. W., and Hotchin, J. (1963). Increased susceptibility of mice to lymphocytic choriomeningitis after peripheral inoculation. Virology, *21:*309–316.

11. Severin, H. H. P. (1946). Longevity and life history of leaf-hopper species on virus-infected and healthy plants. Hilgardia, *17:*121–123.

12. Shope, R. E. (1935). Experiments on the epidemiology of pseudo-rabies: mode of transmission of the disease in swine and their possible role in its spread to cattle. J. Exp. Med., *62:* 85–99.

13. Van Loghem, J. J. (1928). An epidemiological contribution to the knowledge of respiratory diseases. J. Hyg. (Camb.), *28:*33–54.

14. Work, T. H. (1958). Russian spring-summer virus in India: Kyasanur forest disease. Progr. Med. Virol., *1:*248–279.

# Chapter 19

# THE ULTRASTRUCTURE OF THE HOST CELL IN VIRAL INFECTION

COUNCILMAN MORGAN

*Department of Microbiology, Columbia University*
*College of Physicians and Surgeons,*
*New York, New York*

Anyone faced with the task of deciding how best to discuss the structural changes observed in electron microscopic studies of virus-infected tissue must contend with a vast and constantly increasing volume of literature. Consider, for example, that in 1960, when the last comprehensive review of this subject appeared,[50] 172 papers were cited, of which five concerned the herpesvirus group. At last count 31 additional papers discussing viruses of this group alone had been published. Not only are there now numerous studies of long-established agents but new viruses have been isolated and investigated. It is perfectly clear that any systematic, inclusive review at the present time would become a tedious catalogue of observations. How then to proceed? One of the unfortunate aspects of this flood of papers is that much of the early work is buried and forgotten beneath the alluvium. It might be of passing interest, therefore, to examine thin sectioning from an archeological standpoint. A few flights of fancy and even one personal anecdote will be interjected more for amusement than for anything else. Following this a brief discussion of the general effects of viruses on cells will be presented. It will be seen that when all is said and done the lesions produced in the host cells are, with a few interesting exceptions, disarmingly similar. Lastly, a concluding paragraph will contain some perfectly obvious recommendations for future study. Thus if the opening of the chapter seems eccentric, the conclusion, at least, will be traditional.

Although the first biological specimen, a fragmented plant root cell,[34] had been examined in the electron microscope 14 years previously and although the silhouette of tobacco mosaic virus from a purified preparation was seen 9 years before,[29] Dr. Keith Porter and his colleagues were the first to observe a virus within its host cell. They hit upon the idea of simply growing tissue culture cells on formvar and transferring this substrate with the attached cells to a specimen grid. It was hoped that after fixation and dehydration the thin peripheral portion of the cells would permit transmission of a sufficient number of electrons to form an image. This proved to be the case,[9, 48] and it was possible to observe small, spherical, viral particles interspersed between lamellar structures, which were later to be called endoplasmic reticulum.

A significant advance was provided by Newman, Borysko, and Swerdlow,[44] who reported that a transparent plastic, methacrylate, could be used to embed tissue for thin sectioning. The next step took place in the laboratory of R. W. G. Wyckoff at the National Institutes of Health, for it was here in 1949 that infected cells were first sectioned so as to reveal the presence of tobacco mosaic virus[5] and fowl pox virus[42] (Fig. 1). The crude technique consisted of cutting formalin-fixed, methacrylate-embedded tissue with a steel knife mounted on a modified Spencer microtome. Since there was neither a bypass mechanism nor a trough on which to float the sections, relatively thick sections were transferred by means of a dissecting needle from the knife edge to a glass slide. To allow penetration of the electron beam the embedding plastic was dissolved in acetone. The slide was then coated with collodion, which could be floated off with the adherent tissue, and mounted on a specimen grid. Before examination it was

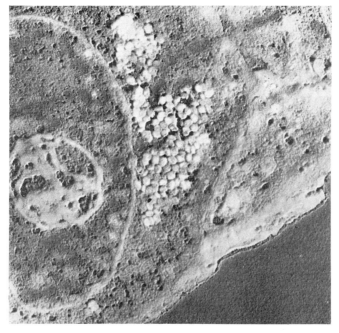

*Figure* 1.   Fowl pox virus in the cytoplasm of an epithelial cell from the chorioallantoic membrane of a chicken embryo. The nucleus with a nucleolus is visible on the left. In this and the following two examples the embedding plastic was dissolved out and the specimens were metal shadowed. They are reproduced as negative prints in conformity with the custom of the times. This electron micrograph was taken by R. W. G. Wyckoff in 1950. ×8200. (From Morgan, C., and R. W. G. Wyckoff. 1950. The electron microscopy of fowl pox virus within the chorioallantoic membrane. J. Immun. *65*:285–295.)

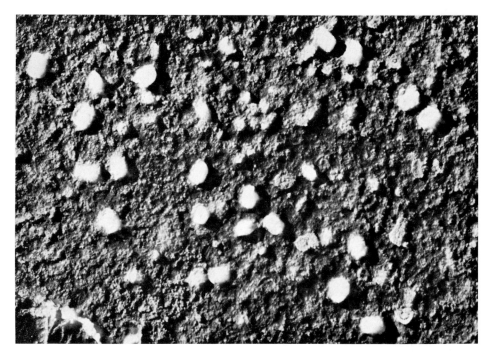

*Figure 2.* Vaccinia virus in the cytoplasm of an epithelial cell. Despite virtually complete destruction of cytoplasmic structure the brick-like shape of the virus is evident. ×25,000. (From Morgan, C., et al. 1954. Structure and development of viruses observed in the electron microscope. II. Vaccinia and fowl pox viruses. J. Exp. Med. *100*:301–310.)

shadowed with metal to enhance contrast and detail. In view of the extreme extraction and distortion inflicted upon the cell by removal of the embedding plastic, one can have nothing but admiration for the resolute manner in which the virus particles maintained recognizable shape (Fig. 2) and to some extent even internal structure (Fig. 3).

While this work was in progress, however, remarkable advances in sectioning were being made. A bypass mechanism and a boat or trough for floating the sections off the knife edge were developed by Claude,[8] while fractured glass knives[31] replaced the steel blades, which could never be adequately sharpened. By 1953, with the development and manufacture of a simple and practical microtome,[47] and with the recognition of osmium tetroxide as an excellent fixative of fine structure,[45] the modern era of thin sectioning had arrived. During the next five years much excitement prevailed, for everywhere there was something new to be seen. The only comparable event in the study of structure had been the development of the light microscope itself, and this, together with the necessary ancillary techniques, required a very much longer period of time.

In the years from 1952 to 1957 the basis of biologic fine structure was established, and it soon became apparent that the organelles were remarkably similar in all cells examined. The endoplasmic reticulum and mitochondria of a frog and a mouse were similar, as was the arrangement of myofibrils in a cockroach and a dog or the appearance of nuclei in pigeons and silkworms. Even the flagellae of bacteria and the cilia of man were found to exhibit a close resemblance. Presumably in the course of evolution the pressures of a changing environment, which resulted in different species acquiring different gross morphology, were not reflected at the fine structural level, and one is led to suggest that cellular components had early achieved such a high state of efficiency that little alteration was subsequently necessary or indeed possible. One may further surmise that this state of efficiency was reached so far back in evolution that the same basic structure was carried as a common denominator by all the diverse species which subsequently developed. It then becomes an intriguing question as to why viruses differ so markedly, for to a large extent they adapt the machinery of the cell to their own reproduction. For example, the pox viruses and herpesviruses, although they afflict a wide variety of hosts, develop in cells that are virtually identical so far as structural and biochemical features are concerned. If one accepts the universality of the genetic code as currently propounded then there is no reason why herpesviruses should not be synthesized at the same sites in the cell as vaccinia virus. Why, then, does the former have to go to all the trouble of differentiating in the nucleus and what is the nature of the message that can stipulate whether DNA is to be made in the

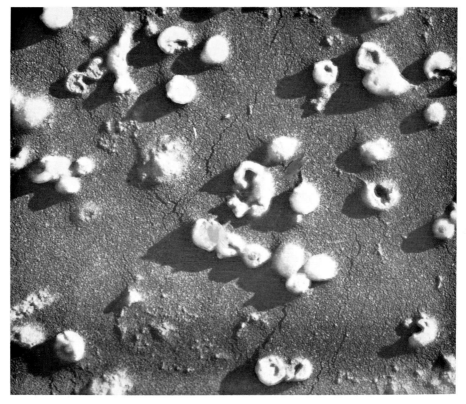

*Figure 3.* Herpes simplex virus in the cytoplasm. Again the cellular architecture has been lost. Several particles are disrupted. At the lower left the core of one particle is clearly visible where the envelope was torn off and at the lower right a core is lying free. The micrograph was taken in 1952. ×47,000. (From Morgan, C., et al. 1954. Structure and development of viruses as observed in the electron microscope. I. Herpes simplex virus. J. Exp. Med. *100:*195–202.)

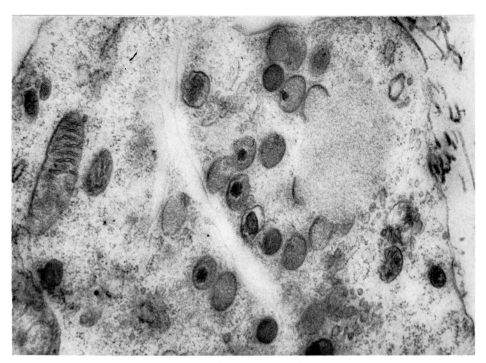

*Figure 4.* A micrograph (published in 1954) showing fowl pox virus in process of formation within the cytoplasm. Note incomplete membranes adjacent to the finely granular matrix at the upper right. ×38,000. (From Morgan, C., et al. 1954. Structure and development of viruses observed in the electron microscope. II. Vaccinia and fowl pox viruses. J. Exp. Med. *100*:301–310.)

nucleus or in the cytoplasm? Answers to these questions cannot be provided at present, but considering the differences between viruses and also the fact that viruses are notoriously inefficient, requiring the synthesis of chemical constituents greatly in excess of the amounts actually utilized in the process of differentiation, it is interesting to speculate that viruses arrived so early in the course of biological history that they still reflect their origin in host cells which may formerly have differed greatly in structure, in pathways of synthesis, and in efficiency. Of course a basic requirement for the survival of viruses in nature is that the composition of the proteins of one type of virus differ sufficiently from another to avoid stimulation of cross-neutralizing antibodies, for, from the standpoint of the virus at least, it would be a sorry state of affairs if infection of an organism by any one virus resulted in the formation of protective antibodies, which precluded subsequent infection by any other. However it was achieved, one cannot but be impressed by the way with which viruses have satisfied this requirement.

But to return to our brief annotated history, the first paper illustrating viruses in ultra-thin sections of infected cells was published by Gaylord and Melnick in 1953.[16] There next appeared a breathless note in *Nature* showing the fine structure of herpes simplex virus and indicating that vaccinia and influenza viruses exhibited markedly different structure.[35] This was followed by publication of detailed studies of herpes simplex virus[36] and then vaccinia

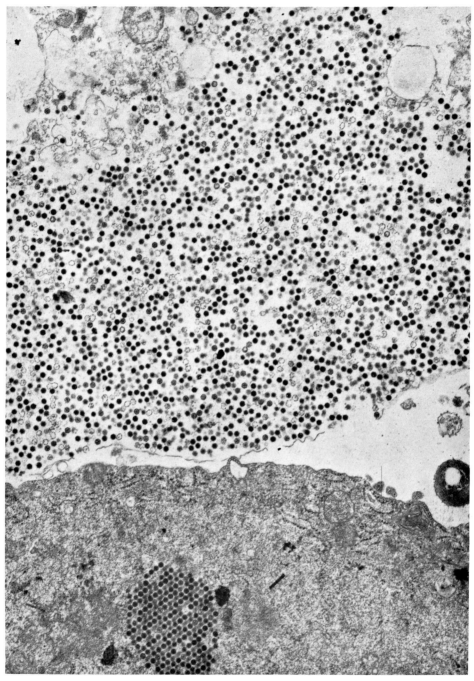

*Figure 5.* A cell at an advanced stage of autolysis but containing innumerable particles of adenovirus. At the lower margin the cellular membrane has ruptured, and virus is about to be released. At the bottom of the micrograph a cell at an earlier stage of infection contains a crystal composed of viral particles. ×26,000.

and fowl pox viruses.[37] The anatomy of these viruses was illustrated and templates or sites of synthesis were shown (Fig. 4). Regarding the manner of replication, it is fundamental to all viruses that a protective wall enclose and protect the infectious nucleic acid, which otherwise is unstable and easily subject to degradation. The extraordinary success of this accomplishment is well demonstrated by the capsid of adenoviruses. It is the rule at advanced stages of infection to encounter cells which have become bags devoid of architecture but containing masses of virus. The disintegration of the fine structure is accompanied by release of enzymes with resulting autolysis of cellular components, and yet the virus appears to be untouched (Fig. 5). Unfortunately the manner in which this essential viral barrier or capsid actually forms cannot be visualized in the great majority of cases simply because the process is too rapid. Considering the large number of studies now extant, differentiation must be almost instantaneous, since it has escaped detection. Poliovirus or adenovirus is either there or it is not; sequential steps in its formation have not been reported. The chief exception to this rule is the pox group, for these elephantine viruses are very slow and deliberate in their maturation. Granular and filamentous matrix appears to aggregate at multiple sites within the cytoplasm of infected cells. Along the margins of such foci numerous viral membranes can be seen at all stages in the process of growth (Fig. 6), and one is prompted to ask whether the membranes are formed in such a way as only to enclose the proper matrix or whether the process is less specific, thus resulting in the enclosure of any material which happens to be in the vicinity. The latter appears to be the case, for in cells doubly infected with vaccinia and herpes simplex viruses numerous herpes capsids come to lie in close proximity to sites where vaccinia virus is differentiating. The unsuspecting vaccinia membrane then proceeds to incorporate the hapless herpes particle quite by accident (Fig. 7). Recognizable cellular components are not similarly engulfed because they are invariably displaced to the periphery and never lie within the template site itself. The actual manner in which such membranes form continues to be one of the basic unsolved questions. It is surprising, for example, that despite the very considerable advances in resolution and structural preservation which have been made since the phenomenon was first described absolutely no sign of molecular orientation precedes the advancing edge of the differentiating membrane (Fig. 8). In other words, one cannot discern any orientation in the arrangement of the finely granular matrix which would suggest that the proteins of the membrane are in process of assembly. Considering the complexity of the structures involved, the extraordinary similarity in size of the viral particles produced, and the fact that the whole process evolves within a cytoplasmic matrix in constant motion, it is difficult not to believe that a very high degree of order indeed must exist at a level beyond the resolution obtainable by current methods. Of course the cell is adept at assembling membranes so that it is not surprising that the virus could utilize the machinery at its disposal, but having said this we are no further along in understanding the basic mechanism.

Just as thin sectioning was well on its way the extraordinary technique of negative staining appeared, and thereby hangs a tale. It is a tale of prejudice, and it illustrates the simple fact that prejudice is as dangerous to reason in science as it is in human relations. The prejudice derived from the

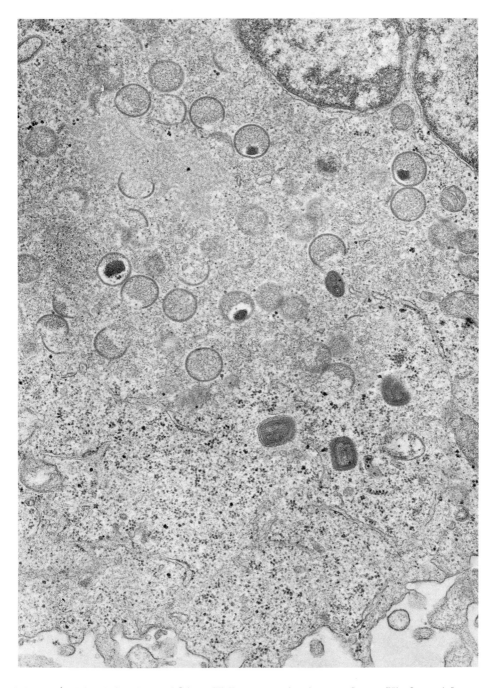

*Figure 6.* Vaccinia virus within a HeLa grown in tissue culture. Viral particles at various stages of differentiation are evident. At the lower right is a mature, infectious virus. Ribosomes, endoplasmic reticulum, and mitochondria have been displaced by the aggregate of viral components. Note the beautiful, detailed preservation afforded by glutaraldehyde-osmium fixation and epon embedding when compared with the early micrograph shown in Figure 4. ×40,000.

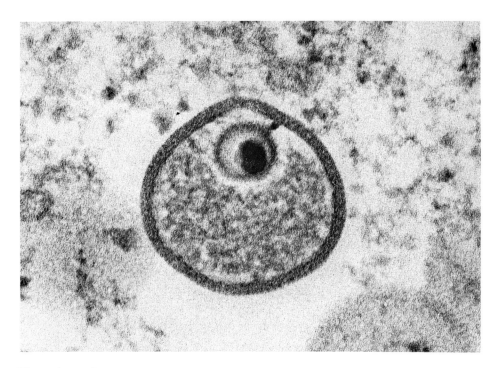

*Figure 7.*    A herpes viral core and capsid which has been enclosed within a particle of vaccinia virus. ×200,000.

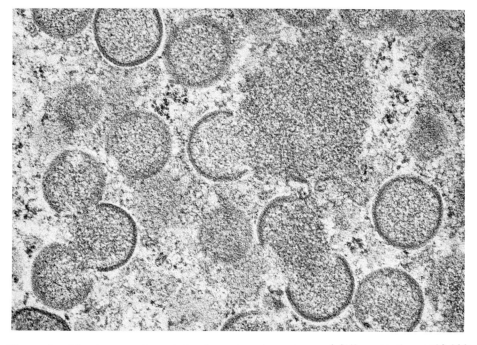

*Figure 8.*    Membranes of vaccinia virus at various stages of differentiation. ×82,000.

simple assumption that mammalian viruses, with the exception of the pox group, were spherical in shape. There were cogent reasons for not thinking this was so but none seemed to reach the clouded mentality of many then engaged in thin sectioning. Crick and Watson,[10] for example, suggested in 1956 that the shell of small viruses was built up of repeating subunits packed in a regular arrangement. A year previously Kjellén et al.[30] and Harford et al.[20] had reported the presence of crystals composed of adenovirus in thin sections of infected cell nuclei. Anybody with a grain of sense, or let us say of unclouded sense, would have immediately deduced that such viral particles in order to crystallize must each possess a regular array of surface charges and hence were probably themselves crystalline in shape. Then in 1957 additional evidence appeared in two independent reports which showed that adenoviruses fixed and dried down on specimen grids were polyhedral in shape.[57, 58] Finally, if I may descend to the level of personal anecdote, for I do not know specifically what others in the field were privately thinking at the time, inspection of our own pictures showed that occasional particles, at least, did not appear spherical. In 1959 arrived an invitation to present our work at the Ninth Symposium of The Society for General Microbiology in London.[41] In the paper, which concluded the published *Symposium*, the following paragraph appears. (Since I am responsible for having written it I will quote it.)

### Shape of Adenoviruses

In preparations of virus fixed with osmium and dried from suspension the particles have a polyhedral shape. The surface forces accompanying the process of drying, however, make these observations difficult to evaluate. It appears unlikely that the procedures of embedding or sectioning would obliterate a preexisting polyhedral shape. . . . We are inclined, therefore, toward the belief that the spherical shape of adenoviruses in thin sections does not represent an artifact.

Not more than 10 minutes after the echoes of this ringing declaration had died Robert Horne quietly rose to present the first definitive picture of negatively stained adenovirus capsids, 252 in number and arranged in the form of a perfect icosahedron.[23] So much for prejudice.

Negative staining with phosphotungstic acid is the chief technique whereby the details of viral structure have been demonstrated, and accordingly much attention has been devoted to this method in recent years. Oddly enough, little is known even now concerning the exact way in which the image is formed. It is not always clear when a suspension of virus is mixed with phosphotungstic acid and subsequently dried down on a specimen grid whether the top and (or) the bottom of the virus is visualized. Müller and Meyerhoff[43] reported the interesting observation that crystals of magnesium oxide embedded in phosphotungstic acid appeared less dense to the electron beam than crystals devoid of stain, and they postulated that since a deposit of phosphotungstic acid can be shown to develop a positive charge and hence bend the beam, the stain was acting as a micro lens at the specimen level. No further work on this interesting problem has appeared.

The drawback to negative staining is that it is difficult to apply not only to the

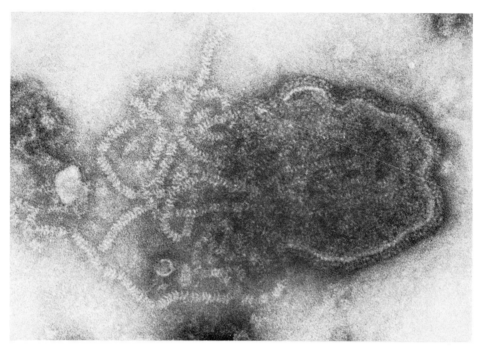

*Figure 9.* Parainfluenza virus negatively stained with phosphotungstic acid. The particle disrupted during preparation of the specimen, and the helical nucleocapsids in process of release stuck to the supporting film. ×200,000. (From Howe, C., et al. 1967. Morphogenesis of type 2 parainfluenza virus examined by light and electron microscopy. J. Virol. *1:*215–237.)

interior of the virus but also to the interior of the cells, and hence the process of viral assembly cannot be visualized. Although the myxoviruses lend themselves well to the technique because their nucleoproteins possess helical symmetry and maintain configuration upon disruption of the particle (Fig. 9), the nucleoproteins of other viruses cannot be so well seen. To view the interior of the cell Horne and Nagington[24] attempted to use pellets of infected cells. After freezing and thawing, the disrupted cells were suspended in ammonium acetate and potassium phosphotungstate. The suspension was sprayed on specimen grids and dried. Fragments of membranes and cell organelles were found in association with the virus, but preservation was so poor that their interpretation of the micrographs as showing virus "in various stages of assembly" is open to considerable doubt. Another procedure involved negative staining of cryostat sections.[1] Although preservation of fine structure was somewhat better, dislocation of cellular components made interpretation of viral development difficult. More recently Prose et al.[49] succeeded in staining the nucleocapsids of parainfluenza virus within the cytoplasm of frozen and thawed cells, but here again cellular architecture was disrupted. Unpublished attempts by the author to remove the embedding plastic from thin sections before negative staining also resulted in severe dislocation of fine structure, although viral capsids were preserved. It is to be hoped that the technique for thin-sectioning unembedded, hydrated, frozen tissue developed by Bernhard and his colleagues[4] will provide

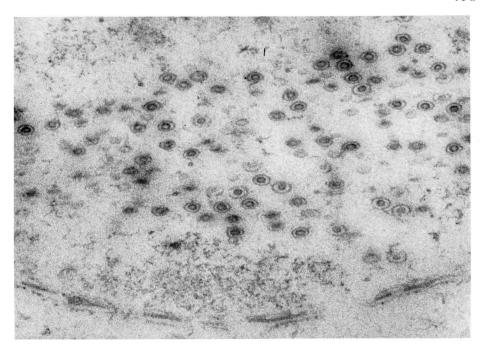

*Figure 10.* A micrograph obtained in 1953. There has been severe extraction of the cell and compression of the virus. This and the following two pictures illustrate intranuclear herpes simplex virus. ×65,000. (From Morgan, C., et al. 1954. Structure and development of viruses as observed in the electron microscope. I. Herpes simplex virus. J. Exp. Med. *100*:195–202.)

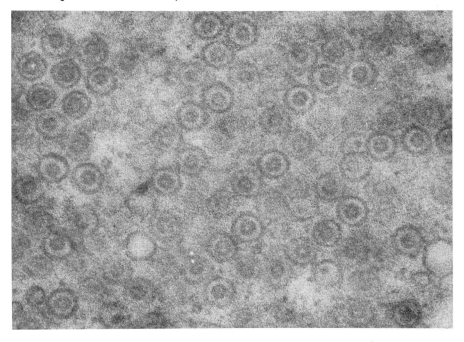

*Figure 11.* Micrograph made in 1959. The virus is better preserved and there is virtually no compression, but the contrast in this thin section is low. ×85,000.

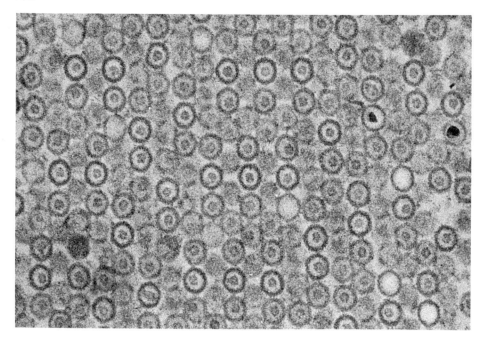

*Figure 12.* Part of a large crystal of herpes simplex virus fixed in glutaraldehyde-osmium and embedded in epon. The section was stained with uranyl acetate and lead citrate. Micrograph taken recently by Dr. Shiro Nii as a postgraduate Fellow from Osaka University, Japan. ×85,000.

the opportunity to apply negative staining more successfully than has hitherto been possible to virus in situ.

As for thin sectioning, the recent adoption of glutaraldehyde followed by osmium tetroxide for fixation and the use of new plastics, such as epoxy resin,[14, 32] araldite,[18] and vestopal,[33, 51] for embedding has resulted in considerably improved preservation of fine structure. Comparison of the results of current methods with those of former years leaves little doubt as to the degree of improvement (Figs. 4, 6, and 10 to 15). There is reason to suspect that, in contrast to the repeated modification of procedures, which characterized the first decade of thin sectioning, a more stable phase in methodology has now been reached. Whether this reflects closer proximity to perfection or simply the advancing age of the trail blazers is, of course, another question.

Turning next to the lesions of host cells, it is important to establish one point at the outset. A virus—any cytopathogenic virus—blocks and (or) preempts the normal metabolic pathways of the cell with the end result that the cellular architecture collapses. Initially the cell is capable of synthesizing viral components and of assembling viral particles, which it can eject by a clever reversal of the phagocytic mechanism, but sooner or later, depending upon the virulence of the virus, there is disruption of the complex membranes which confine the diverse enzymes in appropriate compartments. With autolysis the cell dies and the residual virus, wrapped in its protective coat, is released. There is, however, nothing specific in all this, for cells differ little in how they look as they die. The word that best sums up the appearance of death is "disorganization." Thus it is important to recognize that many of the structural changes we associate with viral invasion of cells are nonspecific.*

As noted at the outset of this chapter, however, there are exceptions. In the case of herpesviruses the cell is provoked to synthesize an extraordinary number of membranes. Presumably these are made initially to enclose the capsid in a protective coat but the process seems to get quite out of hand and membranes are made in great excess (Fig. 16). Another remarkable response by herpes-infected cells is alteration of their surface so that segments not only contain viral antigen but resemble very closely in structure the surface of the virus (Fig. 17). The reason for this is not clear because, unlike influenza and parainfluenza viruses, which bud from the surface of cells and hence need viral antigen at this site to incorporate into their coat (Fig. 18), herpesvirus differentiates deep within the cell. One can only surmise that the syncytia produced by fusion of cells, which seems to result from the contact of the altered portions of the surface with the surface of normal cells, is important to certain strains of herpesvirus since it permits virus to pass from cell to cell even in the presence of neutralizing antibodies.

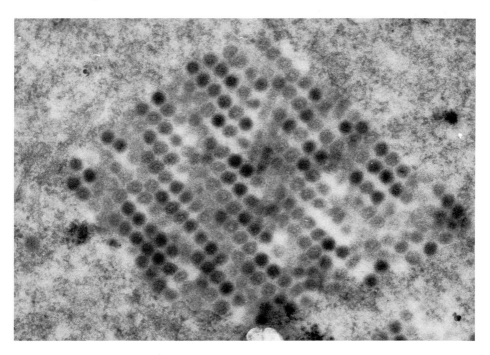

*Figure 13.* An intranuclear crystal composed of adenoviral particles. There are defects in the crystalline lattice. The virus is not sharply defined and there is little suggestion of its crystalline shape. The internal structure is obscure. Micrograph taken in 1955. ×55,000. (From Morgan, C., et al. 1956. Structure and development of viruses observed in the electron microscope. IV. Viruses of the RI-APC group. J. Biophys. Biochem. Cytol. *2*:351–360.)

---

* What then about oncogenic viruses, which instruct cells to multiply in a disordered fashion without regard for the controls and checks exerted by the host upon normal cells? Here again there is little to discuss, for most malignant cells are indistinguishable from normal cells at the fine structural level. A recent report, however, does describe bundles of fibrils in the cytoplasm of hamster tumor cells, which had been induced by adenovirus 12.[28] These fibrils could be tagged with ferritin-conjugated antibodies specific for the T (tumor) antigen.

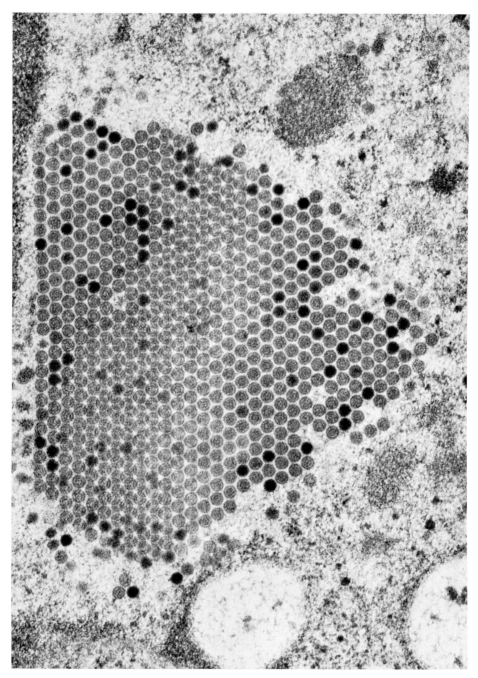

*Figure 14.* A recent micrograph of adenovirus. In the left-hand portion of the crystal can be seen overlapping particles where the section passes between rows of virus. The specimen was prepared in the same manner as was described for Figure 12. The preservation speaks for itself. ×55,000.

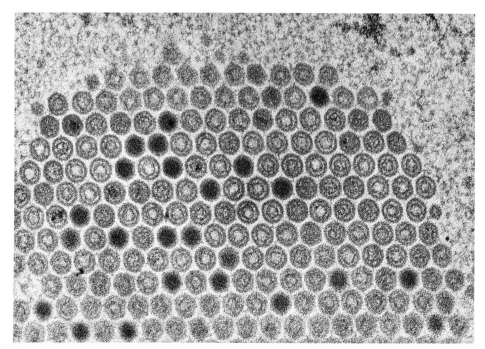

*Figure 15.* Part of another crystal of adenovirus at higher magnification. Particles eccentric to the plane of section are poorly defined. It is believed that only the virus with dense cores is infectious. ×92,000.

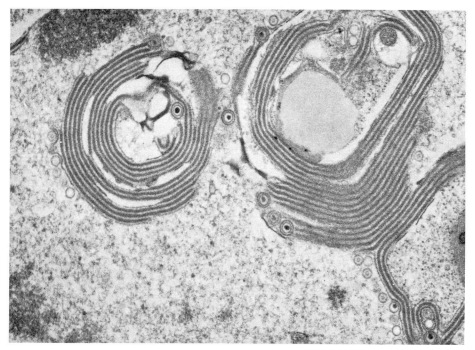

*Figure 16.* Excessive membrane synthesis in the nucleus of a cell infected with herpes simplex virus. Both enveloped and naked capsids are visible. ×35,000.

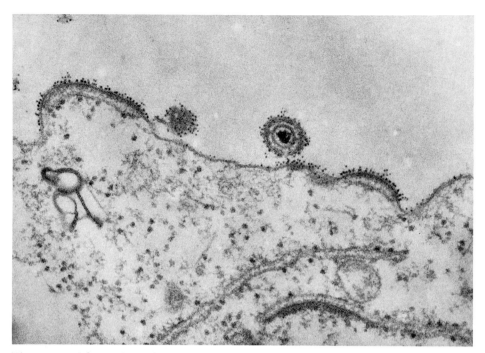

*Figure 17.* The surface of a cell infected with herpes simplex virus. At several sites the cellular membrane has been altered so as to contain viral antigen, which is identified by the presence of ferritin-conjugated antibodies specific for the virus. ×82,000.

A somewhat analogous situation to that described for herpesvirus is found in the case of cells infected with adenoviruses, wherein membrane synthesis likewise occasionally runs wild (Fig. 19). In addition, with type 5 adenovirus[38] and canine hepatitis virus[17] at least, intranuclear protein crystals are formed (Fig. 20). These apparently are not composed of viral protein, for they do not stain with fluorescein-labeled specific antibody,[7] and presumably represent a crystallized byproduct of viral development. It is not unusual for viral components also to accumulate in the course of viral synthesis. Initially the differentiation of a virus is an ordered, integrated, and to some extent, at least, economical process, but as infection proceeds this process seems to become more and more out of phase. Numerous viral particles are found to be devoid of dense internal components, which are presumed to be the nucleoprotein (Figs. 12, 14, and 15). The nucleoprotein may accumulate within the nucleus, as in the case of influenza virus (Figs. 21 and 22), or within the cytoplasm, as in the case of parainfluenza virus (Fig. 23).

One particularly interesting example of cytopathic change has been encountered in studies of the picornaviruses. Approximately four hours after infection (depending upon the type of virus) the nucleus shrinks and there is margination of chromatin. The space separating the double membrane of the nucleus becomes distended and numerous smooth-walled vacuoles appear in the perinuclear areas. As infection proceeds, the shrunken nucleus, as well as vesicles, ribosomes, and vacuolated or distorted mitochondria, assumes a central position and becomes surrounded by a broad zone of finely granular cytoplasmic matrix (Fig. 24). Gabriel C. Godman, in his excellent and thorough review,[19] makes a convincing argument that all the manifestations of the cytopathic effect are brought about by viral proteins, of which the coat protein is probably the most influential. However this may be, these alterations of the host cell provide one of the few examples of an extensive, specific, cytopathic effect produced by a single large group of viruses, which, although similar in size and general mode of replication, differ markedly in antigenic composition and in the clinical syndromes they evoke.

The last example of a cytopathic effect to be mentioned here is the appearance of filaments or microtubules within the nuclei of cells infected with measles virus (Fig. 25). Originally reported by Kallman, Adams, and Williams,[27] and subsequently described by Baker et al.[3] and Tawara et al.,[53] their nature remains unknown. Although probably not viral particles they are stigmata of infection by measles virus. At present considerable interest has been aroused by several reports of similar structures in the nuclei of cells of the central nervous system from patients afflicted with subacute sclerosing leukoencephalitis,[6, 12, 15, 21, 22, 46, 52, 54] a disease characterized by a progressive, fatal panencephalitis predominantly affecting school-age children. The electron microscopic observations (together with immunologic studies) have been advanced as evidence that a measles-like virus is the etiologic agent. This would

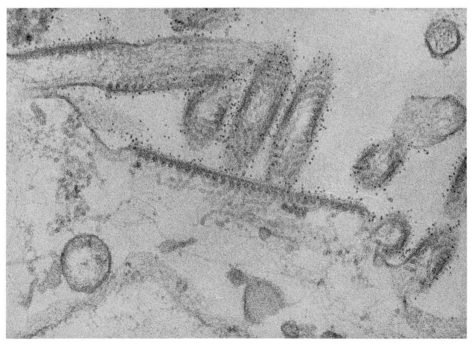

*Figure 18.* An altered segment of the wall of a cell infected with parainfluenza virus. Filaments are in process of extrusion. Ferritin-conjugated antibody specific for the virus was applied. ×100,000. (From Howe, C., et al. 1967. Morphogenesis of type 2 parainfluenza virus examined by light and electron microscopy. J. Virol. *1*:215–237.)

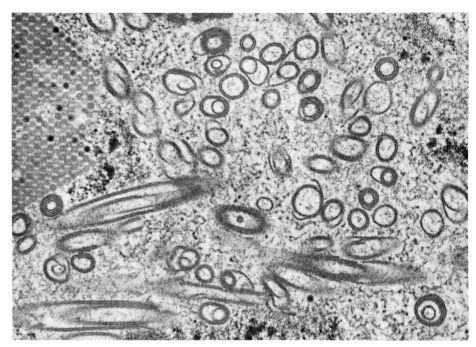

*Figure 19.* Numerous intranuclear tubules composed of concentric lamellae and sectioned at various angles. Part of an adenoviral crystal is visible at the upper left. ×38,000.

seem to be a valid inference because such structures have not been encountered to date either in normal cells or in cells infected with any other virus. It is of interest that cells infected with reovirus contain filaments and tubules in close proximity to the viral particles. These appear, however, in the cytoplasm rather than the nucleus.[2, 11, 26, 55, 56]

With the accelerating use of autoradiography, histochemical staining, enzyme digestion, and labeled antibodies we may confidently expect that further insight will be gained in the quest to correlate anatomy with biochemistry and physiology or, said more simply, structure with function. There remains, however, an unexplored area of critical importance. Up to the present time virtually all our attention has been directed toward experiments using virus-infected tissue culture cells. And this has been quite correct because initially some understanding had to be gained as to how the isolated host cell responded to viral infection. But the time is arriving when attention must be paid to the response of the intact host to the course of viral infection *in vivo*. This is going to be an enormously difficult and complex undertaking. Consider for a moment the technical problems confronting the electron microscopist. It is virtually impossible to cut a section even a square millimeter in area, the average being only about one fourth this size. The sections approximate 100 to 200 Å in thickness and thus 400 to 500 would be necessary to examine all parts of a single cell. In addition, the 200-mesh copper screens generally used to support the specimen obscure 35 per cent of the total area and seriously impair continuity of scanning. In light of the foregoing it must be remembered that

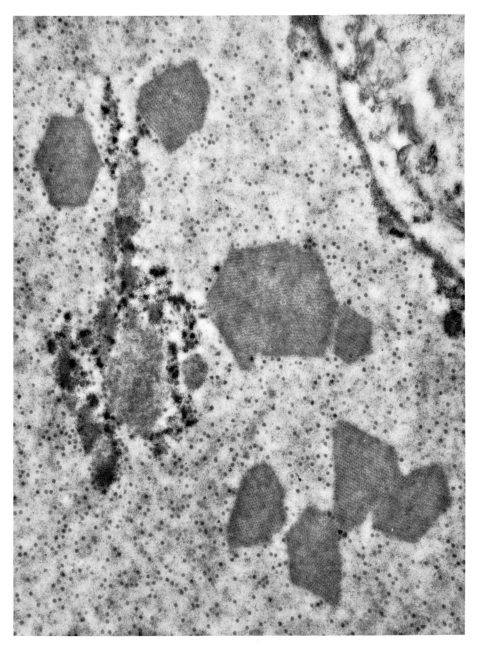

*Figure 20.* Nonviral protein crystals in the nucleus of a cell infected with type 5 adenovirus. ×27,000.

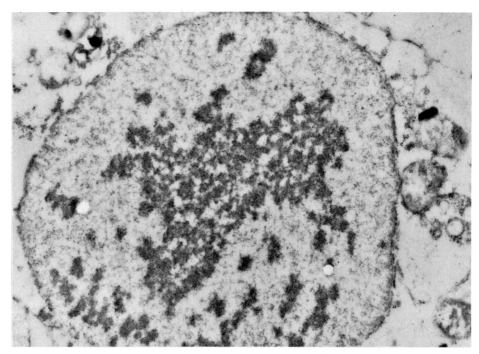

*Figure 21.*    The nucleus of cell infected with influenza. Dense granular material has accumulated. ×28,000. (From Morgan, C., et al. 1961. The application of ferritin-conjugated antibody to electron microscopic studies of influenza virus in infected cells. II. The interior of the cell. J. Exp. Med. *114*:833–836.)

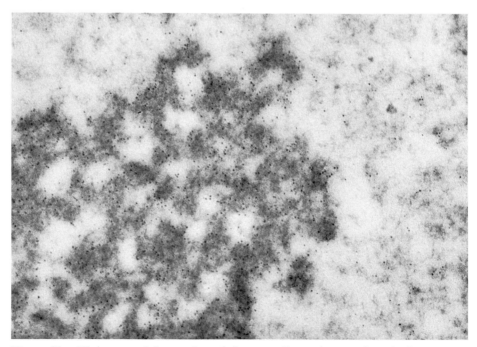

*Figure 22.*    The upper right portion of the preceding micrograph at higher magnification. The dense material is shown to be viral antigen by virtue of the tag with ferritin-conjugated antibody. ×85,000. (From Morgan, C., et al. 1961. The application of ferritin-conjugated antibody to electron microscopic studies of influenza virus in infected cells. II. The interior of the cell. J. Exp. Med. *114*:833–836.)

almost every cell of a tissue culture can be infected, whereas in the animal circumscribed foci of infection are buried in a welter of inflammatory cells and edema fluid, which constitute the host response. An inquiry into this kind of problem was made a few years ago in association with Dr. Harry M. Rose. Mice infected with influenza virus by the respiratory route were sacrificed at intervals, and portions of the trachea, bronchi, and lungs were examined. No virus was found despite gross and microscopic evidence of clearly defined, focal areas of pneumonia.

Renewed and greater efforts must be made to examine the virus in its natural haunts. The response of host cells constituting the interrelated components of functioning organs must be observed. The inflammatory reaction with particular attention to the role of phagocytic cells in disposing of (or possibly spreading) the virus must be studied. All this must finally be correlated with the multiple effects of antibodies on the virus and on the affected tissue if we are to improve our understanding of viruses in their role as etiologic agents of disease.

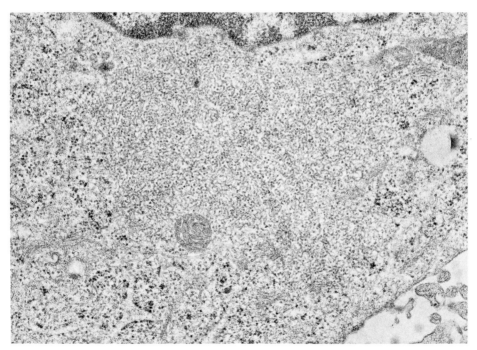

*Figure 23.* An aggregate of filamentous nucleoprotein within the cytoplasm of a cell infected with parainfluenza virus. ×40,000.

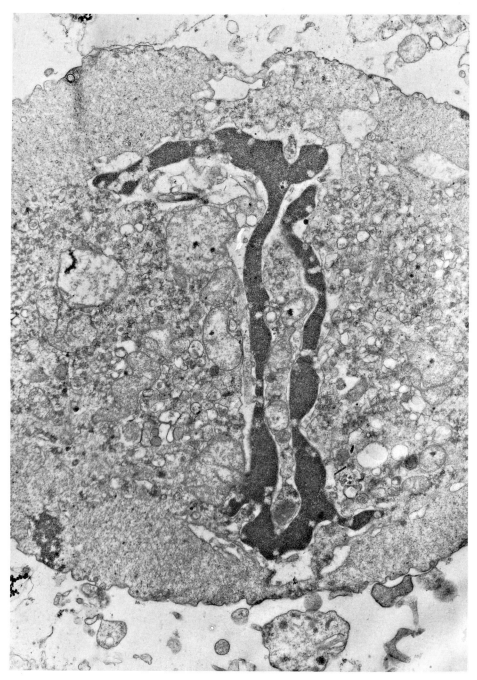

*Figure 24.* A tissue culture cell infected with a picornavirus. Although no viral particles can be identified in this field the cytopathologic appearance is characteristic. ×15,000.

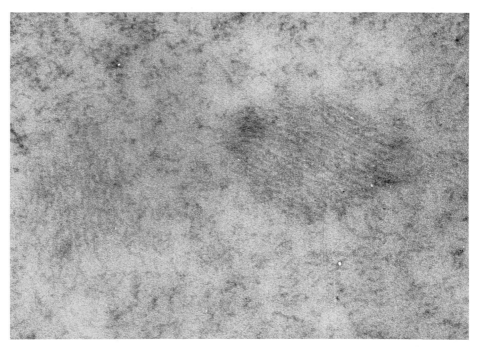

*Figure 25.* Filaments in the nucleus of a cell infected with measles virus. This micrograph is of historic interest, for shortly after Enders and Peebles succeeded in isolating and cultivating measles virus in tissue culture in 1954,[13] we fixed and embedded some infected cells in Dr. Enders' laboratory. This micrograph, taken in 1954, was never published because at that time we did not succeed in identifying the virus and could not be sure whether the filamentous structures were specific, and hence encountered solely within infected cells, or whether they reflected an unusual, but nonspecific type of reaction. ×110,000.

# References

1. Almedia, J. D., and A. F. Howatson. 1963. A negative staining method for cell-associated virus. J. Cell Biol. *16:*616–620.
2. Anderson, N., and F. W. Doane. 1966. An electron-microscope study of reovirus type 2 in L cells. J. Path. Bact. *92:*433–439.
3. Baker, R. F., I. Gordon, and F. Rapp. 1960. Electron-dense crystallites in nuclei of human amnion cells infected with measles virus. Nature *185:*790–791.
4. Bernhard, W., and E. H. Leduc. 1967. Ultrathin frozen sections. I. Methods and ultra-structural preservation. J. Cell Biol. *34:*757–771.
5. Black, L. M., C. Morgan, and R. W. G. Wyckoff. 1950. Visualization of tobacco mosaic virus within infected cells. Proc. Soc. Exp. Biol. Med. *73:*119–122.
6. Bouteille, M., C. Fontaine, C. Vedrenne, and J. Delarue. 1965. Sur un cas d'encéphalite subaiguë à inclusions. Etudie anatomo-clinique et ultrastructurale. Soc. Franç. Neurol. *113:*454–458.
7. Boyer, G. S., F. W. Denny, and H. S. Ginsberg. 1959. The sequential cellular changes produced by types 5 and 7 adenoviruses in HeLa cells and in human amniotic cells. Cytological studies aided by fluoroscein-labelled antibody. J. Exp. Med. *110:*827–844.
8. Claude, A. 1948. Studies on cells: morphology, chemical constitution and distribution of biochemical functions. Harvey Lect. *43:*121–164.
9. Claude, A., K. R. Porter, and E. G. Pickels. 1947. Electron microscope study of chicken tumor cells. Cancer Res. *7:*421–430.

10. Crick, F. H. C., and J. D. Watson. 1956. The structure of small viruses. Nature *177*:473–475.

11. Dales, S. P. J. Gomatos, and K. C. Hsu. 1965. The uptake and development of reovirus in strain L cells followed with labeled viral ribonucleic acid and ferritin-antibody conjugates. Virology *25*:193–211.

12. Dayan, A. D., J. V. T. Gostling, J. L. Greaves, D. W. Stevens, and M. A. Woodhouse. 1967. Evidence of a pseudomyxovirus in the brain in subacute sclerosing leucoencephalitis. Lancet *1*:980–981.

13. Enders, J. F., and T. C. Peebles. 1954. Propagation in tissue cultures of cytopathogenic agents from patients with measles. Proc. Soc. Exp. Biol. Med. *86*:277–286.

14. Finck, H. 1960. Epoxy resins in electron microscopy. J. Biophys. Biochem. Cytol. *7*:27–30.

15. Freeman, J. M., R. L. Magoffin, E. H. Lennette, and R. M. Herndon. 1967. Additional evidence of the relation between subacute inclusion-body encephalitis and measles virus. Lancet *1*:129–131.

16. Gaylord, W. H., and J. L. Melnick. 1953. Intracellular forms of pox viruses as shown by the electron microscope (vaccinia, ectromelia, molluscum contagiosum). J. Exp. Med. *98*:157–172.

17. Givan, K. F., C. Turnbull, and A. Jézéquel. 1967. Pepsin digestion of virus particles in canine hepatitis using epon-embedded material. J. Histochem. Cytochem. *15*:688–694.

18. Glauert, A. M., and R. H. Glauert. 1958. Araldite as an embedding medium for electron microscopy. J. Biophys. Biochem. Cytol. *4*:191–194.

19. Godman, G. C. 1966. The cytopathology of enteroviral infection. Int. Rev. Exp. Path. *5*: 67–110.

20. Harford, C. G., A. Hamlin, and E. Parker. 1955. Electron microscopy of HeLa cells infected with ARD virus. Trans. Assoc. Amer. Physicians *68*:82–86.

21. Harter, D. H., and I. Tellez-Nagel. 1968. Attempts to isolate SSPE agent in cell culture. Neurology *18*:(part 2)133–137.

22. Herndon, R. M., and L. J. Rubinstein. 1968. Light and electron microscopy observations on the development of viral particles in the inclusions of Dawson's encephalitis (subacute sclerosing panencephalitis). Neurology 18:(part 2)8–18.

23. Horne, R. W., S. Brenner, A. P. Waterson, and P. Wildy. 1959. The icosahedral form of an adenovirus. J. Molec. Biol. *1*:84–86.

24. Horne, R. W., and J. Nagington. 1959. Electron microscope studies of the development and structure of poliomyelitis virus. J. Molec. Biol. *1*:33–338.

25. Howe, C., C. Morgan, C. de Vaux St. Cyr, K. C. Hsu, and H. M. Rose. 1967. Morphogenesis of type 2 parainfluenza virus examined by light and electron microscopy. J. Virol. *1*:215–237.

26. Jenson, A. B., E. R. Rubin, C. A. Phillips, and J. L. Melnick. 1965. Reovirus encephalitis in newborn mice. An electron microscopic and virus assay study. Amer. J. Path. *47*:223–239.

27. Kallman, F., J. M. Adams, R. C. Williams, and D. T. Imagawa. 1959. Fine structure of cellular inclusions in measles virus infections. J. Biophys. Biochem. Cytol. *6*:379–382.

28. Kalnins, V. I., H. F. Stich, C. Gregory, and D. S. Yohn. 1967. Localization of tumor antigens in adenovirus-12-induced tumor cells and adenovirus-12-infected human and hamster cells by ferritin-labeled antibodies. Cancer Res. *27*:1874–1886.

29. Kausche, G. A., E. Pfankuch, and H. Ruska. 1939. Die Sichtbarmachung von pflänzlichem Virus im Übermikroskop. Naturwissenschaften *27*:292–299.

30. Kjellén, L., G. Lagermalm, A. Svedmyr, and K. G. Thorsson. 1955. Crystalline-like patterns in the nuclei of cells infected with animal virus. Nature *175*:505–506.

31. Latta, H., and J. F. Hartmann. 1950. Use of a glass edge in thin sectioning for electron microscopy. Proc. Soc. Exp. Biol. Med. *74*:436–439.

32. Luft, J. H. 1961. Improvements in epoxy resin embedding methods. J. Biophys. Biochem. Cytol. *9*:409–414.

33. Maaløe, O., and A. Birch-Andersen. 1956. On the organization of the "nuclear material" in Salmonella typhimurium. In Sixth Symposium, Society for General Microbiology. New York, Cambridge University Press, pp. 261–278.

34. Marton, L. 1934. Electron microscopy of biologic objects. Bull. Acad. Roy. Med. Belg. *20*: 439–446.

35. Morgan, C., S. A. Ellison, H. M. Rose, and D. H. Moore. 1954. Internal structure in virus particles. Nature *173*:208.

36. Morgan, C., S. A. Ellison, H. M. Rose, and D. H. Moore. 1954. Structure and development of viruses as observed in the electron microscope. I. Herpes simplex virus. J. Exp. Med. *100*:195–202.

37. Morgan, C., S. A. Ellison, H. M. Rose, and D. H. Moore. 1954. Structure and development of viruses observed in the electron microscope. II. Vaccinia and fowl pox viruses. J. Exp. Med. *100*:301–310.

38. Morgan, C., G. C. Godman, P. M. Breitenfield, and H. M. Rose. 1960. A correlative study by electron and light microscopy of the development of type 5 adenovirus. I. Electron microscopy. J. Exp. Med. *112*:373–382.

39. Morgan, C., C. Howe, H. M. Rose, and D. H. Moore. 1956. Structure and development of viruses observed in the electron microscope. IV. Viruses of the RI-APC group. J. Biophys. Biochem. Cytol. *2*:351–360.

40. Morgan, C., K. C. Hsu, R. A. Rifkind, A. W. Knox, and H. M. Rose. 1961. The application of ferritin-conjugated antibody to electron microscopic studies of influenza virus in infected cells. II. The interior of the cell. J. Exp. Med. *114*:833–836.

41. Morgan, C., and H. M. Rose. 1959. Electron-microscopic observations on adenoviruses and viruses of the influenza group. In Ninth Symposium, Society for General Microbiology. New York, Cambridge University Press, pp. 256–272.

42. Morgan, C., and R. W. G. Wycoff. 1950. The electron microscopy of fowl pox virus within the chorioallantoic membrane. J. Immun. *65*:285–295.

43. Müller, G., and K. Meyerhoff. 1964. Anomalous contrast in electron micrographs of negative stained specimens. Nature *201*:590–591.

44. Newman, S. B., E. Borysko, and M. Swerdlow. 1949. Ultra-microtomy by a new method. J. Res. Nat. Bur. Standards *43*:183–199.

45. Palade, G. E. 1952. A study of fixation for electron microscopy. J. Exp. Med. *95*:285–298.

46. Perier, O., J. J. Vanderhaeghen, and S. Pelc. 1967. Subacute sclerosing leuco-encephalitis. Electron microscopic finding in two cases with inclusion bodies. Acta Neuropath. *8:* 362–380.

47. Porter, K. R., and J. Blum. 1953. A study in microtomy for electron microscopy. Anat. Rec. *117*:685–710.

48. Porter, K. R., and H. P. Thompson. 1948. A particulate body associated with epithelial cells cultured from mammary carcinomas of mice of a milk-factor strain. J. Exp. Med. *88:* 15–24.

49. Prose, P. H., S. D. Balk, H. Leibhaber, and S. Krugman. 1965. Studies of a myxovirus recovered from patients with infectious hepatitis. II. Fine structure and electron microscopic demonstrations of intracytoplasmic internal component and viral filament formation. J. Exp. Med. *122*:1151–1160.

50. Rose, H. M., and C. Morgan. 1960. Fine structure of virus-infected cells. Ann. Rev. Microbiol. *14*:217–240.

51. Ryter, A., and E. Kellenberger. 1958. L'inclusion au polyester pour l'ultramicrotomie. J. Ultrastruct. Res. *2*:200–214.

52. Shaw, C. M., G. C. Buchan, and C. B. Carlson. 1967. Myxovirus as a possible etiologic agent in subacute inclusion-body encephalitis. New Eng. J. Med. *277*:511–515.

53. Tawara, J. 1965. Fine structure of filaments in dog kidney cell cultures infected with measles virus. Virology *25*:322–323.

54. Tellez-Nagel, I., and D. H. Harter. 1966. Subacute sclerosing leukoencephalitis: Ultrastructure of intranuclear and intracytoplasmic inclusions. Science *154*:899–901.

55. Thomas, J. A., and E. Delain. 1966. Développement, in vitro, du réovirus associé à la souche cancéreuse H 22 b; évolution des structures cytoplasmiques en fibres et en tubules. C. R. Acad. Sci. *262*:1028–1031.

56. Tournier, P., and M. Plissier. 1960. Le développement intracellulaire du réovirus observé du microscope électronique. Presse Méd. *68*:683–688.

57. Tousimis, A. J., and M. R. Hilleman. 1957. Electron microscopy of type 4 adenovirus strain RI-76. Virology *4*:499–508.

58. Valentine, R. C., and P. K. Hopper. 1957. Polyhedral shape of adenovirus particles as shown by electron microscopy. Nature *180*:928.

# Chapter 20

# THE BIOCHEMICAL BASIS OF ADENOVIRUS CYTOPATHOLOGY

HAROLD S. GINSBERG

*Department of Microbiology, School of Medicine,*
*University of Pennsylvania, Philadelphia, Pennsylvania*

Human miseries and economic wastes resulting from diseases of man, animals, and plants induced the birth and stimulated the development of virology. But today, although these prodding stimuli continue to receive attention, the major thrust of virology is felt in a newer and not yet so practical scientific field, molecular biology. At present relatively few virologists consider the host cell and its response to viral infections, aside from the development of malignancies—perhaps examination of the infected cell is too old-fashioned since morphologic pathology is now out of vogue. Nevertheless, at the risk of being considered "not with it," I must note that the biochemical studies in which we have been engaged for the past decade developed from the cytologic observation that adenoviruses produce striking lesions in the nuclei of infected cells.[2, 4–6] It seemed apparent that profound biochemical lesions must be the basis for the cellular damage that appeared and that an understanding of the molecular processes involved should provide an insight into the pathogenesis of the diseases produced. An extensive review of the subject will not be attempted, but rather this chapter will summarize our multidisciplinary approach to the problem using methods bearing the stamp of the "old" (e.g., light microscopy and complement-fixation assays) and the seal of approval of the "new" (e.g., RNA-DNA hybridizations and density-gradient centrifugations).

Adenoviruses were particularly suitable for these investigations since in cell cultures, and possibly in man, their invasion of cells under various circumstances results in: productive or abortive infection; cell death or cell survival; cell destruction or cell transformation. Investigation of productive infections with the consequent replication of infectious virus and development of characteristic cytopathology has been the foundation of our labors, since these virus-cell interactions seem to be the basis of acute diseases induced by adenoviruses. Moreover, under conditions which yield a productive infection, all cells in a culture could be uniformly infected and thus concurrent cytologic and biochemical studies were possible.

The experiments to be described employed methods developed in several disciplines: cytologic and cytochemical procedures utilized by pathologists; quantitative assays and biochemical techniques employed by students of bacteriophages; biochemical and physical chemical methods used by molecular biologists and chemists; immunologic techniques developed by immunologists; and cell cultures and biologic procedures employed by virologists. The concurrent utilization of this variety of techniques has resulted in a description of the characteristic intranuclear cell lesions induced by adenoviruses and the biochemical events which lead to their formation. It might be of interest to a few if we were to recount our studies in the sequence in which they were done. But it is realized by most that the order followed in experimentation is as often dictated by the methods and equipment and the knowledge available at the moment as by the precise demands of a logical development of ideas. It therefore seems more appropriate and certainly more readable now to summarize our studies according to the biologic and biochemical sequence of reactions in the infected cell.

First, however, to facilitate a consideration of the mechanism of the cell injury induced by adenoviruses, of which there are at least 44 immunologically distinct types which infect man and other animals, the structure of the virion and the process of infection will be briefly discussed.

# THE VIRION AND ITS MULTIPLICATION

## MORPHOLOGICAL AND CHEMICAL STRUCTURE

The virions are beautifully formed naked icosahedrons 650 to 800 A in diameter (Fig. 1), composed of a protein capsid consisting of 252 capsomers[33] and a nucleoprotein core containing the DNA viral genome[13] and one or more internal proteins.[39, 40, 41, 58, 62, 71, 71a] Although it was originally predicted that the capsid of an isometric virion would be assembled from numerous structural subunits of a single type of protein,[11] the capsids of adenoviruses consist of several different macromolecular structures: (1) The *hexons* are polygonal hollow structures 70 to 85 A in diameter; the central hole is approximately 40 A in diameter; they are distributed on the faces and edges of the triangular surfaces; and each hexon has six neighbors.[25, 78] (2) The *pentons* consist of a base 70 to 85 A in diameter and a fiber of variable length; they are the 12 vertex units of the icosahedron; each penton has five neighbors; and each therefore is the center of a fivefold axis of symmetry.[75] (3) The penton fiber[25, 75, 78] varies in length depending upon the adenovirus type; and it appears on morphologic[18, 25, 50, 52, 57, 75, 78] and immunologic grounds[50, 51, 55] to consist of at least two distinct proteins, the string-like structure and a terminal knob.

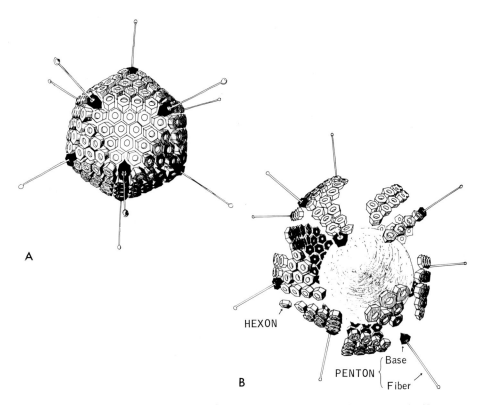

A

HEXON

Base

PENTON

Fiber

B

*Figure 1.* Morphology of a type 5 adenovirus particle diagrammatically represented: *A*, intact virion; *B*, partially disrupted virion demonstrating the structure and position of the known capsid units and the viral core. The *hexons* are the major capsid structures and each has six neighbors; the *pentons* are the corner units and each is composed of a *base* and a *fiber*; each penton has five neighbors; the core contains a molecule of DNA and two basic proteins. (From Ginsberg, H. S., L. J. Bello, and A. J. Levine. 1967. Control of biosynthesis of host macromolecules in cells infected with adenovirus. *In:* Colter, J. S., and W. Paranchych (eds.). The Molecular Biology of Viruses. Academic Press, Inc., New York, pp. 547–572.)

The hexons[25a, 56] and fibers[43, 57] of type 5 adenovirus have been purified adequately to permit physical and chemical analyses. The hexon has the following characteristics: (1) it is a multimeric protein consisting of 12 probably identical polypeptide chains with molecular weights of approximately 25,400 daltons;[25a] (2) its polypeptide chains are linked through noncovalent bonds;[25a] (3) it is an acidic protein with an isoelectric point of about 5.5;[25a] and (4) its amino acid analyses reveal a high content of hydrophobic amino acids.[25a, 56] Chemical characterization of the fiber suggests that it is composed of several identical polypeptides,[45] in contrast to the morphologic and immunologic evidence that it is made from two or more proteins.[50, 51, 55, 57, 75, 78]

The DNAs extracted from purified virions are characteristic double-stranded linear molecules of 20 to 25 × 10[6] daltons.[12, 28, 30, 59] In the 31 human adenoviruses studied, the DNAs range from 11.6 to 13.5 per cent of the weight of the viral particle, and their guanine + cytosine contents vary from 48 to

60 per cent of the total base composition.[28, 59] Other than DNA, protein appears to be the sole remaining constituent.

### PROCESS OF INFECTION

Continuous cell lines of human epithelial cells such as HeLa or KB cells furnished convenient susceptible hosts for the biologic, pathologic, and biochemical studies to be described.

Virions attach to uncharacterized receptors of susceptible cells over a period of 2 to 6 hours depending upon the relative concentration of the virions and the cells.[21, 27, 41, 58] The penton fiber of the vertex subunits is probably the virion's attachment organ since the fiber but not the hexon can combine with susceptible cells.[43, 58] After attachment, the virions are rapidly engulfed, and eclipse of infectivity associated with shedding of the capsid, i.e., "uncoating," follows almost immediately. The process of uncoating, which occurs in cytoplasmic vacuoles, is measured by conversion of the viral DNA from deoxyribonuclease (DNase)-resistant (i.e., intact virus) to DNase-sensitive.[41, 58] Displacement of the pentons with a loss of 5 to 6 per cent of the virion's protein appears to be the initial process to expose the viral genome.[74] After maximum DNase sensitivity is achieved in 60 to 90 minutes, and approximately 85 per cent of the viral DNA has become DNase-sensitive, the viral DNA is still associated with 25 to 50 per cent of the viral protein.[41, 58] Hence, the viral genome is uncovered so that it is susceptible to nuclease, but it is not clear whether it can be transcribed or replicated while still associated with what is probably the internal protein.[41, 58] It is possible that the DNA-protein complex, which remains after the capsid proteins are shed, may undergo a second step in uncoating, similar to poxviruses,[35, 36] and that this final event may transpire in the nucleus where viral DNA synthesis ensues.[21a]

Adenoviruses multiply relatively slowly (Fig. 2). The representative one-step growth curve of type 5 virus shown in the figure is similar in its general features for all adenoviruses studied: (1) the eclipse period ranges from 12 to 18 hours depending upon the virus examined, the host cell em-

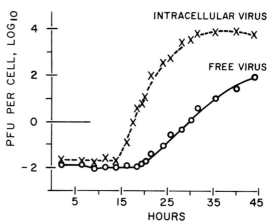

*Figure 2.* Initial cycle of multiplication of type 5 adenovirus. KB cells in spinner cultures were infected at an input multiplicity of $10^{1.7}$ PFU per cell and incubated at 37°C.

ployed, and the method of cell propagation (fundamental differences in the mechanism of multiplication of the different adenoviruses do not appear to exist); (2) the incremental period is comparatively short, i.e., about 12 hours, and maximal viral yield is attained 24 to 30 hours after infection; and (3) more than 90 per cent of the virions remain intracellular, even after cytopathic changes have become extensive.[5, 11a, 21] When monolayer cell cultures are infected, the eclipse period of the multiplication cycle is 2 to 3 hours longer and the maximum viral yield is 1 to 10 per cent of that observed in spinner cell cultures.[11a, 21, 27]

# CYTOPATHOLOGY

### GROSS OBSERVATIONS

Even a casual study of unfixed and unstained monolayer cultures infected with adenoviruses reveals a characteristic enlargement, rounding, and clumping of affected cells. Although many viruses cause cells to round up and fall from the glass surface, few viruses produce the formation of grape-like clusters effected by adenoviruses. The relative size of the cell clumps varies with the viral type: for example, types 3, 4, and 7 produce large clusters, whereas infection with type 1, 2, 5, or 6 results in formation of small clumps and many single rounded cells.[21a] It is particularly striking that the affected cells, although obviously injured and unable to divide, continue to metabolize and do not lyse, at least not until long after they have fallen from the glass.[15, 20] The continued intracellular abode of the virions provides particular evidence for the absence of cell lysis.[20, 21]

It seems likely that the gross cytopathic effects described are due to surface alterations of the infected cells, although experimental evidence on this point has not yet been obtained. Central to this hypothesis are the findings that the penton alone can produce similar cytopathic changes in the absence of viral multiplication,[14, 53, 76] and that those viruses whose synthesis results in the greatest excess accumulation of penton (e.g., types 1, 2, 5, and 6) effect the most widespread cytopathic changes, and evince the early appearance of many single rounded cells and small rather than large cell clusters.[21a]

### MICROSCOPIC AND CYTOCHEMICAL OBSERVATIONS

Nuclear lesions which are the hallmark of adenovirus infections invariably accompany the processes of productive infections. As in viral multiplication, however (cf. Fig. 2), there is an apparent "quiet" period, when the cell retains its normal appearance. Then, beginning 8 to 12 hours after infection, characteristic morphologic changes appear in the nuclei[2, 4-6] at a time when early events in viral synthesis also occur (to be discussed later). Cytopathologic studies have been carried out with a number of adenoviruses, but since types 2 and 5 have been studied biochemically in greatest detail emphasis will be placed on the cellular lesions these viruses induce.[4-6] After type 5 adenovirus infection, the first changes are evident in 8 to 10 hours when multiple small collections of eosinophilic granules appear within the nuclei (Fig. 3). Accumulations of eosinophilic granules soon form well defined, Feulgen-negative inclusion bodies, although the outer rims of a few of the inclusions are basophilic and Feulgen-positive, indicating the presence of DNA. Immunofluorescent staining reveals that the early lesions contain specific viral antigens,[4-6] implying that the inclusions correspond to the factories for synthesis of viral subunits—in this early stage the eosinophilic material probably consists of the early proteins whose syntheses precede and are required for the subsequent biosynthesis of viral DNA. By 14 hours after infection the eosinophilic inclusions begin to acquire basophilic, Feulgen-positive cores; this further identifies the inclusions with the site for accumulation of viral proteins and DNA. Concomitant with these latter changes, the nuclear chromatin becomes rearranged and the affected nuclei enlarge.

About 17 hours after infection small angular, eosinophilic, Feulgen-negative, crystal-like masses appear in the spaces among the rounded inclusions and perturbed chromatin. The sharply demarcated crystal-like structures become long and bar-shaped and more brightly stained with eosin than when they first appeared. These crystalline structures, which contain protein,[47] remain Feulgen-negative, and fail to stain in immunofluorescent studies, although bright, sharp-edged streaks of antigen are present, possibly representing the basophilic material found alongside the eosinophilic crystals.[4] Concurrent with the developments described, the rounded inclusions become more intensely basophilic and Feulgen-positive, and more brightly fluorescent.[4]

In the final stages of cell injury the cells become round and clump, the cell sheet disrupts, and many cells detach from the glass. Much of the intranuclear material merges into a dense, darkly stained mass which is intensely Feulgen-positive, and the eosinophilic crystals appear far less prominent or are absent. The basophilic masses contain material which stains brightly with fluorescent antibodies, and many cells show diffuse intranuclear fluorescence. Fluorescent staining is confined to the nuclei, whose membranes remain intact until the terminal stages when they often become beaded. In the final phases the cytoplasm shows severe degenerative changes, and diffuse cytoplasmic immunofluorescence appears, particularly in areas adjacent to the nucleus.[4, 5]

Electron microscopic observations, which are detailed by Morgan in Chapter 19, show that the viral particles assemble and accumulate, often in crystalline arrays, in the nuclei, and that the eosinophilic crystals are devoid of virions.[46, 47]

Fundamentally the changes are similar in nuclei of cells infected with all adenoviruses studied; i.e., there is enlargement of nuclei and development of large basophilic masses which contain viral proteins, DNA, and intact virions. However, the multiple, well defined eosinophilic intranuclear inclusions are most characteristic of types 1, 2, 5, and 6, whereas the large basophilic intranuclear crystals, which are composed of a crystalline lattice of virions, are observed consistently in cells infected with types 3, 4, and 7.[4] The sharp, eosinophilic, crystalline, virion-free structures just described are most prominently noted in type 5-infected cells, although an occasional cell infected with type 6 adenovirus may contain similar formations.[4]

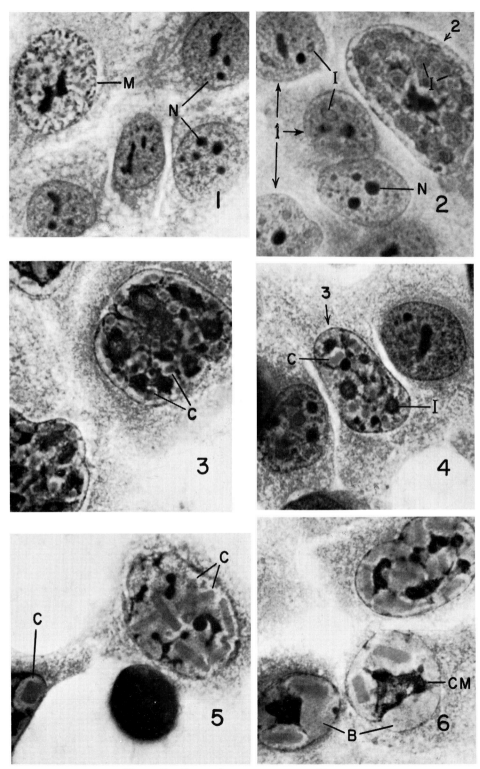

*Figure 3.*    Legend appears on opposite page.

# BIOCHEMICAL EVENTS IN THE SYNTHESIS OF THE VIRION

Observation that the profound cell alterations described here were accompanied by and associated with viral propagation suggested that a detailed investigation of the biochemistry of infected cells would (1) provide data at the molecular level on the biosynthetic pathways leading to the production of infectious viral particles, and (2) reveal the mechanism of cell damage. The discussion in this section and the following one will summarize the data which prove these predictions.

## VIRUS-SPECIFIC RNA

Today every junior high school biology student knows that a specific messenger RNA (mRNA) must be transcribed from a DNA genome to provide the biochemical information essential for the synthesis of a special protein. However, when these investigations were initiated mRNA had not yet been identified and the essential role of RNA was not self-evident.

By the use of the specific inhibitors of RNA synthesis, 6-azauridine and 5-fluorouridine, it was discovered that biosynthesis of RNA was obligatory for production of viral proteins and for the propagation of a DNA-containing virus.[17] These pyrimidine analogues, when added at varying intervals after infection, also furnished a sensitive technique to measure the period of biosynthesis of the *last* RNA species essential for viral propagation. RNA thus identified is associated with the synthesis of viral capsid proteins and is made during the last half of the eclipse period; final synthesis of this species of

---

*Figure 3.* Photomicrographs of HeLa cells infected with type 5 adenovirus. Cells cultured on coverslips were fixed in 95 per cent ethyl alcohol and stained with hemotoxylin and eosin. ×1050.

*1,* Uninfected cells, including mitotic figure (*M*) in early prophase. Nuclei contain multiple nucleoli (*N*).

*2,* 16 hours after infection. Nuclei showing early changes (labeled *1*) contain numerous round eosinophilic intranuclear inclusions (*I*). Nucleus, having undergone greater alterations (labeled *2*), is enlarged, its chromatin is rearranged, and the inclusions (*I*) now have basophilic cores.

*3,* 22 hours after infection. The enlarged nucleus contains early, small, eosinophilic, crystal-like structures (*C*).

*4,* 20 hours after infection. Nucleus labeled *3* contains early, eosinophilic, crystal-like structures (*C*) and darkly stained inclusions (*I*) in which core, rim, and surrounding "chromatin" are no longer distinct.

*5,* 30 hours after infection. Nucleus contains prominent, long, bar-shaped eosinophilic crystal-like structures (*C*). The basophilic inclusions are shrunken and lacking in detail.

*6,* Cells in the latest stages of infection contain elongated eosinophilic crystals, and the basophilic inclusions have merged into central masses (*CM*). The two nuclei in the lower portion of the figure contain homogeneously stained background material (*B*) which gives a positive Feulgen reaction. (From Boyer, G. S., F. W. Denny, Jr., and H. S. Ginsberg. 1959. Sequential cellular changes produced by types 5 and 7 adenoviruses in HeLa cells and in human amniotic cells. Cytological studies aided by fluorescein-labelled antibody. J. Exptl. Med: *110*:827–844.)

RNA is completed shortly after the assembly of infectious viral particles begins.[17]

The period during which virus-specific RNA is synthesized was determined by direct biochemical procedures. The RNA newly made during any period of infection may be marked by incorporation of a radioisotope, e.g.,[32]P orthophosphate, during short labeling periods. The pulse-labeled RNA was found to have the following characteristics: (1) its base composition approaches that of viral DNA during the latter portion of the eclipse period;[38] (2) it hybridizes to denatured viral DNA;[3a, 22, 29a, 67] (3) its synthesis, as measured by the hybridization techniques, can first be detected just before replication of viral DNA and about 6 to 7 hours before the assembly of virions;[29a] and (4) it has a rapid rate of synthesis which continues for 8 to 9 hours before it begins to decline.[3a]

The species of RNA detected with pyrimidine analogues[17] and the majority of the pulse-labeled RNA identified by hybridization with denatured viral DNA[3a, 22, 29a, 67] is associated with the synthesis of viral capsid proteins, i.e., "late" proteins, and may be considered late mRNA. Green and his associates have also identified "early" mRNA, and demonstrated, with the use of competition experiments, that "early" mRNA is made throughout the period of viral propagation, whereas "late" mRNA is predominantly transcribed when viral capsid proteins are synthesized.[29a]

A low molecular weight, 5S RNA, is also synthesized in cells infected with type 2 adenovirus,[65] but its role in infection is obscure. Indeed, although DNA synthesis is required for production of the 5S RNA, there is no evidence which bears upon the question whether it is transcribed from the host or the viral genome—it does not hybridize with either DNA species.[65]

## "Early" Proteins

Several proteins are made after synthesis of "early" messenger RNA is initiated and prior to replication of the viral genome. At least some of these "early" proteins are required for the synthesis of viral DNA and hence for the production of complete virions. It was anticipated that adenoviruses and other DNA-containing animal viruses would require synthesis of virus-specific enzymes since a number of virus-encoded enzymes appear early in the eclipse period of T-even bacteriophage multiplication.[7]

The need for and the biosynthesis of "early" proteins were established by several procedures.

1. Replication of the viral genome is blocked and formation of infectious virus is prevented when p-fluorophenylalanine, an analogue of phenylalanine, is added to infected cells before the synthesis of viral DNA.[77] These data strengthened the concept that the early production of functional proteins is essential for subsequent synthesis of viral subunits.

2. Infection of monolayers of HeLa or monkey kidney cells results in increased activity of aspartic transcarbamylase,[9, 42] thymidine kinase,[37, 42] deoxycytidylate deaminase,[42] and DNA polymerase[37, 42] during the viral eclipse period. Protein synthesis is required for the increase in enzyme activities to

be manifest. The heightened enzyme activities, however, cannot be detected in spinner cultures of infected cells[29, 44]—perhaps because the enzymes are being made at close to their maximal rates in cells dividing exponentially prior to infection. It is generally considered that the enzymes which increase are products of the viral genome, and different from the host enzymes. But the aspartic transcarbamylase (ATCase) is not a virus-coded enzyme even though the purified enzyme from infected cells has a pH optimum, maximal velocity (Vmax), and Michaelis-Menten constant (Km) for aspartate distinctly different from the ATCase from uninfected cells: these altered characteristics follow allosteric changes in the enzyme released from feedback inhibition owing to depletion of the intracellular pyrimidine pool.[8, 9] The other enzymes measured have not been characterized biochemically or immunologically, and therefore it is not known whether the information to synthesize these enymes in infected cells is encoded in the viral or the host genome.

3. Infection of monolayer or suspension cells cultures results in the appearance of immunologically unique "early" proteins which have been termed T antigen[19, 32, 61] and P antigen.[71] These designations, however, imply that each is a single antigen, and therefore the names may be misleading since they have been defined only in terms of their reactions with antisera which could contain antibodies to more than one protein. Sera from hamsters bearing tumors induced by type 12, 18, or 31 adenovirus detect the so-called T antigen as follows: (1) complement fixation permits identification of a protein in tumors induced by or in cells infected by the same viruses;[19, 32, 34, 61, 70] and (2) with immunofluorescence, utilizing the same antisera, not only is the protein measured by complement-fixation assay detected but also a protein appearing as flecks and spots in cells infected with any other adenovirus.[34, 61, 66] To identify the P antigen, antiserum was obtained from a rabbit immunized with an extract of cells infected with type 5 adenovirus in the presence of an arabinosylcytosine to stop DNA biosynthesis and reduce synthesis of capsid antigens.[71] With the use of P antiserum, the following results were obtained: (1) with complement fixation a protein was detected that emerged from disrupted type 5 adenovirus;[71] (2) immunofluorescence permitted visualization of fine flecks and spots early in the eclipse period whereas balls and rings appeared later in the infectious process;[31] and (3) with immunofluorescence of cells infected in the absence of arginine only the early flecks and spots were detected.[69] These data suggest that the T antigen and the P antigen each consist of at least two distinct proteins and that the following early proteins can be identified immunologically: (1) a specific T antigen similar to that present in tumors produced by types 12, 18, and 31 adenoviruses; (2) an adenovirus group antigen identified either with sera from tumor-bearing hamsters or with P antiserum; and (3) a protein that is detected with P antiserum and requires arginine for its synthesis. The time when the latter protein is synthesized has not been determined; it appears to be an arginine-rich macromolecule[71a] which serves as an internal virion protein[71] and which may be identical with the "maturation factor" described by Rouse and Schlesinger.[68, 71b] Functions have not yet been ascribed to the other two immunologically detectable proteins.

## Viral DNA

When a critical level of early proteins is attained, 6 to 10 hours after infection, replication of the viral DNA begins in the nucleus.[16, 21a, 24, 26, 27] In the absence of protein synthesis, production of viral DNA does not commence, and if protein synthesis is stopped, biosynthesis of DNA rapidly halts.[22, 77] Although synthesis of host DNA stops at approximately the same time replication of the viral genome begins, the host cell's DNA remains intact, and the *de novo* synthesis of viral DNA draws its nucleotides from pools of the cell and the medium.[24, 44]

Direct biochemical measurements[24, 27] and utilization of the fluorodinated pyrimidine 5-fluoro-2-deoxyuridine (FUdR) to stop DNA synthesis permit a description of the period and rate of synthesis of viral DNA.[16, 26] Once synthesis of the viral DNA is initiated it proceeds at the previous maximum rate established for cellular DNA in dividing cells.[22, 27] Replication of the viral genome continues for 8 to 12 hours and when synthesis stops the total content of DNA in the infected cells is approximately doubled.[23, 24, 27] Hence, a large number of viral DNA equivalents is made, but strangely only about 10 per cent is packaged into virions.[23] The unused DNA accumulates in the characteristic central basophilic bodies of adenovirus-infected cells.[6]

## Capsid "Late" Proteins

Just as planting must be a prelude to the harvest, replication of the infecting viral genome must precede the synthesis of adenovirus capsid proteins. It is striking that mRNA for the capsid proteins cannot be transcribed from parental DNA;[3a] hexons, pentons, and fibers can be detected only after synthesis of viral DNA begins and an adequate pool of progeny DNA molecules accumulates.[3a, 16] Thus, biosynthesis of the capsid proteins is initiated about 2 hours after replication of viral DNA commences and approximately 2 hours before assembly of new virions can be detected.[16, 60, 77]

Like viral DNA, the capsid proteins accumulate in nuclei of infected cells.[4, 54, 72] But in contrast to DNA, the cytoplasm is considered to be the customary site for protein synthesis. Since there is still uncertainty whether the nucleus can serve as a site for protein synthesis, a study of the synthesis of the easily identifiable adenovirus proteins appeared to offer a unique opportunity to investigate this problem. Contrary to expectation, however, the following evidence indicates that adenovirus capsid proteins are synthesized on cytoplasmic polyribosomes: (1) autoradiographic studies demonstrated that 20 to 24 hours after infection, when over 85 per cent of the proteins being synthesized are viral,[3] proteins are made in the cytoplasm within 1 minute, and then rapidly transported to the nuclei;[75a] and (2) direct measurements showed that polypeptide chains of about 3S are made on 200S polyribosomes,[75a] that they rapidly become immunologically reactive with specific viral antibodies,[75a] and that they aggregate into macromolecules of the size of hexons, pentons, and fibers.[75b]

A lag of 2 to 3 hours intervenes between the initial synthesis of capsid proteins and the final assembly of mature virions.[77] This delay in assembling the completed viral DNA and capsid proteins may result from the late synthesis of a limiting protein such as the penton base,[31] which is required for completion of the capsid, or of the arginine-rich "maturation protein," which may serve as an internal protein and thus be essential for folding of the viral DNA.[39, 40, 62, 68, 69, 71, 71a] It is particularly pertinent to the subject of this essay that the utilization of the capsid proteins produced, like the newly made viral DNA, is wholly inefficient since only 10 to 15 per cent is assembled into virions; the wasteful excess accumulates as a constituent of the intranuclear inclusion bodies.[6, 76, 78] The ineffectual utilization of the structurally normal viral proteins and DNA may result because: (1) an essential protein constituent of the virion, such as the "maturation protein" or penton base, is made in limiting amounts; or (2) the viral DNA may be incorrectly complexed with hexon and fiber proteins[1, 44] so that only a small proportion of these reactants are available for efficient utilization when the last essential protein becomes available.

## CONSEQUENCES OF INFECTION ON BIOSYNTHESIS OF HOST MACROMOLECULES

The viral genome, upon entrance into the cell nucleus, assumes its instructive role to provide information and to direct the production of proteins which serve as catalysts for the biosynthesis of DNA replicates. The progeny viral genomes in turn lead to the fabrication of proteins, which protect and assist in the assembly of the newly made viral DNA. These biosynthetic events subsequently result in the development of inclusion bodies[2, 4-6] and profound alterations of the cell's capacities to make its own macromolecules.[3, 3a, 22] Examination of the total accumulation of RNA, DNA, and protein

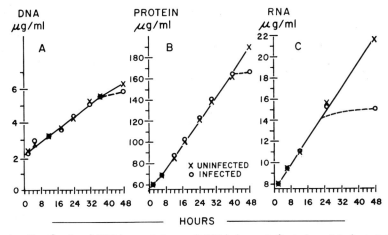

*Figure 4.* Synthesis of DNA, protein, and RNA in uninfected and infected KB cells in spinner cultures. Cells were infected with type 5 adenovirus at an input multiplicity of 50 PFU per cell.

TABLE 1.   *Synthesis of Cellular and Viral DNA in KB Cells Infected with Type 5*
*Adenovirus*

| TIME AFTER INFECTION * HOURS | PER CENT INHIBITION KB CELL DNA† | SYNTHESIS OF VIRAL DNA‡ |
|:---:|:---:|:---:|
| 6 | 6 | 0 |
| 8 | 66 | + |
| 10 | 91 § | +++ |
| 12 | 96 § | ++++ |

    * 200 PFU per cell.
    † Measured after a 2 hour period of incorporation of ³H-thymidine. KB cell DNA was separated from viral DNA by chromatography on methylated albumin-kieselguhr column.
    ‡ Only semiquantitative estimations could be made owing to presence of excess unlabeled viral DNA as marker. + = approximately 20 per cent of maximum.
    § Minimal values of inhibition; no peak of radioactivity corresponding to KB cell DNA was detectable.

in spinner cultures of cells, which are dividing exponentially before infection with type 5 adenovirus, reveals that infection must hinder the biosynthesis of host macromolecules: syntheses of DNA and protein continue at unchanged linear rates for about 40 hours after infection (Fig. 4) despite the production and accumulation of viral DNA and protein during this period;[22, 27] synthesis of total RNA is also linear and unaltered for 20 to 24 hours (Fig. 4) after which its production rapidly decreases;[3a, 22] and although division of infected cells stops 10 to 12 hours after infection, the cell mass increases and the total DNA and protein per cell approximately doubles in 48 hours.[22, 27]

A remarkable degree of selectivity regulates the replication of host and viral DNAs since the switch-off of host DNA synthesis begins just before or when biosynthesis of viral DNA commences.[22] It is possible to measure simultaneously the biosyntheses of host and viral DNAs: the two species can be separated by chromatography on methylated albumin-kieselguhr (MAK) columns or equilibrium centrifugation in cesium chloride density gradients.[22, 26] Application of these techniques reveals that replication of host DNA begins to diminish 6 to 10 hours after infection with type 5 adenovirus, depending upon the multiplicity of infection (Table 1), and its synthesis is almost completely blocked 2 to 4 hours later.[22] But the synthesis of neither host nor viral DNA is essential for the inhibition of host DNA replication. Thus, at the onset of infection, if 5-fluoro-2-deoxyuridine (FUdR) is added to stop DNA synthesis in uninfected and infected cells, and 10 hours later the block is reversed with excess thymidine, viral but not host DNA is made immediately in the infected cells; host DNA synthesis resumes without delay in uninfected cells.[21a]

Production of host proteins is undisturbed until about 15 hours after infection.[3] The process which then inhibits synthesis of host proteins but permits viral proteins to be produced without restraint expresses another remarkable degree of selective control. Host protein synthesis (measured by immunologic precipitation of ¹⁴C-labeled proteins and the assay of six host enzymes*) begins to decrease about 15 hours after infection and is retarded

    * The increase of six normal cell enzymes (phosphoglucose isomerase, fumarase, deoxyribonuclease, lactic dehydrogenase, acid phosphatase, and alkaline phosphatase) is proportionate to the linear increase in proteins.

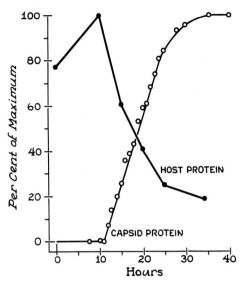

*Figure 5.* Synthesis of host and viral capsid proteins in spinner cultures of KB cells infected with 200 PFU per cell of type 5 adenovirus. Valine-[14]C was added to cultures for 2 hour periods after infection. Viral capsid proteins were precipitated with specific anti-serum, and the number of acid-precipitable counts remaining in the super-natant fluid was considered to be labeled host protein (data on protein synthesis from Bello and Ginsberg[3a]). Capsid proteins were also measured by complement-fixation assays.

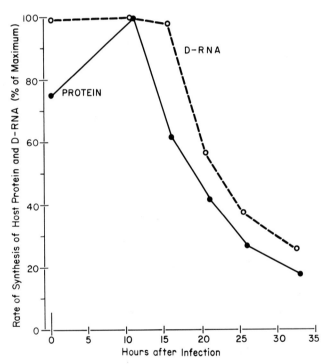

*Figure 6.* Comparison of rates of syntheses of host protein and D-RNA. A suspension culture of KB cells was infected with type 5 adenovirus at an input multiplicity of 200 PFU per cell. At various times after infection two samples were taken: one was for determination of protein synthesis as described in Figure 5; to the second culture [3]H-uridine was added for 1 hour and the amount incorporated into D-RNA was determined by hybridization with denatured KB cell DNA. The values are plotted at the midpoint of each pulse period. (From Bello, L. J., and H. S. Ginsberg. 1969. Relationship between deoxyribonucleic acid-like ribonucleic acid synthesis and inhibition of host protein synthesis in type 5 adenovirus-infected KB cells. J. Virol. 3:106–113.)

70 to 80 per cent within an additional 8 hours (Fig. 5), while viral proteins are made maximally until about 25 hours after infection.[3] In contrast to the process which blocks host DNA synthesis, already noted, if viral DNA replication is prevented, viral mRNA and viral capsid proteins are not made, and host protein synthesis is not interrupted.[3]

Obviously, the highly specific control over the syntheses of host proteins must be directed at either the transcription of the host genome or the translation of host mRNAs. The two possibilities were easily distinguished, by measuring the synthesis of host RNA which specifically hybridized with denatured host DNA. Clearly the synthesis of the hybridizable host DNA-like RNA (dRNA), which includes mRNA, is inhibited at approximately the same time that protein synthesis is hindered (Fig. 6), and the rates of reduction in syntheses of both macromolecules are approximately parallel.[3a, 22] Thus, the interruption of biosynthesis of host proteins follows an inability to utilize the dRNA (which for the purpose of this discussion will be assumed to reflect the mRNA) which is made. Although the mechanism of this highly selective process is unknown, the discrimination may result because the viral mRNA is made at a rate five to ten times greater than the synthesis of host dRNA. Thus, the viral mRNA has a quantitative advantage over the host mRNA, and therefore may compete successfully with host mRNAs for a limited supply of intranuclear ribosomal subunits. Consequently, only viral mRNA is translated.

## SUMMATION

From the data that have been described it is now possible to relate the molecular events to the cytopathology observed in cells infected with adenoviruses. But the mechanisms of the reactions which stop cell division, halt the biosyntheses of host macromolecules, and result ultimately in cell death are still ambiguous. It seems desirable, nevertheless, to identify the biochemical reactions responsible for the characteristic intranuclear lesions and to utilize the data available to speculate upon the direct mechanisms of cell death just as is done by a morphologic pathologist after he has completed a necropsy.

A diagrammatic representation of the developing nuclear lesions and the sequential biosynthetic events which yield infectious virus (Fig. 7) graphically correlates the morphologic and biochemical processes. The nuclear changes[2, 4-6] appear to be the direct consequence of abundant synthesis and wasteful under-utilization of virus-specific macromolecules: (1) the early eosinophilic bodies are the "store houses" for the early proteins; (2) the basophilic, Feulgen-positive rims around the eosinophilic bodies represent morphologic evidence for the first synthesis of viral DNA; (3) the prominent central basophilic masses are formed from the great excess of viral DNA and viral capsid proteins which are made but not assembled into virions; (4) the hyaline-like, basophilic, Feulgen-positive material, which appears as a diffuse background in the affected nuclei, denotes additional unused viral DNA; (5) the unique basophilic, Feulgen-positive crystals are crystalline arrays of virions; and (6) the eosinophilic needle-like crystals are made of nonvirion protein, whose origin and function are unknown.

Interruption of the host's DNA synthesis about the middle of the eclipse period (Fig. 7) unquestionably accounts for the subsequent inability of infected cells to divide. But the molecular event or events which account for this selective control remain obscure. It may be pertinent that purified fiber protein accomplishes the same effect when added to cell cultures,[43] and that the fiber and hexon proteins inhibit both DNA and DNA-dependent RNA polymerases *in vitro*.[44] It is unlikely, however, that the relatively small amounts of hexon and fiber proteins which enter the cell as components of infecting virions could directly inhibit replication of the comparatively large quantity of host DNA which possesses numerous loci for initiation of replication. It is possible, however, that the viral capsid proteins act as inducers of the inhibitory reaction either at the nuclear membrane or at some other site.

A block in synthesis of host DNA alone cannot promote the subsequent

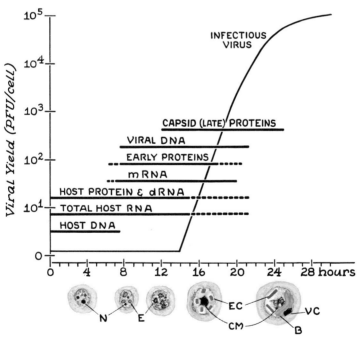

*Figure 7.* Diagrammatic correlation of the development of nuclear alterations in cells infected with type 5 adenovirus with the biosynthesis of host and virus-specific macromolecules and the appearance of infectious virus. Nucleoli (*N*); round, eosinophilic inclusions (*E*); elongated eosinophilic crystal-like structures (*EC*); central basophilic, Feulgen-positive mass (*CM*); lightly basophilic, homogeneously stained, Feulgen-positive background material (*B*); and basophilic viral crystal (*VC*).

cytopathic effects (i.e., rounding and clumping of cells) since interruption of DNA replication with FUdR does not induce these changes.[21a] Central to this problem, however, is the observation that pentons, the capsid corner units, when added to cell cultures can initiate similar cytopathic effects in 6 to 8 hours.[14, 53] Furthermore, gross cytopathic changes of infected cells do not begin until 20 to 24 hours following infection—after production of the penton and accumulation of the complex morphologic units have begun. It should be noted that production of host protein and RNA is likewise blocked just prior to the appearance of gross cytopathic changes (Fig. 7). It seems reasonable to presume that interruption of the biosyntheses of these macromolecules is unhealthy for the cell since chemical inhibition of protein synthesis with cyclohexamide or puromycin results in marked damage of KB cells in a few hours.[21a]

At this juncture the processes producing cytopathic changes and biochemical lesions seem to converge. The fiber and hexon, which are major components of the prominent nuclear basophilic masses (inclusion bodies) in adenovirus-infected cells (see Fig. 3), can inhibit DNA polymerase and DNA-dependent RNA polymerase *in vitro.*[44] No direct proof is available, but it is reasonable to suppose that the accumulation of large amounts of these viral proteins would have a profound intracellular effect, and stop biosyntheses of all RNAs, host and viral, as well as viral DNA.

Frequently hypotheses may be tested and biologic functions may be proved using genetic mutants. This cannot yet be accomplished formally with adenoviruses. Nature, however, has provided the virologist with a model in which adenoviruses, by analogy, play the role of conditionally lethal mutants. Thus, primary monkey kidney cells serve as nonpermissive hosts for adenoviruses, whereas KB or HeLa cells permit productive infections. In contrast to the productive infection, under restrictive conditions adenoviruses initiate an abortive infection in which a normal complement of viral DNA equivalents is made but only a limited amount of capsid proteins is produced.[44a, 63, 64] It follows, if the hypotheses and correlations made above are correct, that because capsid proteins do not accumulate the abortive infection should not induce characteristic nuclear lesions. This prediction proved to be correct.[44a] An abortive infection may thus permit the viral genome to replicate and persist in a viable cell, and cell transformation with unrestricted division and even malignant growth of some cell types may then follow. But frequently, even in abortive infections, severe chromosomal aberrations may follow association of the viral genome with the host chromosome, and the damaged cell does not survive.[10, 48, 49, 73, 79, 80]

The reader must now find himself in a position similar to that of one who observes an unfinished portrait—the artist's subject can easily be recognized but some important features are obscure. So it is with a consideration of the biochemical basis for the cell injury induced by adenoviruses: the basic causative factors of the intranuclear lesions can be identified, and the fundamental basis for the observed cytopathic effects can be suggested from the general picture as outlined. To complete the picture, however, i.e., to explain the molecular mechanisms which underlie all features of adenovirus cell damage, additional genetic and biochemical studies are required.

## ACKNOWLEDGMENTS

Deep gratitude and appreciation go to my outstanding colleagues who contributed so much to these studies (the parts which each played are shown in the bibliographic score). I wish also to thank Drs. M. Green, W. C. Russell, and R. W. Schlesinger who supplied preprints of important papers before publication.

The investigations summarized were supported by Public Health Research Grants AI-03620, AI-05731, and 2 TI AI-203 of the National Institute of Allergy and Infectious Diseases and conducted under the sponsorship of the Commission on Acute Respiratory Diseases, Armed Forces Epidemiological Board (supported by the Office of the Surgeon General, Department of the Army).

# *References*

1. Allison, A. C., H. G. Pereira, and C. P. Farthing. 1960. Investigation of adenovirus antigens by agar gel diffusion techniques. Virology, *10:*316–328.
2. Barski, G. 1956. Caractère spécifique de la lésion cellulaire causée *in vitro* par les virus du groupe A.P.C. et sa valeur diagnostique. Ann. Inst. Pasteur *91:*614–622.
3. Bello, L. J., and H. S. Ginsberg. 1967. Inhibition of host protein synthesis in type 5 adenovirus-infected cells. J. Virol. *1:*843–850.
3a. Bello, L. J., and H. S. Ginsberg. 1969. Relationship between deoxyribonucleic acid-like ribonucleic acid synthesis and inhibition of host protein synthesis in type 5 adenovirus-infected KB cells. J. Virol. *3:*106–113.
4. Boyer, G. S., F. W. Denny, Jr., and H. S. Ginsberg. 1959. Sequential cellular changes produced by types 5 and 7 adenoviruses in HeLa cells and in human amniotic cells. Cytological studies aided by fluorescein-labelled antibody. J. Exptl. Med. *110:*827–844.
5. Boyer, G. S., F. W. Denny, Jr., I. Miller, and H. S. Ginsberg. 1960. Correlation of production of infectious virus with sequential stages of cytologic alteration in HeLa cells infected with adenoviruses types 5 and 7. J. Exptl. Med. *112:*865–882.
6. Boyer, G. S., C. Leuchtenberger, and H. S. Ginsberg. 1957. Cytological and cytochemical studies of HeLa cells infected with adenoviruses. J. Exptl. Med. *105:*195–216.
7. Cohen, S. S. 1968. Virus-Induced Enzymes. Columbia University Press, New York.
8. Consigli, R. A., and H. S. Ginsberg. 1964. Control of aspartate transcarbamylase activity in type 5 adenovirus-infected HeLa cells. J. Bacteriol. *87:*1027–1033.
9. Consigli, R. A., and H. S. Ginsberg. 1964. Activity of aspartate transcarbamylase in uninfected and type 5 adenovirus-infected HeLa cells. J. Bacteriol. *87:*1034–1043.
10. Cooper, J. E. K., H. F. Stich, and D. S. Yohn. 1967. Viruses and mammalian chromosomes. VIII. Dose response studies with human adenoviruses types 18 and 4. Virology *33:*533–541.
11. Crick, F. H. C., and J. D. Watson. 1956. Structure of small viruses. Nature *177:*473–475.
11a. Denny, F. W., Jr., and H. S. Ginsberg. 1961. Certain biological characteristics of adenoviruses types 5, 6, 7 and 14. J. Immunol. *88:*567–574.
12. Eb, A. J. van der, and L. W. van Kesteren. 1966. Structure and molecular weight of the DNA of adenovirus type 5. Biochim. Biophys. Acta *129:*441–444.
13. Epstein, M. A., S. J. Holt, and A. K. Powell. 1960. The fine structure and composition of type 5 adenovirus: An integrated electron microscopical and cytochemical study. Brit. J. Exptl. Pathol. *41:*567–576.
14. Everett, S. F., and H. S. Ginsberg. 1958. A toxinlike material separable from type 5 adenovirus particles. Virology *6:*770–771.
15. Fisher, T. N., and H. S. Ginsberg. 1957. Accumulation of organic acids by HeLa cells infected with type 4 adenovirus. Proc. Soc. Exptl. Biol. Med. *95:*47–51.
16. Flanagan, J. F., and H. S. Ginsberg. 1962. Synthesis of virus-specific polymers in adenovirus-infected cells: Effect of 5-fluorodeoxyuridine. J. Exptl. Med. *116:*141–157.
17. Flanagan, J. F., and H. S. Ginsberg. 1964. Role of ribonucleic acid biosynthesis in multiplication of type 5 adenovirus. J. Bacteriol. *87:*977–987.
18. Gelderblom, H., H. Bauer, H. Frank, and R. Wigand. 1967. The structure of group II adenoviruses. J. Gen. Virol. *1:*553–560.
19. Gilead, Z., and H. S. Ginsberg. 1965. Characterization of a tumorlike antigen in type 12 and type 18 adenovirus-infected cells. J. Bacteriol. *90:*120–125.

20. Ginsberg, H. S. 1957. Biological and physical properties of the adenoviruses. Ann. N. Y. Acad. Sci. 67:383–391.

21. Ginsberg, H. S. 1965. Characterization of adenoviruses. III. Reproductive cycle of types 1 to 4. J. Exptl. Med. 107:133–152.

21a. Ginsberg, H. S. Unpublished data.

22. Ginsberg, H. S., L. J. Bello, and A. J. Levine. 1967. Control of biosynthesis of host macro-molecules in cells infected with adenovirus. In: Colter, J. S., and W. Paranchych (eds.). The Molecular Biology of Viruses. Academic Press, Inc., New York, pp. 547–572.

23. Ginsberg, H. S., and M. K. Dixon. 1959. Deoxyribonucleic acid (DNA) and protein altera-tions in HeLa cells infected with type 4 adenovirus. J. Exptl. Med. 109:407–422.

24. Ginsberg, H. S., and M. K. Dixon. 1961. Nucleic acid synthesis in types 4 and 5 adenovirus-infected HeLa cells. J. Exptl. Med. 113:283–299.

25. Ginsberg, H. S., H. G. Pereira, R. C. Valentine, and W. C. Wilcox. 1966. A proposed terminology for the adenovirus antigens and virion morphological subunits. Virology 28:782–783.

25a. Ginsberg, H. S., R. Scherz, and M. K. Dixon. Unpublished data.

26. Green, M. 1962. Studies on biosynthesis of viral DNA. Cold Spring Harbor Symp. Quant. Biol. 27:219–235.

27. Green, M., and G. E. Daesch. 1961. Biochemical studies on adenovirus multiplication. II. Kinetics of nucleic acid and protein synthesis in suspension cultures. Virology 13:169–176.

28. Green, M., and M. Pina. 1964. Biochemical studies on adenovirus multiplication. VI. Proper-ties of highly purified tumorigenic human adenoviruses and their DNA's. Proc. Natl. Acad. Sci. U.S. 51:1251–1259.

29. Green, M., M. Pina, and V. Chagoya. 1964. Biochemical studies on adenovirus multiplica-tion. V. Enzymes of deoxyribonucleic acid synthesis in cells infected by adenovirus and vaccinia virus. J. Biol. Chem. 239:1188–1197.

29a. Green, M., M. Pina, K. Fujinaga, S. Mak, and D. Thomas. 1968. Transcription of viral genes in adenovirus-infected and transformed cells. In: Pollard, M. (ed.). Perspectives in Virology VI. Academic Press, Inc., New York, pp. 15–38.

30. Green, M., M. Pina, R. Kimes, P. C. Wensink, L. A. MacHattie, and C. A. Thomas, Jr. 1967. Adenovirus DNA. I. Molecular weight and conformation. Proc. Natl. Acad. Sci. U.S. 57:1302–1309.

31. Hayashi, K., and W. C. Russell. 1968. A study of the development of adenovirus antigens by the immunofluorescent technique. Virology 34:470–480.

32. Hoggan, M. D., W. P. Rowe, P. H. Black, and R. J. Huebner. 1965. Production of "tumor-specific" antigens by oncogenic viruses during acute cytolytic infections. Proc. Natl. Acad. Sci. U.S. 53:12–19.

33. Horne, R. W., S. Brenner, A. P. Waterson, and P. Wildy. 1959. The icosahedral form of an adenovirus. J. Mol. Biol. 1:84–86.

34. Huebner, R. J., W. P. Rowe, H. C. Turner, and W. T. Lane. 1963. Specific adenovirus complement-fixing antigens in virus-free hamster and rat tumors. Proc. Natl. Acad. Sci. U.S. 50:379–389.

35. Joklik, W. K. 1964. The intracellular uncoating of poxvirus DNA. I. The fate of radio-actively-labeled rabbitpox virus. J. Mol. Biol. 8:263–276.

36. Joklik, W. K. 1964. The intracellular uncoating of poxvirus DNA. II. The molecular basis of the uncoating process. J. Mol. Biol. 8:277–288.

37. Kit, S., L. J. Piekarski, D. R. Dubbs, R. A. de Torres, and M. Anken. 1967. Enzyme induc-tion in green monkey kidney cultures infected with simian adenovirus. J. Virol. 1:10–15.

38. Köhler, K., and T. Odaka. 1964. Zeitpunktk der Synthese und Zusammensetzung der Messenger-RNS bei KB-Zellen nach Adenovirus-Infektion. Z. Naturforsch. 19b:331–336.

39. Laver, W. G., H. G. Pereira, W. C. Russell, and R. C. Valentine. 1968. Isolation of an internal component from adenovirus type 5. J. Mol. Biol. 37:379–386.

40. Laver, W. G., J. R. Suriano, and M. Green. 1967. Adenovirus proteins. II. N-terminal amino acid analysis. J. Virol. 1:723–728.

41. Lawrence, W. C., and H. S. Ginsberg. 1967. Intracellular uncoating of type 5 adenovirus deoxyribonucleic acid. J. Virol. 1:851–867.

42. Ledinko, N. 1966. Changes in metabolic and enzymatic activities of monkey kidney cells after infection with adenovirus 2. Virology 28:679–692.

43. Levine, A. J., and H. S. Ginsberg. 1967. Mechanism by which fiber antigen inhibits multi-plication of type 5 adenovirus. J. Virol. 1:747–757.

44. Levine, A. J., and H. S. Ginsberg. 1968. Role of adenovirus structural proteins in the cessation of host-cell biosynthetic functions. J. Virol. 2:430–439.

44a. Lyons, M. J., M. P. Friedman, and H. S. Ginsberg. In preparation.
45. Maizel, J. V., Jr., D. O. White, and M. D. Scharff. 1968. The polypeptides of adenovirus. II. Soluble proteins, cores, top components and the structure of the virion. Virology *36:*126–136.
46. Morgan, C., G. C. Godman, P. M. Breitenfeld, and H. M. Rose. 1960. A correlative study by electron and light microscopy of the development of type 5 adenovirus. I. Electron microscopy. J. Exptl. Med. *112:*373–382.
47. Morgan, C., G. C. Godman, P. M. Breitenfeld, and H. M. Rose. 1960. A correlative study by electron and light microscopy of the development of type 5 adenovirus. II. Light microscopy. J. Exptl. Med. *112:*383–402.
48. Nichols, W. W. 1966. Studies on the role of viruses in somatic mutation. Hereditas *55:*1–27.
49. Nichols, W. W., M. Peluse, C. Goodheart, R. McAllister, and C. Bradt. 1968. Autoradiographic studies on nucleic acid chromosomes of cultured leukocytes after infection with tritium-labeled adenovirus type 12. Virology *34:*303–311.
50. Norrby, E. 1966. The relationship between the soluble antigens and the virion of adenovirus type 3. I. Morphological characteristics. Virology *28:*236–248.
51. Norrby, E., and P. Skaaret. 1967. The relationship between the soluble antigens and the virion of adenovirus type 3. III. Immunological identification of fiber antigen and isolated vertex capsomer antigen. Virology *32:*489–502.
52. Norrby, E., and G. Wadell. 1967. Soluble components of adenovirus type 4. Virology *31:*592–600.
53. Pereira, H. G. 1958. A protein factor responsible for early cytopathic effect of adenoviruses. Virology *6:*601–611.
54. Pereira, H. G., A. C. Allison, and B. Balfour. 1959. Multiplication of adenovirus type 5 studied by infectivity titration and by the fluorescent antibody technique. Virology *7:*300–314.
55. Pereira, H. G., and M. V. T. de Figueiredo. 1962. Mechanism of hemagglutination by adenovirus types 1, 2, 4, 5, and 6. Virology *18:*1–8.
56. Pettersson, U., L. Philipson, and S. Höglund. 1967. Structural proteins of adenoviruses. I. Purification and characterization of adenovirus type 2 hexon antigen. Virology *33:*575–590.
57. Pettersson, U., L. Philipson, and S. Höglund. 1968. Structural proteins of adenoviruses. II. Purification and characterization of the adenovirus type 2 fiber antigen. Virology *35:*204–215.
58. Philipson, L. 1967. Attachment and eclipse of adenovirus. J. Virol. *1:*868–875.
59. Pina, M., and M. Green. 1965. Biochemical studies on adenovirus multiplication. IX. Chemical and base composition analysis of 28 human adenoviruses. Proc. Natl. Acad. Sci. U.S. *54:*547–551.
60. Polasa, H., and M. Green. 1965. Biochemical studies on adenovirus multiplication. VIII. Analysis of protein synthesis. Virology *25:*68–79.
61. Pope, J. H., and W. P. Rowe. 1964. Immunofluorescent studies of adenovirus 12 tumors and of cells transformed or infected by adenoviruses. J. Exptl. Med. *120:*577–588.
62. Prage, L., U. Pettersson, and L. Philipson. 1968. Internal basic proteins in adenovirus. Virology *36:*508–511.
63. Rapp, F., L. A. Feldman, and M. Mandel. 1966. Synthesis of virus deoxyribonucleic acid during abortive infection of simian cells by human adenoviruses. J. Bacteriol. *92:*931–936.
64. Reich, P. R., S. G. Brown, J. A. Rose, W. P. Rowe, and S. M. Weissman. 1966. Nucleic acid homology studies of adenovirus type 7-SV$_{40}$ interactions. Proc. Natl. Acad. Sci. U.S. *55:*336–341.
65. Reich, B. R., B. G. Forget, S. M. Weissman, and J. A. Rose. 1966. RNA of low molecular weight in KB cells infected with adenovirus type 2. J. Mol. Biol. *17:*428–439.
66. Riggs, J. L., N. Takemori, and E. H. Lennett. 1968. Cross-reactivity between T antigens of adenoviral immunotypes of proved and currently unproved oncogenic potential. J. Immunol. *100:*348–354.
67. Rose, J. A., P. R. Reich, and S. M. Weissman. 1965. RNA production in adenovirus infected KB cells. Virology *27:*571–579.
68. Rouse, H. C., and R. W. Schlesinger. 1967. An arginine-dependent step in the maturation of type 2 adenovirus. Virology *33:*513–522.
69. Russell, W. C., and Y. Becker. 1968. A maturation factor for adenovirus. Virology *35:*18–27.
70. Russell, W. C., K. Hayashi, P. J. Sanderson, and H. G. Pereira. 1967. Adenovirus antigens —a study of their properties and sequential development in infection. J. Gen. Virol. *1:*495–507.
71. Russell, W. C., and B. E. Knight. 1967. Evidence for a new antigen within the adenovirus capsid. J. Gen. Virol. *1:*523–528.

71a. Russell, W. C., W. G. Laver, and P. J. Sanderson. 1968. Internal components of adenoviruses. Nature *219:*1127–1130.

71b. Schlesinger, R. W. 1969. Adenoviruses: The nature of the virion and of controlling factors in productive or abortive infection and tumorigenesis. Adv. Virus Res. *14:*1–62.

72. Stich, H. F., V. I. Kalnins, E. MacKinnon, and D. S. Yohn. 1967. Electron microscopic localization of adenovirus type 12 antigens. J. Ultrastructure Res. *19:*556–562.

73. Stich, H. F., G. L. Van Hoosier, and J. J. Trentin. 1964. Viruses and mammalian chromosomes. Chromosome aberrations by human adenovirus type 12. Exptl. Cell Res. *34:*400–403.

74. Sussenbach, J. S. 1967. Early events in the infection process of adenovirus type 5 in HeLa cells. Virology *33:*567–574.

75. Valentine, R. C., and H. G. Pereira. 1965. Antigens and structure of the adenovirus. J. Mol. Biol. *13:*13–20.

75a. Velicer, L. F., and H. S. Ginsberg. 1968. Cytoplasmic synthesis of type 5 adenovirus capsid proteins. Proc. Natl. Acad. Sci. *61:*1264–1271.

75b. Velicer, L. F., and H. S. Ginsberg. Unpublished data.

76. Wilcox, W. C., and H. S. Ginsberg, 1961. Purification and immunological characterization of types 4 and 5 adenovirus-soluble antigens. Proc. Natl. Acad. Sci. U.S. *47:*512–526.

77. Wilcox, W. C., and H. S. Ginsberg. 1963. Protein synthesis in type 5 adenovirus-infected cells. Effect of p-fluorophenylalanine on synthesis of protein, nucleic acids, and infectious virus. Virology *20:*269–280.

78. Wilcox, W. C., H. S. Ginsberg, and T. F. Anderson. 1963. Structure of type 5 adenovirus. II. Fine structure of virus subunits. Morphologic relationship of structural subunits to virus-specific antigens from infected cells. J. Exptl. Med. *118:*307–314.

79. zur Hausen, H. 1968. Chromosomal aberrations and cloning efficiency in adenovirus type 12 infected hamster cells. J. Virol. *2:*915–917.

80. zur Hausen, H. 1968. Persistence of the viral genome in adenovirus type 12-infected hamster cells. J. Virol. *2:*918–924.

# Chapter 21

# SMALLPOX

ALLAN W. DOWNIE

*Visiting Professor, Department of Pediatrics, University
of Colorado Medical Center, Denver, Colorado*

Smallpox has existed in the world for centuries. Because of its striking clinical picture of severe illness associated with a generalized pustular eruption and the occurrence of epidemics with high mortality, the records of its incidence during the past three or four centuries are probably more complete than for most other infectious diseases. Nor does the disease, in its major form, seem to have altered in its lethality during this period. The advent of the antibiotics, though this has lessened the occurrence of septic complications, has as yet had comparatively little effect on the mortality rate. In the present century, a milder form of smallpox, variola minor or alastrim, has been prevalent in certain areas of the world, particularly in the Americas and parts of Africa. But this form of smallpox is clinically and epidemiologically distinct from the more severe form, variola major, which has figured so prominently in past records of severe pestilences.

Smallpox was the first disease for which prophylactic immunization was practiced. In the eighteenth century immunization was effected by variolation or inoculating the smallpox, but after Jenner's publication in 1798 this was replaced by vaccination or inoculating the cowpox—a relatively mild disease of cows that occasionally affected farm workers, who in consequence were immune to smallpox. For many years, vaccination was effected by transfer of vesicle fluid from arm to arm, but because the virus tended to become less virulent by such passage, fresh materials from affected cows or farm workers were occasionally brought into use. Human "lymph" was widely distributed throughout the country in vials or dried on cotton threads, so that by 1868 Ballard records that it was uncertain whence vaccine lymphs in current use were derived. The production of vaccine lymph by inoculation of virus on the skin of calves, was practiced in Italy from 1863 and in France from 1866.[2] From that time the practice has altered little until recent years. The origin of current vaccinia strains used in the preparation of smallpox vaccine is no more easy to trace today than the genealogy of lymph stocks of 100 years ago.

In this chapter consideration is given chiefly to those reactions of the host to invasion by the infectious agent which are manifest as disease. The physical and biochemical nature of variola virus and the intracellular changes associated with its multiplication are not discussed. However, because of the influence that vaccination has had on the incidence, severity, and clinical picture of smallpox as seen today, some space is devoted to a discussion of the biological characters of the viruses of variola, vaccinia, and cowpox.

## HISTORY

It is generally stated that smallpox was present in India and China before the Christian era, but the first recorded epidemic further west was apparently in Arabia in 568[72] or 569,[94] possibly introduced from Africa by an Abyssinian army. According to Moore,[72] smallpox reached Europe in the ninth century; its spread was promoted by the invasion of Europe by the Saracens and the return of crusaders in the twelfth and thirteen centuries. According to Creighton,[18] the first clear account of smallpox appears early in the sixteenth century. At this time, too, the disease was common among African natives brought by slave ships to the West Indies and on its introduction to the mainland produced devastating epidemics among the Mexicans. In England smallpox was the most serious epidemic and endemic disease in the seventeenth and eighteenth centuries. In the latter half of the eighteenth century the smallpox mortality in some years was approximately one-sixth of the birth rate. In the town of Chester from 1772 to 1777, one-third of all deaths in children under ten years of age was caused by smallpox,[45] and in London over a period of 30 years, smallpox was responsible for one-eighth of all deaths in those over two years of age.[21] Although the disease was endemic in the large towns, rural areas often remained free for years but were apt to suffer epidemic outbreaks when smallpox was introduced from the towns. In America the disease was not endemic, even in the towns, at this time. The density of population was perhaps too low to sustain smallpox as an endemic disease. In Boston, Massachusetts, for example, there was no serious epidemic of smallpox between 1730 and 1752. In the latter year one-third of the population suffered from it and all ages were attacked.[18] The urban endemic prevalence in Britain may have been maintained in part by the practice of variolation which was widespread in the second half of the eighteenth century.

The inoculation of smallpox was introduced in England in 1721. (For a detailed account of the history of inoculation in England and France the reader may consult the scholarly work of Genevieve Miller.[70]) While the disease resulting from inoculating smallpox matter into the skin by incision or puncture had a shorter incubation period and was generally milder than smallpox as usually acquired, this was not always so. In the first eight years of the practice of variolation in England, 17 of 897 persons inoculated died of the subsequent disease.[94] The practice was introduced in Boston, Massachusetts, soon after the first trials in London, and the apparent success of the measure in halting an epidemic in Charleston, South Carolina, in 1738 did much to popularize the method. Most western Europe countries, however, did not adopt variolation until 1750 or later. With more careful selection of the material for inoculation, for example, the use of clear fluid from the early vesicle at the site of inoculation, more superficial insertion by skin puncture or scarification, and better care of the patients there was less risk associated with the practice than in the years immediately after its introduction. However, even at the end of the eighteenth century the death rate from inoculated smallpox was reported to be 1:200 to 1:500. It was appreciated as early as 1722 that the inoculated disease was contagious but not until many years later was the practice introduced of inoculating whole communities at one time and isolating those who had not had smallpox or for one reason or another were not to be inoculated. The experience of Boston, Massachusetts, when variolation was practiced because of outbreaks of smallpox is illustrated in Table 1.

TABLE 1.  *Boston: Smallpox**

| YEAR | POP. | NATURAL SMALLPOX Cases | % Mort. | INOCULATED SMALLPOX Cases | % Mort. | % INOCULATED SMALLPOX | HAD SMALLPOX BEFORE |
|------|------|------|------|------|------|------|------|
| 1721 | 11,000 | 5759 | 14.6 | 287 | 2.0 | 2 | |
| 1730 | 13,000 | 3600 | 13.9 | 400 | 3.0 | 10 | |
| 1752 | 15,684 | 5545 | 9.7 | 2124 | 1.4 | 28 | 5998 |
| 1764 | 15,700 | 699 | 17.7 | 4977 | 0.9 | 87 | ca. 8370 |
| 1776 | – | 304 | 9.5 | 4988 | 0.6 | 90 | |
| 1778 | – | 122 | 32.8 | 2121 | 0.9 | 95 | |
| 1792 | 19,300 | 232 | 29.8 | 9152 | 2.0 | 97 | ca. 10,300 |

* Data from Blake, J. B. 1953. J. Hist. Med. 8:284–300.

It is possible that the relatively high mortality attributed to inoculated disease in 1792 was occasioned by the inoculation of persons already incubating the disease.

In the nineteenth century the incidence of smallpox slowly declined in western Europe and in North America. This was coincident with the widespread practice and legal enforcement of vaccination; but better housing conditions, better provision for the isolation of patients, and the development of public health services probably contributed to the decline. Smallpox, however, did not cease to be an endemic disease in Britain until the 1930's and in America, not until the following decade. In the meantime, variola major has retained its lethal qualities in those areas of the world where it is endemic; and in western countries where epidemics have resulted from its importation, the overall case mortality has remained around 20 per cent. On the other hand, the mortality from variola minor has been low. Between 1920 and 1930, years of high incidence of variola minor in the United States and in Britain, the case mortality rate was less than 1 per cent.

# THE VIRUSES OF VARIOLA, COWPOX, AND VACCINIA— BIOLOGICAL AND ANTIGENIC RELATIONSHIPS

A description of the physical and chemical structure of these viruses is to be found elsewhere.[25, 48] The discussion here is limited to those features which distinguish the three viruses and may have some bearing on their possible origin.

Electron microscopic study of the physical structure of the three viruses has revealed no differences between them, although the variola viruses have not been as intensively studied by this and by other techniques as have cowpox and vaccinia. Also, detailed analysis of chemical structure has not revealed differences between vaccinia and cowpox viruses but again, perhaps for obvious reasons, data are scarce for variola viruses. On the other hand, the antigenic structure and serological relationships have been more fully investigated. The protective value of vaccination against smallpox is evidence of close immunological relationship, and in the years immediately following the introduction of vaccination, when variolation was also practiced, many individuals vaccinated with cowpox virus were found to be immune to subsequent variolation. Cross immunity experiments in monkeys, such as those of Horgan and Haseeb,[50] show fairly complete immunity to variola and alastrim following infection with vaccinia and cowpox strains. Immune sera prepared against strains of variola major, variola minor, vaccinia, and cowpox showed almost complete cross reactivity in neutralization and complement fixation tests with antigens prepared from these viruses, although the sera after absorption with pure elementary body suspensions show minor differences between cowpox and variola-vaccinia viruses.[24, 26, 61] No differences were detected between the viruses of variola major, variola minor, and the strains of vaccinia used in these tests. Subsequent work has shown, however, that the differences demonstrable between vaccinia and cowpox were no greater than have subsequently been shown to exist between strains of vaccinia from different sources. Comparative neutralization tests against vaccinia and variola viruses using human postvaccination sera, convalescent sera from unvaccinated cases of variola minor and variola major, and sera prepared against variola major and vaccinia viruses in rabbits show slightly higher titres against the homologous virus (unpublished observations). It should be emphasized, however, that the differences are of a minor nature compared to the great serological overlap shown by viruses of the group.

The antigenic study of cowpox and vaccinia strains by the method of gel diffusion seemed to show a qualitative difference in their antigens.[39, 73] However, careful analysis of these antigens by the Ouchterlony method of gel diffusion by Rondle and Dumbell[81] showed that the differences were quantitative only, and that the eight or nine antigens demonstrable were present in both viruses. On the other hand, the white variant of cowpox appeared to lack an antigen present in both wild cowpox and vaccinia viruses. McCarthy and Helbert[64] could detect no differences in the hemagglutinins produced by the viruses under consideration.

The differences between cowpox, vaccinia, and variola viruses which are constant and used in their identification in the laboratory depend on differences in host range, the appearance of the lesions produced on the chick chorioallantois, their rate of growth in tissue culture, and their ceiling temperatures, i.e., the highest temperature at which macroscopic lesions are produced on the chorioallantois.[5]

The host range of variola viruses is fairly limited. Apart from man, disease can be produced regularly only in monkeys or in suckling mice infected by the intracerebral route. Cowpox and vaccinia viruses, on the other hand, have a wide range and regularly produce lesions in the common laboratory animals and domestic ungulates (vaccinia, however, produces lesions in the skin of fowls while cowpox does not).[48] On the chick chorioallantois variola strains regularly produce much smaller lesions than do vaccinia and cowpox strains. In this tissue the ceiling temperature of vaccinia is 41°C., of cowpox 40°C., of variola major 38.5°C., and of variola minor 38.5°C.[5] Vaccinia viruses grow and produce cytopathic effects in tissue culture more quickly than do variola viruses.[67, 74] Wild cowpox virus strains regularly produce hemorrhagic lesions in animals and on the chick chorioallantois as a result of more ready growth in mesodermal tissue and particularly in vascular endothelium. Strains of vaccinia virus vary in the degree of hemorrhage associated with experimental infections in animals and in the chick chorioallantois, but this is never as obvious as in the lesions produced by wild cowpox strains. The lesions produced by cowpox virus show typical large homogeneous, cytoplasmic, strongly acidophilic inclusions while the inclusions produced by vaccinia and variola are diffuse, granular, and weakly acidophilic. These differences are more constant than those demonstrable between strains of vaccinia virus which have been passed repeatedly in different animal hosts or by different routes of inoculation, and between mutants of vaccinia and the parent strains from which they have been derived.[36] The close relationship between these viruses is, however, readily demonstrated by recombination experiments with the production of hybrid viruses under suitable experimental conditions.[6, 35]

It has been suggested by Burnet[13] that from an evolutionary viewpoint

TABLE 2.  *Characteristics of Variola, Vaccinia, and Cowpox Viruses Used in Identification*

|  | VARIOLA VIRUSES | VACCINIA VIRUS | COWPOX VIRUS |
|---|---|---|---|
| Host Range | Man, monkeys | Wide; man, many domestic and laboratory animals | Wide; man, many domestic and laboratory animals |
| Lesions on Chorioallantois in 3 days | Small, raised, white, 1 mm. | Large, flatter, white, 2–4 mm. | Large, red, 2–3 mm. |
| Growth in Tissue Culture | Grows slowly; C.P.E., 2–6 days | Grows quickly; C.P.E., 1–3 days | Grows quickly; C.P.E., 1–3 days |
| Ceiling Temperature Chick Embryo | V. major 38.5°C. V. minor 38°C. | 41°C. | 40°C. |
| Cytoplasmic Inclusions | Granular, diffuse, faintly eosinophilic | Granular, diffuse, faintly eosinophilic | Homogeneous, strongly eosinophilic |

smallpox is more likely to have been derived from a pox disease of animals than that the pox diseases of animals were derived from smallpox in man. Animals probably existed in herds, which would favor transmission and endemic infection before man became gregarious. Burnet has suggested that variola may have evolved from a pox disease in wild ungulates or in African monkeys. The characteristics of monkey pox virus and the clinical and pathological features of the disease[40] make the latter alternative an attractive one.

It has been suggested that cowpox is a relatively recent disease acquired by bovines from smallpox in man.[23] However, the absence of records of cowpox before Jenner's description does not necessarily imply that the disease had not existed for many centuries, for exact descriptions of animal diseases generally are lacking in early records. The virus of cowpox differs so markedly in many biological properties from that of variola that it seems unlikely to be a recent derivative from variola. The relatively mild nature of the disease in cattle is more in keeping with a long association of host and parasite.

## Origin of Vaccinia

The origin of strains of vaccinia virus has been much in dispute and it poses a question for which there is no certain answer. The hypotheses put forward are: (1) that vaccinia strains have been derived from variola virus by transfer to the cow and adaptation by passage in that host, presumably by selective growth of mutants; (2) that by continuous passage in human skin through variolation in the eighteenth and early nineteenth centuries variola virus became gradually attenuated for man until it produced the mild disease now characteristic of vaccinia in man, and presumably lost its strict host specificity;[77] (3) that vaccinia represents a hybrid derived from simultaneous infection of man with cowpox and variola in the years immediately after the introduction of vaccination by Jenner when cowpox was used to vaccinate patients in smallpox hospitals;[6] (4) that vaccinia is the original pox virus from which other specialized pox viruses have evolved;[48] and (5) that vaccinia has been derived from cowpox and by repeated passage in vaccine institutions on the skin of cows, sheep, and other animals has become altered in certain of its characters.

The origins of most strains of vaccinia available throughout the world are unknown, as exact records of their passage histories are not available. Early lymphs were distributed from England to countries in Europe and to America by Jenner and other English physicians of his day. Strains now used in different countries vary somewhat in the severity of infection produced in man and laboratory animals; this may be related to different origins but may equally reflect differences in their animal passage histories.

1. The view that vaccinia has been derived by adaptation of variola virus to the cow is based on reported successful experimental transfer of smallpox material to cows with the emergence of vaccinia. As Herrlich et al.[47] point out, the positive results reported were more than counterbalanced by many negative attempts and most of the reported successes were achieved when contamination by established strains of vaccinia could not be ruled out. During the past 30 years all attempts to produce vaccinia from variola under strict

isolation conditions have failed. Of these investigations the most exhaustive were those reported by Herrlich and his colleagues[47] carried out over a period of six years in many different animal species using a variety of approaches including those reportedly successful in the past. Moreover, the biological properties of the viruses of vaccinia and variola are so different that a change from one virus to the other by a few animal passages seems unlikely.

2. The second hypothesis differs from the first in that it postulates the change from variola to vaccinia through continuous propagation of variola by arm to arm inoculation in man. Attenuation by this kind of transfer is not usually associated with broadening of host range, which is one of the characteristic properties of vaccinia strains. Indeed, continuous passage in one kind of host tends to lessen host range, a phenomenon used today in the development of live virus vaccines.

3. There is no direct evidence for or against the view that vaccinia is a hybrid produced by recombination between variola and cowpox. Some strains of vaccine lymph were developed from naturally occurring infection in cattle or in horses after the practice of variolation had ceased; but the increase in vaccination with cowpox lymph at times of epidemic prevalence of smallpox might conceivably have provided opportunities for concomitant infection of human beings with both viruses.

4. The suggestion that vaccinia, because of its wide host range, is the original pox virus from which all others have evolved is perhaps attractive. But then the question arises, in what animal species has it been perpetuated over the centuries? It is true that vaccinia strains have been recovered from outbreaks of cowpox in cattle, especially on the Continent, but in most instances there is evidence that such outbreaks originated through contact with recently vaccinated humans. In those outbreaks where cowpox virus has been isolated—and this includes practically all reported in England and many in Holland—no such origin has been suggested. These observations suggest that true cowpox is an endemic disease peculiar to cows which has probably existed for centuries in England and parts of Europe.

5. The properties of vaccinia strains currently available make the last hypothesis most acceptable to the writer. After many passages of cowpox virus on the chick chorioallantois the large solid type of inclusion characteristic of cowpox infection becomes less numerous and inclusions of the granular type typical of vaccinial lesions become more common in the infected ectodermal cells (personal observation and Berger[7]). By repeated passage of cowpox virus by scarification on the skin of calves and sheep and occasional passes in the rabbit, the virus may have lost its "affinity" for mesodermal tissue and, consequently, the hemorrhagic character of the lesions has lessened. Strains of vaccinia virus passed repeatedly in rabbits by the intratesticular or intracerebral route produce more hemorrhagic lesions in the rabbit skin and in the chorioallantois than do strains which have been passed repeatedly by skin scarification. The alternation of hosts used in passing cowpox strains for the production of lymph may have broadened their host range. Vaccinia then, in this view, is a laboratory virus probably derived from the natural pox virus of cows by continuous propagation in laboratories and vaccine institutes during the last century.

# CLINICAL FEATURES OF SMALLPOX

## *Variola Major*

For a detailed and comprehensive description of the clinical features of smallpox, the works of Ricketts and Byles,[78] Dixon,[23] and Herrlich et al.[48] should be consulted. These three books contain many excellent clinical photographs, some in color. Here the main clinical features are noted to facilitate discussion of pathology and pathogenesis.

The incubation period of smallpox, i.e., the time from infecting contact to the onset of illness, is usually between 10 and 14 days. Twelve days is the common incubation period although in rare instances it may be as short as 8 or 9 days and occasionally as long as 16 or even 17 days. The onset is often acute, with fever, malaise, and some degree of prostration. There is often severe headache, backache, pains in the limbs, and sometimes vomiting. This initial or toxemic phase lasts for 4 to 6 days in the ordinary case. In about 10 per cent of cases there may be in this initial phase a toxemic rash which is quite separate from the focal rash that is shortly to appear. The toxemic rash has a predilection for the groins, axillae, and flanks. It may be erythematous in character when it has no grave prognostic significance and occurs more often in previously vaccinated persons. In other cases the rash may be petechial or purpuric and in the worst cases petechial hemorrhages may appear over much of the body surface. On the third or fourth day the focal eruption appears and in the average case within 2 days thereafter the temperature drops to near normal and the patient feels much better.

The focal rash usually appears first on the buccal and pharyngeal mucosa, the face, or the forearms and hands and then spreads to the trunk and lower limbs. For the first few days of the eruption, the lesions on the face and arms may be a day in advance of those on the legs. In the average case, however, the lesions on any one area of skin are all at the same stage of development. The macules become firm papules within 24 hours and in two days fluid has collected in the papules and the resulting vesicles enlarge and quickly become opaque from the periphery inward owing to the accumulation of inflammatory cells. In the average case the pustules are usually markedly raised from the skin, are tense, and feel firm to the touch. About 8 or 9 days after the onset of the eruption, the pustules may show umbilication as they begin to dry up, and crusting is usually complete by 14 to 16 days from the onset of illness. By the end of three weeks most of the crusts have separated except for those on the palms of the hands and soles of the feet.

As stressed by Ricketts, the distribution of the rash, as much as its character and homogeneity, is important in arriving at a clinical diagnosis. Although there is a certain amount of variation from case to case, the focal eruption is usually most profuse on the face, which may be swollen and edematous. The forearms and hands are usually more affected than the upper arms, the extensor surface of the limbs more than the flexor, the back more than the front of the trunk, the chest more than the abdomen. More lesions are usually present on the feet and legs below the knee than on the thighs.

The eruption is typically centrifugal in distribution. Hollows such as the axillae, the groins, the front of the elbow and the popliteal areas, the skin of the neck under the jaw, and the orbital hollow tend to have fewer lesions; prominences such as forehead, malar eminences on the cheek, the wrists, the knees, and skin over the malleoli may be markedly affected. Areas of pressure, as by a belt, garter, or collar, or old scars may be selected by the eruption. In all except the mild cases there is usually some increase in fever associated with the stage of pustulation, but in patients who recover the temperature falls to normal as the lesions begin to dry up.

This brief account is applicable to the majority of smallpox patients but there are cases which show marked deviation from this general picture.

*In the fulminating or early hemorrhagic case* there is usually fever of moderate degree, although it may be marked, intense headache and backache, sometimes pain in the chest or abdomen, restlessness, marked flushing or erythema of the face, and extreme prostration. In two or three days petechiae appear in the skin, there may be subconjunctival hemorrhage and bleeding

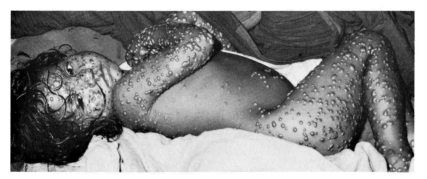

*Figure 1.* Smallpox with discrete eruption. (Courtesy of Dr. V. A. Fulginiti.)

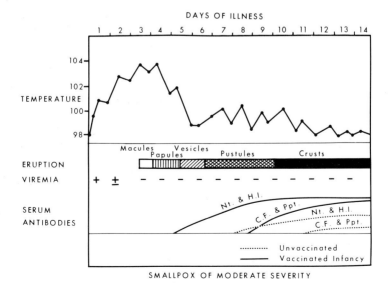

*Figure 2.*

from the gums, the nose, rectum and, in women, the vagina. There is a complete loss of muscle tone and the face may have a masklike appearance. In the most acute cases, death may occur on the fourth or fifth day before any focal rash has appeared, and in such cases a diagnosis of acute septicemia, especially meningococcal, or acute leukemia may be made. If the patient survives beyond the fourth day, a few early soft papular lesions or early flat vesicles may be found on the hands, forearms, or elsewhere.

*In the flat or malignant variety* there is again a severe initial illness with fever persisting throughout the eruptive phase. The appearance of the focal lesions may be delayed; they are slow to mature, and the vesicles are flat and soft and velvety to the touch. The lesions may show considerable variation and the centrifugal distribution may not be obvious. Umbilication of the vesicles may be present. Hemorrhages often appear at the base of the lesions and sometimes in the skin between them (Rao's late hemorrhagic cases). Death usually occurs between the tenth and fourteenth days. In the patients who recover, the vesicular lesions slowly dry up, often without going through the stage of pustulation, and convalescence is prolonged.

*The ordinary variety* (Dixon's types 4 to 7)[22] comprises the majority of cases, both in the vaccinated and unvaccinated, and conforms to the usual description of smallpox. The severity of the clinical illness is generally related to the extent of the eruption.

*The modified variety* is seen mostly in vaccinated patients. The modification relates to the character and development of the focal eruption, for the initial illness may be severe and not necessarily of short duration. The skin lesions tend to evolve quickly and may lack the uniformity of ordinary cases. The lesions may vary considerably in size, many being quite small, so that there is an appearance of cropping. The lesions may be few in number and even when numerous they tend to heal quickly so that scabbing may be complete by the tenth day. There is usually no secondary fever during the eruptive phase. It is in these cases that an erroneous diagnosis of chickenpox is often made.

*In variola sine eruptione,* after a normal incubation period, there is the usual initial febrile illness lasting two or three days, but no eruption follows. This type of illness is uncommon but occurs occasionally in well vaccinated contacts and is associated with a well marked rise in serum antibodies.[27] Variolous conjunctivitis is sometimes seen in ordinary cases of smallpox but can occasionally occur as the only clinical evidence of infection in vaccinated contacts.[19] Occasionally there is a slight rise in temperature associated with the conjunctivitis and in the few cases in which examination has been made there has been an increase in serum antibody following the conjunctivitis. Table 3 (page 509) shows the relative incidence and case fatality rate of the major varieties of smallpox in over 6000 vaccinated and unvaccinated smallpox patients admitted to the Infectious Diseases Hospital in Madras between 1961 and 1967.

Another type of illness is seen among well vaccinated contacts of smallpox patients 7 to 12 days after contact. This illness is usually of virus pneumonia type, with fever, malaise, headache, muscular and joint pains, and lassitude with subsequent dyspnea on exertion.[16] The illness may last for two or more weeks but is unaccompanied by skin eruption. Radiological examination of the chest usually shows some diffuse mottling, usually over the lower lobes,[51] and the radiological changes may persist for some time.[33] The observations of Leroux et al.[59] in the Vannes outbreak of variola major suggest that this type of illness in contacts is more common than is generally realized. It seems likely, as suggested by Dixon, that these changes are the result of an allergic reaction in the lungs occurring perhaps in response to the viremia of an infection which, however, gives rise to no cutaneous eruption. The term "smallpox allergic pneumonitis" might be a more suitable designation for this condition than "smallpox pulmonary allergy," suggested by Dixon, or "smallpox handler's lung," used by Evans and Foreman.[33] In the cases of Evans and Foreman repeated nasopharyngeal washings yielded no virus. There is no evidence that individuals suffering from this condition are infectious for their contacts.

### SMALLPOX AND PREGNANCY

It has long been recognized that the pregnant woman is particularly apt to suffer from the most severe forms of variola major. Rao and his colleagues[76] compared the severity of smallpox in 254 pregnant women with much larger numbers of male and nonpregnant female patients in the same age group (15 to 44 years). In the pregnant women the hemorrhagic variety of smallpox was seven time more common in the vaccinated and five times more common in the unvaccinated as compared with the same categories in males and nonpregnant females. The incidence of severe infections was considerably higher in the unvaccinated as compared to vaccinated pregnant women; but even in the latter group the incidence of hemorrhagic cases was about three times that in unvaccinated males or nonpregnant females. In the earlier months of pregnancy, abortion was common. Of those women contracting smallpox in the seventh or eight month of pregnancy, less than half had live births, whereas when smallpox was contracted near full term, there were 90 per cent of live births. The reason for the greater susceptibility of pregnant women to severe smallpox infection is unknown, but it has been suggested by Rao that it is related to high levels of circulating corticosteroids.

## Variola Minor (Alastrim)

This kind of smallpox, though milder, presents the same clinical picture as variola major. The initial or toxemic illness lasts usually from three to five days and during this period there may be toxemic rashes of erythematous or even hemorrhagic character.[68] In Marsden's series of 13,686 cases, three cases were toxic or hemorrhagic and 19 had confluent eruptions. The focal eruption usually appeared by the third or fourth day of illness. The great majority showed discrete eruptions with fewer than 100 lesions on the face. The eruption went through the same phases of development as those seen in the major disease although many lesions were small and superficial; the distribution of the eruption was similar, but umbilication of the lesions was uncommon and scabbing tended to occur rather earlier. Secondary fever at the pustular stage of the eruption occurred in over 5 per cent of the cases. Thirty-four of Marsden's patients died. Smallpox was the direct cause of death in 5 patients whose ages ranged from two days to three weeks; it was the immediate exciting cause in 11 patients and a definite contributory cause in 3. Among 150 pregnant women there were only six abortions and there was little evidence that pregnancy had such an adverse effect on the course of the disease as in variola major. However, it is generally agreed that in any single case it is impossible, on clinical grounds alone, to distinguish a case of variola minor from a case of variola major with a discrete or modified eruption.

### INOCULATION SMALLPOX

This type of smallpox as described by writers in the eighteenth century was generally milder than the disease as usually acquired. The lesion at the site of inoculation usually developed in three or four days; its appearance was followed by axillary adenitis, fever, and general malaise about the seventh day and the generalized eruption a day or two later. Occasionally acute fulminating infections occurred, although some of these severe attacks may have been in persons inoculated during the incubation period of smallpox. The incubation period, from inoculation to the onset of constitutional symptoms, was several days less than in the "naturally" acquired disease. The disease acquired by contact with inoculated cases appeared to be of normal severity. The practice of inoculating smallpox may still be carried on in remote parts of Asia or Africa; the outbreak in Kweilin, Kwangsi, in 1940–1941 was believed to have originated from inoculated cases.[84] Smallpox is occasionally transmitted by accidental inoculation through the skin and in such cases the disease conforms in type to that described following inoculation in the eighteenth century.

### CONGENITAL SMALLPOX

As noted earlier, variola major occurring in the early months of pregnancy is likely to lead to abortion and in later months to stillbirths. In some of the stillborn, variolous eruptions may be present on the skin. In variola major or minor occurring near term the baby may be born during the smallpox attack in the mother. In some of the instances recorded by Marsden and Greenfield[69] and Dixon,[22] the interval between the onset of illness in the mother and the appearance of the eruption on the baby after birth was 9 to 12 days. These observations indicate that when infection is transmitted from mother to baby, presumably through the placenta, the incubation period in the baby is several days shorter than in smallpox acquired after birth and approximates that seen in inoculated smallpox.

### COMPLICATIONS OF SMALLPOX

Septic complications in the form of boils or subcutaneous abscesses are not uncommon in variola major, although the incidence in Marsden's cases of variola minor was low. Bacterial bronchopneumonia was a common postmortem finding in Councilman's 54 cases[17] and was present in all 9 cases autopsied by Sweitzer and Ikeda.[85] In Bras's series of 177 autopsies, in only 25 was bronchopneumonia sufficiently developed to be considered a cause or concurrent cause of death.[12] In this outbreak in Djakarta, however, most of the patients had received antibiotic treatment. Only seven of Marsden's patients with variola minor suffered from bronchopneumonia. A relatively high incidence of osteomyelitis in smallpox has recently been reported from Nigeria and the Congo. The condition has usually been seen in unvaccinated children under five years old in whom this complication may occur in 2 to 5 per cent of smallpox cases.[11, 15, 32] The signs of bone and joint involvement usually appear in the second or third week of illness, the bones near the wrists, elbows, knees, or ankles being most often affected. The condition appears radiologically to be a juxtametaphyseal osteoporosis and although there may be some subsequent interference with growth, the immediate prognosis is good. Encephalomyelitis may be a complication associated with either type of smallpox. In Marsden's series of variola minor there were seven cases with three deaths. Eye complications occur in 5 to 10 per cent of cases in the form of simple blepharitis, conjunctivitis, or keratitis.

### Blood Changes in Smallpox

The blood picture in smallpox varies to some extent according to the nature of the case. In the ordinary case with a discrete pustular eruption there is little change in the red blood cells. At the early stage of the disease the total leukocyte count may be normal or slightly increased, but in the eruptive phase there may be a leukopenia with a marked decrease in granular leukocytes and a relative and absolute increase in lymphocytes. In the late pustular stage there is frequently a return to normal counts or some degree of leukocytosis. Lymphocytosis is seen in other virus infections but is particularly marked in smallpox, caused perhaps by the severe involvement of the lymphoid tissue. In hemorrhagic cases, especially in fulminating cases, the blood picture may be very striking—so much so that Ikeda considered it of definite diagnostic value.[52] Pathological forms of normoblasts with basophil stippling or polychromatophilia were common; the total leukocyte count was markedly increased, with a low polymorph count (30 to 40 per cent), a marked increase in lymphocytes and mononuclear cells, and the presence of myelocytes, metamyelocytes, and myeloblasts, suggesting intense stimulation of the bone marrow. This leukoerythroblastic picture in acute hemorrhagic smallpox has been noted by others and has been responsible for erroneous diagnoses of acute leukemia.

The blood sedimentation rate is often within normal limits, and platelet counts may not be greatly diminished except in hemorrhagic cases when there is a progressive decrease often to a very low figure (20,000). The clotting time is not increased in ordinary cases of smallpox but in all hemorrhagic cases studied by Roberts et al.[80] and McKenzie et al.[65] there were marked defects in the clotting mechanism. There was a marked deficiency of platelets, prothrombin, and accelerator globulin (factor V) and an increase in circulating antithrombin.

## MORBID ANATOMY OF SMALLPOX

The pathological changes described in the internal organs in smallpox are necessarily based on studies in the more severe types of disease. The pathological changes seen in the 54 cases studied by Councilman and his colleagues[17] were complicated by secondary bacterial sepsis. In the 177 autopsies which provided Bras's material superadded septic complications were uncommon because most of the patients had been treated with antibiotics.[12] Bras emphasized that the changes in hemorrhagic smallpox were not essentially different from those of other cases. The basic pattern was the same, with differences in development and intensity.

The changes described in skin biopsies from alastrim cases by de Jong[54] were not essentially different from those seen in the skin of variola major cases by Councilman et al.[17] and Bras.[12] The earliest change to be observed in the skin is dilation of the capillaries in the papillae of the corium with swelling of the lining endothelium and an infiltrate of lymphocytes and histiocytes. Changes then appear in the overlying epidermis. At first a few cells in the middle layer of the epidermis become enlarged, and vacuoles appear in the cytoplasm, which stains poorly. The nucleus condenses and later disappears. There is proliferation of cells in the malpighian layer, and this, together with the swelling of cells, leads to great thickening of the epithelial layer. As the process of degeneration spreads to neighboring cells in the middle layer, there is intercellular edema, the cell membranes rupture, and a vesicle is formed. The vesicle tends to be loculated with septa formed by the remains of incompletely destroyed cells. The epithelial cells beneath the vesicle are at first compressed and disorderly, but individual cells or groups of cells get detached and become rounded off. The nuclei shrink, and the cytoplasm becomes more eosinophilic. In the fully developed vesicle the roof is formed of compressed cells of the stratum spinosum, the keratohyaline layer, and the horny layer. The base is formed of degenerate rounded cells of the malphighian layer which may later disappear, so that the pock cavity extends to the corium. Pustules form when polymorphonuclear leukocytes enter the vesicle from the dermis, and the septa which previously crossed the vesicle disappear. In the healing stage, fluid is absorbed from the pustule and the contents dry up. Epithelial cells from the sides of the cavity encroach upon it and proceed to grow under the residual mass of the exudate so that finally a crust is left of degenerated epithelial cells, leukocytes, and debris. The pitting, which is most severe on the face, is caused by destruction of sebaceous glands followed by organization and subsequent shrinking of granulation tissue.[12] In cases of fulminating smallpox extravasated blood cells are present in the corium; and even when no skin lesions have been obvious to the naked eye at the time of death, areas of degeneration with commencing vesicle formation are to be seen in the epithelial layer.

Lesions are found in the mucous membrane of the mouth, tongue, pharynx, larynx, and upper part of the esophagus concurrent with those in the skin. Vesicles are not usually seen but necrosis of the epithelium occurs in small focal or more extensive areas of the mucosa. Because of the absence of an impervious keratin layer the damaged epithelial cells are shed from these lesions at an early stage of the disease.

In the heart, apart from subendothelial hemorrhages and occasional collections of mononuclear cells around small vessels, pathological changes are not frequent, in spite of clinical signs of myocardial involvement seen in severe cases of smallpox. Councilman and his colleagues[17] commonly found bronchitis and bronchopneumonia at autopsy, but in Bras's series, while hyperemia of the lungs was common, bronchopneumonia was seen in a small proportion of the cases.

The liver is constantly enlarged, but apart from occasional small hemorrhages, gross changes are not obvious. The endothelial cells lining the sinusoids, like those in the spleen and bone marrow, show hyperplasia and degenerative changes, more pronounced in the early stages. The spleen is usually enlarged and congested; the follicles appear to be hyperplastic and in the pulp a few neutrophilic granulocytes are to be seen. Numerous large lymphoid cells are present, similar to those found also in the sinusoids of the liver, in the lymph nodes, and in the capillaries in the kidney and other organs. In the kidneys dilatation of vessels and degeneration of tubular epithelium is found, particularly in the outer pyramidal zone. Focal necrotic lesions were frequently observed in the testes by Councilman, and Bras noted that focal lesions, not readily visible with the naked eye, were seen regularly in patients dying in the pustular stage and frequently in the crusting stage. Such lesions were not seen in the ovaries. No specific findings were noted in the gastrointestinal tract except occasional hemorrhages in the ascending colon. In fulminating cases, hemorrhages were noted under the serosa in the pericardium, pleura, and peritoneum, in the lungs, liver, kidneys, bladder, and uterus, and occasionally in the bone marrow.

Cytoplasmic inclusions are characteristic of infections with variola and vaccinia viruses. In the early lesions in the skin and mucous membranes they are readily found in sections stained by hematoxylin and eosin as round or oval, faintly basophilic or acidophilic bodies lying in the cytoplasm usually close to the nucleus (Guarnieri bodies). In more advanced lesions, suitably stained sections (Mann's stain) show faintly acidophilic granular inclusions occupying a large part of the cytoplasm of infected cells. They are particularly well seen in the epithelial cells at the base of vesicles or pustules. These inclusions consist of masses of elementary bodies with a variable amount of matrix. Intranuclear inclusions have been described in the lesions of smallpox by Magrath and Brinkerhoff[66] and by Torres[87] but they are not a conspicuous feature of the lesions. They are not mentioned by Bras[12] but have been seen by the writer in sections of skin from two of nine fatal cases of variola major examined.

## PATHOGENESIS

The virus is believed to enter the body through the respiratory tract, except in the rare instances of accidental inoculation through the skin or of

infection of the baby in utero. It is not known whether the virus is inhaled
in the form of minute droplets expelled from the mouth and nose of the patient,
in the form of infected dust from the vicinity of the patient, or whether virus
is carried to the mouth or nose by contaminated fingers. Infection is transmitted most commonly to close contacts of the patient when any of these
modes of transfer might be operative. The resistance of the virus dried in dust
or bedclothes has often been demonstrated and has been responsible for the
infection of laundry workers.

## INCUBATION PERIOD

It is not known whether the virus multiplies at the initial site of entry
in the mucosa of the respiratory tract; but during the incubation period of
12 days patients are not infectious to their contacts. This suggests that a
primary lesion is unlikely in the mucosa of the upper respiratory tract, but
does not exclude the possibility that the virus might multiply in mucosal cells
of the lower respiratory tract. A small amount of virus liberated into the
lumen of the lower air passages might not be expelled in the secretions from
the respiratory tract. The observations of Duguid[31] suggest that dissemination
to the environment of bacteria in the trachea or bronchi does not readily take
place unless inflammatory changes and excess secretion induce bouts of
coughing. On the other hand, there is evidence from fluorescent antibody studies
on distemper in ferrets and dogs[60] and in mouse pox[79] that virus introduced
by the respiratory route may pass through the respiratory mucosa without
producing lesions in the lining epithelium and be carried by phagocytic cells
to neighboring lymph nodes. In rabbits exposed by contact to rabbit pox[4] and
in cattle exposed to rinderpest[86] virus may be recovered one to three days
after contact from draining lymph nodes but not from overlying respiratory
mucosa. Further multiplication of virus goes on in these and other tissues
during the incubation period to produce viremia which is demonstrable at the
onset of illness and on which the further progress of the infection depends.
But the sites of virus multiplication in the incubation period of smallpox have
not been determined directly, and can only be surmised from the study of
experimental infections with other pox viruses in their natural animal hosts.
The first of extensive studies of this kind were made by Fenner in ectromelia
or mouse pox,[34] and his results have been for the most part confirmed by
observations on rabbit pox,[4] on fowl pox,[92] and on monkey pox.[89] The studies
of Westwood and his colleagues[58, 91] and Hahon and Wilson[42] on experimental
variola in monkeys are not so informative in relation to the pathogenesis of
smallpox in man. The virus strains were not very pathogenic for the monkeys
used, for large doses of virus had to be administered by aerosol to produce
clinical infection and the disease produced was not exactly comparable to
human smallpox in its clinical or pathological aspects. In the studies of the
pox infections in their natural hosts just mentioned, virus reached regional
lymph nodes within one or two days after infection and soon thereafter was
found in the spleen, borne there presumably by the blood. This early viremia
may not be detectable by blood culture and the virus appears to be rapidly
removed from the blood by cells of the reticuloendothelial system and does

not localize in the skin to produce lesions at this time. Virus increased in lymph nodes, spleen, liver, bone marrow, and other internal organs and at the time fever was observed was readily found in the blood.

It seems likely that in smallpox, virus multiplies in reticuloendothelial cells in lymph glands, spleen, liver, bone marrow, and probably the lung during the incubation period. Councilman et al.[17] noted in smallpox patients who died after a few days illness destruction of the Kupfer cells in the liver, and Bras[12] records similar findings in the liver, spleen, and bone marrow; in patients dying later there was marked proliferation of these cells which he regarded as evidence of earlier severe damage. These observations support the idea that multiplication of virus in the incubation period of smallpox takes place in these organs.

## CLINICAL PERIOD

The onset of the initial illness seems to coincide with the second massive viremia. The release of virus at this time from cells in which it has been multiplying is presumably associated with cellular damage. The work of Barry Wood[93] suggests that cellular pyrogens may be responsible for the onset of fever. In milder cases of smallpox the viremia may be of short duration; in the confluent and fulminating cases it is greater in extent and lasts much longer.[28, 48, 71]

Although the virus must be disseminated by the circulation throughout the body, it is mainly in the skin and mucous membranes of the mouth and upper respiratory tract that further evidence of virus multiplication appears. As noted previously, the earliest changes seen histologically are in the capillaries in the papillae of the corium. The swelling of the lining endothelial cells and neighboring cellular infiltration suggests that the virus first infects these cells. Possibly this occurs through the adhesion of infected leukocytes or cell fragments at the time of initial fever; the injection of pyrogen in experimental animals has been shown to lead to margination of leukocytes in peripheral capillaries.[93] From infected dermal capillaries virus spreads to the overlying epithelium. By the time macules and papules are visible in the skin, extensive infection of the epithelium has taken place, for scrapings of the lesions at this time reveal large numbers of virus particles and suitably stained sections show inclusion material in the epithelial cells. By the time the skin lesions have reached the vesicular stage, histological studies suggest that in the average case further extension of infection in the epithelium does not occur. It is uncertain whether local extension is inhibited by local production of interferon or by the action of antibody, which is usually detectable in the blood serum about this time (Fig. 2, p. 495), or by other unknown factors. The further development of the vesicle to pustule is evidence of the inflammatory response of the tissues to necrosis of epithelial cells produced by the growth of virus within them. This inflammatory response may be absent in malignant cases of smallpox in which, even after ten days of illness, pustulation has not followed the flat vesicular stage. The appearance of new skin lesions, sometimes over a period of two or three days, might be caused by the prolongation of viremia over the first day or two of initial illness through the fresh release of virus into the circulation from the damaged skin capillaries infected at the onset of fever.

It has already been noted that in contrast to the skin, internal organs examined post mortem usually show no evidence of focal areas of necroses such as might be expected to result from multiplication of virus disseminated by the initial viremia. There is no satisfactory explanation for this apparent selective local virus activity. Smallpox virus may have a special predilection for stratified epithelium, whatever that may involve; but obviously during the incubation period, before there is fever, the virus multiplies in tissues other than surface epithelium, and, as noted previously, seems to grow in vascular endothelium in dermal capillaries soon after the onset of fever. It may be that the circulation of blood in the skin capillaries is subject to more fluctuation than that in internal organs, and localization of virus may be determined by such differences. The work of Bedson and Dumbell[5] on the ceiling temperature of pox viruses shows that under their experimental conditions (growth on the chick chorioallantois) the virus of variola produced lesions only at temperatures up to 38.5°C., alastrim had a ceiling temperature even lower (37.5°C.), while vaccinia strains produced lesions at temperatures up to 41°C. If the growth of variola virus in the human body is inhibited by temperatures near the ceiling temperature determined in chick embryos, then the onset of fever in smallpox might limit growth in the internal organs while permitting such growth in the skin and in mucous membranes of the mouth and upper respiratory tract, where temperatures may be a degree or two less. The occurrence of clinical evidence of orchitis[48] and the finding of focal lesions in the testes and their absence in the ovaries[12] lend a little suport to the suggestion that fever at the onset of illness might be in part responsible for the apparently selective localization of lesions in the skin and certain mucous membranes. In experimental generalized infections of rabbits with vaccinia virus, in rabbit pox, in mouse pox, and less frequently in monkey pox, focal lesions are to be found in the internal organs, but the causal viruses have higher ceiling temperatures than the viruses of smallpox. In severe and fatal chickenpox, lesions are not uncommon in the internal organs and this virus also has a higher ceiling temperature in tissue cultures of human cells than has variola virus.[14]

It may be concluded from these considerations that multiplication of variola virus during the incubation period takes place in the internal organs; but after the onset of illness, growth of virus is mainly restricted to the skin and mucous membranes. The reason for the centrifugal distribution of the eruption, the sparing of flexures, and the greater involvement of extensor than flexor surfaces of the limbs and trunk remain unexplained. Possibly the low ceiling temperature of variola virus may contribute, as the eruption tends to be most profuse where skin temperatures are lower. Ricketts suggested that the rash tended to occur in those areas most subject to slowing or fluctuation of the flow of blood in skin capillaries; he thus sought to explain the predilection of the rash for areas over prominent tendons and bones, sites of recent injuries to the skin, and places where there is pressure from bandages, belts, ill fitting boots, and so forth. Such factors may occasionally determine local concentration of the eruption in chickenpox, but no satisfactory explanation is available for the difference in general distribution of the eruption in this disease as compared to smallpox.

The fulminant hemorrhagic cases of smallpox have often a short incubation period and from the onset of illness these patients show virus in the blood, often in large quantity, which may persist to the time of death.[28, 48, 71] The degree of viremia at onset presumably reflects great multiplication of virus in the internal organs during the incubation period. Its persistence during the febrile illness may be derived from extensive infection of vascular endothelium in capillaries of the skin and mucous membranes, and of the overlying epithelium. Histological examination of the skin and stained smears shows enormous amounts of virus in the skin in spite of the absence of macroscopically visible lesions. The hemorrhages in the skin and mucous membranes are characteristic of the severe type of disease and are presumably caused by severe damage to vascular endothelium associated with virus multiplication. The prolonged viremia in these cases is associated with the presence of soluble antigen in the blood. In a recent study of early and late hemorrhagic cases (to be published) soluble antigen was detectable in the serum of 34 of 47 patients. These patients show little evidence of resistance to their infection and neutralizing antibody is usually not detectable in the blood.[27, 82] The relatively high incidence of this variety of smallpox in pregnant women and the possible importance of hormonal factors in its genesis has been discussed by Rao et al.[76] The blood picture and severe disturbances of coagulation factors appear to result from severe involvement of the bone marrow and vascular endothelium. It has been suggested by Westwood[90] that in these acute fulminating infections death is due to a shock syndrome induced by direct toxic damage to the vascular endothelium. Clinical evidence of myocardial involvement has been noted in severe cases of smallpox[1] although Bras[12] found little evidence of this on histological examination. Little information is available from metabolic or biochemical studies on smallpox patients; patients are generally in isolation hospitals where the necessary facilities are lacking.

It was suggested by earlier workers that death in acute fulminating infections was caused by combined virus and bacterial septicemic infections. The postmortem findings of Councilman et al.[17] and the recovery of bacteria in blood cultures made during life[85] lent support to this view. However, the frequent failure to find bacteria by blood culture, the absence of evidence of concomitant bacterial infection in postmortem studies in patients treated with antibiotics,[12] and the failure of antibiotic therapy to influence the mortality in severe cases indicate that in the acute fulminating infections death is a consequence of the severe generalized virus infection alone. The occasional finding of bacteria in the blood is incidental to the general lowered resistance of the patient, and the blood invasion is a terminal event. In malignant cases of smallpox, including late hemorrhagic cases, death usually occurs in the second week of the disease. In these severe infections there is extensive involvement of the skin and little reactive inflammatory response in the tissues, for pustulation is often absent or delayed. This is often associated with a poor or delayed antibody response.[46] It seems likely that the outcome of this type of infection, as in the early hemorrhagic cases, is determined in part by the extent of virus proliferation in the tissues in the later stages of the incubation period. The mechanism by which extensive cell destruction with involvement of large skin areas determines a fatal issue is not clear. Late deaths occurring after the second week are associated with septic and other complications favored by the lower resistance induced by the virus infection.

## IMMUNITY

The resistance to smallpox varies considerably in different individuals, independently of specific immunity induced by vaccination or previous small-pox infection. This has been emphasized particularly by Dixon,[22] who notes that even in the unvaccinated all degrees of severity of illness may be encountered. It is apparent from Rao's data from Madras shown in Table 4 (p. 509) that severity may vary with age and that discrete cases in the unvaccinated patients are most likely to occur in the age group 5 to 14 years. This apparent variation in natural resistance may depend on the infecting dose of virus, which is impossible to ascertain in smallpox patients. The severity may depend on the "physiological activity" of the tissues, which may also determine the speed and magnitude of response to the virus infection. Nonspecific factors in serum or tissue fluid and production of interferon may also be concerned in resistance in the absence of specific antibody, but the importance of these factors in "natural" resistance has not been determined.

Before considering the role of specific antibody in resistance to and recovery from infection, it may be well to look for a moment at the methods used for its detection and measurement. Antibody is produced by certain cells of the lymphocyte-plasma series, and for its proper functioning in the destruction of bacteria, and probably viruses, the cooperation of cells is usually necessary. This is illustrated in the treatment of vaccinia gangrenosa with vaccinia immune globulin. This treatment is effective only in patients who have functionally active cells of the lymphoid series.[37] It is true that antibody may combine with virus and prevent its replication in susceptible cells, but active virus can be dissociated from antibody by various procedures. Heat-stable antibody by itself is not virucidal. The specific antibody activity which is measured by laboratory tests represents only the activity of the antibody-forming cells and the methods we use for its titration are at best crude. The measurement of neutralizing activity of serum, which is the best index we have of effective antibody, is usually carried out with heat-inactivated serum. It has been shown that certain nonspecific labile factors in fresh serum may greatly enhance the virus-inhibitory effect of heat-stable antibody.[63] These heat-labile factors are absent in neutralization tests as usually carried out, but may be important in the potentiation of antibody in the intact animal. Neutralization tests with variola and vaccinia viruses are usually carried out on the chick chorioallantoic membrane or in some form of tissue culture. In such systems there is usually complete absence of phagocytic cells, which may be concerned in the intact animal with the destruction and disposal of virus "sensitized" by combination with antibody; therefore our failure to detect antibody by the tests usually employed does not necessarily mean that it is not present in the serum or tissue fluids of the animals from which they were obtained. We find that in an actively immunized animal resistance to infection,

for example by intradermal challenge in skin of a rabbit or a second vaccination a week after a primary vaccination, may be apparent a day or two
earlier than antibody activity may be detectable in its blood. However, in
spite of the limitations of our techniques for measuring antibody, the use of
these techniques provides a useful indication of an immune response to the
virus under study.

In considering the immune response to vaccinia and variola viruses it can
be readily demonstrated by serum antibody titrations that the speed and
extent of antibody rise varies considerably in different individuals. Moreover,
there is also marked individual variation in the length of time that such
antibody persists. The variation in the duration of immunity can be more
directly demonstrated by the variation in susceptibility to revaccination years
after a primary take. It should perhaps not be overlooked that revaccination
may be a more severe test of immunity to smallpox than exposure to a case
of the disease. Vaccination with a primary-type take may be encountered
in persons who have suffered from clinical smallpox within ten years. A local
variolous eruption has been seen on the skin of a mother where there had been
physical contact with the eruption on a variolous child; the mother had herself
suffered from smallpox in childhood and in consequence had well marked
pitted scars on her face. The once-vaccinated person may have lost much of
his measurable serum antibody, but nonetheless is usually more resistant to
infection than the unvaccinated person. Not only does revaccination produce
a more rapid reaction and quicker healing of the local lesion, but neutralizing
antibody increases or appears more rapidly in the serum than after primary
vaccination (Fig. 3).[62]

These observations have relevance to the significance of antibody in
modifying the course of the disease. There has been a tendency in recent
years to minimize the importance of antibody in recovery from infection, and
there is no doubt that other nonspecific mechanisms may play a part. The
demonstrable effect of vaccinia immune gamma globulin, given to close family

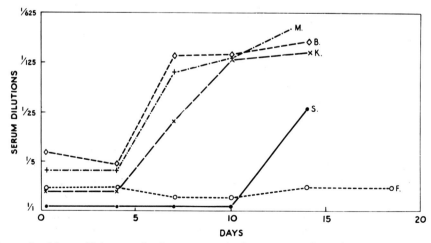

*Figure 3.* Neutralizing antibody response in five young adults following revaccination. M, B, K, and F had accelerated vaccinoid-type reaction. S had primary-type
reaction.

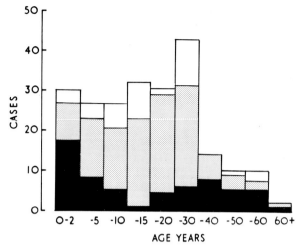

*Figure 4.* Age distribution and severity of smallpox in 220 unvaccinated persons of different ages, in Liverpool, 1902–1903. White blocks, mild cases; gray blocks, severe cases; black blocks, fatal cases. (From Hanna: Studies in Smallpox and Vaccination. J. Wright & Sons, Bristol, 1913.)

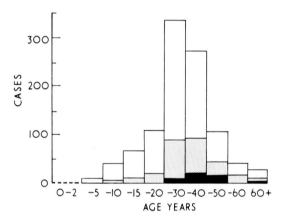

*Figure 5.* Age distribution and severity of smallpox in 943 vaccinated persons of different ages, in Liverpool, 1902–1903. (From Hanna: Studies in Smallpox and Vaccination. J. Wright & Sons, Bristol, 1913.)

contacts after exposure, in preventing or modifying the disease is evidence of its usefulness in defense against infection.[56, 57] Once the clinical illness has developed, antibody appears to have less effect. By this time virus is widely disseminated to cells in the skin and mucous membranes where it is inaccessible to the action of antibody. Antibody can act only on cell-free virus and if present in the incubation period may prevent dissemination by the blood or tissue fluids. It may be noted, however, that in experimental rabbit pox infections with a highly virulent virus, the intravenous injection of high-titred rabbit immune serum after the onset of fever saved animals which had been infected with many lethal doses of virus.[10] The effects of vaccination in protecting against smallpox is shown in the age distribution of smallpox in the vaccinated and unvaccinated (Table 4 and Figs. 4 and 5). For a variable number of years vaccinated individuals have enough antibody to protect against clinical illness. As specific immunity wanes, some individuals exposed to infection develop clinical disease which is generally milder than in the unvaccinated. In these patients the immunity response occurs more quickly after the onset of illness than in the unvaccinated. This is reflected in the earlier appearance of neutralizing antibody in the vaccinated patients.[27] Indeed the speed of antibody response may be such that following the viremia of onset, localization and growth of virus in the skin may not occur (variola sine eruptione). The diminution in the extent of the rash and the more superficial nature and rapid evolution of the lesions characteristic of modified smallpox in vaccinated persons may be attributed to the rapid production of antibody by cells "sensitized" by previous vaccination. It seems likely that in some vaccinated contacts who fail to develop the disease virus may multiply in the tissues for some days before the secondary antibody response occurs; but such response may be sufficiently rapid to inhibit virus growth before the onset of the initial illness. Recent antibody studies in smallpox contacts (unpublished) suggest that such subclinical infections do occur. Persons with these infections are of no importance in the spread of disease to their contacts.

At the other extreme some vaccinated individuals may lose their antibody completely and also the capacity of their antibody-forming tissue to respond rapidly to the stimulus of acquired infection with variola virus. Such individuals are those who respond to revaccination with a primary-type take and who develop unmodified smallpox of confluent or even hemorrhagic type on exposure. The figures in Table 3 suggest that vaccination does not protect against the hemorrhagic forms of smallpox.[75] However, when one examines

TABLE 3. *Frequency of Different Types of Smallpox in Vaccinated and Unvaccinated Patients in Madras, 1961–1967*\*

|  | VACCINATED PATIENTS | | | UNVACCINATED PATIENTS | | |
|---|---|---|---|---|---|---|
| CLINICAL VARIETY | No. Cases | Frequency % | Case Mortality % | No. Cases | Frequency % | Case Mortality % |
| Haemorrhagic | 112 | 3.3 | 93.7 | 84 | 2.4 | 96.4 |
| Flat | 46 | 1.4 | 72.5 | 230 | 6.5 | 96.5 |
| Ordinary | 2355 | 69.8 | 2.8 | 3126 | 88.9 | 30.2 |
| Modified | 862 | 25.5 | 0 | 78 | 2.2 | 0 |
| Totals | 3375 | 100.0 | 6.0 | 3518 | 100.0 | 35.5 |

\* From Smallpox Eradication, World Health Organization Technical Report Series, No. 393, 1968.

TABLE 4. *Frequency of Clinical Types with Reference to Age and Vaccinial Status in Madras, 1961–1967*\*

|  | AGE | No. OF CASES | % DISTRIBUTION OF CASES BY AGE | % INCIDENCE OF CLINICAL TYPES | | | |
|---|---|---|---|---|---|---|---|
|  |  |  |  | Haemorrhagic | Flat | Ordinary | Modified |
| Vaccinated | 0–4 | 94 | 2.8 | 1.1 | 5.3 | 57.4 | 36.2 |
|  | 5–14 | 387 | 11.5 | 1.8 | 0.5 | 59.2 | 38.5 |
|  | 15–44 | 2677 | 79.3 | 3.6 | 1.2 | 71.1 | 24.1 |
|  | 45+ | 217 | 6.4 | 3.7 | 3.2 | 77.9 | 15.2 |
| Unvaccinated | 0–4 | 2077 | 59.0 | 1.1 | 8.1 | 87.9 | 2.9 |
|  | 5–14 | 851 | 24.2 | 0.9 | 3.9 | 94.3 | 0.9 |
|  | 15–44 | 525 | 14.9 | 8.0 | 4.2 | 86.3 | 1.5 |
|  | 45+ | 65 | 1.9 | 16.9 | 10.8 | 70.8 | 1.5 |

\* From Smallpox Eradication, World Health Organization Technical Report Series, No. 393, 1968.

the data in Table 4, it is obvious that in the unvaccinated group the great majority of patients were under 4 years of age, while in the vaccinated group they were in the age group 15 to 44, when the immunity from primary vaccination in childhood had waned. The hemorrhagic forms of smallpox were much more common in the patients over the age of 15 years than in the younger age group. Table 4 shows that in the older age group the incidence of hemorrhagic smallpox, as indeed of the flat or malignant type at all ages, was greater in the unvaccinated than in the vaccinated.

There would appear to the writer to be no need to postulate the existence of three separate and distinct components of immunity—anti-invasion, antidissemination, and local skin immunity[23]—to explain the various manifestations of smallpox encountered in vaccinated and unvaccinated persons. The features of the different clinical types may be explained by the variation in the speed and extent of the immune response in the infected individual. At the moment the best measurement of this response, although it is a crude one, is obtained by the titration of neutralizing antibody in the blood of the patient.


## TRANSMISSION OF INFECTION

As there is no known animal reservoir for smallpox and chronic carriers do not exist, the source of infection is the person suffering from the disease. Transmission occurs by direct contact or indirectly through utensils, clothing, or dust infected by the patient. Spread most commonly occurs by household contact within families, although infection of laundry workers and others handling the soiled clothing or bedclothes of a patient, usually undiagnosed, has occurred in a number of outbreaks. Infected persons do not transmit the disease during the incubation period. From the public health point of view patients are regarded as potentially infectious from the onset of illness until the last scabs have separated. But epidemiological evidence suggests that patients are not usually infectious until the eruption appears, a view held by epidemiologists in the past.[44, 78] Virus could not be recovered from mouth washings of smallpox patients in the first two days of fever and was most frequently recovered from the sixth to the ninth day of illness,[30] the stage of the disease which Haygarth[44] regarded as most infectious. However, recovery of virus before the appearance of the eruption or in its absence has occasionally been reported.[8, 67, 88] From swabs of circumoral skin and pillows of smallpox patients virus usually could be recovered from the sixth to the fourteenth day of illness.[29] By the time the eruption appears on the skin large amounts of virus are present in the lower epithelial layers of skin but the impermeable nature of the upper layers of the epidermis prevents virus from reaching the surface until rupture of vesicles or pustules occurs at a later stage. In the mouth, nose, and nasopharynx there is no such impermeable covering of mucous membranes and the early erosion of lesions ensures heavy contamination of the saliva and mucous secretions. Patients with the acute fulminating form, in whom bleeding from mucous membranes may occur soon after the onset of illness, may be infectious throughout the febrile illness.[83] In the early eruptive phase of the disease, infection is derived from virus in the saliva and upper respiratory secretions, and only later from the skin lesions. Because of its resistant nature, potentially infective virus may persist in clothing or dust for weeks. Immune contacts may possibly carry virus on their clothing but the more dangerous source of virus dissemination is the vaccinated person whose immunity has waned and whose smallpox infection is so mild that medical help is not sought or the illness is mistaken for varicella. This has been a feature of several of the outbreaks which have occurred since the war in several European countries as a result of importations from abroad. The outbreak in London, 1957, is illustrative.[49] Diagnosis of smallpox was first established on June 28. Extensive enquiries were made to trace the source of infection and the following facts were elicited. *Case 1:* Well vaccinated male returned from Nigeria on March 29 and became ill on April 11 of an illness diagnosed as chickenpox. *Case 2:* His daughter, aged 8, vaccinated in infancy, became ill on April 25, and this was diagnosed as chickenpox (second attack). *Case 3:* Unvaccinated brother of Case 1, whom he visited on May 1, became sick on May 13 and died four days later of acute illness diagnosed as acute leukemia—necropsy in hospital (? May 18) and specimens sent to laboratory. *Case 4:* Laboratory cleaner at this hospital, vaccinated in childhood, became sick June 8 of illness diagnosed as chickenpox. *Case 5:* Grandson of Case 4, unvaccinated, became ill June 22; the diagnosis of smallpox was made June 26, and the patient died July 5. *Case 6:* Daughter of Case 4, vaccinated in childhood, became ill June 25 and later was confirmed as a case of smallpox. By the time the diagnosis of smallpox was confirmed in Case 5, and subsequently in Cases 4 and 6, it was impossible to establish with certainty that Cases 1, 2, and 3 were indeed smallpox, but the careful epidemiological inquiries and clinical histories strongly indicated that the spread of infection was as noted here. Not only does the outbreak illustrate how modified smallpox may be wrongly diagnosed as chickenpox and fulminating cases as leukemia, but it also indicates how slowly the disease may spread. In the greater London area between April 11 and June 27 there were apparently four undetected cases of smallpox, each one apparently giving rise to only one other case. Smallpox does not have the epidemic potential of influenza and is less contagious than measles or chickenpox. The incubation period of 12 days and the low infectivity of the patient during the preeruptive illness are features that facilitate control of spread in the community by isolation of cases, surveillance and vaccination of contacts, and other preventive measures.

In variola minor the spread of infection from cases occurs in the same manner as in variola major. But control of the milder disease is not so readily effected; notification is apt to be less complete and missed cases, ambulant while still infectious, tend to prolong outbreaks. Many outbreaks of variola major which resulted in Britain after World War II through importations from endemic areas in Asia and Africa were fairly quickly controlled by energetic preventive measures, so that outbreaks were limited in extent. On the other hand, the outbreak of variola minor in Lancashire in 1951–1952 lasted for four and a half months with over 140 cases.

## CONTROL OF SMALLPOX

It is not intended here to go into detail but merely to indicate, in general, the methods which are being followed to control the spread of the disease. As in other infections liable to epidemic spread, control measures may be directed to interrupting the chain of transmission or to rendering a population immune by immunization with an effective vaccine. Both methods are used to a varying extent depending on the situation in a particular country, i.e., whether the disease is endemic or not.

The countries of Europe, North and Central America, Africa north of the Sahara, Australia, New Zealand, and some countries of Asia are presently free from endemic smallpox (Fig. 9, p. 515). In these nonendemic countries, control may be effected by attempting to exclude the disease by quarantine measures and by requiring valid vaccination certificates of all those entering from countries where smallpox is known to exist. This by itself is rarely effective, for vaccination certificates may be fraudulently obtained, and while examination for vaccination scars is more useful in determining whether an immigrant has been vaccinated or not, it is not possible to tell from such scars the approximate date of vaccination. Moreover, the history of outbreaks in Europe during the last 30 years has clearly shown that vaccinated persons may enter a country from an endemic area and develop illness some days later. The control of smallpox introduced to a smallpox-free country in this way depends on an efficient public service and is based on (1) the detection and isolation of cases which occur, (2) the vaccination of contacts and their surveillance for a period of at least 16 days following last contact, and (3) disinfection of the patient's room or house after his removal to an isolation hospital. Vaccination should be carried out by the expanding-ring method,[95] attention being given primarily to close family and household contacts. Some of the nonendemic countries require by law that all children be vaccinated against smallpox and some countries require that this vaccination be repeated at intervals of five to 10 years to maintain the level of immunity in the general population. This is difficult administratively and is expensive. Moreover, the complications that may result from universal vaccination of children and adolescents may be more serious than the risks of imported smallpox.[55] As shown in Table 3, about half the patients with smallpox admitted to the infectious diseases hospital in Madras bore scars from vaccination in infancy; to ensure a protective immunity in any population would require revaccination every three or five years. It has been argued that vaccination in infancy only is of limited value in preventing the spread of smallpox[20] and that in nonendemic areas free from the constant risk of importation of the disease from neighboring countries the disease can be effectively controlled by the preventive measures, including vaccination of contacts, just outlined. It has been suggested by those who favor universal vaccination that the disease might spread explosively in a completely unprotected population, but we have no evidence to support this. In the years prior to the introduction of prophylactic inoculation against smallpox in England the disease did not occur in explosive epidemic fashion.

In the endemic areas of the world the situation is rather different and much effort, supported by the World Health Organization, is now being directed toward the eradication of smallpox on a global basis. If such a fortunate result were finally achieved, vaccination with its associated risks would no longer be necessary anywhere. In the endemic areas, because of the high risk of infection and usually poorly developed public health services, universal vaccination and revaccination of all the population is necessary every five years, special attention being paid to the vaccination of nomadic or migrant groups and vaccination of all new additions to the population through births or immigration. This is a very large undertaking in the heavily populated endemic areas, such as India, Pakistan, and Indonesia. It requires a well organized program carried out by teams of well trained public health officers, vaccinators, and inspectors and a plentiful supply of active freeze-dried vaccine of high potency. It requires further a complete registration of the population and of births in each area and this is often lacking. This program of vaccination has to be supplemented by a good detecting and reporting system so that the occurrence of smallpox cases can be quickly known and containment measures quickly taken to stamp out local outbreaks as they occur. A program of eradication was started in most of the Indian states in 1963 and 1964 but the reported incidence of smallpox has not fallen since then. Many of the defects in the carrying out of the program have been pointed out by Gelfand[38] and steps to remedy past deficiencies are now being planned with the help of

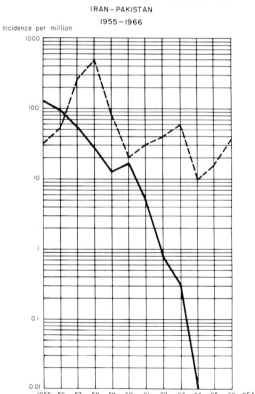

*Figure 6.* Graph showing virtual abolition of smallpox from Iran following well planned and well executed smallpox eradication campaign.

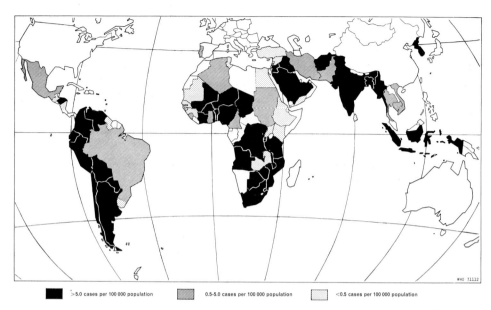

>5.0 cases per 100 000 population    0.5-5.0 cases per 100 000 population    <0.5 cases per 100 000 population

\* No reports received from China (mainland), Kuwait, Liberia, Morocco, Muscat and Oman, Nepal, Panama, Qatar, South-West Africa, Trucial Oman, and Yemen.

*Figure 7.* Smallpox incidence in endemic countries in 1950. (From W.H.O. Chronicle, 1968, *22*:134–141.)

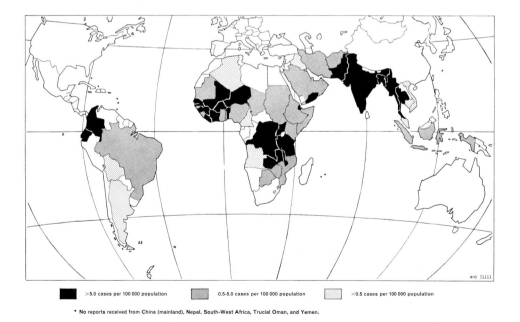

>5.0 cases per 100 000 population    0.5-5.0 cases per 100 000 population    <0.5 cases per 100 000 population

\* No reports received from China (mainland), Nepal, South-West Africa, Trucial Oman, and Yemen.

*Figure 8.* Smallpox incidence in endemic countries in 1959. (From W.H.O. Chronicle, 1968, *22*:134–141.)

W.H.O. That smallpox may be controlled and virtually abolished from a country by a well planned program energetically carried through has been demonstrated by the dramatic fall in incidence of smallpox in Iran (Fig. 6) following a vigorous nationwide vaccination campaign begun in 1955, and repeated in 1960. Success has also been achieved in certain other countries in South America, Asia, and parts of Africa where endemic smallpox has been absent for the last few years (Figs. 7, 8, and 9). The administration of vaccinia immune gamma globulin[56, 57] or methisazone[3] to close family contacts who have not recently been vaccinated may be of value in preventing the occurrence or lessening the severity of disease in such contacts. Insofar as these measures prevent secondary cases they may lessen the sources of infection and so contribute to control of spread, but they must be regarded as ancillary to and not a substitute for energetic vaccination of contacts.

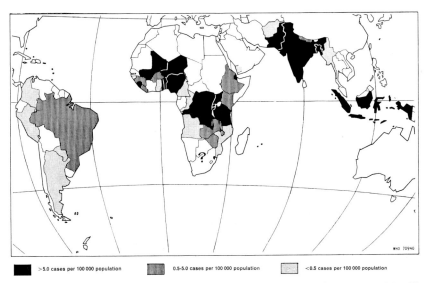

■ >5.0 cases per 100 000 population    ▦ 0.5-5.0 cases per 100 000 population    ▨ <0.5 cases per 100 000 population

*Figure 9.*  Smallpox incidence in endemic countries in 1966. (From W.H.O. Chronicle, 1968, *22:*134–141.)

# References

1. Anderson, T., M. A. Foulis, N. R. Grist, and J. B. Landsman. 1951. Clinical and laboratory observations in a smallpox outbreak. Lancet *1:*1248–1251.
2. Ballard, E. 1868. On Vaccination. Its Value and Alleged Dangers. Longmans, Green & Co., London.
3. Bauer, D. J. 1965. Clinical experience with the antiviral drug Marboran (1-methylisatin β-thiosemicarbazone) Ann. N.Y. Acad. Sci. *130:*110–117.
4. Bedson, H. S., and M. J. Duckworth. 1963. Rabbit pox: An experimental study of the pathways of infection in rabbits. J. Path. Bact. *85:*1–20.
5. Bedson, H. S., and K. R. Dumbell. 1961. The effect of temperature on the growth of pox viruses in the chick embryo. J. Hyg. *59:*457–469.
6. Bedson, H. S., and K. R. Dumbell. 1964. Hybrids derived from the viruses of variola major and cowpox. J. Hyg. *62:*147–158.
7. Berger, K. 1956. Kuhpockenvirus und Vaccinevirus. Z. Hyg. *143:*151–158.
8. Bingel, K. F., and F. Kruse. 1959. Methoden und Ergebnisse des virolgischen und serologischen Untersuchungen bei der Pockenerkrankungen in Heidelberg (Dezember 1958–Januar 1959). Medizinische No. 20, pp. 961–969.

9. Blake, J. B. 1953. Smallpox inoculation in colonial Boston. J. Hist. Med. *8:*284–300.

10. Boulter, E. A., J. C. N. Westwood, and H. B. Maber. 1961. Value of serotherapy in a virus disease (rabbit pox). Lancet *2:*1012–1015.

11. Braband, H. 1964. Pocken-osteomyelitis. Zbl. Bakt. [Orig.] *195:*35–40.

12. Bras, G. 1952. The morbid anatomy of smallpox. Docum. Med. Geog. Trop. *4:*303–351.

13. Burnet, F. M. 1945. Virus as Organism. Harvard University Press, Cambridge, Mass., p. 80.

14. Caunt, A. E., C. J. M. Rondle, and A. W. Downie. 1961. The soluble antigens of varicella-zoster virus produced in tissue culture. J. Hyg. *59:*249–258.

15. Cockshott, W. P. 1965. Osteomyelitis variolosa. Z. Tropenmed. Parasit. *16:*199–206.

16. Conybeare, E. T. 1939. Illness occurring in contacts with confluent smallpox. Lancet *1:*813–815.

17. Councilman, W. T., G. B. Magrath, and W. R. Brinkerhoff. 1904. The pathological anatomy and histology of variola. J. Med. Res. *11:*12–135.

18. Creighton, C. 1894. A History of Epidemics in Britain. Vol. 2. Cambridge University Press, Cambridge, pp. 434–631.

19. Dekking, F., A. R. Rao, L. St. Vincent, and C. H. Kempe. 1967. The weeping mother, an unusual source of variola virus. Arch. Ges. Virusforsch. *22:*215–218.

20. Dick, G. W. A. 1962. Prevention of virus diseases in the community. Brit. Med. J. *2:*1275–1280.

21. Dimsdale, T. 1781. Tracts on Inoculation Written and Published at St. Petersburg, 1768, with Additional Observations. James Phillips, London.

22. Dixon, C. W. 1948. Smallpox in Tripolitania, 1946; an epidemiological and clinical study of 500 cases, including trials of penicillin treatment. J. Hyg. *46:*351–377.

23. Dixon, C. W. 1962. Smallpox. Churchill, London, p. 512.

24. Downie, A. W. 1939. The immunological relationship of the virus of spontaneous cowpox to vaccinia virus. Brit. J. Exp. Path. *20:*158–176.

25. Downie, A. W. 1965. The Poxvirus Group. In Viral and Rickettsial Diseases of Man, Eds. Horsfall, F. L., and I. Tamm. J. B. Lippincott Co., Philadelphia, pp. 932–964.

26. Downie, A. W., and K. McCarthy. 1950. The viruses of variola, vaccinia, cowpox and ectromelia. Neutralization tests on the chorio-allantois with unabsorbed and absorbed immune sera. Brit. J. Exp. Path. *31:*789–796.

27. Downie, A. W., and K. McCarthy. 1958. The antibody response in man following infection with viruses of the pox group. Antibody response in smallpox. J. Hyg. *56:*479–487.

28. Downie, A. W., K. McCarthy, A. Macdonald, F. O. MacCallum, and A. D. Macrae. 1953. Virus and virus antigen in the blood of smallpox patients. Their significance in early diagnosis and prognosis. Lancet *2:*164–166.

29. Downie, A. W., G. Meiklejohn, L. St. Vincent, A. R. Rao, B. V. Sundara Babu, and C. H. Kempe. 1965. The recovery of smallpox virus from patients and their environment in a smallpox hospital. Bull. WHO *33:*615–622.

30. Downie, A. W., L. St. Vincent, G. Meiklejohn, N. R. Ratnakanan, A. R. Rao, G. N. V. Krishman, and C. H. Kempe. 1961. Studies on the virus content of mouth washings in the acute phase of smallpox. Bull. WHO *25:*49–53.

31. Duguid, J. D. 1946. The size and the duration of air-carriage of respiratory droplets and droplet-nuclei. J. Hyg. *44:*471–479.

32. Eeckels, R., J. Vincent, and V. Seynhaeve. 1964. Bone lesions due to smallpox. Arch. Dis. Child. *39:*591–597.

33. Evans, W. H. M., and H. M. Foreman. 1963. Smallpox handlers lung. Proc. Roy. Soc. Med. *56:*274–275.

34. Fenner, F. 1948. The clinical features and pathogenesis of mousepox (infectious ectromelia of mice). J. Path. Bact. *60:*529–552.

35. Fenner, F. 1962. The Leeuwenhoek Lecture. Interactions between pox viruses. Proc. Roy. Soc. [Biol.] *156:*388–414.

36. Fenner, F., and B. M. Comben. 1958. Genetic studies with mammalian pox viruses. 1. Demonstration of recombination between two strains of vaccinia viruses. Virology *5:*530–548.

37. Fulginiti, V. A., C. H. Kempe, W. E. Hathaway, D. S. Pearlman, O. Sieber, J. J. Eller, J. W. Joyner, and A. Robinson. 1968. Progressive vaccinia in immunologically-deficient individuals. Proceedings of Third Developmental Immunology Workshop on Immunologic Deficiency Diseases of Man, National Foundation Birth Defects Series, 1968.

38. Gelfand, H. M. 1966. A critical review of the Indian smallpox eradication program. Amer. J. Public Health *56:*1634–1651.

39. Gispen, R. 1955. Analysis of pox virus antigens by means of double diffusion. A method for direct serological differentiation of cowpox. J. Immun. *74:*134–141.

40. Gispen, R., J. D. Verlinde, and P. Zwart. 1967. Histopathological and virological studies on monkey pox. Arch. Ges. Virusforsch. *21*:205–216.
41. Hahon, N. 1958. Cytopathogenicity and propagation of variola virus in tissue culture. J. Immun. *81*:426–432.
42. Hahon, N., and B. J. Wilson. 1959. Pathogenesis of variola in *Macaca iris* monkeys. Amer. J. Hyg. *71*:69–80.
43. Hanna, W. 1913. Studies in Smallpox and Vaccination. J. Wright & Sons, Bristol.
44. Haygarth, J. 1785. An Enquiry How to Prevent Smallpox. J. Johnson, Chester, pp. 42 and 43.
45. Haygarth, J. 1793. A Sketch of a Plan to Exterminate the Casual Smallpox from Great Britain. Vol. 1. J. Johnson, London, pp. 138–142.
46. Herrlich, A., A. Mayr, and H. Mahnel. 1959. Das Antikörperbild der Variola-Vaccineinfektion. 2. Serologische Untersuchungen an Variolapatienten. Zbl. Bakt. [Orig.] *175*: 163–182.
47. Herrlich, A., A. Mayr, H. Mahnel, and E. Muntz. 1963. Experimental studies on transformation of the variola virus into the vaccinia virus. Arch. Ges. Virusforsch. *12*:579–599.
48. Herrlich, A., A. Mayr, and E. Muntz. 1967. Die Pocken. Ed. 2. G. Thieme, Stuttgart, pp. 1–360.
49. Hogben, G. H., G. D. W. McKendrick, and C. G. Nicol. 1958. Smallpox in Tottenham 1957. Lancet *1*:1061–1064.
50. Horgan, E. S., and M. A. Haseeb. 1939. Cross immunity experiments in monkeys between variola, alastrim and vaccinia. J. Hyg. *39*:615–639.
51. Howat, H. T, and W. M. Arnott. 1944. Outbreak of pneumonia in smallpox contacts. Lancet *2*:312.
52. Ikeda, K. 1925. The blood in purpuric smallpox. Clinical review of forty-eight cases. J.A.M.A. *84*:1807–1813.
53. Jenner, E. 1798. An enquiry into the causes and effects of the variolae vaccinae, a disease discovered in some of the western countries of England, particularly Gloucestershire, and known by the name of cowpox. Reprinted by Cassell and Co. Ltd., London, 1896.
54. de Jong, M. 1956. The alastrim epidemic in the Hague, 1953–1954. Docum. Med. Geog. Trop. *8*:207–235.
55. Kempe, C. H., and A. S. Benenson. 1965. Smallpox immunization in the United States. J.A.M.A. *194*:161–166.
56. Kempe, C. H., T. O. Berge, and B. England. 1956. Hyperimmune vaccinal gamma globulin. Source, evaluation and use in prophylaxis and therapy. Pediatrics, *18*:177–188.
57. Kempe, C. H., C. Bowles, G. Meiklejohn, T. O. Berge, L. St. Vincent, B. V. Sundara Babu, S. Govindarajan, N. R. Ratnakanan, A. W. Downie, and V. R. Murthy. 1961 . The use of vaccinia hyperimmune gamma globulin in the prophylaxis of smallpox. Bull. WHO *25*:41–48.
58. Lancaster, M. C., E. A. Boulter, J. C. N. Westwood, and J. Randles. 1966. Experimental respiratory infection with pox viruses. II. Pathological studies. Brit. J. Exp. Path. *47*: 466–471.
59. Leroux, Amphoux, Billaud, Bouillaud, G. Cadoret, Delord, Y. Duhamel, Lobrichon, Baldrich, and Audouy. 1955. Epidémie de variole à Vannes de décembre 1954-mars 1955. Presse Méd. *63*:639–642.
60. Liu, C., and D. L. Coffin. 1957. Studies on canine distemper infection by means of fluorescein-labelled antibody. The pathogenesis, pathology and diagnosis of the disease in experimentally infected ferrets. Virology *3*:115–131.
61. McCarthy, K., and A. W. Downie. 1948. An investigation of immunological relationships between the viruses of variola, vaccinia, cowpox and ectromelia by neutralization tests on the chorioallantois of chick embryos. Brit. J. Exp. Path. *29*:501–510.
62. McCarthy, K., A. W. Downie, and W. H. Bradley. 1958. The antibody response in man following infection with viruses of the pox group. 2. Antibody response following vaccination. J. Hyg. *56*:466–478.
63. McCarthy, K., and W. D. Germer. 1952. Two heat-labile factors in normal sera which neutralize variola virus. Brit. J. Exp. Path. *33*:529–536.
64. McCarthy, K., and D. Helbert. 1960. A comparison of the hemagglutinins of variola, alastrim, vaccinia, cowpox and ectromelia viruses. J. Path. Bact. *79*:416–418.
65. McKenzie, P. J., J. H. Githens, M. E. Harwood, J. F. Roberts, A. R. Rao, and C. H. Kempe. 1965. Haemorrhagic smallpox. 2. Specific bleeding and coagulation studies. Bull. WHO *33*:773–782.
66. Magrath, G. B., and W. R. Brinkerhoff. 1904. On the occurrence of Cytorrhyctes variolae, Guarnieri, in the skin of the monkey inoculated with variola virus. J. Med. Res. *11*:173–179.

67. Marennikova, S. S., E. B. Gurvich, and M. A. Yumasheva. 1963. Laboratory diagnosis of smallpox and similar viral diseases by means of tissue culture methods. 1. Sensitivity of tissue culture methods in the detection of variola virus. Acta Virol. *7:*124–130.

68. Marsden, J. P. 1948. Variola minor. A personal analysis of 13,686 cases. Bull. Hyg. *23:*735–746.

69. Marsden, J. P., and C. R. M. Greenfield. 1934. Inherited smallpox. Arch. Dis. Child. *9:*309–314.

70. Miller, G. 1957. The adoption of inoculation of smallpox in England and France. University of Pennsylvania Press, Philadelphia.

71. Mitra, A. C., S. N. Chatterjee, J. K. Sarkar, P. Manji, and A. K. Das. 1966. Viraemia in haemorrhagic and other forms of smallpox. J. Indian Med. Assoc. *47:*112–114.

72. Moore, J. 1815. The History of the Smallpox. Longeman, Hurst, Rees, Orme and Brown, London.

73. Nicoli, J., and C. Jolibois. 1964. Antigènes solubles des "Pox virus". Etude des antigènes solubles variolique et vaccinal. Ann. Inst. Pasteur *107:*374–383.

74. Pirsch, J. B., L. A. Mika, and E. H. Purlson. 1963. Growth characteristics of variola virus in tissue culture. J. Infect. Dis. *113:*170–178.

75. Rao, A. R. 1964. Haemorrhagic smallpox. A study of 240 cases. J. Indian Med. Assoc. *43:*224–229.

76. Rao, A. R., I. Prahlad, M. Swaminatham, and A. Lakshmi. 1963. Pregnancy and smallpox. J. Indian Med. Assoc. *40:*353–363.

77. Razzell, P. E. 1965. Edward Jenner. The history of a medical myth. Med. Hist. *9:*216–229.

78. Ricketts, T. F., and J. B. Byles, 1908. The Diagnosis of Smallpox. Cassell & Co., London, p. 154.

79. Roberts, J. A. 1962. Histopathogenesis of mousepox. 1. Respiratory infection. Brit. J. Exp. Path. *43:*451–461.

80. Roberts, J. F., G. Coffee, S. M. Creel, A. Gaal, J. H. Githens, A. R. Rao, B. V. Sundara Babu, and C. H. Kempe. Haemorrhagic smallpox. 1. Preliminary haematological studies. Bull WHO *33:*607–613.

81. Rondle, C. J. M., and K. R. Dumbell. 1962. Antigens of cowpox virus. J. Hyg. *60:*41–49.

82. Sarkar, J. K., S. N. Chatterjee, A. C. Mitra, and A. Mondal. 1967. Antibody response in haemorrhagic smallpox. Indian J. Med. Res. *55:*1143–1149.

83. Stallybras, C. O. 1931. The Principles of Epidemiology and the Process of Infection. Routledge & Son, London, pp. 329 and 339.

84. Su, T. L. 1944. Smallpox in Kweilen, Kwangsi, 1940–41. An epidemiological and clinical study. Indian Med. Gaz. *79:*332–337.

85. Sweitzer, S. E., and K. Ikeda. 1927. Variola. A clinical study of the Minneapolis epidemic of 1924–25. Arch. Dermat. Syph. *15:*19–29.

86. Taylor, W. P., W. Plowright, R. Pillinger, C. S. Rampton, and R. F. Staple. 1965. Studies on the pathogenesis of rinderpest in cattle. 4. Proliferation of the virus following contact infection. J. Hyg. *63:*497–506.

87. Torres, C. M. 1935–36. Further studies on the pathology of alastrim and their significance in the variola-alastrim problem. Proc. Roy. Soc. Med. *29:*1525–1540.

88. Verlinde, J. D., and H. A. E. Van Tongeren. 1952. Isolation of smallpox virus from the nasopharynx of patients with variola sine eruptione. Antonie Leeuwenhoek *18:*109–112.

89. Wenner, H. A., F. D. Macasaet, P. S. Kamitsuka, and P. Kidd. 1968. Monkey pox. 1. Clinical, virologic and immunologic studies. Amer. J. Epidem. *87:*551–566.

90. Westwood, J. C. N. 1963. Virus pathogenicity. In Mechanisms of Virus Infection. Ed. Smith, W. Academic Press, New York, pp. 255–307.

91. Westwood, J. C. N., E. A. Boulter, E. T. W. Bowen, and H. B. Maber. 1966. Experimental respiratory infection with pox viruses. 1. Clinical, virological and epidemiological studies. Brit. J. Exp. Path. *47:*453–465.

92. Wittmann, G., and A. Mayr. 1960. Experimentelle Untersuchungen über die Immunität bei Hühnerpocken und bei Berücksichtigung der Schutzimpfung. Zbl. Bakt. [Orig.] *177:*518–541.

93. Wood, W. B. 1959. The genesis of fever in infectious disease. In Immunity and Virus Infection. Ed. Najjar, V. A. John Wiley & Sons, New York, pp. 144–162.

94. Woodville, W. 1796. The History of the Inoculation of the Smallpox in Great Britain. James Phillips, London.

95. World Health Organization Expert Committee on Smallpox. 1964. WHO Technical Report Series No. 283. Geneva.

# Chapter 22

# POLIOMYELITIS

(Infantile Paralysis)

JOHN R. PAUL

*Yale University School of Medicine,*
*New Haven, Connecticut*

No account of poliomyelitis[1] would be adequate today without mention of the decline in the incidence of this disease in the United States and many another civilized country, to the extent that it has now almost reached the vanishing point (Figs. 1 and 2). Indeed, when and where inactivated or attenuated poliovirus vaccines have been used efficiently, the reduction in the incidence of paralytic poliomyelitis has been little short of miraculous. From the time that the inactivated (Salk-type) poliovirus vaccine was first introduced in 1955, this incidence has undergone a sharp decline so that from a maximum of about 25,000 paralytic cases a year in the United States, the total has dropped to less than 100 in recent years (Fig. 2). No wonder the public has felt that this is a cause for relief, and the parents of young children would be happy if they never heard about "polio" again.

This does not mean that this disease has promptly gone the way of diphtheria and scarlet fever, for it is still common in certain parts of the world. And yet, if only because the advances recently made in poliomyelitis were achieved with such difficulty, and because so many false leads were followed before the right path was found, a description of sorts would seem indicated.

The main feature which has dominated the public image of poliomyelitis from the beginning is the disability which this infection has sometimes caused. The spectacle illustrated on many a fund-raising campaign of a brave but paralyzed little child, boldly attempting his first steps with steel braces attached to his legs, is a familiar one, and this picture has had a well-nigh irresistible

---

1. A more detailed description of polioviruses and the disease poliomyelitis, with a far more complete list of references, will be found in Bodian, D., and Horstmann, D. M.: Poliomyelitis. *In:* Viral and Rickettsial Infections of Man, 4th edition, edited by Horsfall and Tamm. Philadephia, J. B. Lippincott Co., 1965.

ANNUAL POLIOMYELITIS INCIDENCE RATES
UNITED STATES, 1935-1965.  CASES PER 100,000 POPULATION

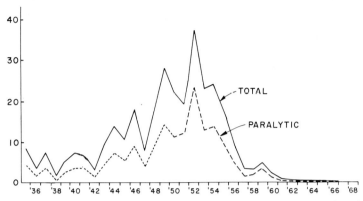

*Figure 1.* Annual poliomyelitis incidence rates, United States, 1935–1965. Source: National Morbidity Reports. (Data recorded from Poliomyelitis Surveillance Reports, National Communicable Disease Center, Atlanta, Georgia.)

PARALYTIC  POLIOMYELITIS  CASES  U.S.A. , 1961-1965

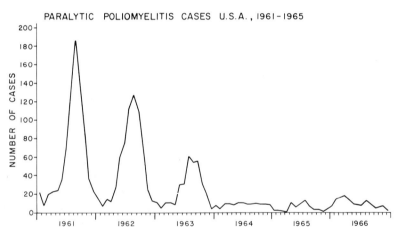

*Figure 2.* Numbers of paralytic poliomyelitis cases in the United States, 1961–1966. Source: National Morbidity Reports. (Data recorded from Neurotropic Viral Diseases Surveillance—Poliomyelitis, National Communicable Disease Center, Atlanta, Georgia, July 31, 1967.)

appeal. Thus the erroneous idea was built up that *all* poliomyelitis patients suffer in this manner. Almost every name descriptive of poliomyelitis or its causative viruses has been derived from the debility with which the disease has been inextricably associated. And yet, by paying too close attention to lesions in the central nervous system and to neuromuscular disability, it was inevitable that the true nature of the disease was overlooked. Thus the fact that 95 per cent of human poliovirus infections begin and end as systemic (generally inapparent) infections was for a long time obscured. By far the majority of infections seldom reach beyond the alimentary tract and the lymphatic system; extensive damage to the central nervous system occurs only in a very small fraction. But naturally enough, by continued application to the details of the lesions in the central nervous system, their neuropathology and neurophysiology, and the resultant paralysis and atrophy of muscles, too much emphasis has been placed on these, the most serious features of the disease. It was not surprising that this resulted in a loss of perspective about poliomyelitis and considerable confusion about the actual nature of the infection.

Indeed it was not until clinical and microbiological investigators began to realize that in order to deal with the true pathogenesis of the infection caused by polioviruses they must examine its systemic aspects. This was what led eventually to the control of the disease; and this is what will be the concern of this article, which deals essentially with systemic host reactions between poliovirus and the individual as well as reactions between the virus and the community.

Incidentally, an account of poliomyelitis as a specific disease is no longer completely accurate, for in recent years the enterovirus family (which includes polioviruses) has been enlarged to include Coxsackie viruses and echoviruses, and it has become apparent that these agents can also on rare occasions cause a clinical *syndrome* resembling poliomyelitis. It thus seems reasonable to deal with poliomyelitis in terms of polioviruses, but at the same time with an awareness that other agents may behave similarly and induce identical clinical signs and symptoms.

# HISTORY OF POLIOVIRUSES[2]

Although the question as to whether poliomyelitis is an infectious disease was challenged prior to 1900, history was made in 1908, when Landsteiner and Popper[3] discovered the etiological agent to be a virus. This occurred at a time when very few viruses related to human diseases had been identified. The main reason that Landsteiner and Popper were so quickly convinced of the validity of their discovery was that the experimental infection in the monkey provided such an extraordinary resemblance to paralytic poliomyelitis in man. However, this comparison was not without its drawbacks, because for more than 25 years investigators were so captivated by experimental poliomyelitis in the monkey as something they could work upon in the laboratory that they almost completely abandoned attempts to pursue clinical investigation and to study poliovirus infections in man. Furthermore it was during this period that investigators became obsessed with the idea that the virus penetrated the brain early in the disease, having supposedly invaded directly via a nasal portal of entry; as a result they abandoned all consideration that the alimentary or other routes of infection might be involved. Also they were convinced that the poliovirus family existed in the form of only one strain,

---

2. The term *poliovirus* as an unhyphenated word was introduced by the Virus Subcommittee of the International Nomenclature Committee in 1955. (see von Magnus, H., Gear, J. H. S., and Paul, J. R.: Virology, *1*:185–9, 1955).

3. Landsteiner, K., and Popper, H.: Wien. Klin. Wschr., *21*:1830, 1908.

although differences in virulence and neurotropism for the monkey were admitted. The idea that there was a family of three types of poliovirus was not fully established until 40 or more years after the initial discovery of the virus. Needless to say, this caused an immense amount of confusion among microbiologists and immunologists during the first part of the twentieth century.

It was not until the work of Burnet and Macnamara in 1931 that this situation began to be clarified.[4] By 1933, at least two types of antigenically different polioviruses had been recognized, but not until 1949 was the classification into three types established by a Committee on Typing set up by the National Foundation for Infantile Paralysis. All so-called wild strains so far recovered from patients in nature have been shown to belong to serotype I, II, or III. Indeed it is fortunate that the family of polioviruses is so small, compared with the size of some viral tribes, such as the rhinovirus and adenovirus families. Some degree of crossing or heterogeneity exists between the three types; this indicates a common antigen within the poliovirus family, at least between types I and II, and II and III, but it is insufficient to affect the concept of type-specific human immunity. Second paralytic attacks caused by different serotypes have occurred, but second paralytic attacks of poliomyelitis in man due to the same type of poliovirus must be very rare indeed. Repeated inapparent infections due to the same type may occasionally occur.

The type-specific portion of polioviruses resides in the RNA moiety but the property of type-specificity has a more complicated structure. Two distinct antigens have been identified for each poliovirus serotype: the "D" antigen which sediments at 160S and is associated with the complete virus particle, and the "C" antigen which sediments at 80S and is associated with particles lacking RNA.

Until about 1940 it was maintained that viruses never or only very rarely invaded the intestinal tract of man. This was obviously an erroneous idea, and was repudiated when it gradually became clear that poliomyelitis is an infection which involves *primarily* the alimentary tract. When, in 1948, the huge family of enteroviruses other than poliovirus[5] began to enter the picture, it was found that the number of agents which inhabit the alimentary tract transiently, but strangely enough produce no lesions of any major significance there, is larger than was previously thought. These enteroviruses and the illnesses they cause are described in Chapter 24 of this book. They share a common epidemiology with poliovirus infections.

Details of the physical and chemical properties of polioviruses can be found in accounts in *Viral and Rickettsial Infections of Man* (see footnote 1) or in other reliable texts on virology. Suffice it to say here that in material purified to the crystalline state the virus particles are of small size, being of the order of 29 m$\mu$ in diameter. A further analysis of purified polio-

---

4. Burnet, F. M., and Macnamara, J.: Brit. J. Exp. Path., *12*:57, 1931.

5. In recent years the enteroviruses—poliovirus, Coxsackie virus and echoviruses—have been combined by taxonomists into one group and classified along with the rhinoviruses under the name *picornaviruses*, which is where they will rest for the present. The derivation of this word is from *pico* implying small size, followed by the initials RNA to indicate that these are RNA viruses.

virus has revealed a composition of 20 to 25 per cent RNA, which forms the core of the virus particle, the shell being composed of protein. The absence of lipid, a property shared by all enteroviruses, accounts for the fact that these agents resist the action of ether, chloroform, bile, and detergents. This property has been put to practical use countless times as a means of differentiating polioviruses from certain other families of viruses.

## Host Range in Vertebrates Other than Man

This biologic property is of less importance than it was once thought to be. Originally man and some of the other primates were considered to be the only animals susceptible to infection by polioviruses, but in 1939 Armstrong made a signal advance when he adapted the Lansing strain of poliovirus (subsequently identified as a Type II strain) to the cotton rat and thence to mice. This was an accomplishment which enormously increased the usefulness of this strain in immunological research and in the study of experimental poliomyelitis. Subsequently laboratory strains of all three serotypes were adapted to rodents; a Type II strain has also been adapted to suckling hamsters and even to embryonated hen's eggs. But there is no escaping the fact that the basic and natural host of polioviruses is man. The questionable privilege of high susceptibility is shared to a certain degree by the chimpanzee and to a lesser extent by a number of species of monkeys; but the proper subject, and the most difficult one, for the study of host reactions to the poliovirus family remains *Homo sapiens,* and this is the subject on which the author has tried to concentrate his attention in this article.

## Poliomyelitis-like Diseases of Animals

A number of viruses exist in native mammalian hosts which resemble human poliovirus in their behavior, although not one of them has a cross-immunity reaction with the human poliovirus family. The most famous of these agents is the virus of *encephalomyelitis of mice* discovered by Theiler in 1934 (the TO virus). This murine virus has been cleverly used by Dr. Herdis von Magnus of Copenhagen, Denmark, as a model for investigating the epidemiology and pathogenesis of poliovirus infections,[6] although the significance of her contributions has been largely overlooked. She found that all mouse colonies she tested were naturally contaminated with TO virus, and, correspondingly, a great majority of mice acquired their immunity to this infection at an early age. But she took pains to build up a colony which was free from TO virus and discovered that in such a virus-free colony the young mice were 10 to 250 times more susceptible to TO infection than young mice in the ordinary TO-infected colony. This observation provides abundant food for thought, if one is given the privilege of switching from mice to men. To substitute the human scene at the dawn of the sanitary age, a time when the slogan prevailed that "cleanliness is next to godliness," perhaps it was the "most godly" populations that became relatively virus-free and

6. von Magnus, H.: Acta Path. Microbiol. Scand. (Separatum), *27*:605–610, 611–624, 1950.

therefore had their resistance lowered in much the same manner as did the mice in the TO-free colonies which von Magnus established experimentally. It is possible that increased susceptibility so derived was the basic reason that such a sharp increase in the incidence of human poliomyelitis occurred in countries where sanitary methods were no longer primitive. The rising incidence began in the early years of the twentieth century and went on to increase mightily until halted by vaccination. Such behavior was not necessarily due to an enhancement in virulence of polioviruses, but to a shift in host resistance, brought on by man's changing habits. Of this we shall hear more later.

Another virus, similar in its behavior to polioviruses, and peculiar to its own mammalian species, is the agent of Teschen disease, an encephalomyelitis of hogs. This is an infection which is limited largely to southeastern parts of Europe and for a time bore the name of "pig polio."

## Tissue Culture

Early in 1949, poliomyelitis research was given a new direction and a new lease on life through the monumental discovery by Enders, Weller, and Robbins[7] that the viruses could be grown *in vitro* in tissue cultures of non-neural cells. The story is familiar. Its special and timely impact was in the field of poliovirus infections but it has had far ranging implications besides for many another viral infection. The limits of its potential have yet to be explored. A most exciting and also most practical feature about this finding was that polioviruses could be detected in tissue culture by their characteristic cytopathic effects. In other words, it was no longer necessary to induce the experimental disease in the monkey in order to demonstrate the presence of the virus. Added to this, high titers of polioviruses, from 100- to 1000-fold higher than those previously achieved, could be obtained in tissue culture, thus yielding concentrations of such density that the preparations could be used to advantage in various immunological tests: neutralizing, complement fixing, precipitin tests, and so forth. Furthermore, the availability of methods of growing the three types of virus in high concentration, in relatively pure suspension, and in large volumes brought the development of poliovirus vaccines to within the realm of possibility.

Tissue culture methods have also enormously enhanced the facility with which intracellular development of polioviruses could be studied. It was found that the viruses attach to host cells at an exponential rate which is influenced by various factors, including temperature, pH, and high salt content of the media. Synthesis of the infectious poliovirus RNA actually begins within two hours after the virus has become attached to the cell. For a description of the intracellular details of this process, not only in tissue culture cells but in the motor neurons of the spinal cord as well, the reader can again be referred to the excellent account by Bodian and Horstmann, to which I have already referred (see footnote 1).

In addition, although tissue culture-adapted poliovirus strains with

---

7. Enders, J. F., Weller, T. H., and Robbins, F. C.: Science, *109:*85–87, 1949.

reduced neurovirulence were developed by Enders in 1952, the plaque technique developed by Dulbecco and used by Sabin (1957) for the selection of individual clones was a major feature which eventually led to the development of attenuated vaccine strains with greatly reduced neurovirulence.

The property of neurovirulence is, in general, correlated well with the temperature marker—the so-called rct/40°, which indicates reproductive capacity at 40°C. High degrees of neurovirulence are associated with good growth in tissue culture at 40°C., whereas strains with diminished neurovirulence show optimal growth at 34° to 36°C. and fail to propagate at temperatures as high as 40°. A number of other genetic markers which characterize different strains of polioviruses have also been described (see footnote 1).

# PATHOLOGY AND PATHOGENESIS

Knowledge of the manner in which polioviruses leave their mark on the human host, i.e., the clinical consequences, and of the gross and microscopic *pathology* of poliomyelitis is obviously essential to a proper understanding of the overall picture of this infection. These features deserve particular attention in an age in which most interest seems to be on molecular biology or on the minutiae of the infection of a single cell.

## PATHOLOGY

As I have already emphasized, only in a small percentage of patients does poliovirus infection ever proceed far enough to cause lesions in the central nervous system and to affect the motorneurons sufficiently to cause weakness or paralysis of muscle groups. More common is a generalized systemic response with such symptoms as fever, vomiting, and listlessness, in which the only visible clinical signs appear in the form of a dusky red throat, and perhaps enlarged tonsils; in the rare patient who undergoes an abdominal operation in this stage, enlargement of the regional or mesenteric lymph nodes has also been noted. And outnumbering the mild cases by far are inapparent infections in which viremia and virus shedding from the throat and intestinal tract nevertheless occur. Thus poliomyelitis is primarily a *systemic* infection (or at least it always has a primary systemic phase) rather than an infection which goes straight into the central nervous system and inflicts its initial damage there.

The pathological changes in the central nervous system, which have always received a large share of attention, exist chiefly in the motor neurons of the gray matter of the cord. Here most of the serious lesions are produced. The permanence of the damage inflicted is largely due to the fact that these cells, unlike most others in the body, cannot regenerate themselves. The CNS lesions consist of primary neuronal changes wrought by intracellular multiplication of the polioviruses, followed by an inflammatory reaction of variable degree, which acts as a secondary response to the nerve cell injury. And yet some neurons pass through the various destructive stages without evidence of surrounding inflammation. It is clear that when a motor neuron is involved extensively, dissolution of the cytoplasmic Nissl substance occurs, and changes in the nucleus appear. When irreversible damage has taken place, the necrotic cell may be removed by leukocytes or macrophages, or it may simply undergo lysis. The secondary inflammatory reaction which immediately follows may rapidly reach marked proportions. The principal types of cells found in the early stage of inflammation are: polymorphonuclear leukocytes, mononuclear leukocyctes, and macrophages. Subsequently lymphocytic cells predominate in the CNS tissue for two or three weeks where they persist in the form of perivascular accumulations for many months.

### Pathogenesis

Today it is universally agreed that the usual portal of entry for polioviruses is the mouth; rarely they may be introduced parenterally, as for example in the accidental injection of a vaccine which contains virulent polioviruses. The important feature is that in both the inapparent and the symptomatic infection the virus settles first in the oropharynx and in the intestinal tract. It multiplies in these sites and is shed from the pharynx for approximately two weeks, and from the intestinal tract for four to six weeks or longer.

The manner in which polioviruses penetrate beyond the alimentary tract, travel, and gain access to the CNS, whether by way of the nerves or nerve fibrils, or mainly by way of the blood, would seem to be a problem of basic importance. It is suspected that the reticuloendothelial tissues and lymphatic vessels may be the source of virus in the blood. The occurrence of a stage of viremia, analogous to that which occurs in other acute viral infections, in the incubation period or minor illness phase of poliomyelitis suggests that primary invasion of the central nervous system may be by way of the blood. Sabin[8] maintains that no significant viremia occurs unless the virus so distributed by the blood can multiply in a variety of extraneural tissues—this is a property possessed to a varying degree by some strains and not by others. As far as attenuated strains of virus are concerned, recent experimental evidence in man tends to reaffirm the importance in Type II infections. The effectiveness of antibodies in blocking the virus in the blood is an all-important point.

# CLINICAL FEATURES

Clinical aspects of poliomyelitis have been well and continuously documented over a period of 50 years or more. Indeed, so much has been written about not only the acute aspects but also the subacute and the residual effects that it would be more appropriate to refer the reader to the wealth of data contained in current textbooks of medicine or pediatrics.

8. Sabin, A. B.: Science, *123*:1151–1157, 1956.

These clinical accounts, of which only two are mentioned here,[9] are devoted mainly to descriptions of the more serious cases which, as I have repeatedly stressed, represent only some 5 per cent of poliovirus infections, a feature illustrated in Figure 3. But they are certainly the cases of most concern to the pediatrician or internist. This is understandable enough since these are the cases which require the most skill in diagnosis and the most clinical judgment in selecting the appropriate methods of care. It would be particularly true of patients with serious respiratory difficulties or those who require expert orthopedic treatment. The rank and file of internists consider the inapparent or insignificant "cases," illustrated diagrammatically in Figure 3, as "healthy carriers," and therefore of no consequence, but they are all individuals in whom the infection runs its course and all develop antibody responses in the same manner as the patient with clinically recognizable poliomyelitis. The age-specific pattern of inapparent infections is also the same as that which frank poliomyelitis follows within a given geographical area. To the clinical epidemologist or student of the natural history of polio-

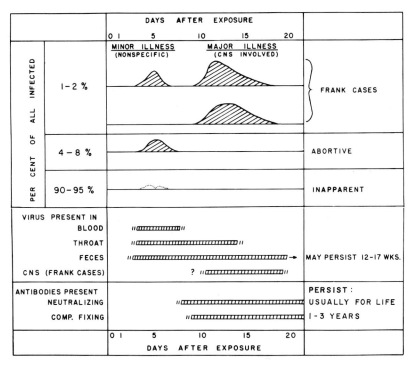

*Figure 3.* Schematic diagram of the clinical and subclinical forms which poliovirus infections may assume, showing the presence of the virus and the development of antibodies in relation to the course of the infection (Redrawn from Paul, J. R., WHO Monograph Series, No. 26, 1955, p. 23.)

9. Weinstein, L.: Poliomyelitis. *In:* Cecil-Loeb Textbook of Medicine, 12th edition, edited by Beeson and McDermott. Philadelphia, W. B. Saunders Co., 1967.

Horstmann, D. M.: Poliomyelitis. *In* Pediatrics, 14th edition, edited by Holt, McIntosh, and Barnett. New York, Appleton-Century-Crofts, Inc., 1968.

myelitis, mild or inapparent infections have a special importance for they are the prime source of virus dissemination.

Patterns of the clinical responses to poliovirus infection are separated into two general types: the nonspecific *minor illness* which follows a few days after infection is established; and the less common *major illness*, in which signs of CNS involvement appear some 10 to 14 days after exposure. Either form may occur alone, or the patient may exhibit a diphasic course in which the minor illness is followed by several days of well-being before the major illness (frank poliomyelitis) develops. Figure 3 illustrates diagrammatically the relationships of the several clinical forms, the times at which virus is present in different anatomical sites, and the development of antibodies during the course of infection.

The *minor illness* is of short duration, often 24 to 48 hours. The symptoms are those common to the nonspecific illnesses associated with other enteroviral infections: low grade fever, slight sore throat, vomiting, and listlessness. The first sign of real trouble may come with the onset of the *major illness*. Usually the symptoms of the major illness, whether they appear unheralded or follow immediately after the minor illness, or after a latent period of a few days, consist of a repetition of the earlier symptoms in more severe form, with added features amounting to evidence that the virus has invaded and begun to damage the central nervous system. Fever, severe headache, and stiff neck and back are characteristic. If no further signs develop the illness is classified as nonparalytic, or, more accurately, as aseptic meningitis due to poliovirus. However, in patients destined to develop the paralytic disease, there is evidence of progressive CNS involvement consisting of loss of power in muscles supplied by nerves of the brain stem, medulla, and most commonly, spinal cord.

There are no abnormalities of the spinal fluid in the minor illness, but the major illness is generally accompanied by an increase of white cells (predominantly mononuclear) in the cerebrospinal fluid in the range of 50 to 300, and by a modest increase in protein, which reaches a peak after several weeks and declines to normal after four to six weeks.

## ANTIBODY RESPONSES

These are also illustrated in Figure 3. Type-specific neutralizing antibodies (the most reliable means of determining whether an individual has been infected with a given serotype) are detectable seven to ten days after infection is established, which is about the time that CNS signs appear. The titers have reached maximum levels in approximately half the patients by the time of hospital admission. High levels ($> 1:512$) are maintained in 60 to 70 per cent during the first few months following infection, but the height of the antibody is not related to the severity of the clinical response: it makes no difference whether the infection was accompanied by extensive paralyses or remained mild or inapparent. Obviously the level of neutralizing antibodies and the level of immunity in an individual are not one and the same, but by and large, they can be assumed to be closely related. Neutralizing antibodies decline somewhat over the years immediately following infection but remain at appreciable levels for life, and, accordingly, are a valuable index of permanent immunity.

Other kinds of antibodies, such as complement fixing (CF), are demonstrable in significant titers in some 80 or 90 per cent of patients, but after two or three years they usually sink to undetectable levels. This makes their presence an index of *recent* infection. Antibodies demonstrable by precipitin methods (the agar-gel method, for example) follow the same pattern as do CF responses. The evidence to date indicates that neutralizing and other antibodies which appear after attenuated poliovirus infections, *i.e.*, Sabin-type vaccination, persist in the same manner as they do following wild poliovirus infections. However, observations have been carried out for only 10 to 12 years and the long-term persistence of immunity remains to be demonstrated.

## EPIDEMIOLOGY

Epidemiological aspects could be spoken of as the *community* host response, a most important one according to sociological or public health points of view. Apparently the virus of poliomyelitis is one of those which, like measles virus, is always ready to spread into and circulate among a susceptible population if the opportunity arises. But unlike measles, with polioviruses by far the majority of infections lie below the clinical horizon. Nevertheless, today there are few unvaccinated communities, no matter how remote, that can hope to escape poliovirus infection for long; and when "wild" virus spreads among susceptibles, there are almost bound to be some paralytic cases. Epidemics are particularly apt to occur in isolated communities where the interepidemic period has been protracted, for the risk of a potentially severe outbreak increases annually as a population composed of unvaccinated infants, children, and even young adults is built up. Such a susceptible population is like a growing vacuum into which the virus may surge when the opportunity presents itself. There are few more striking examples of this train of events than the poliomyelitis epidemics which have occurred in the Pacific Islands and in remote Arctic regions. In these virgin soil populations not only has the incidence of the disease been extraordinarily high, but there have been many adult cases, indeed in people far beyond the usual age limit. As with other infections, with an increase in the age of patients, a greater severity of clinical manifestations is observed. For instance, in an epidemic among Canadian Eskimos in 1948–1949, almost 60 per cent of the entire population was involved and the paralytic disease was accompanied by an appalling death rate. The virus infected all age groups, but the *lowest* clinical attack rate was in those up to four years old! One is reminded of that famous epidemic of measles in the Faeroe Islands in which the same epidemiological principles were involved; viz., (1) introduction of the virus into an isolated population in which all age groups were susceptible; (2) high infection rates in the total population; and (3) most severe clinical response and highest mortality in young adults. Indeed one virgin soil epidemic of poliomyelitis which occurred on Tahiti in 1951 suggested that in communities in which young and older age groups are equally susceptible, infection sweeps through and involves virtually all susceptibles, but the diagnosed cases and the cases with severe paralysis and death occur much more commonly in young adults, whereas young children are more apt to have mild or in-apparent infections.

Differences in age-specific attack rates are also characteristic of poliomyelitis in urban and rural environments. In urban settings crowding and closer contact results in earlier acquisition of poliovirus infections than is the case in rural areas where the population density is lower and opportunities for exposure are correspondingly reduced. That poliomyelitis, particularly urban poliomyelitis, was originally an endemic disease of infancy and early child-hood had been recognized from earliest times and yet this age distribution is linked closely to the habits of the population and to the sanitary environment. When these features change, the susceptible age groups change accordingly.

An appreciation of this concept contains the roots of an explanation as to why at the end of the nineteenth century, poliomyelitis suddenly began to appear in epidemic form. This shift from endemic to one of periodic epidemics is generally considered to have been associated with the dawn of the sanitary age. Anyway, the two events took place more or less simultaneously. The theory assumes that virulent strains of polioviruses had begun to circulate freely throughout the cities and rural areas of Scandinavia and northern Europe, perhaps because of increasing facility of transportation. This occurred at a time when infants were just beginning to be partially protected from bacterial infections such as typhoid fever and other enteric diseases by the imposition of certain principles of sterility in the handling of milk, water, and food, and by the improvement of the sanitary environment generally. Thus by partially reducing exposure to enteric pathogens there was a post-ponement of the age at which infants and young children became infected with polioviruses. Accordingly, in places where endemic infantile poliomyelitis had once flourished and induced immunizing infections early in life, now that children were allowed to reach a slightly older age before being exposed a pool of susceptibles was built up, and periodic introduction of the virus resulted in rapid epidemic spread with hundreds—even thousands—of frank infections.

An inverse relationship between *infant mortality* and the incidence of poliomyelitis also reflects this close tie between epidemics and social and sanitary conditions. Poliomyelitis is relatively rare in populations with high infant mortality rates and poor sanitary environments. When sanitation improves, infant mortality rates are apt to fall to lower and lower levels. When they reach about 75 per thousand, experience has shown that not only are first epidemics of poliomyelitis likely to occur within a few years, but this often leads to a general increase of cases as well as to an increase of the age of the patients (see Fig. 4).[10]

---

10. Payne, A. M.-M.: Papers and Discussions Presented at the 3rd International Poliomyelitis Conference, Rome, 1954. Philadelphia, J. B. Lippincott Co., 1955.

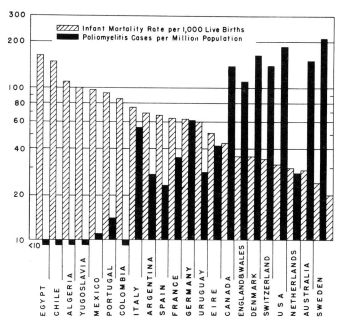

*Figure 4.* Infant mortality rates vs. simultaneous rates of the incidence of poliomyelitis in different countries showing an inverse relationship. (Data from Payne, A.-M.-M., Papers and Discussions Presented at 3rd International Poliomyelitis Conference, Rome, 1954. Philadelphia, Lippincott, 1955, pp. 393–400.)

With respect to the age distribution of poliomyelitis, when the infection is restricted to the infantile group (birth to two years), it is estimated that more than 99 per cent of such infections are inapparent. On the other hand, when a sizeable percentage of schoolchildren also fall within the ranks of the susceptibles, then the percentage of inapparent infections may decline, perhaps to 95 per cent. This means that when older children, adolescents, and young adults become infected, they are more and more likely to develop clinical evidences of disease which are recognizable as poliomyelitis.

But still, in the great majority of circumstances infants and young children represent the most susceptible members of the population, and experience the highest infection rates. It is this age group which forms the main but hidden reservoir of infection in the community. Thus the unpleasant truth is that children six months to two or three years old are the real but usually unsuspected miscreants in spreading polioviruses. Before about 1940 this fact was less appreciated. In recent years, however, Dr. Sven Gard[11] of Sweden, has reemphasized the point that infants can be regarded as so-called "dangerous carriers"; he demonstrated that children between the ages of 6 and 18 months who have not been "toilet trained" are the most effective disseminators of polioviruses. They are therefore a far greater menace to young parents and to nursemaids who may be susceptible than are older children.

Today it is not necessary to rely on retrospective age-specific case rates

---

11. Gard, S.: Second International Conference on Live Poliovirus Vaccines. Washington, Pan American Sanitary Bureau, 1960, p. 187.

to estimate the experience of a population with polioviruses, for measurements can actually be made in advance of an epidemic, using serological methods. Thus the epidemiologist can assay the immune status of a given population from time to time by measuring age-specific patterns of antibodies. In most unvaccinated populations living in primitive sanitary environments, the youngest children, being the most susceptible, acquire infection with polioviruses and develop antibodies and immunity at a very early age. Thus by the time they are five, children in such populations have neutralizing antibody rates of 80 or 90 per cent to all three types of poliovirus. In contrast, before vaccination was introduced, in populations living under conditions of good sanitation and hygiene, serological surveys revealed that children often reached the age of 15 before a comparably high percentage had acquired antibodies to all three types. Even in places where effective vaccination has been practiced, antibody rates may not equal those achieved by natural processes; but it is to be remembered that in the absence of vaccination such high rates of antibodies (and immunity) have been achieved in infancy at the price of a considerable number of paralytic cases.

Although poliomyelitis has been characterized as an endemic tropical disease which occasionally strayed into northern or southern temperate zones, it has become practically worldwide in distribution and there is no reason to doubt that it has penetrated to every inhabited part of the globe. Its epidemiological behavior has varied in different places from moderate endemicity and low incidence to a pattern of severe recurrent epidemics and, accordingly, high incidence. As already mentioned, these trends can be followed by periodical serological surveys which can reveal how things are going in a given population. Such surveys are particularly valuable in tropical and subtropical countries where poliomyelitis, owing to its sporadic occurrence, has been previously unrecognized and regarded as uncommon. But, as an unpleasant reminder that polioviruses actually have been present in such areas all the time, the disease regularly comes to the surface when groups of young foreign visitors such as soldiers enter the country as "susceptible immigrants," and acquire poliomyelitis at far higher rates than would have been expected if they had remained in their homeland.[12]

The effect of climate and season on the epidemiology of poliomyelitis, though profound, is curiously enough still poorly understood. No satisfactory reason has as yet been given to explain the summer incidence of the disease in temperate climates. It is particularly puzzling why this effect should be so sharp and dramatic, and produce epidemics at such a high rate during the summer and early autumn, since the infection is obviously spread by human contact. The explanation remains something of a mystery. Some poorly understood factor, conditioned by summer weather, must introduce large amounts of poliovirus into the community at certain times. The idea that human susceptibility sinks to low levels at certain times is less tenable.

Although the *direct contact* explanation for the spread of poliomyelitis is the most important one, it may not be the complete answer at all times and in all places. In any event, it does seem that man can contaminate not only his

12. Paul, J. R.: Amer. J. Hyg., 50:57–62, 1949.

fellow associates, but also his immediate and intimate environment. Polio-viruses, like enteric bacteria, have been found not only in human feces, but in fecal material collected in open privies and, under natural circumstances, in urban sewage. Yet the mere presence of poliovirus in sewage at certain periods of the year does not indicate that sewage is *the* avenue, or even *an* avenue, of infection at all. It is merely evidence that the community is con-taminated. Seldom, if ever, has there been evidence to incriminate poliomyelitis as a water-borne disease. In only a few outbreaks has there been reason to believe that milk was a source of infection.

A variety of arthropods from time to time have been suspected of spread-ing the viruses, because of the seasonal incidence, but such an explanation must be of only minor significance in the overall picture. Many varieties of insects have been tested for the presence of polioviruses. The tests have yielded no positive results except in the case of flies and cockroaches, but the role of these insects would seem to be only that of mechanical vectors. The word "mechanical" is used here advisedly. There is evidence that poliovirus, present in flies artificially infected, lasts in or on these insects for about 15 days, whereas in cockroaches, on the other hand, the virus has been found 51 days after infection. It is the author's opinion that in certain areas where sanitary conditions are substandard and flies are exceedingly common, such as in some villages and cities in the Middle East, Asia, and Africa where flies are seen constantly on the faces and about the eyes and lips of young children, under these circumstances they might possibly play a role as disseminators of virus.

## COMMENT

It would seem that poliovirus owes its success as a self-sustaining para-site to the ability of wild strains of the agent to maintain themselves in the human alimentary tract where they have been accustomed to being passed from child to child in most parts of the inhabited world. The infinitesimally small percentage of infections which result in crippling deformities are but a drop in the bucket when one considers the enormous human reservoir of infections in the childhood population. It might almost seem that it would have been a slight advantage from the point of view of this microbial agent if naturally occurring poliomyelitis viruses could have *all* been attenuated. The species might then have flourished as harmless inhabitants of the intestinal tract; and they probably would not have been discovered until the mid-twen-tieth century when tissue culture methods came into common use. But when it comes to an explanation of why polioviruses were endowed with the property of virulence and neurotropism as well as enterotropism, this defeats the imagination. But here I am getting into a philosophical area where I doubt if anyone yet has the answers.

As for the parasites' relationship to the community from the *sociological* standpoint, the idea has been stressed that poliomyelitis viruses behave differ-ently in different environments. In communities where sanitation is primitive and living conditions are crowded and poor, facilities for the spread of such a virus are better than elsewhere, and infants have the opportunity of coming in contact with all three types of polioviruses early in life. Few of them reach the age of five without having been infected with at least one strain although clinically these infections are largely inapparent. Immunity is acquired early and silently in such areas and no large group of susceptibles is built up among children or young adults. As a seemingly paradoxical consequence, the infection continually smolders and epidemics of poliomyelitis among natives are unlikely to occur. This results in a highly immune population in which only the youngest children are susceptible and the sporadic paralytic cases are therefore limited to children aged six months to four years old. Epidemics are almost unknown in these areas. In contrast, in unvaccinated populations where sanitary arrangements are no longer primitive, the so-called developed populations, the risk of exposure and contact with virus at an early age is diminished, but just as the situation is in measles, the ever present virus awaits that time when a sizeable group of susceptibles is built up, and periodically an epidemic situation ensues.

## CONTROL MEASURES

Regardless of the changing patterns of poliomyelitis in different parts of the world, in no juvenile population has the need for vaccination been reduced. Profound alterations in incidence and in the ages of patients have been brought into the epidemiological picture by the use of two different poliovirus vaccines during the past 12 years and no doubt more changes will come in the future. Both vaccines are considered here from the standpoint of their effectiveness and the degree to which they have contributed to the techniques of artificial immunization, as well as to knowledge of human immunity in poliomyelitis and other viral infections. Another feature in the control of poliomyelitis is the importance of local epidemiological factors in making the choice of different approaches to immunization.

### Inactivated Poliovirus (Salk-type) Vaccine

A primitive poliovirus vaccine, inactivated by formalin, was tried by Brodie and Park in 1935 but it was soon abandoned. It was not until 20 years later that Salk was able to use this same method, greatly improved thanks to the availability of quantitative techniques, in developing the vaccine which he introduced in 1955, and which bears his name. It had an immediate and profound effect. Rates of paralytic cases in the United States fell from 13.9 per 1000 in 1954, to 0.5 in 1961 (see Figs. 1 and 2). Not only was the incidence reduced after 1954, but the epidemiological picture was altered so that outbreaks were largely urban and localized to lower socioeconomic groups living in crowded substandard areas. Most of the cases occurred in inadequately vaccinated individuals in the age group under six years.

Previous experience of the host with infection by any of the three types of poliovirus has a marked influence on the antibody responses to inactivated vaccine. Children or adults who have never had any natural infection and who therefore lack antibodies for all three types require a greater antigenic stimulant to induce significant antibody levels than do those who have had one or more infections and possess antibodies to at least one type. Persistence of immunity following immunization with inactivated vaccine depends on such variables as the potency of the injected antigenic component, the number of doses received, previous experience of the host with polioviruses, and whether the environment provides opportunity for many or few natural infections which result in antibody booster effects.

It is known that antibodies from inactivated poliovirus vaccine occasionally do not prevent subsequent infection with either homotypic or heterotypic polioviruses. And yet there is evidence that among some populations which have been well vaccinated with the inactivated (Salk-type) vaccine marked suppression of wild virus prevalence has occurred. This has been especially prominent in Sweden where potent vaccines have been used. Thus, there has been a decline in incidence of paralytic cases in nonvaccinated persons in that country as well as in those who have been adequately vaccinated, and the circulation of wild polioviruses has been reduced almost to the vanishing point.

In spite of the remarkable record of effectiveness of the inactivated virus vaccine, it has become apparent that it has certain limitations in terms of the ultimate control of paralytic poliomyelitis as a world problem. In primitive rural areas, for instance, a major drawback is the difficulty in reaching a large enough segment of the population, particularly the highly susceptible preschool children, with the four or more doses of this vaccine which must be *injected*. While such vaccination campaigns may be feasible in small, economically advanced countries, in developing countries the economic and logistic problems of adequate distribution are virtually insurmountable.

Also, difficulties associated with the vaccine itself include the tendency for antibody levels to decline to undetectable levels in young, previously triple-negative children who have never experienced natural infection. Unless continued reinforcement is employed these children will tend to slip back into their previously susceptible state.

## LIVE ATTENUATED POLIOVIRUS VACCINE

Much is now known about the immunizing capacity of the live attenuated poliovirus vaccine, which is administered orally, and it has permitted, as a result of human experimentation with attenuated strains, the accumulation of new knowledge concerning the pathogenesis of poliovirus infection in the individual and in the community.

Koprowski and his associates[13] in 1952 were the first to vaccinate humans with laboratory manipulated strains of poliovirus of reduced neurovirulence. Subsequently a more sophisticated method of attenuation was used by A. B. Sabin. And it was his strains which were accepted and licensed in the United States as the officially approved live virus vaccine in the early 1960's. Although the Sabin vaccine strains currently in use measure up well, no strain of attenuated poliovirus has yet been shown to lack neurovirulence for the monkey completely, nor has any strain been found which is completely stable on continued or prolonged passage in the human intestinal tract. The attenuated vaccine strains, which immunize as a result of their capacity to be implanted

---

13. Koprowski, H., Jervis, G. A., and Norton, T. W.: Amer. J. Hyg., *55:*108–126, 1952.

and induce infection in the alimentary tract, undergo significant multiplication in the pharynx and gut within 24 to 48 hours after the vaccines are ingested. Evidence has also accumulated that *viremia* occurs during this same period with considerable frequency following the ingestion of Type II (Sabin) poliovirus vaccine but rarely has it been demonstrated with the Sabin strains of the other types.

The protective effect induced by live attenuated virus vaccine has at least two components, one from humoral antibody formation, and the other apparently associated with a mechanism of local resistance in the alimentary tract. The most recent evidence suggests that this involves locally produced gamma A antibody, which is secreted onto the mucous surface of the gut. Whether there is also a cellular element to postinfection resistance of the alimentary tract is not known. However, it would seem likely that, as in other infections, the development of delayed hypersensitivity might well be involved in clearing the tissues of virus during the infection and in maintaining subsequent resistance to reinfection.

One drawback of oral vaccine is that extensive dissemination of non-poliovirus enteroviruses in a population can block its effectiveness. In temperate climates vaccination campaigns have been carried out in the winter or spring to avoid such interference, but in tropical and subtropical areas the problem is more complicated because enteroviruses are apt to circulate the year round.

The safety of oral vaccine has been established by its extensive use. In the United States some 400 million doses had been given as of 1968. Only with extreme rarity have postvaccinal or contact "vaccine-associated" paralytic cases occurred following use of the attenuated strains of Sabin vaccine; this hazard, while theoretically reasonable, has not been shown to be of much practical significance. It is currently estimated that such accidents occur approximately once for every 3 million doses administered.

That the community is protected as well as the individual is clear. As for the duration of immunity induced by the Sabin-type vaccine, the height of antibody levels (and their persistence) appears to be similar to the responses following natural infections, and these are of considerably greater magnitude than those which result from one, two, or sometimes three or more injections of inactivated (Salk-type) vaccine.

The dissemination of attenuated vaccine strains of poliovirus in the community has been viewed by some as an advantage because it increases the immunization of susceptibles; others view it as a disadvantage since repeated human passage might conceivably enhance the virulence of the previously attenuated strains. Nevertheless in many countries in which millions of persons have been vaccinated there has been no evidence of such reversion.

## SUMMARY

I have said little about the treatment of the acute disease and the use of mechanical aids to respiration, or of orthopedic measures to be taken, and of the provision of after-care. This does not mean that these therapeutic measures are unimportant; in fact, quite the opposite. But they have all been so adequately reviewed in various medical texts that further discussion would seem unnecessary here. And furthermore, treatments are very likely to undergo rapid change from time to time. Indeed it would be interesting to know how many of the features described in this article as truths will still hold 100 years hence. My guess is that where adequate immunization of infants with attenuated poliovirus vaccine is carried out on a continuous basis, clinical poliomyelitis will be an all but forgotten disease.

I say this in conclusion because in the past two or three generations ideas about this disease have undergone such a complete right about face. Originally, in the nineteenth century, at least, it was regarded as an endemic disease limited to infants, but it is now known to affect all age groups and characteristically to attack in periodic epidemics. From being considered mildly contagious or infectious, it is now regarded as highly infectious. From being considered an infection in which the outcome usually was marked by acute paralysis, it is now known that only one person in a hundred or a thousand or more of those infected with wild poliovirus becomes paralyzed. A disease that was for a time considered a respiratory affection which had a nasal portal of entry is now regarded as one of the alimentary tract. And, most of all, a disease which for a long time defied all efforts at prevention has now been brought almost completely under control in many parts of the world.

# Chapter 23

# ARBOVIRUSES: EPIDEMIOLOGICAL CONSIDERATIONS

WILBUR G. DOWNS

*Yale University School of Medicine,
New Haven, Connecticut*

Epidemiological teaching makes extensive use of models, employing as much factual information as may be available and applying stochastic reasoning to fill in the gaps. Once a mathematical model has been constructed, modern computing technics can be applied to attack each variable in succession, explore the variable over a considerable range, and generate a series of curves of epidemic expectancy. It may be initially important to recognize and to use the variable, even though its limits in the natural scene cannot be accurately assessed.

Certain diseases that involve essentially a microorganism or virus and man—for example, measles, poliomyelitis, and influenza—can be studied with relatively simple models, although the problem of controlling the variables connected with the host, man, is always formidable.

When one takes a further step and considers a disease such as malaria, many fresh complexities are introduced. In addition to man and the microorganism, there is an invertebrate vector. The problem fascinated several generations of malariologists, beginning with Sir Ronald Ross, and several attempts were made to construct mathematical models that would take the numerous parameters into account. A model for malaria has been developed[19] that considers the variables introduced by the parasite, the anopheline vector, and the human host. For each species of malaria parasite, and for each species of anopheline vector, adjustments must be made to the corresponding parameters. Similarly, the various aspects of the life of the human host must be accounted for, including living habits, working habits, sleeping habits, and clothing customs, since these may affect the exposure of the host to the vector. A single parameter for a mosquito—for example, length of life—may require protracted field studies of the anopheline mosquito in question. The data carefully collected may not be applicable to another species, or even to the same species in a different environment. Nonetheless, the equations are very useful. Once the variables have been recognized, and their importance in influencing the epidemic model determined, they may occupy positions as arithmetical, or exponential, modifiers of the final statement. Values for a given variable can be juggled, and the effect on the computer-generated epidemic observed. Such manipulations permit the epidemiologist to decide what points in the epidemic cycle may be most vulnerable to attack and whether control measures should be, for example, directed against the parasite, the vector, or the human host: to shield the human against the vector; to attack the parasite in the human; to protect the human by prophylactic drugs against invasion by the parasite; or to protect the human by vaccines.

The epidemiology of arbovirus infections is even more complicated than that of diseases such as malaria or filariasis, and furthermore follows no standard pattern. Before we consider this problem in detail, basic definitions must be carefully made.

The concept of an arbovirus is carefully explained in the 1967 W.H.O. publication "Arboviruses and Human Disease,"[43] and a direct quotation follows: "Arboviruses are viruses which are maintained in nature principally, or to an important extent, through biological transmission between susceptible vertebrate hosts by haematophagous arthropods; they multiply and produce viremia in the vertebrates, multiply in the tissues of arthropods, and are passed on to new vertebrates by the bites of arthropods after a period of extrinsic incubation."

The phrase "multiply in the tissues of arthropods" is important in excluding certain viruses. The virus of myxomatosis, for example, in its life cycle certainly uses an insect, the flea, as vector in the virus passage from rabbit to rabbit; however, the virus does not multiply in the flea, and the transmission can be regarded as mechanical. This has been called the "flying needle" or "flying pin" concept when applied to mosquitoes, Simuliidae, Tabanidae, and similar aeronauts. For the flea, we should use "jumping needle" and for the tick, "crawling needle." It would be a mistake, however, to assume that mechanical transmission need not be considered in arbovirus epidemiology. One of the most efficient arbovirus vectors, *Aedes aegypti*, is notorious for its habit of interrupted feeding. It is an extremely wary mosquito, easily disturbed when biting, but returning again and again to the same or a nearby person for yet another attempt at engorgement. If such a mosquito happens to be infected, it may transmit the infection to several new hosts. On a typical evening in *Aedes aegypti*-infested quarters in the tropics, one or more mosquitoes may assault the ankles of all the people in a room within the space of an hour or two. Should one of these people be circulating yellow fever virus, dengue virus, or Chikungunya virus, the stage is set for direct transfer of virus via mosquito minus the usual incubation period in the mosquito. In the same way the ubiquitous *Culex quinquefasciatus* also might serve as a mechanical vector for certain arboviruses—dengue, for example, for which it demonstrably does not serve as a true biological vector. What we do not know is how important the mechanical vector possibilities actually are.

Within recent years, several of the accepted arboviruses have been observed with electron microscope technics and estimates made of size and structure. Among investigators oriented toward structural morphology, physics, and chemistry, and seeking a common denominator, there has been some concern when certain arboviruses (for example, the viruses of vesicular stomatitis) have been found strikingly different morphologically from other arboviruses (for example, Western equine encephalitis virus or Sindbis), and the suggestion has been made that the former therefore are not "arboviruses." Holmes and Warburton[15] point out that rubella virus has many of the characteristics of arboviruses and query whether this agent should be considered an arbovirus. If the epidemiological definition remains the accepted one, such incongruities or similarities simply serve to stimulate interest and attention, without affecting the basic concept. The epidemiological definition does not attempt to describe the physical, chemical, or morphologic characteristics of the virion itself, and the gate is left conveniently open for any viruses that satisfy the biological criteria.

There are several properties shared by most currently recognized arboviruses which can be invoked to assist in evaluation of a candidate virus. Although very useful, such considerations nevertheless do not replace the biological definition. One of these properties, susceptibility of the virus to inactivation by diethyl ether, chloroform, or sodium desoxycholate (DCA), is routinely employed for initial screening in many laboratories. In carefully controlled experiments, in which the amount of nonvirus contamination of the suspension is minimal, results with all three chemical agents are in close agreement, and probably represent the expression of action against lipid components of the virus capsule.

The biological "need" for such a property is an interesting subject for speculation. In the case of DCA sensitivity, it is easy to concede that an enterovirus must be resistant, so as to withstand the onslaught of bile compounds in the gut, and that an arbovirus, circulating in the blood, does not need this protection. This argument loses some of its force, however, when one considers the blood circulation of polioviruses and Coxsackie viruses. Incidentally, there are several reported instances of isolation of Coxsackie viruses from mosquitoes. In such cases, the assumption is that the mosquitoes in question have recently ingested viremic blood and that the isolation represents detection merely of a passive transport state.

Scherer and Hurlbut[36] have described Nodamura virus, isolated from mosquitoes in Japan and quite resistant to inactivation, multiplying to a limited degree in mosquitoes. Corriparta virus is another possible instance of a resistant arbovirus,[39] and African horse sickness viruses and bluetongue disease of sheep viruses have long been known to be quite resistant to inactivation. Moreover, it has been established that varying degrees of susceptibility to inactivation by ether, chloroform, or DCA exist among viruses of the major arbovirus groups. Group B arboviruses are without exception very susceptible, while group A arboviruses are perhaps somewhat less so. The experimental conditions may be of considerable importance, and susceptibility may go unrecognized if the virus preparation has not been adequately purified initially, before treatment with the inactivating reagent. Certain of the arboviruses, including those of African horse sickness and bluetongue disease of sheep, show only a minor, but reproducible, degree of inactivation under the best of conditions. Parenthetically, many of the enteroviruses will show some increase in amount of virus detectable on titration after treatment with the chemical agents in question.

Many viruses that are not arboviruses are inactivated by these chemical procedures, among them the myxoviruses and the poxviruses. This point is of more than minor interest to the arbovirologist. There have been instances where failure to keep this consideration in mind has resulted at the least in a great deal of unnecessary work, and at the worst in very costly mistakes. In one instance, a virus isolated from humans in Europe and readily inactivated by DCA was studied extensively in several laboratories before it was found to be a strain of Newcastle disease virus. The field and laboratory details of the isolation of this agent and the possibility of a laboratory contamination at some point in the virus passage history have not been clarified.

To take another instance, Myers and co-workers[22] in Vellore, India, have reported a smallpox case seen early in the course of infection, before the characteristic eruption had appeared. This case was encountered during routine studies on unclassified fevers in clinics of the Christian Medical College. A virus was isolated from the serum specimen inoculated into mice, and this virus behaved on initial passages in mice much like an arbovirus. Eventually it was identified as smallpox virus. Similar episodes have happened at the Belém Virus Laboratory.

One other instance may be mentioned. The Yale Arbovirus Research Unit (YARU) recently received an unknown "arbovirus" from a European laboratory, with accompanying information that it was DCA-sensitive and had a high-titered homologous complement-fixation system. After months of work at YARU had shown that the new agent was not serologically related to any known arbovirus, it was discovered to be a poxvirus, ectromelia (mouse pox). Unfortunately, by this time ectromelia had become established in the mouse colony—an event which has since seriously hampered laboratory operations. Concurrently, it was determined that several strains of ectromelia were included in a series of virus preparations which several years earlier had been sent to the then Rockefeller Foundation Virus Laboratories in New York from eastern Europe. These strains were being studied in mice at the time, but a laboratory "escape" apparently did not occur.

The technics for laboratory study of arboviruses have undergone considerable development over the years. In the instance of technics for virus isolation and study in the mouse system, Theiler[40] first described intracerebral inoculation of adult white mice with the virus of yellow fever. For over 20 years, and with numerous arboviruses, intracerebral inoculation of adult mice remained the commonly used method, both for virus isolation attempts and for virus titrations, neutralization tests, and preparation of virus stocks. Dalldorf's studies of Coxsackie viruses stimulated a reexamination of this position, with the result that over the past 15 years the infant mouse has been widely used for primary virus isolation, for preparation of viral stocks and antigens, and for neutralization tests. In addition, various tissue culture systems have been extensively employed in recent years. Not only are there several viruses for which a specific tissue culture system and technique may be superior to the infant mouse, but also specific types of studies for which the infant mouse cannot be employed satisfactorily. Moreover, Sawyer and Lloyd[34] showed long ago that different mouse strains varied in susceptibility for certain arboviruses. Given the present greatly expanded scope of arbovirus investigations, this question has not received the further attention it merits.

For general field work concerned with isolation of viruses of several different types and ranges of pathogenicity, coming from human, vertebrate, and arthropod sources, it continues to be true that infant mice, inoculated intracerebrally, will detect a much greater total of arboviruses than any other single system yet developed. There have, however, been specific instances in which the use of infant mice for virus isolation has not been successful. In the 1964 dengue outbreak in the West Indies, for example, the dengue 3 strain involved was most difficult to detect in any system, mouse or tissue culture, and was finally recognized only after indirect tests in tissue culture. The question thus arises, "How many arboviruses are around for which we have as yet no system adequate for isolation and detection?" No answer is possible.

Before 1950, arbovirus research was limited to a few teams of investigators working on specific disease problems: Eastern, Western, and St. Louis encephalitis in the United States, yellow fever in South America and Africa, the tick-borne encephalitides in the U.S.S.R., Japanese encephalitis in the Orient, and Murray Valley encephalitis in Australia. Dengue and the sandfly fevers received some attention during the World War II years, but attracted relatively little after that. The number of recognized arboviruses was small.

The 1950's witnessed a greatly accelerated worldwide program of arbovirus research, with many laboratories participating. Scores of previously unrecognized virus agents were uncovered from human, animal, and arthropod sources. The few laboratories with facilities permitting work with agents from all over the world were glutted—and indeed still are—with new isolates awaiting definitive study. Technics for preparation of hemagglutinins from arboviruses, first elaborated by Sabin and Buescher,[31] were progressively modified, and Clarke and Casals[9] at the Rockefeller Foundation Virus Laboratories in New York established technical fundamentals that are still basic. Technics for complement fixation were also modified and improved, and are now widely used. These two tests, plus the neutralization test and virus challenge, were employed by Casals to establish the base for the current system of classification for arboviruses.

The 1967 W.H.O. Report[43] gives a listing of presently recognized groups, and a similar listing can be found in the recently published *Catalogue of Arthropod-Borne Viruses of the World*[39] which contains detailed information, virus by virus, on most of the world's arboviruses. Discrepancies between the W.H.O. list and the *Catalogue* are minor and of no import in a field undergoing rapid change.

The arbovirus classification generally adopted is based on the demonstration of serological relationships, according to which all related viruses constitute an antigenic group. The tests principally used, hemagglutination inhibition (HI), complement fixation (CF), and virus neutralization (N test), are in close agreement in general terms. However, the pattern varies considerably from virus group to virus group. Among the group B arboviruses, the HI test is most sensitive in detecting relationships, whereas in the Bunyamwera group the CF test serves better. Shope and Causey[38] showed that among the group C viruses (in the Bunyamwera supergroup) the pattern of relationship varies with the type of test used.

Major groupings of arboviruses comprise groups A and B and the Bunyamwera supergroup (which contains the Bunyamwera group, Bwamba group, group C, the California group, and the Capim, Guama, and Simbu groups, and an unassigned category). There also are a number of smaller groups, some with only two virus members. Frequently mentioned small groups are those designated phlebotomus fever, Tacaribe, vesicular stomatitis, African horse sickness, and bluetongue disease of sheep.

The 1967 W.H.O. Report[43] lists 252 arboviruses, an approximate number at best. Of these, 19 are in group A, 39 in group B, 65 in the Bunyamwera supergroup, 9 in the African horse sickness group, 12 in the bluetongue group, and 12 in the phlebotomus fever group. Forty viruses fall in 16 other small groups.

Of very particular interest are 56 viruses listed as "ungrouped." "Ungrouped" signifies that the agent in question, as far as has been determined, shows no serological relationship to any other arbovirus, or indeed to any other virus whatsoever. Some of the ungrouped viruses have been isolated from mosquitoes, some from ticks, some from vertebrates. While most of these viruses are obscure agents, several are quite well known, among them the viruses of Colorado tick fever, Crimean hemorrhagic fever, Nairobi sheep disease, and Rift Valley fever. The latter two agents cause important diseases of livestock in Africa. As detailed serological study of the ungrouped agents continues, relationships undoubtedly will be uncovered for some of them. The task of cross comparison of 56 viruses, virus by virus, first with all the known grouped viruses and then with each of the other 55, is an enormous one. The origin and the phylogenetic position of each such lone-wolf biologic moiety remain to be explained.

Among the grouped viruses, there are further considerations which present riddles for those with the insatiable urge to classify. In group B, for example, are agents such as Modoc and Montana myotis leukoencephalitis (MML) for which a definite serologic relationship can be shown to other members of the group that are certainly arthropod transmitted. To date, however, no evidence exists that Modoc and MML are arthropod transmitted.

Scattered through many of the groups are other instances where certain viruses are in the group on the basis of serological relationship, and thus are listed as arboviruses even though the evidence to complete the definition may be quite incomplete. Since there is no other spot in the realm of viruses in which to place such outriders, it seems expedient to leave them where they are until someone proposes a better plan. At the present stage of knowledge, any course followed is arbitrary.

In still other instances, consideration of an agent as being an arbovirus rests on even more tentative grounds. Viruses of the Tacaribe group, including Tacaribe, Junin, Machupo, and Amapari, are found in South America and Trinidad. Tacaribe virus was recovered only once from a mosquito in Trinidad, and was isolated several times from the tissues of bats. Junin has been reported isolated from mites in Argentina, whereas the majority of isolations are from humans, and some from small rodents. Amapari has been isolated from mites combed from the fur of rodents in Brazil, whereas the majority of the isolations are from the tissues of rodents themselves.[27] Machupo virus, the causative agent of Bolivian hemorrhagic fever, has been recovered from the tissues of small rodents but not from either mosquitoes or ectoparasites. The observation that Machupo is excreted in the urine of chronically infected rodents for long periods of time[16] has led to speculation that the viruses of the Tacaribe group may have a means of spread through contact with contaminated environment, and not have an arthropod transmission cycle at all.

The possibilities that some viruses which do fulfill the criteria for acceptance as arthropod-borne viruses may also upon occasion utilize other means of transport than arthropods to infect vertebrates must be considered. It has been demonstrated in eastern Europe that the virus of tick-borne encephalitis, which infects goats, can be spread to man in the milk, and outbreaks generated by this type of transmission have been described.[3] In a recent outbreak of Venezuelan equine encephalomyelitis in Venezuela, recovery of the virus from throat washings of humans has been reported.[5] It has already become evident, from frequent laboratory-acquired infections, that VEE virus can readily infect humans with minimal apparent direct contact, and laboratory studies indicate that the virus can be disseminated by aerosol route.[17] The possibility must be entertained that epidemics started by one mechanism, arthropod transmission, may secondarily swing into a human to human cycle (as indeed does the bacterial infection, plague). Information deriving from direct observation as to how many viruses might be able to adopt means of spread outside of the normal transmission cycle is simply nonexistent for all but a very few viruses.

Once an epidemic is well started by natural cycle mechanisms, there is also the possibility that the normal vector arthropod—or other arthropods in no way a part of the normal vector cycle—may cause extensive virus dissemination among vertebrates by serving as a mechanical vector, passing rapidly from vertebrate to vertebrate as feeding is interrupted. This was mentioned earlier and must not be forgotten.

Diagrams serve to illustrate the several transmission cycles that have been determined.

Figure 1 illustrates the transmission cycle for yellow fever. In the jungles of the New World tropics, the tree-hole-breeding and treetop-dwelling mosquitoes of the genus *Haemagogus* maintain a virus cycle in monkeys. In Africa, *Aedes africanus* serves as a sylvan vector. Some species of monkeys, *Alouatta* ssp. (howlers), suffer heavy mortality as yellow fever virus moves through their populations, and they may be nearly exterminated from a region in the wake of an epidemic.[4] Other monkey species, *Cebus* ssp., for example, become infected but experience low mortality. And although *Haemagogus* mosquitoes in the New World certainly play the major role, other mosquitoes, including aedine and sabethine species, have been encountered naturally infected and may in some cases have significance as vectors.

Humans fall into the trap in accidental fashion—through a forest expo-

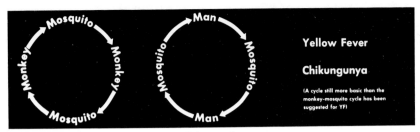

*Figure 1*

sure of some sort. It is when the infected human returns to his dwelling, or his village or city, that the second half of the diagram becomes operative. If *Aedes aegypti*, a mosquito exquisitely tooled to serve as a virus vector to humans, is present in the community, it may pick up the virus and start an epidemic cycle which can proceed quite independent of the forest cycle. The mechanics of the human cycle in Africa differ in some details. The mosquito-monkey-mosquito cycle may go on in the forest moderated by *Aedes africanus* (and possibly some other African aedine mosquitoes and mosquitoes of other genera), and man may become infected as he invades the forest. However, monkeys may play a more direct part by invading the human habitat, raiding agricultural crops on the plantations, and providing a virus source for *Aedes simpsoni*, a mosquito common in the plantation locale, where it breeds in the leaf axils of banana plants and in other containers of small accumulations of water. *Aedes simpsoni* in turn can pass the virus on to man, and at this point *Aedes aegypti*, if present, can assist or replace *A. simpsoni* in further development of an epidemic.

Each new generation of epidemiologists attacking the yellow fever endemic-epidemic situation wrestles with the complexities of attempting to determine whether a cycle still more basic than the mosquito-monkey cycle exists, to explain puzzling features of yellow fever maintenance and persistence in forest areas. No such cycle, involving birds, small rodents, cold-blooded vertebrates, invertebrates other than arthropods, transovarial transmission of virus in arthropods, virus contamination of mosquito breeding sites, reactivation of latent virus infection in the vertebrate, and so forth, has yet passed beyond a conjectural stage.

Another virus which may have a pattern like that in Figure 1 is Chikungunya. In recent years, this virus has been responsible for huge epidemics in both Africa[29] and Asia.[14] The illness can be characterized in broad terms as "dengue-like" but is further known to cause more painful involvement of joints than does dengue. It is reported in Asia to be associated with hemorrhagic manifestations in a small proportion of cases.[33] That *Aedes aegypti* is associated with the epidemics in humans is quite clear. While an extra-human cycle is not nearly as well established as in the instance of yellow fever virus, enough evidence has been accumulated in Africa from serological studies of monkeys to make it a good guess that a cycle occurs in nature which involves primates other than man.

A third virus, Mayaro, a group A agent closely related to Chikungunya, fills the New World niche. Outbreaks in humans have been described[1, 8]

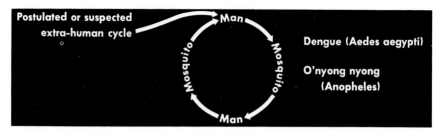

*Figure 2*

and, judging from antibody surveys, the virus is very prevalent as a human infection over a vast area of the Amazon and Orinoco basins, and presumably has a forest cycle. Repeated isolation of Mayaro virus from *Haemagogus* mosquitoes in Brazil lends support to the hypothesis.

Oropouche virus, a member of the Simbu group and first isolated from man in Trinidad, has been associated with epidemics in humans in Amazonian towns.[26] It has been recovered in Brazil from a forest animal and from forest mosquitoes. The cycle may resemble that in Figure 1. The urban outbreaks of Oropouche infection have been carefully studied through the agency of the nearby Belém Virus Laboratory but, despite extensive search, the vector for such outbreaks has not been determined.

Figure 2 illustrates the pattern for the dengue viruses, transmitted from man to man by *Aedes aegypti* and, in some more special cases, by other aedines such as *Aedes albopictus*. The cycle is simpler than that shown in Figure 1. An extra-human cycle for the dengue viruses has long been sought. It has been established that the viruses can infect monkeys. Monkeys in nature have been shown to have antibodies that neutralize dengue virus.[30] The serological complexity of the antibody patterns that develop in response to infection by one or more members of arbovirus group B (which includes the dengues) is so formidable that the interpretation of serological dengue-positive reactions in vertebrates such as monkeys and bats[23] must be approached with great caution.

Dengue (sensu latu) has long been recognized as an annoying affliction of mankind, but not a major scourge. Events in recent years, however, have provided mounting evidence that various of the currently recognized dengue viruses can produce, particularly in small children, a very severe illness, with hemorrhagic manifestations and sometimes shock, collapse, and death. Serious annual epidemics are now reported for some of the large cities in the Orient—Manila and Bangkok,[14] Singapore,[18] Calcutta,[32] and Penang.[24] Halstead and co-workers[13] have suggested that serious illness in humans follows infection with more than one dengue strain, sequentially and after an appropriate interval, and that serious complications ensue as the result of hyperimmunization and sensitization phenomena rather than as expressions of primary virus assault on host tissue.

The African virus, o'nyong-nyong, a close relative of Chikungunya and Mayaro, has been responsible for one major outbreak in humans, in East Africa.[12] The virus was isolated repeatedly from anopheline mosquitoes. No information exists on possible extra-human cycles, and the interpretation of

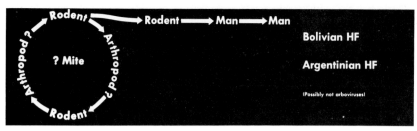

*Figure 3*

serological findings in African animals is complicated by the serological overlap between the agent and the related Chikungunya and Semliki Forest viruses. The virus is widespread in East, West, and Central Africa, if serological evidence from human surveys can be viewed with confidence.

Figure 3 presents a possible cycle for viruses of the Tacaribe group: Junin, the causative agent of Argentinian hemorrhagic fever, and Machupo, the causative agent of Bolivian hemorrhagic fever. Other agents in the group, including Tacaribe from Trinidad and Amapari from Brazil, have not yet been shown to involve humans. As mentioned earlier, further studies are needed to settle the position of this virus group. Possibly the viruses are not arboviruses at all. Relationships between members of this group can be demonstrated—sometimes readily, sometimes with more difficulty—by the complement-fixation reaction. Cross-neutralization testing reveals very minimal overlap, and thus far it has not been possible to prepare hemagglutinating antigens with the viruses.

Figure 4 is at best a guess about the cycle for the phlebotomus fever group of viruses. A significant feature of the cycle shown here is the transovarial passage of virus from *Phlebotomus* (Diptera: Psychodidae) to *Phlebotomus*, a mechanism that might permit maintenance of virus in nature for protracted periods of time without need for passage through vertebrates. Transovarial passage actually has not been conclusively proven. An extrahuman cycle for the *Phlebotomus*-transmitted arboviruses has not been demonstrated. However, in both the Old World and the New World, several viruses have recently been added to the original pair of Neapolitan sandfly fever and Sicilian sandfly fever viruses, solely on the basis of serological cross-reactivity. The fact that some of these new additions have been isolated from small vertebrates provides some reinforcement to the hypothesis of an extra-human cycle for these viruses.

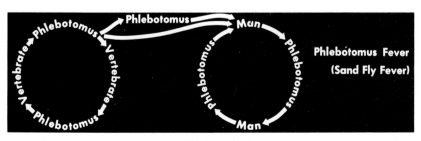

*Figure 4*

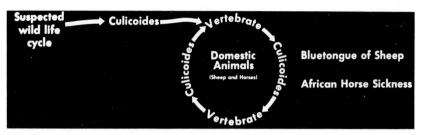

*Figure 5*

Figure 5 illustrates still another cycle, which is possibly operative for both African horse sickness viruses and the viruses of bluetongue disease of sheep. The vectors in both cases are "sandflies" of the genus *Culicoides* (Diptera: Heleidae). These viruses are not typical of the majority of arboviruses since they are inactivated by treatment with DCA only to a modest degree. Both the African horse sickness and bluetongue groups comprise a number of recognizably different agents, easily distinguished one from the other, yet producing a similar clinical disease and transmitted by the same vectors. They constitute small complexes of agents that are less closely related inter se than are, for example, a number of the group B arboviruses, such as the several dengues and West Nile.

Figure 6 illustrates the cycle typical of many of the common and most important arboviruses, including several of the agents responsible for encephalitis outbreaks in domestic animals and man. Among these are Eastern equine encephalitis (EEE), Western equine encephalitis (WEE), and Venezuelan equine encephalomyelitis (VEE), all group A arboviruses; and St. Louis encephalitis, Murray Valley encephalitis, and Japanese encephalitis, all group B arboviruses. Other, less well known agents include Mucambo, Sindbis, and Whataroa in group A, and such group B viruses as Bussuquara, Ilheus, Uganda S, West Nile, and Zika. Probably most of the agents in the Bunyamwera supergroup, agents in many of the smaller groups (Anopheles A, Anopheles B, Bakau, Changuinola, Koongol, Nyando, Piry, Turlock), and many viruses in the ungrouped category also have transmission cycles that conform to this general type. Broadly speaking, the representation is of a basic zoonosis. In some instances the vertebrates may be birds, in others small mammals, while apparently in some, both birds and small mammals may be involved.

For any given virus, the basic cycle may be quite specific, both as to ver-

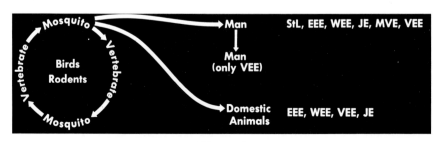

*Figure 6*

tebrate host(s) and to mosquito vector(s). As an example, in the northeastern United States *Culiseta melanura* is a major vector of the virus of EEE. This mosquito is of limited distribution, particularly favoring deep-swamp locations with acid waters. It feeds largely on birds and rarely attacks large animals and man. The major virus cycle is thus limited to this mosquito and birds, and to localized areas. However, there are other mosquitoes that feed on birds and that can be infected by EEE virus. Certain of these mosquitoes have less restricted feeding habits than *Culiseta melanura*, and may serve to move the virus out into equines and even to man. EEE virus, as it affects man, is particularly to be feared, since there is a high case fatality rate.

Western equine encephalitis (WEE) virus in the irrigated regions of the western United States has a cycle quite different from that of EEE virus. *Culex tarsalis*, a ubiquitous mosquito in the irrigated fields, nearby river bottoms, and swamps, feeds freely on both birds and mammals. It serves to infect the bird population and also small mammals, and transmits virus readily both to horses and to man. Mortality among equines may be high. Fortunately for man, the case fatality rate in humans is low, with convincing evidence of many subclinical, unrecognized human infections detected only in surveys for prevalence of antibodies, but relatively few cases of clinically recognizable encephalitis. In the eastern United States, WEE has a cycle involving principally *Culiseta melanura* and small birds. Although the virus is widespread from Florida to Massachusetts, cases of WEE in humans and horses are apparently very rare, if seen at all.

VEE virus appears to follow a pattern closer to that of WEE virus than of EEE virus, at least as far as human disease is concerned, and there is evidence accumulating from several sources to indicate that the virus may utilize small mammals rather than birds for basic virus maintenance. Birds, however, have been found naturally infected. As mentioned earlier, VEE virus can be detected in throat swabs from human cases, which raises the possibility of transmission without arthropod mediation.

In considering the epidemiology of Japanese encephalitis (JE) virus, possibly the single most important arbovirus with respect to impact upon humans, Scherer and co-workers[35, 37] advanced an important epidemiological concept of amplifier host. They showed that at the Shinhama heronry on the Kanto Plain near Tokyo, at the time when fledgling birds were in the nests, there was a high proportion of infected fledglings that could serve as virus source to the abundant mosquito, *Culex tritaeniorhynchus*, thus elevating the infection rates in mosquitoes. Since these mosquitoes feed freely on man, the rookery could be regarded as a focus for amplification of virus, with extension to humans. In the same region are large pig farms. Pigs are infected with JE virus with no apparent illness, circulate virus, also infect large numbers of mosquitoes, and serve as important amplifiers. A control approach, based on vaccination of pigs or even outright infection of pigs in the winter months when mosquitoes are not active, is being tried, the intent being to diminish the sources of circulating virus available to mosquitoes.

Quite possibly, nestling birds of other species, in other localities and with other viruses, may similarly serve as virus amplifiers. This possibility would be enhanced in a locality where some concentration factors are at work—for example, redwing blackbirds in a marsh. It also has been suggested in California that virus amplification can occur when large flocks of nonimmune birds in late-summer migrations southward from regions where virus has not been active settle down in regions where an endemic virus cycle is already operative. Probably, examples of amplification will be found for many arboviruses. The concept is important as illustrating a method whereby a basic low-grade endemic cycle may break out of bounds and give rise to an epidemic.

It seems characteristic of the cycles illustrated by Figure 6 that the vertebrate hosts usually are not affected by the virus in question. Exceptions do occur; for example, there is considerable mortality in the white-crowned sparrow, *Zonotrichia* sp., experimentally infected with WEE virus (J. L. Hardy, 1968, personal communication). Such seem to be special cases, however, and it is not likely that such a vertebrate represents a true endemic host. But when the virus is carried out of the basic endemic cycle and infects larger vertebrates, horses or man, serious disease may follow. This is certainly the case with the viruses of EEE, WEE, SLE, JE, Murray Valley encephalitis, and others. The large vertebrate is commonly regarded as an accidental victim, and is unlikely to be other than a dead end (figuratively and sometimes literally) for the virus. Levels of viremia in such hosts are often (but not always) low, the period of viremia short, and the amount of actual contact with the vector often limited.

Recently there have been reports[6, 11, 41] of infection of cold-blooded vertebrates, particularly snakes, with the virus of WEE; of persistence of the virus for long periods of time in such hosts, in the case of snakes even over the period of winter hibernation; of recovery of the virus from snakes infected in nature; and of infection of mosquitoes by feeding on viremic snakes. Such a cycle could explain the persistence of virus in a region from year to year, it having earlier been shown by several teams of investigators that overwintering of infected mosquitoes, with resumption of virus transmission in the spring, is a very unlikely possibility. Studies on the role of cold-blooded vertebrates in the endemic cycles, not only of WEE but also of other arboviruses, certainly need to be extended.

The pressure that nature puts on the virus cycle in temperate climates, with protracted periods of winter and with lessened or absent vector activity in winter, may have its counterpart in the tropics, at least in those regions that have severe and prolonged dry seasons.

Since so many of the arboviruses do infect birds, and since viremic birds often do not appear to suffer ill effects from the infection and can presumably still fly considerable distances, it is tempting to explain the virus outbreaks that suddenly crop up in localized areas as being secondary to introduction of virus by birds. There are instances where such introduction by birds almost certainly has taken place, an example being the EEE outbreak in Jamaica in 1962.[2] However, strong doubts exist as to whether this theory is the universal explanation for virus occurrence in a region. In the case of EEE virus, which is found from Argentina to Massachusetts and has been shown to be present in the jungles of the Amazon, the Rupununi Savannah region of interior British Guiana (Guyana), and the forests of Trinidad and Panama as well as in temperate regions, Casals[7] demonstrated serological differences between the strains in North America and those in South America. Although migrating birds make the passage twice annually by the millions, there is no direct evidence that they serve to transport virus intercontinentally, from north to south and vice versa. So little is really known regarding this important question that generalizations simply may not apply as one considers first one virus and then another. Reeves and co-workers[28] have shown that occasionally virus can be recovered from a bird infected many months earlier. It is tempting to postulate virus reappearance in a region through a reactivation of virus in an earlier-infected vertebrate, with resultant virus dissemination through vectors. Such an occurrence has not been demonstrated. Along similar lines, certain insectivorous bats, when infected with Japanese encephalitis or Venezuelan equine encephalomyelitis virus, would circulate virus over a long period of time and maintain virus over a period of hibernation.[10]

An enormous amount of further information is needed to help clarify basic epidemiological concepts—information that can come only from observations in the field correlated with laboratory studies and involving team efforts of ornithologists, mammalogists, and general ecologists as well as virologists.

Figure 7 illustrates still another extremely important cycle, wherein the vector arthropods are ticks. Several viruses very important in human and animal disease are among the tick-transmitted viruses. These include the virus of tick-borne encephalitis (TBE) (often earlier known as Russian spring-summer encephalitis and Central European tick-borne encephalitis) in Europe and the U.S.S.R; its three close relatives, the viruses of louping ill, affecting sheep in the British Isles, and of Kyasanur Forest disease in India, predominantly involving man and monkeys, plus Powassan virus which infects small mammals and man in the northern United States and Canada; and the unrelated virus of Colorado tick fever, involving man and small mammals in the Rocky Mountain region. In addition, there is a long list of tick-associated agents for which little if anything is yet known of vertebrate involvement.

Extensive studies, particularly in the U.S.S.R., Czechoslovakia, Finland, and Austria, have shown the involvement of small animal and bird populations with the virus of TBE, and the concept of "nidality" of infection has been advanced. Pavlovsky[25] clearly enunciated the theory of "nidality" or natural focality, and an English translation from a recent book provides a statement in ecological language: "A natural focus is a section of terrain marked by a definite biogeocenosis which is characterized by more or less clearly defined biotopes, and the presence of biocenoses which, apart from indifferent components, include animals serving as hosts for the causative agent and as donors for blood-sucking Acarina or other insects that may

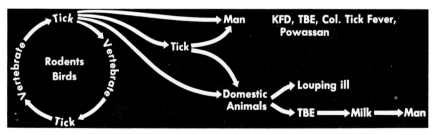

*Figure 7*

become vectors and transmit the pathogen to susceptible animals (recipients)." In a region characterized by large expanses with generally similar physiogeographic details and vegetation, there may be circumscribed areas where a focus of infection with TBE can be demonstrated and shown to remain active over many years. Within the area of the focus, one can at any time, with diligent enough search, encounter infected ticks and infected small mammals. An explanation as to why rather similar territory close by may remain uninvolved is not advanced.

Kyasanur Forest disease (KFD) in India is caused by a virus closely related to TBE virus. The area of infection is a region of less than 100 square miles in Mysore State. Monkeys are important sentinel animals in this region. Virus activity in a restricted area appears to die down as the monkey population becomes seriously reduced, only to reappear in a nearby region where the monkey population has become reestablished. Human involvement is a secondary dead-end phenomenon. The role of small mammals in maintenance of a KFD virus cycle is still not clearly defined. They certainly do become infected, but the quantitative relationships of ticks, monkeys and small mammals—and birds also—are not yet well enough known to permit a clear understanding of the dynamics of the cycle and the relative importance of the different components.

For both TBE and KFD viruses, certain ixodid ticks serve as vectors. *Ixodes ricinus* in the U.S.S.R. is the principal vector of TBE. This tick feeds freely on many hosts, including man, and man is infected when he invades regions where the natural cycle of tick-small mammal or tick-bird is established. *Haemaphysalis spinigera* in Mysore is the hard tick that is principally involved in KFD transmission, and again man becomes infected when he invades the region where the tick-monkey cycle is in progress. *Haemaphysalis spinigera* will readily attack man. A tick amplifying mechanism appears to be operative in India, since the cattle are pastured in the same forests where monkeys dwell. The ticks feed readily on cattle, and the tick populations in regions where the cattle graze may become very high.

In the New World, Powassan virus is the representative of the tick-borne encephalitis complex in arbovirus group B. This virus was recovered from the brain of a child infected in Ontario.[20] Further studies by McLean and Larke [21] in Canada and by Whitney[42] in New York State show an endemic cycle for this virus in small mammals (woodchucks, squirrels, and so forth) and a vector tick, *Ixodes marxi*. The major importance of TBE virus as a human disease agent in the U.S.S.R. is in sharp contrast to the distinctly minor role played by Powassan in the New World. The initial fatal human case of Powassan virus infection remains so far the only case on record, and human immunes are distinctly uncommon, although the virus is widespread and probably not uncommon at all if looked for. The explanation for this contrast may be very simple, and may simply be that *Ixodes marxi* does not feed readily on hosts other than its preferred hosts (small mammals), whereas *Ixodes ricinus* does.

Transovarial transmission of TBE and KFD viruses in ticks has been reported. It is not an easily demonstrated phenomenon, but one that must nonetheless be considered in connection with long-term virus maintenance in nature. Also ticks are, of course, much more long-lived than mosquitoes, and some tick life cycles can extend over a couple of years. Long-term trans-stadial virus persistence in ticks has repeatedly been demonstrated for several viruses. Certain ticks may have very distinct feeding preferences, wherein feeding in the larval and nymphal stadia is restricted to small mammals or birds, and feeding of the adults to large mammals. Other species may not show such restrictive feeding. Still other ticks may feed exclusively on a single vertebrate species.

For the tick-borne viruses, such biological facts raise many questions in connection with virus epidemiology, which will be solved only by close collaborative work between laboratory and field. One valuable contribution by the laboratory has been the demonstration, with the serologically related viruses of group B (the mosquito-borne agents on the one hand and the tick-borne agents on the other), that mosquitoes are not readily infected with the tick-borne viruses, indeed are strikingly resistant, and that ticks are not readily infected with the mosquito-borne viruses. Recent development of insect tissue cultures, both mosquito and tick, may provide valuable tools for study of virus-vector specificities.

## DISCUSSION

The foregoing discussion of arbovirus epidemiology is based upon an accumulation of factual material and a very considerable extrapolation from fact. This is necessary and justifiable, but the worker, and the reader, must remain constantly aware of the need for proof. Casals was responsible for an interesting section in the 1967 W.H.O. Report[43] which pointed out that at present only three examples exist of observation and reproduction under controlled conditions of a complete natural cycle of an arbovirus, each case including identification of the natural host and natural vector and demonstration of extrinsic incubation and of viremia in the vertebrate. These viruses are the viruses of yellow fever, dengue, and sandfly fever. The Report goes on to state that numerous examples exist of a virus's being accepted as arthropod borne, even though the complete natural cycle has not been reproduced exactly. In these, the association in nature between arthropod and disease or virus plus the experimental demonstration of laboratory transmission provides overwhelming evidence, and it can be confidently assumed that the natural cycle is adequately established.

There are numerous other viruses tentatively accepted as arboviruses and included in the *Catalogue of Arthropod-Borne Viruses*[39] for which evidence is far from complete. The position of these viruses can be resolved only by further investigation.

## ACKNOWLEDGMENT

The figures accompanying this article were elaborated by Dr. Max Theiler, who kindly gave permission for their use.

# References

1. Anderson, C. R., W. G. Downs, G. H. Wattley, N. W. Ahin, and A. A. Reese. 1957. Mayaro virus: A new human disease agent. II. Isolation from blood of patients in Trinidad, B. W. I. Am. J. Trop. Med. & Hyg. *6*:1012–1016.
2. Belle, E. A., L. S. Grant, and M. V. Thorburn. 1964. An outbreak of eastern equine encephalomyelitis in Jamaica. II. Laboratory diagnosis and pathology of eastern equine encephalomyelitis in Jamaica. Am. J. Trop. Med. & Hyg. *13*:335–341.
3. Blaskovic, D. 1967. The public health importance of tick-borne encephalitis in Europe. Bull. W.H.O. *36*(Suppl. 1):5–13.
4. Boshell, J. 1955. Yellow fever in Central America. *In* Yellow Fever—a Symposium in Commemoration of Juan Carlos Finlay, Jefferson Medical College of Philadelphia, pp. 61–69.
5. Briceño Rossi, A. L. 1964. Estudios del virus encefalomielitico equino Venezolana. Rev. Venez. Sanid. Asist. Social *29*:351–437.
6. Burton, A. N., J. McLintock, and J. G. Rempel. 1966. Western equine encephalitis in Saskatchewan garter snakes and leopard frogs. Science *154*:1029–1031.
7. Casals, J. 1964. Antigenic variants of eastern equine encephalitis virus. J. Exptl. Med. *119*: 547–565.
8. Causey, O. R., and O. M. Maroja. 1957. Mayaro virus: A new human disease agent. III. Investigation of an epidemic of acute febrile illness on the River Guama in Para, Brazil, and investigations of Mayaro virus as causative agent. Am. J. Trop. Med. & Hyg. *6*: 1004–1011.
9. Clarke, D. H., and J. Casals. 1955. Improved methods for hemagglutination studies with arthropod-borne viruses. Proc. Soc. Exptl. Biol. & Med. *88*:96–99.
10. Corristan, E. C., L. C. LaMotte, Jr., and D. G. Smith. 1956. Susceptibility of bats to certain encephalitis viruses. Federation Proc. *15*:584.
11. Gebhardt, L. P., and D. W. Hill. 1960. Overwintering of western equine encephalitis virus. Proc. Soc. Exptl. Biol. & Med. *104*:695–698.
12. Haddow, A. J., C. W. Davies, and A. J. Walker. 1960. O'nyong-nyong fever—an epidemic of virus disease in East Africa. Trans. Roy. Soc. Trop. Med. & Hyg. *54*:517–522.
13. Halstead, S. B., S. Nimmannitya, C. Yamarat, and P. K. Russell. 1967. Hemorrhagic fever in Thailand, newer knowledge regarding etiology. Jap. J. Med. Sci. Biol. *20*(Suppl.): 96–103.
14. Hammon, W. M., A. Rudnick, and G. E. Sather. 1960. Viruses associated with epidemic hemorrhagic fevers of the Philippines and Thailand. Science *131*:1102–1103.
15. Holmes, I. H., and M. F. Warburton. 1967. Is rubella an arbovirus? Lancet *2*:1233–1236.
16. Johnson, K. M., R. B. Mackenzie, P. A. Webb, and M. L. Kuns. 1965. Chronic infection of rodents with machupo virus. Science *150*:1618–1619.
17. Kuehne, R. W., W. D. Sawyer, and W. S. Gochenour, Jr. 1962. Infection with aerosolized attenuated Venezuelan equine encephalomyelitis virus. Am. J. Hyg. *75*:347–350.
18. Lim, K. A., and Y. C. Chan. 1966. Studies of hemorrhagic fever in Singapore. Bull. W.H.O. *35*:78.
19. Macdonald, G. 1957. The Epidemiology and Control of Malaria. Oxford University Press, London.
20. McLean, D. M., and W. L. Donohue. 1959. Powassan virus: Isolation of virus from a fatal case of encephalitis. Canad. Med. Assoc. J. *80*:708–711.
21. McLean, D. M., and R. P. B. Larke. 1963. Powassan and Silverwater viruses: Ecology of two Ontario arboviruses. Canad. Med. Assoc. J. *88*:182–185.
22. Myers, R. M., D. E. Carey, and E. S. Jesudass. 1967. Virus isolation by inoculation of mice with blood serum from a presumptive case of variola. Indian J. Med. Res. *54*:746–751.
23. O'Connor, J. L., L. C. Rowan, and J. J. Lawrence. 1955. Relationships between the flying-fox (genus *Pteropus*) and arthropod-borne fevers of North Queensland. Nature *176*:472.
24. Paramaesvaran, N. 1966. Hemorrhagic fever in Penang: A report on 41 cases. Bull. W.H.O. *35*:40.
25. Pavlovsky, E. N. 1939. Vestnik Acad. Nauk, U.S.S.R. *10*:98–108.
26. Pinheiro, F., M. Pinheiro, G. Bensabath, O. R. Causey, and R. E. Shope. 1962. Epidemia de virus Oropouche em Belém. Rev. Serv. Esp. Saude Publ. *12*:15–23.
27. Pinheiro, F. P., R. E. Shope, A. H. Paes de Andrade, G. Bensabath, G. V. Cacios, and J. Casals. 1966. Amapari, a new virus of the Tacaribe group from rodents and mites of Amapa Territory, Brazil. Proc. Soc. Exptl. Biol. & Med. *122*:531–535.
28. Reeves, W. C., G. A. Hutson, R. E. Bellamy, and R. P. Scrivani. 1958. Chronic latent infections of birds with western equine encephalomyelitis virus. Proc. Soc. Exptl. Biol. & Med. *97*:733–736.

29. Robinson, M. C. 1955. An epidemic of virus disease in Southern Province, Tanganyika Territory in 1952–53. Trans. Roy. Soc. Trop. Med. & Hyg. *49:*28–32.
30. Rudnick, A. 1965. Studies of the ecology of dengue in Malaysia: A preliminary report. J. Med. Entomol. *2:*203–208.
31. Sabin, A. B., and E. L. Buescher. 1950. Unique physico-chemical properties of Japanese B encephalitis virus hemagglutinin. Proc. Soc. Exptl. Biol. & Med. *74:*222–230.
32. Sarkar, J. K. 1966. Virological studies of hemorrhagic fever in Calcutta. Bull. W.H.O. *35:*59.
33. Sarkar, J. K., S. N. Chatterjee, S. K. Chakravarti, and A. C. Mitra. 1965. Chikungunya virus infection with hemorrhagic manifestations. Indian J. Med. Res. *53:*921–925.
34. Sawyer, W. A., and W. Lloyd. 1931. Use of mice in tests of immunity against yellow fever. J. Exptl. Med. *54:*533–555.
35. Scherer, W. F., E. L. Buescher, and H. E. McClure. 1959. Ecologic studies of Japanese encephalitis virus in Japan. V. Avian factors. Am. J. Trop. Med. & Hyg. *8:*689–697.
36. Scherer, W. F., and H. S. Hurlbut. 1967. Nodamura virus from Japan: A new and unusual arbovirus resistant to diethyl ether and chloroform. Am. J. Epidemiol. *86:*271–285.
37. Scherer, W. F., J. T. Moyer, T. Izumi, I. Gresser, and J. McCown. 1959. Ecologic studies of Japanese encephalitis virus in Japan. VI. Swine infection. Am. J. Trop. Med. & Hyg. *8:*698–706.
38. Shope, R. E., and O. R. Causey. 1962. Further studies on the serological relationships of group C arthropod-borne viruses and the application of these relationships to rapid identification of types. Am. J. Trop. Med. & Hyg. *11:*283–290.
39. Taylor, R. M., ed. 1968. Catalogue of Arthropod-Borne Viruses of the World. Public Health Service Publication No. 1760. U. S. Department of Health, Education, and Welfare.
40. Theiler, M. 1930. Studies on action of yellow fever virus in mice. Ann. Trop. Med. & Parasitol. *24:*249–272.
41. Thomas, L. A., C. M. Eklund, and W. A. Rush. 1958. Susceptibility of garter snakes (*Thamnophis* ssp.) to western equine encephalomyelitis virus. Proc. Soc. Exptl. Biol. & Med. *99:*698–700.
42. Whitney, E. 1963. Serologic evidence of group A and B arthropod-borne virus activity in New York State. Am. J. Trop. Med. & Hyg. *12:*417–424.
43. World Health Organization. 1967. Technical Report Series No. 369, Arboviruses and Human Disease. Geneva.

# Chapter 24

# THE COXSACKIE
# AND ECHO VIRUSES

GILBERT DALLDORF

*Sloan-Kettering Institute for Cancer Research,*
*Donald B. Walker Laboratory, Rye, New York*

Twenty years ago it was learned that our late-summer epidemics of "poliomyelitis" are usually mixed epidemics, epidemics of poliomyelitis complicated by a spectrum of viruses that in their diversity represent Bronowski's "wild variety of nature." More than 60 have been recognized since 1948 when the first was identified. All share the known physical and chemical properties of the polioviruses, their seasonal and geographic distribution and many of the characteristics of poliovirus infections.

These "cousins"* of the polioviruses fall into two families, the Coxsackie and echo viruses. The Coxsackie viruses are pathogenic for immature mice and induce in them distinctive lesions that permit identification and subdivision into two groups, A and B. The Group A viruses cause extensive hyalin degeneration of the skeletal muscles, the Group B strains cause encephalitis, a remarkable lesion of the brown fat, and focal muscle degeneration. The echo viruses are not pathogenic for newborn mice and must be isolated and characterized in tissue cultures. The identification of the various *types* is serologic.

A considerable number of the viruses are now firmly established as the etiologic agents of well known diseases. For others the evidence is inconclusive. A few appear to be of little or no pathogenicity. It is clear that a number of types have, at times, caused paralytic poliomyelitis, that the Group B Coxsackie viruses are responsible, probably solely responsible, for epidemic pleurodynia and myocarditis neonatorum, that particular Group A viruses are the etiologic agents of herpangina, and that other Coxsackie and echo types have accounted for several rather distinctive illnesses marked by lesions of the throat or skin and that most, if not all, can induce aseptic meningitis or "nonparalytic poliomyelitis."

---

* The title of an editorial in the January 21, 1950, issue of Lancet was "Polio's Cousins from Coxsackie."

Proof of etiologic relationships has sometimes been difficult. The illnesses are seldom fatal and the associated virus is therefore rarely identified with the essential lesions. During late summer and fall infection with Coxsackie and echo viruses is commonplace and many patients may be presumed to be infected with enteroviruses unrelated to their illnesses. Multiple infections may cause serious technical difficulties and uncertainties implicit in all complex infections. The methods of isolating the viruses are relatively cumbersome and have serious limitations. We know too little about the *pathogenesis* of the disease associated with the Coxsackie and echo viruses, and since serologic classification is wholly arbitrary and the known chemical and physical properties provide no clues to their activity as infectious agents, our understanding of the diseases remains incomplete. Moreover these agents are characteristically plastic as regards their pathogenicity and strains of a given type vary greatly in virulence and almost invariably represent mixed populations. There are no satisfactory laboratory tests of human pathogenicity, although among the polioviruses the responses to bicarbonate and antigenic analysis have been helpful in separating virulent and avirulent strains. And finally, multiplicity of infection and demonstrated enhancing and antagonistic effects among various combinations imply that the enteroviruses are a promising field for ecologic studies.

## THE VIRUSES

The Coxsackie viruses were identified in 1948 after a search prompted by the study of an unusual epidemic of paralytic disease in the Battle Hill section of White Plains, New York, in 1943.[1] The agent associated with that epidemic, MM virus, is now recognized to be a member of the EMC (encephalomyocarditis) group of viruses. It induces, in mice, a disease that resembles poliomyelitis but is itself quite different from the polioviruses in important respects. The study of MM virus prompted a search for other mouse pathogenic agents in specimens from poliomyelitis patients and this was encouraged and continued when it was noted that an occasional specimen that was not pathogenic for monkeys, and therefore presumably free of poliovirus, did, in fact, induce minor signs of motor weakness in mice, and, more significantly, distinctive, if minute, poliomyelitis-like lesions in their central nervous systems.

Efforts were made to find a more responsive test animal or to increase the susceptibility of mice. Eventually suckling mice were inoculated. Their use was prompted by Ørskov and Andersen's use of newborn animals in the study of Theiler's virus (mouse encephalomyelitis).[2] Two fecal specimens from young poliomyelitis patients were promptly demonstrated to contain viruses that caused weakness and paralysis in suckling mice.[3] In one of the specimens poliovirus was also present; this was the forerunner of an oft-repeated observation.

Immature animals had been used in the study of various virus infections but not in the *isolation* of viruses. Their greater susceptibility to many (but not all) viruses has since been used to advantage in the isolation of many arboviruses and mouse leukemia virus.

The discovery of the echo viruses inevitably followed the success of Enders, Weller, and Robbins in cultivating poliovirus in cells grown *in vitro*.[4] While testing fecal specimens in tissue cultures they encountered a virus[5] serologically different from the polioviruses which proved to be only the first of a long series of agents of no known clinical significance. They were considered to be "orphans" and were later labeled echo viruses, *e*nteric *c*ytopathogenic *h*uman *o*rphans.

Both Coxsackie and echo viruses are characterized by their smallness —the diameter of the virions is 28 m$\mu$—and their ribonucleic acid content. Like the polioviruses, they are *picorna*viruses, *pico* meaning very small and *rna* for their nucleic acid character. Exhaustive study of many Coxsackie viruses, echo viruses, and polioviruses has shown striking similarities and so far no chemical or structural differences that might explain their striking biological properties. The occasional disparity that has been demonstrated applies to a very few echo viruses and may reflect the miscellany included in that group which seems to occupy the end of the enterovirus spectrum.

All members of the three groups are unusually stable as regards infectivity. They may be preserved for long periods at $-20°C$. and at higher temperatures in the presence of molar magnesium chloride.[6] They are insensitive to ether, 70 per cent alcohol, and many disinfectants and detergents but are inactivated by formaldehyde and chlorine. These properties are helpful in handling specimens but required rigid laboratory practices to prevent cross infection and to protect laboratory personnel.

The identification and documentation of antigenic types has become steadily more laborious and complex as the number of recognized types has grown and has led to a few difficult and, at times, arbitrary decisions. The prototype of echo 9, for example, was isolated from a healthy child and was not mouse pathogenic. Only later when epidemic strains were found were the Coxsackie characteristics evident. The epidemic strains were submitted for typing to a Coxsackie virus reference laboratory where they were identified as typical Group A viruses and assigned the type number 23.[7] While the original designation has been maintained by some authors, echo 10 virus, also isolated from a healthy carrier, has been dropped from the echo family and assigned to a new one, the reovirus group. A more recently described virus, presumably a new picornavirus type, has renewed this problem. It was recovered from four children with respiratory infection among a large group in which parainfluenza virus type 1 was prevalent. One of the four strains so far characterized induced Group A Coxsackie lesions in suckling mice.[8] In view of past experience the nature of additional strains should be helpful in properly classifying this new candidate.

The antigenic relationships as well as the number of antigenic types limit the usefulness of serologic diagnosis of human infections. Serologic tests are sometimes helpful in surveys but diagnosis usually requires the isolation of virus and this can be laborious and equivocal. Common practice today is to inoculate tissue cultures. A variety of cells should be used, for the differences between cell lines are as marked as between cells and animals. A typical example was provided by an investigation of an outbreak of echo 6 virus infection. Of the 11 isolates, 3 were cytopathogenic for both monkey

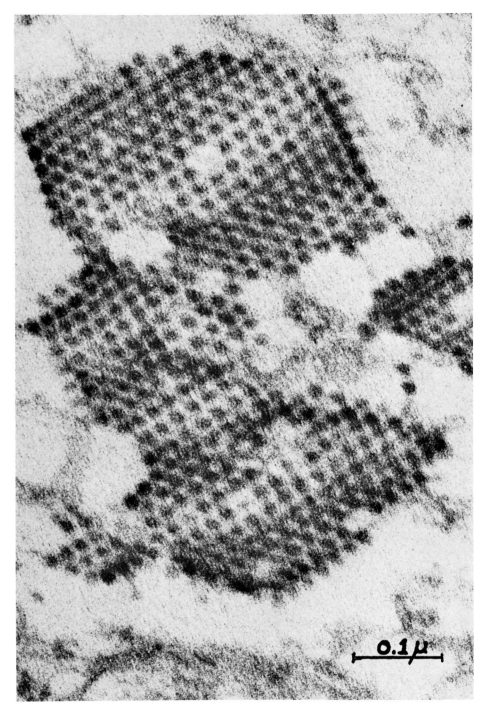

*Figure 1.*    Coxsackie virus, Group B, type 5. (Photograph courtesy of Dr. Jørgen Fogh.)

kidney and human uterine cells, 7 for the uterine cells alone, and 1 for the monkey kidney but not the uterine cells.[9]

Mouse tests also involve several variables. The route of inoculation may be critical as well as the number of animals at test. There are differences in susceptibility between mouse strains. Experience is required to recognize the responses in the mice, to judge when to harvest and pass the tissues. Histologic examination is invaluable in identifying subclinical infection in mice. Histologic examination is frequently much more sensitive than observation of the animals.

The possibility of multiple infection must always be kept in mind. "New" serologic types have often turned out to be mixtures of two known types, and one strain that was extensively studied some years ago proved to be a mixture of three Group A types. The use of several test systems affords a good deal of protection against errors of this kind. Tissue culture tests may disclose one virus and mouse tests a second, or different cell lines may afford a clue to a mixture. In critical cases it is necessary to type the first isolate and retest the original specimen in the presence of antiserum to the agent first isolated. This should be done whenever the laboratory results are at variance with the clinical findings. Laboratory results are *aids* to diagnosis.

The problem of etiology is often clouded by the nature of the specimen. Isolation of a virus from a fecal specimen is much less significant than isolation from blood or cerobrospinal fluid and these are less conclusive than recovery from the *lesion;* this might be called Koch's fourth postulate. Even in such circumstances the possibility of mixed infection needs to be kept in mind. Gear found both a poliovirus and a Coxsackie virus in the brain stem of a patient who died of paralytic poliomyelitis.[10] These limitations also need to be kept in mind in judging the significance of published reports linking certain enteroviruses with particular diseases.

These pitfalls in proving an etiologic relationship were fully recognized by Huebner and his associates in their investigation of herpangina. The criteria they set were that the association of the virus and the disease should be confirmed at different times and in different places and that only clinically typical cases of herpangina would be included in the evaluation.[11] (These are the rules Koch followed years ago in establishing the etiologic role of cholera vibrio.) By these criteria six Group A Coxsackie viruses (2, 4, 5, 6, 8, and 10) were identified as etiologic agents of herpangina. (Herpangina affords an additional example of the validity of Koch's fourth postulate. The oral blisters are highly infectious.)

Primary cultures of monkey kidney cells are probably the most commonly used in searching for enteroviruses but human uterine (amnion) cells should be used whenever possible and embryonic human kidney cells have been invaluable at times. Isolates are first screened against pooled antisera available from the National Institutes of Health and the World Health Organization. The antisera are pooled to take advantage of the known antigenic relationships. Typing is confirmed by quantitative neutralization tests. A number of prime strains have been documented and variants turn up now and then that require detailed investigation. Much systematic study will be required to provide a comprehensive atlas of the types. Such an effort could possibly throw light on the evolution of the viruses.

In addition to the Group B Coxsackie viruses, types 9, 21, and 23 of Group A are readily recovered in this way, as are all of the echo viruses. In the presence of lesions of the throat the affected areas should be swabbed. Anal swabs or fecal specimens are usually collected as well, and cerebrospinal fluid if meningeal symptoms are present. The specimens are suspended in tissue culture fluid fortified with antibiotics and applied to the sheets of cells and inoculated into newborn mice. Several litters should be used and the infants randomized. Both intracerebral and intraperitoneal routes of inoculation should be tried and an inoculation into the brain via the fat pad between the scapulae is recommended when Group B virus is suspected. The lesions in the brown fat (the hibernating gland) are pathognomonic of the Group B viruses and can easily be recognized with the naked eye once the animal has been skinned.

The tissue cultures are observed for cytopathogenic effects, and the mice for tremors (Group B Coxsackie viruses) or weakness (Group A), and their tissues are harvested for passage. Surviving sick animals often provide an immediate identification. The Group A viruses cause opaque, grayish streaking in the skeletal muscles, the Group B viruses opacities of the intrascapular fat pad. The neutralization test is most reliable in typing mouse strains.


## THE DISEASES

Several distinctive diseases of man are consequence of Coxsackie and echo virus infections.


### Epidemic Pleurodynia

Epidemic pleurodynia was recognized late in the nineteenth century, shortly after Kussmaul identified the common epidemic paralysis of children as "poliomyelitis anterior acuta." The early history of both relate to outbreaks in Scandinavia and north Europe but, like poliomyelitis, epidemic pleurodynia has since been found to be worldwide in its distribution. The disease was first described in North America by Dabney in 1888 and has characteristically and unpredictably appeared since in epidemic form. Well documented outbreaks occurred in the Red Hook section of Brooklyn in 1942,[12] in Boston and New England in 1947,[13] in Great Britain in 1951,[14] and in Hungary in 1958.[15]

The epidemic disease, again like poliomyelitis, affects mainly the young. In Sylvest's classic report[16] of the Bornholm epidemic (many refer to epidemic pleurodynia as Bornholm disease) half the patients were younger than 15 years. Lindberg described an epidemic limited to children.[17] Pickles characterized pleurodynia as "a disease of alarming symptoms but no death rate"[18] but this may not be strictly correct, for fatal cases have been described, although the laboratory evidence leaves something to be desired.

Epidemic pleurodynia is recognized by the sudden onset of severe, localized pain, devil's grip, most common in the chest but frequently in the abdomen, an extremity, or the neck. The pain may be excruciating but often subsides within the day. The fever course is sometimes biphasic in type as is so often true of poliomyelitis. Prodromata, if present, are not distinctive. The chest pains are aggravated by breathing and are at times referred to a shoulder. Chest pain is more common in older children and adults, abdominal pain in younger children. The pain returns with the fever. Numbness of the hands has been noted and headache and stiffness of the neck are relatively common. While recovery is usually uneventful, relapses are not infrequent and persistent fatigue and depression were complained of by young adults affected during the 1947 epidemic.

Orchitis is the commonest complication. It has occurred in as many as a third of all male patients. Ovarian tenderness has not been found. Myocarditis and pericarditis dominate in many epidemics. In the very young the myocarditis is severe and often fatal (vide infra). Involvement of the central nervous system has been an important sequel. In addition to aseptic meningitis, which is relatively common, meningoencephalitis may occur, especially among younger patients. The cerebral complications usually appear several days after the onset.

The muscle pain is at times associated with palpable muscle tumefactions which greatly impressed Sylvest. Direct evidence of the nature of the muscle tumor was provided by Lepine, Desse, and Sautter,[19] who observed degeneration of muscle cells and inflammatory reactions in biopsy specimens.

The etiologic agents of epidemic pleurodynia are the Group B Coxsackie viruses. (There is suggestive but still not conclusive proof that pleurodynia has been caused by other enteroviruses.) All of the known serotypes seem capable of causing pleurodynia. Virus may frequently be recovered from the blood and cerebrospinal fluid and for longer periods from the feces.

## Myocarditis Neonatorum

South African workers first established Group B Coxsackie viruses as the causative agents of acute and frequently fatal myocarditis in infants. Their patients were newborn infants exposed to an epidemic of Bornholm disease in a nursery.[20] A type 4 virus was originally isolated but other Group B types have since been implicated.

Outbreaks of fatal myocarditis in infants and young children had previously attracted the attention of physicians, and Stoeber's review of fatal cases led her to speak of "epidemic myocarditis in infancy" as a nosologic entity.[21] Since her studies were of postmortem material, specimens were not available for testing for viruses but there is circumstantial evidence to suggest the German cases were due to Coxsackie viruses. One of the most thoroughly studied early cases was reported by Kibrick and Benirschke.[22] The infection was thought to have occurred in utero. Destructive lesions were present in the heart and central nervous system. Within a few years similar cases of myocarditis were described by many observers and comparable though less severe myocardial and pericardial lesions were demonstrated in young adults as well.[23]

The disease in newborn infants appears suddenly, in most instances within the first week of life, sometimes a few hours or days after a brief episode of diarrhea and anorexia. Lethargy, grayish pallor, and mild icterus are common features (hepatitis has been demonstrated in fatal cases).

Tachycardia, dyspnea, and cyanosis, which may be present early, disclose the circulatory embarrassment, and cardiomegaly and hepatomegaly can be extreme. The spleen may be palpable, and electrocardiograms confirm the myocardial damage. The cerebrospinal fluid shows pleocytosis, xanthochromia, and increased protein content. The course may be fatal within the hour of onset. The extent of involvement of various organs established myocarditis neonatorum as equivalent to the disease seen in experimentally infected mice. In man and mouse age is the determining factor. Lewes and Lane suggested the term "acute, *benign* pericarditis" for Group B virus cardiac infections in young *adults*.[24] One can only speculate regarding its frequency. In 17 random New York cases of B-5 virus infection Plager identified 5 with pericarditis and found 15 additional citations.[25]

The heart is susceptible to infection by a great variety of viruses, and suggestive changes of myocarditis are sometimes noted in poliomyelitis. Kibrick found evidence of this kind in several instances of echo virus infection[26] but the severity of the disease caused by Group B Coxsackie viruses sets it apart from all others so far reported.

The spectrum of pathogenicity is reflected in the experimental infections. Thus Rabin et al.[27] have described the myocardial lesions induced by a particular Group B (type 3) strain that is pathogenic for mice up to the age of weaning. The report is noteworthy for the electron microscopic and immunofluorescent observations as well. The lesions appear to have been more severe than those Lerner associated with a number of strains of A-9 virus isolated in Boston between 1959 and 1961 which induced focal myocardial lesions in adult mice although the susceptibility of the skeletal muscles disappeared during the second week of life.[28]

It is important to note that Wickman's vital contribution to our understanding of poliomyelitis, the occurrence of nonparalytic illnesses (see Chapter 22), also holds for these "cousins." Epidemics of Group B Coxsackie virus infections may be characterized clinically by pleurodynia or myocarditis but these severe manifestations are usually greatly outnumbered by minor illnesses, pharyngitis being a common expression.

## HERPANGINA

Herpangina is also characteristically a disease of the young. It is caused by at least six of the Group A viruses, including types 2, 4, 5, 6, 8, and 10. The illness begins with fever of several days' duration, anorexia, and dysphagia. Headache and convulsions occur in some of the patients but muscle pains are not common. The characteristic and pathognomonic manifestation is the appearance of discrete oral lesions, usually on the anterior pillars of the fauces, less frequently on the palate, the uvula, the tonsils, or the tongue, but not on the gingival or buccal mucosa. The individual lesion begins as a small white papule (1 to 2 mm. in diameter) surrounded by a red areola which enlarges and becomes more inflamed as the papule ulcerates. Vesicles and ulcers may both be present four to six days after onset. They average five to the patient. Leukocytosis is uncommon, as are complications, the most frequent of which is aseptic meningitis. Parotitis and hemolytic anemia have been noted.

The clinical character of herpangina is sufficiently distinctive that an experienced physician can recognize it without difficulty and the inoculation of suckling mice with an extract of a throat swab only serves to confirm what may be established by inspection alone.

## PARALYTIC DISEASE

There is ample evidence that many of the echo and Coxsackie viruses can induce paralytic poliomyelitis-like syndromes in man, and Coxsackie virus A-7, initially isolated from patients with poliomyelitis, was found responsible by Voroshilova and Chumakov for a severe and quite typical outbreak of paralytic disease in Russia.[29] The Russian workers found this "AB-IV" virus capable of causing poliomyelitis in monkeys as well and proposed it be classified as type 4 poliovirus. Their observations have been confirmed by others.[30] While the experience with A-7 is in many ways the most striking example of the neuropathogenicity of the Coxsackie and echo viruses, there is solid evidence to implicate many of the other types as well. In general, the severity of paralysis associated with the Coxsackie and echo viruses has been less than that caused by the polioviruses, and recovery more rapid and complete, but there are well documented exceptions to the rule.

## ASEPTIC MENINGITIS

Aseptic meningitis is a common manifestation of Coxsackie and echo virus infection and is caused by a variety of other viruses as well. It may occur in combination with more distinctive symptoms or alone in which case it affords no clue to the responsible agent. Headache, fever, stiffness of the neck, and pleocytosis of the cerebrospinal fluid in the absence of bacterial infection are the hallmarks of aseptic meningitis.

## RASHES

The emergence of epidemic strains has frequently been associated with rashes and eruptions as well as intensification of the neurotropism of these viruses. A good example was provided by the echo 9 virus epidemic that swept much of Europe in 1955 and 1956. The epidemic disease apparently evolved in Italy where it is believed to have been endemic for some years before the large-scale outbreaks attracted attention.[31] The epidemics were marked by brief morbilliform rashes and more severe involvement of the central nervous system, radiculomyelitis, and at times encephalomyelitis.

Sporadic cases also appeared in northern European countries, preceding the epidemics,[32] which were seasonally like poliomyelitis, with peak incidence in the late summer and fall. Like poliomyelitis, the fever curves were commonly biphasic. The usual symptoms of headache, stiff neck, and vomiting were commonly combined with a morbilliform rash of the trunk that often faded after a few hours. In severe illnesses the rash occasionally became hemorrhagic. Pharyngitis (but not herpangina) was common and in the severe cases alterations in the reflexes, bladder paralysis, or spotty weakness of skeletal muscles was noted. Diverse rashes have been noted in individual epidemics, petechial, hemorrhagic, and vesicular, and are far more common in those under four years. Horstmann observed an epidemic in which the face was prominently involved.

The heightened pathogenicity of the epidemic strains was associated with pathogenicity for newborn mice, as has already been noted. Thus some European workers first recognized the Coxsackie A characteristics of the virus and referred strains to the Albany laboratory for typing. They were recognized as a "new" type and designated A-23. In those laboratories in which tissue culture methods were favored, the antigenic relationship to echo 9 was noted and the mouse pathogenicity was disregarded.

It should be noted that sporadic echo 9 virus infections have apparently caused both paralysis[33] and cerebellar ataxia.[34] In the former instance poliomyelitis was excluded by serologic tests. In the latter, the echo 9 strain was recovered from the cerebrospinal fluid as well as the throat and feces.

Type A-16 Coxsackie virus has been associated with a maculopapular rash of the hands and feet that characteristically becomes vesicular and has been called "hand, foot, and mouth disease." The oral blisters resemble those seen in herpangina. The prototype virus was isolated in South Africa. The first epidemic strains were recovered in Ontario, in 1957, where some 60 patients were investigated.[35] The illnesses were mild and no sequelae were noted. In affected households half of all the members became ill, usually the youngest children. Similar illnesses have since been associated with this serotype in other parts of the world and in other years.

Maculopapular rashes have been present during illnesses caused by several echo viruses. Neva's studies[36] implicated echo type 16 and others have established relationships to type 4.[37] Indeed there are scattered reports involving many additional echo serotypes. The eruptions have characteristically been associated with symptoms of aseptic meningitis.

### LYMPHADENITIS

Steigman implicated Coxsackie A-10 virus in an epidemic, largely of children, that was characterized by discrete whitish or yellowish nodular lesions of the uvula, the anterior pillars, and the posterior pharynx. In distinction to herpangina the lesions were never vesicular, and histologic examination showed the papules composed of tightly packed lymphocytes. Inclusion bodies were seen in the overlying epithelium (not herpetic).[38] Lymphadenitis, with enlargement of the spleen as well as the cervical and other peripheral lymph nodes, is by no means rare in Coxsackie virus infections.

Melnick suggested that enterovirus infection should be considered in summer epidemics associated with a high incidence of aseptic meningitis but little paralysis, in those associated with rashes, and in outbreaks of diarrheal disease in very young infants in which bacterial infections have been excluded.[39] The evidence regarding enteroviruses and diarrhea is somewhat contradictory and one gains the impression that the known enteroviruses are seldom responsible for severe forms of gastroenteritis or enteritis or major respiratory syndromes. Both conditions have been discussed in terms of the enteroviruses and contrary opinions are held by many.

# PATHOGENESIS AND ANATOMICAL PATHOLOGY

The pathogenesis of infection, certainly of those types associated with significant human disease, is evidently very similar to that of poliomyelitis and the reader should consult Chapter 22. Infection is primarily alimentary: virus spreads and causes responses in alimentary lymphatic structures and is disseminated by the blood. Infection persists longer in the intestinal tract than in the mouth. Infection is much more common among the under-privileged, presumably because of neglect of personal hygiene.

Lesions of the central nervous system may be indistinguishable from those caused by the polioviruses, as Horstmann and Manuelidis concluded in a study of Coxsackie A-7 in monkeys.[40] It will be remembered, however, that this virus is somewhat exceptional in its resemblance to the polioviruses in man. Extensive studies of the central nervous system in primates infected with other Coxsackie and echo viruses have shown many similarities between the lesions of these infections and those of poliomyelitis. In the case of Group B infections the lateral horns of the spinal cord are more conspicuously involved than the anterior horns. Nevertheless the generalization seems justified that there is a significant resemblance between the lesions in the central nervous system caused by the polio viruses and those caused by many of the Coxsackie and echo viruses.

The lesions of the brown fat represent a striking example of likeness. These lesions were originally noted as a conspicuous anatomic feature of Group B Coxsackie virus infection in mice,[41] and Shwartzman and Aronson later found identical lesions in primates infected with polioviruses.[42] While it is true that similar changes occur in mice infected with foot and mouth disease virus, the lesion is otherwise a most unusual one and constitutes another striking resemblance. Persistence of infection in brown fat is exceptional and has been considered of possible importance in the survival of Group B viruses but the experiments have so far failed to show overwintering (in ground squirrels).[43]

Group A Coxsackie viruses cause extensive, destructive lesions of the striated muscles of baby mice which account for the weakness and paralysis. Usually the central nervous system is unaffected but field strains of three types were early encountered that caused a degree of motor neuron damage as well. The lesion of the neurons appeared in 10 to 12 gm. mice, and muscle destruction in immature animals. The lesion of the anterior horns was seen irregularly. One of the three types (A-14) was later adapted to weaned mice by dint of repeated passage of infected spinal cord inoculated intraspinally.

The adapted strain regularly induced lesions similar to those caused by poliovirus.[44] Presumably other Group A strains might be similarly modified, as has now been done with all three of the polioviruses.

Tenderness and pain in the muscles is well known in poliomyelitis but has not been investigated. Muscle biopsy is contraindicated and would intensify paralysis. The lesion responsible for the muscle tumefactions noted in epidemic pleurodynia has, however, been examined microscopically and found to correspond to what is seen in experimental animals.[19] It seems likely that the finer analysis of the lesions of the striated muscles affords an excellent opportunity to explore the pathogenesis of enterovirus infections. Gädeke's observations are noteworthy.[45]

Certain lesions seen in mice have no known counterparts in man. Group B viruses, for example, may cause massive dissolution of the cerebrum of the mouse. If the animals survive, great cysts remain. Pappenheimer found massive lesions of the mouse pancreas as well following Group B virus infection.[46] This tropism is lost after brain to brain passage and is intensified by pancreas transfers.

The myocardial lesions that are so important an expression of Group B infections in infants and young children have their counterpart in experimental animals including monkeys. There is considerable type and strain variability. Adult mice may be infected and develop myocarditis while being dosed with cortisone.[47]

The anatomical pathology, one may conclude, reflects basic properties of the viruses and, in general, holds true for various species. It provides points of reference within which a more fundamental understanding of pathogenesis might be found and supports the concept of a spectrum of pathogenicity within which the morbid effects in man and experimental animals fit very neatly. Much attention has been given to the virus-cell relationships as represented by cells cultivated *in vitro*. Knowledge of greater significance awaits the investigation of the relationships in the animal as a whole.


## THE GENETICS OF THE ENTEROVIRUSES

The variety of the enteroviruses and the frequency of mixed infections might be fruitfully explored in terms of virus genetics. It seems reasonable to suspect that the various types may have evolved from common antecedents. In the years the viruses have been available for study little evidence has been found of change comparable to that which occurs among the influenza viruses, but mutations represented by changes in virulence and behavior in tissue cultures, for example plaque formation, are commonplace. It is quite striking that the types found throughout the world have so far shown no differences other than variations in virulence. Epidemiologic forces have evidently been more important than genetic changes in determining the pattern of disease.

Recombination has been demonstrated in the polioviruses but very little has so far been done to study, in genetic terms, the possible significance of mixed infections. Theoretically cross reactivation and heterozygosis as well as complementation and phenotypic mixing could all be expected to enter into the relationships among these viruses as they occur in nature. All await exploration.

## ECOLOGICAL RELATIONSHIPS

The Coxsackie viruses were identified during the height of the campaign to control the growing epidemics of poliomyelitis that marked the nineteen forties. The viruses were found associated with the polioviruses with which they share many properties. Experimental studies early demonstrated that Group B viruses inhibited the evolution of experimental poliomyelitis (the interference phenomenon)[48] and older records suggested that paralytic polio- myelitis and epidemic pleurodynia had rarely occurred together. The rela- tionship seemed to be a reciprocal one.[49] On the other hand, an unusually severe epidemic of paralytic poliomyelitis was otherwise remarkable for the extent of simultaneous infection with *Group A strains*,[50] and in monkeys com- bined infection with one Group A virus and an attenuated strain of poliovirus resulted in frank paralysis.[51] There was therefore suggestive evidence of inter- ference by certain of the viruses and enhancement by others.

These observations directed attention to the ecologic relationships among the enteroviruses. Not long afterward live virus vaccines were being tested and provided a further example of interference when it was learned that many children who were excreting echo or Coxsackie viruses were refractory to infection with the vaccine viruses.[52] Live virus vaccines should be used during seasons when enterovirus infections are uncommon, because "takes" and therefore immunization are conspicuously subject to this limitation. On the other hand, it seems possible that under other circumstances the introduc- tion of vaccine strains of virus might be expected to displace field strains.

One of the limiting factors in interferences in man seems to be that various viruses favor different portions of the gastrointestinal tract. This is well known among strains of the polioviruses and apparently can provide for simultaneous infection with interfering viruses, one of which may inhabit the throat and the other, part of the bowel. Certainly Group B Coxsackie and poliovirus infections have occurred on occasion in the same individual. The striking interferences in experimental animals are not subject to this limita- tion, the influence of which is difficult to measure.

These intriguing questions remain unanswered, as well as how much paralytic disease is directly caused by polio's "cousins." The questions had arisen with much justification shortly before widespread poliomyelitis vac- cination was undertaken. The massive application of active immunization was therefore a huge biologic experiment as well as a great, organized effort to protect against the three polioviruses. The results thus far have been highly gratifying in the reduction of paralytic poliomyelitis but have not thrown much light on the ecologic relationships.

Among the questions that remain unanswered are whether the greater effectiveness of live rather than inactivated vaccines is due to a higher degree

of active immunization and whether the widespread introduction of the attenuated vaccine strains has also suppressed or displaced field strains to a
significant degree other than by active immunization. The question of whether
paralytic disease in the past has sometimes resulted from an enhancing effect
of combined infection can hardly be answered with complete confidence since
protection against the polio virus component would be expected to protect
against the combined effect as well.

Many other interesting questions remain. Has the massive introduction
of the vaccine viruses displaced certain Coxsackie and echo viruses? There is
evidence that pleurodynia and herpangina have been prevalent during recent
years but the epidemiologic data are inadequate to resolve the issue. The
1956 to 1957 pandemic of Coxsackie B-5 and echo 9 infection has defied
analysis. What would be the behavior of the "cousins" of the polioviruses if
vaccination eradicated the virulent strains? The experience to date has been
too limited to justify any conclusions as to cause and effect. The eventual
outcome may throw light on the importance of the ecologic relationships that
presumably exist.

Translation from theory and managed, experimental observations to
nature and the field is the work of the epidemiologist. The author has sought
the opinion of an epidemiologist thoroughly acquainted with these diseases.
His opinion is that the establishment of an interrelationship on a community-
wide basis will be extremely difficult, in part because of the limitations of
present methods of measurement which are "crude beyond description." He
suspects that the infections in question move in long term cycles for totally
obscure reasons and judges the occasional reciprocal frequency of paralytic
poliomyelitis and particular enterovirus infections as no more conclusive than
the single case.

Possibly the intensive study of individual patients from a holistic point
of view would be rewarding. It would be necessary to stoutly resist the temptation to accept single determinants as wholly responsible and to energetically
search for complex infections in the presence of clinical atypia. It is well
to remember that clinicians suspected the existence of these "cousins" long
before virologists. De Rudder had postulated a pleomorphic variant of poliovirus as the probable cause of epidemic pleurodynia[53] and Zahorsky had
speculated about the relationships between poliomyelitis and herpangina[54] at
a time when virologists were content to accept Landsteiner's virus as solely
responsible for our late-summer epidemics.

# References

1. Jungeblut, C. W., and G. Dalldorf. 1943. Epidemiological and experimental observations
   on the possible significance of rodents in a suburban epidemic of poliomyelitis. Am. J.
   Pub. Health *33:*169–172.
2. Ørskov, J., and E. K. Andersen. 1948. Poliomyelitis in mice. Acta path. et microbiol. Scand.
   *25:*746–754.
3. Dalldorf, G., and G. M. Sickles. 1948. An unidentified, filtrable agent isolated from the
   feces of children with paralysis. Science *108:*61–62.

4. Enders, J. F., T. H. Weller, and F. C. Robbins. 1949. Cultivation of the Lansing strain of poliomyelitis virus in cultures of various human embryonic tissues. Science 109:85–87.
5. Robbins, F. C., J. F. Enders, T. H. Weller, and G. L. Florentino. 1951. Studies on the cultivation of poliomyelitis viruses in tissue culture. Am. J. Hyg. 54:286–293.
6. Ozaki, Y., and J. L. Melnick. 1963. Reaction of poliovirus and formaldehyde in magnesium chloride solution to enhance potency of killed-virus vaccine. J. Immunol. 90:429–437.
7. Sickles, G. M., M. Mutterer, and H. Plager. 1959. New types of Coxsackie virus, Group A, cytopathogenicity in tissue culture. Proc. Soc. Exper. Biol. & Med. 102:742–743.
8. Schieble, J. H., V. L. Fox, and E. H. Lennette. 1967. A probable new human picornavirus associated with respiratory disease. Am. J. Epidemiol. 85:297–310.
9. Plager, H. 1962. The Coxsackie viruses. Ann. New York Acad. Sc. 101:390–397.
10. Gear, J. H. S. Personal communication.
11. Parrott, R. H., S. Ross, F. G. Burke, and E. C. Rice. 1951. Herpangina. Clinical studies of a specific infectious disease. New England J. Med. 245:275–280.
12. Howard, T., et al. 1943. Epidemic pleurodynia in Brooklyn in the summer of 1942. J.A.M.A. 121:925–929.
13. Finn, J. J., T. H. Weller, and H. R. Morgan, 1949. Epidemic pleurodynia: clinical and etiologic studies based on one hundred and fourteen cases. Arch. Int. Med. 83:305–321.
14. Warin, J. F., F. K. Sanders, J. B. M. Davies, and A. D. Vizosa. 1953. Oxford epidemic of Bornholm disease, 1951. Brit. M. J., 1:1345–1351.
15. Dömok, I., and E. Molnar. 1960. An outbreak of meningoencephalomyocarditis among newborn infants during the epidemic of Bornholm disease of 1958 in Hungary. Ann. paediat. 194:102–114.
16. Sylvest, E. 1934. Epidemic Myalgia: Bornholm Disease. Copenhagen, Levin and Munksgaard.
17. Lindberg, G. 1936–1937. Epidemic myalgia in children. Acta Paediat. 19:1–49.
18. Pickles, W. N. 1954. Bornholm disease. Brit. M. J. Nov. 27.
19. Lepine, P., G. T. Desse, and V. Sautter. 1952. Biopsies musculaires, examen histologique et isolement du virus coxsackie chez l'homme atteint de myalgie épidémique (maladie de Bornholm). Bull. Acad. nat. méd. 136:66–69.
20. Montgomery, J., J. H. S. Gear, F. R. Prinsloo, M. Kahn, and Z. G. Kirsch. 1956. Myocarditis in the newborn. An outbreak in a maternity home in Southern Rhodesia associated with Coxsackie Group-B virus infection. South African M. J. 29:608–612.
21. Stoeber, E. 1952. Weitere Untersuchungen über epidemische Myocarditis. Ztschr. Kinderh. 71:319–356, 592–623.
22. Kibrick, S., and K. Benirschke. 1956. Acute aseptic myocarditis and meningoencephalitis in the newborn child infected with Coxsackie virus Group B, type 3. New England J. Med. 255:883–889.
23. Weinstein, S. B. 1957. Pericarditis. New England J. Med. 257:265–267; Cercassi, U., and A. Tuveri. 1959. Due casi di pericardite acute da Coxsackie B2. Aggiorn. mal. infes. 5:1–10.
24. Lewes, D., and W. F. Lane. 1961. Acute benign pericarditis due to Coxsackie virus, Group B, type 3. Lancet 2:1385–1386.
25. Plager, H. Personal communication.
26. Kibrick, S. 1964. Current status of Coxsackie and Echo viruses in human disease. Progr. Med. Virol. 6:27–70.
27. Rabin, E. R., S. A. Hassan, A. B. Jenson, and J. L. Melnick. 1964. Coxsackie B-3 myocarditis in mice. An electron microscopic, immunofluorescent and virus assay study. Am. J. Path. 44:775–797.
28. Lerner, A. M. 1965. An experimental approach to viral myocarditis. Progr. Med. Virol. 7:97–115.
29. Voroshilova, M. K., and M. P. Chumakov. 1959. Poliomyelitis-like properties of Ab-IV-Coxsackie A-7 Group of viruses. Progr. Med. Virol. 2:106–170.
30. Habel, K., and L. N. Loomis. 1957. Coxsackie A-7 Virus and the Russian "poliovirus Type 4." Proc. Soc. Exper. Biol. & Med. 95:97–605; Grist, N. R. 1962. Type A-7 Coxsackie (type 4 poliomyelitis) virus infection in Scotland. J. Hyg. 60:323–332; see also Grist, N. R. 1965. Further studies of Coxsackie A-7 virus infection in the west of Scotland. Lancet 1:261–263.
31. Archetti, I., A. Felici, F. Russi, and C. Fua. 1957. Richerche sulla definizione eziologica della meningonevrassite Marchigiani, 1955. Policlinico 64:224–234.
32. Lennartz, H., G. Maass, and G. Kersting. 1957. Zur Ätiologie der abakteriellen Meningitis. Klin. Wchnschr. 35:327–334; Tyrrell, D. A. J., and B. Snell. 1956. Recovery of a virus from cases of an epidemic exanthem associated with meningitis. Lancet 2:1028–1029; Nihoul, E., and L. Quersin-Thiry. 1957. A new clinical entity? Lancet 1:269–270; also Am. J. Hyg. 66:102, 1957.

33. Plager, H., and F. F. Harrison. 1961. Paralysis associated with Echo virus type 9. New York J. Med. *61:*798–800.
34. McAllister, R. M., K. Hummeler, and L. L. Coriell. 1959. Acute cerebellar ataxia: Report of a case with isolation of Type 9 Echo virus from the cerebrospinal fluid. New England J. Med. *261:*1159–1162.
35. Robinson, C. R., F. W. Doane, and A. J. Rhodes. 1958. Report of an outbreak of febrile illness with pharyngeal lesions and exanthem: Toronto, summer 1957. Isolation of Group A Coxsackie virus. Canad. M.A.J. *79:*615–621.
36. Neva, F. A., R. F. Feemster, and I. J. Gorbach. 1954. Clinical and epidemiological features of an unusual epidemic exanthem. J.A.M.A. *155:*544–548.
37. Karzon, D., G. L. Eckert, A. L. Barron, N. S. Hayner, and W. Winkelstein, Jr. 1961. Aseptic meningitis epidemic due to Echo 4 virus. Am. J. Dis. Child. *101:*610–622.
38. Steigman, A., M. M. Lipton, and H. Braspennick. 1962. Acute lymphonodular pharyngitis: A newly described condition due to Coxsackie A virus. J. Pediat. *61:*331–336.
39. Melnick, J. L. *In:* Horsfall, F. L., Jr., and Tamm, I.: Viral and Rickettsial Infections of Man. 4th ed. Philadelphia, Lippincott, 1965.
40. Horstmann, D. M., and E. E. Manuelidis. 1958. Russian Coxsackie A-7 virus (AB IV strain) —neuropathogenicity and comparison with poliomyelitis. J. Immunol. *81:*32–42.
41. Gifford, R., and G. Dalldorf, 1951. The morbid anatomy of experimental Coxsackie virus infection. Am. J. Path. *28:*1047–1063.
42. Shwartzman, G., and S. M. Aronson. 1954. Participation of brown fat in pathogenesis of experimental poliomyelitis of monkeys. Proc. Soc. Exper. Biol. & Med. *86:*767–771.
43. Dempster, G., G. I. Grodums, and W. A. Spencer. 1961. Experimental Coxsackie B-3 infection in the hibernating squirrel and bat. Canad. J. Microbiol. *7:*587–594; see also later studies in J. Cell. Physiol., vol. 67.
44. Dalldorf, G. 1957. Neuropathogenicity of Group A Coxsackie viruses. J. Exper. Med. *106:*69–76.
45. Gädeke, R. 1952. Vergleichende morphologische und chemische Muskelbefunde bei Säuglingsmäusen und Meerschweinchen nach experimenteller Infektion mit Viren der Coxsackie-A-Gruppe. Klin. Wchnschr. *30:*1040–1041; Gädeke, R., and H. Waltenberger. 1952. Ztschr. Naturforsch. *7b:*524–531.
46. Pappenheimer, A. M., J. B. Daniels, F. S. Cheever, and T. H. Weller. 1950. Lesions caused in suckling mice by certain viruses isolated from cases of so-called nonparalytic poliomyelitis and of pleurodynia. J. Exper. Med. *92:*169–190.
47. Kilbourne, E. D., and F. L. Horsfall, Jr. 1951. Lethal infection with Coxsackie virus of mice given cortisone. Proc. Soc. Exper. Biol. & Med. *77:*135–138.
48. Dalldorf, G. 1951. The sparing effect of Coxsackie virus infection on experimental poliomyelitis. J. Exper. Med. *94:*65–71.
49. Dalldorf, G. 1955. The Coxsackie viruses. Ann. Rev. Microbiol. *9:*277–296.
50. Melnick, J. L., and N. Ledinko. 1951. Social serology: antibody levels during an epidemic of poliomyelitis. Am. J. Hyg. *54:*354–382.
51. Dalldorf, G. 1958. Poliomyelitis as a complex infection. J. Exper. Med. *108:*605–616.
52. Ramos-Alvarez, M., and A. B. Sabin. 1956. Intestinal viral flora of healthy children demonstrable by monkey kidney tissue culture. Am. J. Pub. Health *46:*295–299.
53. de Rudder, B. 1937. Epidemic pleurodynia and poliomyelitis. Klin. Wchnschr. *16:*585–589.
54. Zahorsky, J. 1924. Herpangina (a specific infectious disease). Arch. Pediat. *41:*181–18.

# Chapter 25

# INFECTION WITH ONCOGENIC VIRUSES

BERNICE E. EDDY

*Division of Biologics Standards, National
Institutes of Health, Bethesda, Maryland*

Our current knowledge of cancer is at about the same level as our knowledge of poliomyelitis in the early 1940's. Much information on poliomyelitis was available at that time but the crucial experiments which ultimately led to the control of the disease had not been done. The National Foundation for Infantile Paralysis, Inc., sponsored the preparation of *A Bibliography of Infantile Paralysis* with selected abstracts and annotations covering 8320 papers published between 1789 and 1944.[43] A paper on another subject, which was not included in this bibliography, might have given a clue to the turning point in poliomyelitis research five or six years before Enders, Weller, and Robbins carried out the experiments which made possible the development of vaccines to control the disease. Huang, in 1943,[73] utilized the degenerative changes in cultures of minced skeletal muscles of nine-day-old chick embryos infected with western equine encephalomyelitis virus to titrate and test for neutralization of the virus. Enders and his co-workers reported their epochal experiments on the cytopathic effect of poliovirus in non-neural human embryonic cell cultures in 1949.[39] It is possible that experiments which could give a clue to a solution of the cancer problem have also been done, but if so, the information has not been generally recognized.

The purpose of this communication is to discuss some of the poorly understood observations which have been made concerning cancer. There is little doubt that the interrelationships of these observations will be clarified eventually. At present, however, it is difficult to assess the relative significance of the body of information at hand. Some of the phenomena may relate generally to the infectious process or may be concomitant activities related to the injured host cell, and may not be directly related to oncogenesis.

Tumor-inducing viruses have been known for many years[13, 38, 46, 105, 110, 116, 117] but the surge of information on oncogenic viruses over the past 16 years has been largely due to two discoveries: (1) the pronounced susceptibility of newborn animals to tumor induction by an oncogenic virus, and (2) the demonstration that an oncogenic virus can be grown *in vitro*, and that it may share many of the properties of nononcogenic viruses. A cell-free extract from tissues of a mouse with spontaneous leukemia induced leukemia when injected into newborn mice but not when injected into adult mice.[58, 59] Subsequently, age of the host was found to be an important factor in the induction of tumors by other oncogenic viruses. The polyoma virus was grown in mouse embryo cell cultures and the virus and the antibodies it evoked in animals could be titrated by the same methods used for nononcogenic viruses—cytopathic effect, hemagglutination, and inhibition of these phenomena by specific antiserum or fixation of complement by specific antiserum.[34–36, 107, 127]

The infectious oncogenic viruses are not confined to any one taxonomic group. Their sizes range from diameters of about 48 m$\mu$ (polyoma, simian virus 40 [SV-40] and other members of the papova group) to the large spherical or brick-shaped fibroma or myxoma viruses which measure 200 to 350 m$\mu$ in diameter or length. Some viruses, such as the murine leukemia viruses, the mammary carcinoma virus, and the chicken leukosis viruses, are ribonucleic acid (RNA) viruses, while the papovaviruses and adenoviruses are deoxyribonucleic acid (DNA) viruses. Most of the mature oncogenic RNA viruses contain a lipid fraction. These RNA viruses are easily inactivated by heat and other physical or chemical agents, as are the fibroma and other oncogenic poxviruses. However, the intact polyoma virus or SV-40 or the nucleic acid which can be extracted from these DNA viruses may be quite resistant to formalin, ether, and heat. Six high-titer preparations of SV-40 were sealed in glass and kept in boiling water for 15 minutes. Enough virus remained in four of these lots to induce tumors in one or more animals of each litter of newborn hamsters inoculated.[29]

Nucleic acid extracted from DNA oncogenic viruses grown in cell culture has been shown to be capable of replicating and maturing to infectious virus when incubated with susceptible cells under suitable conditions.[25, 76, 145] Many antiviral antibody reactions depend upon the protein capsid coats of the particles. Empty capsids of polyoma virus have been found to be just as capable of hemagglutinating washed erythrocytes as the intact virus.[17]

The nucleic acid content of some of the oncogenic viruses resemble the nucleic acids of the tumor-susceptible host cells.[5, 57] Among the viruses studied in this respect are the Shope papilloma virus, polyoma virus, SV-40, and the adenoviruses. Studies of the guanine-cytosine ratio in the DNA of the adenoviruses indicate that they fall into three groups. These groups correspond to types which are highly oncogenic, weakly oncogenic, or nononcogenic for newborn hamsters. (It is possible that all adenovirus types are oncogenic under certain circumstances. Adenovirus type 2 frequently infects small children and has been regarded as nononcogenic until recently, when it was shown to be able to transform cultures of rat embryo cells.[45] Transformation is not synonymous with oncogenesis but the two characteristics are often associated.)

The polyoma virus has been shown to contain three different kinds of DNA, separable by sedimentation in a density gradient. These DNA fractions differ in their ability to hybridize with normal mouse RNA.[91, 147] Most of this activity was localized in the slowly sedimenting DNA component while little or none was detectable in the rapidly sedimenting DNA component. This latter component was found to contain most of the infectious DNA. The authors speculate that the slowly sedimenting DNA component may have resulted from the encapsidation of host cellular DNA fragments during the maturation stage of virus development.

Under natural conditions, tumors appear to be the unusual manifestation of infection with an oncogenic virus, just as paralysis is the unusual manifestation of infection with poliovirus. One property shared by all the known oncogenic viruses is the ability to remain in their respective hosts for long periods of time without producing signs or symptoms of disease.

In the laboratory, tumor induction with a number of oncogenic viruses can be increased to almost 100 per cent by injecting newborn, nonimmune animals with a large dose of virus. As in other diseases, the latent period prior to tumor manifestation varies with the particular virus, its titer at the time of infection, and the species of the host animal. When mice are injected with the mammary carcinoma virus, a tumor may appear only after a lapse of five or six months and in some animals tumors make their appearance two or more years following inoculation. A newborn mouse infected with the polyoma virus may develop a tumor 6 to 12 weeks after inoculation or even much later. Newborn hamsters inoculated with the polyoma virus occasionally develop tumors a week later, but the usual time is 25 to 45 days or longer. SV-40, on the other hand, seldom induces tumors in hamsters until 70 to 100 days after inoculation. Some of the animals do not develop tumors until near the end of their two-year life span.

The histological types of virus-induced tumors and the sites of the tumors vary depending upon the virus and the host. The murine leukemia viruses usually induce only leukemias in mice or rats, but can induce lymphomas on rare occasions. The polyoma virus may produce almost any histological type of tumor in mice except leukemias.[126] In many strains of mice, tumors are most frequently induced in the salivary glands. In the A strain of mice, however, bone tumors occur with great frequency.[27, 122] Nontumorous lesions, such as runting, swelling of the convoluted kidney tubules, and anemia, may also occur in mice and rats. In general, tumors induced in hamsters by the polyoma virus are sarcomas or hemangiomas. Polyoma virus-infected rabbits develop multiple benign fibromatous nodules in the skin which regress after a time. However, another strain of polyoma virus has been reported to cause malignant tumors when administered to rabbits intracardially or intravenously.[56]

Tumor development is a poor indicator of infection by oncogenic viruses. Older animals may be infected by large doses of many of the oncogenic viruses, as evidenced by the production of antibodies, and yet fail to develop tumors.

The oncogenic viruses, like other viruses, are antigenic and stimulate the production of antibodies within their hosts. These antigens and the humoral antibodies they elicit may be measured by the same techniques employed for nononcogenic viruses. In some animals the virus does not multiply to any appreciable extent. Hamsters inoculated with SV-40 illustrate such a case. In this instance, the development of detectable antiviral antibodies in the serum depends upon the concentration of the virus or antigenic mass in the inoculum. Antiviral antibody, unless given before inoculation of the virus, does not prevent the development of tumors. Animals bearing tumors induced by the polyoma virus, SV-40, or the adenoviruses may have a high titer of antiviral antibodies in their serum, yet the continued development of the tumor is not hindered.

The transformation of cells, either *in vivo* or *in vitro*, is not fully understood; nevertheless much useful information concerned with this process has been accumulated. A series of changes occur during which the cells become neoplastic and synthesis of infectious virus is lessened or halted.[129, 142] These changes do not necessarily occur simultaneously. *In vitro*, only a few cells, often one in $10^4$ to $10^6$, are transformed and the first evidence is usually the loss of contact inhibition.[1] Normal cells usually form a sheet on a glass surface and the cell surfaces are aligned next to each other in an orderly fashion. After loss of contact inhibition the cells aggregate and grow over each other. The cell surfaces change and apparently become friable. Cytoplasm and nuclear material has been reported to flow out of a cell and form bridges with other cells.[10, 82] Chromosomes have been observed in some of the bridges between two tumor cells or in the bridge from a tumor cell to a normal cell, but not from a normal cell to a tumor cell. Tumor cells in the same culture may vary in a number of their properties. Some form dense clones; others form thin ones.[143] The thin clones are more likely to die out. For some unknown reason, some clones of transformed cells are neoplastic and transplantable to isologous hosts when first observed; others are not transplantable until they are maintained in cell culture for some time. Chromosome breaks and other changes also occur. These changes may take place either before or after the cells have been shown to be transplantable.[19]

The reason why some cells are transformed and others are not is unknown. Nor is it known why the synthesis of infectious virus is slowed or stopped in most virus-induced tumors. Cells from animal species which do not support good growth of infectious virus are often transformed with greater ease than cells of the natural susceptible host. Hamster and rat embryo cells, for example, can be transformed by the polyoma virus with greater ease than cells from mice, the natural host of the virus. SV-40 is malignant for hamsters, but it is not known to cause tumors in its natural host, the monkey. Transformation *in vitro* does not take place readily. Often the infected cells must be held for several weeks before piled-up foci of cells, evidence of transformation, is detected. However, embedding diluted infected cells in agar does permit earlier detection of morphologically different transformed cell colonies.[88] In a mixed culture, the transformed cells multiply faster, produce more acid, and ultimately overgrow the normal cells in the culture. Many apparently normal cells cultivated *in vitro* will, after a period of time, also become transformed,[111] but the change occurs earlier when the cells are purposely infected with an oncogenic virus.

Transformation is reported to be enhanced by (1) infection with a high multiplicity of virus in the inoculum,[132] (2) a high pH,[78, 79] (3) exposure of cells to magnesium ions after virus adsorption,[130, 131] (4) incubation at 24°C. for seven days followed by incubation at 37°C.,[90, 109] (5) a rich culture medium,[124, 125] (6) omission of calcium from the culture medium,[45] and (7) gamma or x-irradiation.[21] Recently cells morphologically normal have been shown to undergo transformation in a shorter period of time when grown in a medium containing 10 per cent horse serum than when grown in 10 per cent calf serum.[41] Some cells grown in calf serum did not become malignant. Bovine lung cells could not be transformed by the polyoma virus when the medium was enriched with bovine serum, but transformation did occur when lamb serum was used.[23, 21] The possibility exists that the horse and lamb serum might have contained other agents. However, more specific information on the effect of nutrient media on cell transformation by viruses is desirable. Work along this line may be rewarding.

Minocha and Consigli[92] found that differences in the nutrient fluids used for mouse embryo cells infected with the polyoma virus influenced the synthesis of viral proteins in the presence of 5-fluorodeoxyuridine (FUDR). Polyoma proteins were not synthesized in cultures maintained in Eagle's medium containing FUDR but were synthesized in similar cultures with Parker's 1066 medium containing FUDR. It was noted that 5-methyl deoxycytidine was a constituent of Parker's 1066 medium but not of Eagle's medium. When 5-methyl deoxycytidine was added to Eagle's medium, the synthesis of specific viral capsid proteins occurred in the presence of FUDR.

Often infectious virus cannot be recovered from transformed or malignant cells. Such cells may contain at least two specific antigens related to the virus, and also two nonspecific substances or antigens. Adult mice or hamsters immunized with the polyoma virus or with tumor cells induced by but free of detectable polyoma virus resist transplantation of a polyoma virus-induced tumor from an isologous host,[60, 123] but do not resist transplantation of an SV-40-induced tumor.[19, 62, 81] This phenomenon is explained by the observation that the virus induces a new cellular antigen, known as a transplantation antigen, which stimulates antibodies that prevent the host from accepting the tumor transplant. The reaction is specific and transplantation antibody is not generally effective against tumor cells induced by another virus.[119–121] It is believed to be located on the host cell surface,[61, 141] and the formation of antibody to it is dependent upon an intact lymphoid system.[22]

Most of the information available on transplantation antigens has been obtained by *in vivo* tests. These tests are often difficult to interpret because the test procedures used are rather insensitive. Furthermore, their completion requires several days to weeks. There are now at least two *in vitro* tests, both based on cytolysis, which can be used to measure the transplantation antigen. These have some disadvantages, but they are more precise than *in vivo* tests and can be carried out within a shorter period of time. One test involves colony growth inhibition in agar of previously mixed and incubated tumor cells, sera, and complement. The colony counts obtained with cells combined with antiserum and complement are reduced as compared to the colony counts of cells combined with normal serum and complement.[70, 121] In the other test, tumor cells are labeled with chromium 51 (sodium chromate) and then mixed with antiserum and complement, and the radioactivity liberated from the disrupted cells is measured by counting an aliquot of supernate in a crystal scintillation counter.[15, 146]

The majority of oncogenic viruses stimulate transplantation antigens. However, some mutant strains of polyoma virus have been described which failed to manifest this property. Moreover, one strain tended to stimulate the development of transplanted tumors.[64] The relationship of the transplantation antigen to defective viruses is poorly understood.

Two strains of polyoma virus were found to be defective in inducing transplant antibody. Cell cultures derived from one such transplantable virus-induced tumor, which contained no infectious virus, but did contain polyoma tumor-specific antigen, could be infected by the other defective virus strain. Virus propagated in these cultures, and also the defective virus strains grown on normal mouse embryo cultures, were used to inoculate three groups of mice. Four weeks later the sera from these groups of mice were shown to contain polyoma virus hemagglutination-inhibition antibodies. The mice were then challenged with virus-free tumor cells. Transplantation was inhibited in mice which had been infected with virus grown on tumor cells induced by the other defective polyoma strain. Mice infected with either of the two defective strains alone did not inhibit transplantation.[137] It is tempting to speculate that the defective polyoma virus particles lacked different components of the transplantation antigen, but when combined the two components were effective in inhibiting tumor transplantation.

Immunization against tumor induction can also be carried out after a newborn animal is infected. Many hamsters inoculated with a single dose of adenovirus type 12 or SV-40, either of which is capable of inducing a tumor in almost every hamster, could be prevented from developing tumors by repeated injections of large doses of the same live virus in the time period between the administration of the initial virus dose and the time of regular tumor development.[37] Repeated injection of virus after a tumor was detected had no effect on the continued development of the tumor. Immunization with virus inactivated by heat, ultraviolet radiation, or formalin was ineffective in protecting against tumor development.[29]

Hamsters infected with SV-40 when newborn and protected from developing tumors by repeated injections of live virus were also resistant to transplantation of an isologous SV-40 tumor, whereas such tumors could be readily transplanted to hamsters already bearing an SV-40-induced tumor.[33]

Newborn hamsters injected daily with adenovirus type 12 for six to ten days developed fewer tumors than hamsters which received a single dose of virus.[30] Thus within the short period of six to ten days, some of the hamsters became competent to produce antibodies which prevented tumor development. The nature of these protective antibodies is unknown but the possibility exists that they are identical with antibodies to the transplantation antigens.

Another specific cell antigen (known as the T, tumor, neo, or ICFA antigen) stimulates an antibody that is found in the serum of some, but not all, tumor-bearing animals, regardless of whether the tumor contains infectious virus.[14, 75, 100] The antigen is produced in the early lytic cycle before the appearance of infectious virus and in the presence of inhibitors of viral DNA synthesis. It can be detected by complement fixation or immunofluorescence. Unlike the transplantation antigen, it is present in the nucleus. Some minor differences have been found in T antigens, but in general those occurring in lytic infection and in transformed cells are the same, and the complement-fixation test and the immunofluorescent tests measure the same antigen. The antigens appear to be proteins. Their activity is destroyed by trypsin and by heat at 56°C. They are not dialyzable, and are not sedimented at speeds which sediment the virus particles. The biological role of the T antigens is obscure. They have been especially useful in studies of viral genomes in "hybrid" viruses and "hybrid" cells. Single cells have been shown to be transformed by two different viruses and the doubly transformed cells retained the tumor antigens induced by both viruses for many transplant generations.[133, 135, 138]

Attempts to identify the causative agent of different human tumors through the use of immunofluorescence or complement-fixation reactions to detect T or tumor antigens for adenoviruses types 7, 12, or 18 or SV-40, or to human neoplastic tissue, have not been successful.[84, 104, 108] Either no immunologically reactive components were revealed, or they occurred infrequently with diverse types of tumors, such as liposarcomas, leukemias, lymphosarcomas, reticulum cell sarcomas, Hodgkin's disease, carcinomas, and melanomas, and in nonmalignant as well as malignant tissues. Among the more provocative studies are those with Burkitt lymphoma. Antibodies against herpes-like viruses present in cultured Burkitt tumor cells have been found in patients with the disease and in normal individuals, but it is not clear whether these are antibodies to the diseases in question or to an adventitious virus.

Two nonspecific substances induced in cells by some of the oncogenic viruses, as well as by nononcogenic viruses, are interferon and Forssman antigen. Interferon is nonantigenic, or weakly antigenic, and is produced subsequent to polyoma virus infection. Polyoma virus-induced interferon in infected cell cultures has been shown to inhibit encephalomyelitis virus and to delay polyoma virus propagation in cell cultures.[2] A weakly oncogenic strain of polyoma virus was more sensitive to this interferon than a highly oncogenic strain.[54] Interferon, like the T antigen, is a protein produced early in the lytic system. It is sensitive to trypsin, moderately heat stable, not sedimentable at $100,000 \times g$ for one hour, and insensitive to nucleases.

Hamster kidney tumors induced by the polyoma virus when tested with rabbit antisheep erythrocyte serum showed an increase in Forssman antigen in comparison with tests using normal hamster kidneys.[44] The antigen was present in seven clones of polyoma-transformed hamster cells grown for 3 to 31 weeks and in cells of a single clone of transformed cells transplanted in adult hamsters for approximately four years. Forssman antigen was not detected in a continuous line of spontaneously transformed uncloned hamster embryo cells or in a culture from a clone of hamster cells treated with x-radiation.

The induction of viral and cellular antigens by an oncogenic virus is not the only phenomenon which affects tumor production. Other factors are operative. A virus may fuse or hybridize with another virus, oncogenic or nononcogenic; a transformed cell may contain genetic material from more than one virus; one microorganism may stimulate or interfere with infection by another virus; cells of different types may hybridize; and infectious virus may be "rescued" under certain circumstances from virus-free transformed or malignant cells containing a portion of the viral genome.

Hanafusa et al.[63] were the first to show that virus could be recovered from certain virus-free chicken tumors after inoculation of the bird with a nononcogenic "helper" virus. The new virus recovered from the tumor retained many of the properties of the virus which was injected into the bird, and in addition it was oncogenic when passed to a new susceptible host. Later a strain of adenovirus type 7, which had been propagated in rhesus monkey kidney cells where it could have been in contact with SV-40, was found to induce tumors in hamsters.[74, 106] This virus showed no evidence of contamination with SV-40. SV-40 could not be recovered, and the strain reacted with adenovirus type 7 antisera. However, some of the tumors it induced in hamsters had the gross appearance of SV-40 tumors and serum from hamsters bearing SV-40-induced tumors reacted with the tumor antigen in the cells both by the complement-fixation test and by immunofluorescence. Other virus combinations have been reported: adenovirus type 3 and SV-40, adenovirus type 2 and SV-40.[45, 95, 103] The explanation of the "hybrid" virus or the defective virus grown with a "helper" virus is that the nucleic acid of the defective virus is encased in the protein coat of a second virus, which is not necessarily an oncogenic virus. The infectious hybrid virus may exhibit many characteristics of the virus whose protein coat it bears, and it is neutralized by antiserum against the virus which provided the protein coat.

The explanation may be more complex. Mattern et al.[89] have described three morphological units of the polyoma virus with diameters of 48, 38, and 22 m$\mu$, in addition to filamentous forms, also described by other investigators. The single particles are believed to have 72, 32, and 12 capsomeres or surface knobs, respectively. These observations suggest that the virus may be constructed from interior to exterior, first as the small particle, 22 m$\mu$ in diameter, followed by other layers of material to form particles 38 m$\mu$ and 48 m$\mu$ in diameter. The 48 m$\mu$ particle is the infectious particle. In addition to the three sizes of particles, some of the virus particles in the cytoplasm were covered by a phospholipid layer, making the total diameters 50 to 60 m$\mu$. Filamentous counterparts of the three spherical particles were seen and small filaments were observed to protrude from some of the larger filaments. The role of the multiple forms of the virus particle in the construction of the infectious virus is, as yet, speculative. Since the filaments disappear after a time, they may be precursors of the spherical forms.

Different sizes of particles were observed in at least two other systems. Particles of different sizes were observed in purified virus preparations of SV-40 grown in primary green monkey kidney cells. However, no filamentous forms were observed in the purified preparations of SV-40 or in sections of monkey kidney cells infected with the virus. Two spherical forms, 50 and 38 m$\mu$ in diameter, have been observed in rabbit papilloma preparations. Herpes-like particles from malignant Burkitt lymphoma cells have been observed to have an extra envelope. The relationship of these particles of different sizes to either the transplantation or the tumor antigens is unknown. Nor is it known whether morphologically different particles occur among the adenoviruses and other known oncogenic viruses.

The presence of empty capsids seen in the electron microscopic preparations of certain viruses, particularly in certain bands following density-gradient centrifugation, invites speculation as to what happens to the inner portions of the particles. It is entirely possible that virus capsids can be made without the nucleic acid cores. If other virus particles, like polyoma or SV-40, are made up of smaller units which fit into the next larger size unit, the core of an infectious virus may not be entirely nucleic acid; it may be nucleic acid plus a capsid layer. Defective viruses are known to induce tumors, but whether the smallest units are oncogenic must await further investigation. Bendich et al.[11] obtained evidence that viral nucleic acid was free in the blood and considered that the distribution of this genetic material could be responsible for metastasis of the tumors.

The activation or inhibition of a virus by another microorganism is not confined to oncogenic viruses. A number of years ago, an avirulent poliovirus was shown to be activated by a Coxsackie virus.[18] The passage of polyoma virus from mouse to mouse by cell-free extracts which also contained the murine leukemia virus could be explained by the activating effect upon the polyoma virus by the leukemia virus.[58, 59] The polyoma virus alone could not be passed from mouse to mouse unless the concentration of virus was increased between passages by propagation in susceptible cell cultures.[127] Chany and Brailovsky have given the name "stimulon" to the substance which enhances the growth of one virus by another virus.[16] The apparent activation of a latent virus in mice by injection of tumor material has been reported by a number of investigators. Heidenhain[69] noted tumors in mice injected with human tumor material ranging from zero to 6.7 per cent of 2029 mice as compared with 1.5 per cent in 2428 control mice. Grace et al.[55] observed tumors in 5 per cent of 1324 mice injected with human tumor material and none in 1900 mice which received only normal cell culture material. Moore[93] injected 3990 mice with material from 208 tumor specimens. Of these, 10.2 per cent developed tumors and these tumors occurred mostly in mice which had received lympho-sarcoma material. Tumors developed in only 4.3 per cent of 784 control mice. Girardi,[51, 52] on the other hand, using sex-segregated animals, failed to induce tumors in mice with human tumor material. Adenoviruses, which failed to replicate in monkey kidney cells, could do so in the presence of SV-40. More-over, the titer of an adenovirus was shown to increase when cultivated with SV-40.[102]

The opposite effect, in which one microorganism inhibits another, also occurs. At least some of the interference is due to the synthesis of interferon, a nonspecific cellular substance which prevents infection of cells but which has no direct action on the virus, but competition for susceptible cell sites may also be a factor.

Certain bacterial infections also have an antagonizing effect on the development of tumors. Tubercle bacilli of the Calmette-Guérin strain (BCG) given to hamsters prior to injection with polyoma virus reduced the incidence of tumors and prolonged survival time, and hemagglutination inhibition, complement fixation, and neutralizing antibodies were augmented.[85] It has been reported that Ehrlich ascites and Yoshida sarcoma cells lose their invasiveness in the mouse and rat after infection with a live group A streptococcus in vitro. The cells infected by other bacteria did not show this activity.[66, 98, 115]

The demonstration of fusion of different somatic cells and the evolution of a new viable cell, differing from the parent cell, is an important tool which may ultimately provide a practical means for identifying the etiological agent or agents of some human tumors. In 1960, Barski, Sorieul, and Cornefert[9] mixed cells from two clones of polyoma virus-transformed mouse cells from high- and low-cancer mice lines. They grew the mixture in cell culture, and also inoculated it into mice. A new cell type evolved and clones of the new cells differed from the parent cells. Moreover, high carcinogenicity was an attribute of the cells. Some morphological and biological features resembled those of the low-cancer lines, but their malignancy approximated that of the high-cancer line. The hybrid cells were stable during an observation period of nearly a year, whether maintained in cell cultures or recovered from tumors induced in mice by mixed cells from the two cancer lines.[7, 8]

Gerber and Kirschstein were able to recover SV-40 from "virus-free" SV-40-induced hamster ependymoma cells when grown together with SV-40-susceptible African green monkey kidney cells.[50] Likewise, Svoboda et al.[134] and Šimkovič et al.[118] recovered the Rous virus from Rous virus-induced rat tumor cells by contact with Rous-susceptible chick fibroblasts *in vivo* or *in vitro*. It is evident now that the "rescue" of the SV-40 and Rous genomes from the virus-free tumor cells was dependent upon cell fusion.

Cell agglutination and cell fusion were shown to be facilitated by the addition of Sendai virus[65, 96] and of Newcastle disease virus.[82] Ultraviolet-irradiated Sendai virus, when added to virus-free tumor cells and indicator cells, was shown to enhance cell fusion[97] and also to enhance the recovery of infectious virus. Recovery of infectious virus was dependent not only on contact of the tumor cells and the indicator cells, but upon the plating efficiency and viability of the tumor cells.[47]

The recovery of infectious SV-40 from virus-free tumor cells was soon confirmed.[83, 139, 144] Not all strains of Sendai virus have been effective in rescue experiments, nor can infectious virus be recovered from all virus-induced tumors. It is obvious that there is much to learn about the defective, noninfectious viral genomes, and more sensitive techniques would facilitate gaining such information.

Much is known about oncogenic viruses in animals, but, with the exception of information concerning the benign human wart and molluscum contagiosum virus, there are no data to establish the viral etiology of cancer in man. The search for viruses in human tumors has been disappointing.[51, 52, 55] In light of knowledge gained from studies of some of the animal viruses, this is not surprising. Although the murine leukemia viruses, the polyoma virus, and a number of other oncogenic viruses were first recovered from tumor-bearing animals, SV-40[31, 32] and the oncogenic adenoviruses[140] were not originally recovered from tumors. They were first propagated in cell cultures and then inoculated into newborn animals. SV-40 can often be recovered from primary SV-40-induced tumors[28] but usually it cannot be recovered from transplanted SV-40 tumors. Even in the primary tumors, so little infectious virus is present that tumors cannot be induced in susceptible animals by injection of cell-free extracts of the tumors. The concentration of virus must be increased by propagation in cell culture before there is enough to induce tumors in another animal. Certain types of adenovirus will induce tumors in every or almost every animal injected, yet the virus cannot be recovered from either a primary or a transplanted tumor. If diagnosis depended upon the recovery of infectious virus from such tumors, the oncogenicity of the adenoviruses would still be unknown.

Burkitt lymphomas and human leukemias are unique in that the tumor cells can be cultivated *in vitro* and almost all of them contain particles which resemble herpesvirus.[40] Similar particles have also been seen in cultures of lymphocytes from normal individuals[48] and from patients with mononucleosis.[12, 72] A herpesvirus has been recovered from cultures of Burkitt lymphoma cells which has induced neurological symptoms in hamsters or rabbits, but it has not been observed to induce either lymphoma or leukemia in an animal.[128] Whether the particles represent a leukemia or lymphoma virus or a passenger virus must await further investigation. Evidence to date is that the particles are widespread in the population and that they are of etiological significance in infectious mononucleosis.

Antibodies against Burkitt lymphoma cells and acute myeloid leukemia cells have been found in the sera of normal individuals. Very young children had no antibodies, but the incidence and mean titers rose gradually with age. In the 14- to 20-year age group, 70 per cent had antibodies against the myeloid leukemia and 40 per cent against different Burkitt lymphoma cell lines.[3]

In another study, in which antigens from at least $10^7$ sonicated or frozen and thawed cells derived from cultures of Burkitt lymphoma tissues were used, tumor antibodies in the sera of 17 patients from Africa with Burkitt lymphoma were demonstrated by immunofluorescence. Complement-fixation antibodies were demonstrated in the sera of 12 of 13 persons tested. The sera of a number of Americans also reacted with the Burkitt antigen; about 30 per cent of sera of 55 children were positive by immunofluorescence and 20 per cent by the complement-fixation reaction. In 58 sera from adults, the percentages were higher—up to 90 per cent by the immunofluorescence test and 60 per cent by the complement-fixation test. The immunofluorescence and complement-fixation tests agreed in 72 per cent of the samples.[4, 71] Antibodies against cultured Burkitt lymphoma cells in sera from Burkitt lymphoma patients, from other cancer patients, and from normal individuals were also shown by the use of an immunodiffusion test.[99] Sera from a number of monkeys and chimpanzees as well as sera from normal humans were shown to contain complement-fixing antibodies for Burkitt lymphoma cells.[49] Klein et al.[80] also demonstrated a reaction between Burkitt lymphoma cells and the patient's sera, and Fink[42] reported immunofluorescence in tests with cells from human leukemias and antiserum prepared in monkeys or rabbits with purified virus-like particles from human leukemic plasma.

Recent studies by Henle et al.[72] indicate that the herpes-like particles are related to, or are the cause of, infectious mononucleosis. Patients with infectious mononucleosis regularly developed antibodies to the herpes-type particles in cultures derived from Burkitt tumors and to other cells of the hematopoietic system. The relationship of the particles to the etiology of Burkitt lymphoma or leukemia remains obscure. The particles may be passenger viruses or they may be the etiological agents of these malignant diseases.

As in other diseases, the host range of the known oncogenic viruses is a characteristic of the particular virus. It was previously believed that each human tumor was species- and even organ-specific. On the hypothesis that human tumors are caused by viruses, there would be little basis for such an assumption today. If tumors are the unusual manifestation of infection with an oncogenic virus, it is not surprising that few of the so-called "clumps" of cancer cases[67, 113] have been observed. On the other hand, the high incidence of cancer suggests that the etiological agent or agents may be widespread in the population.

If viruses cause cancers in man, how might they spread (1) within the individual, and (2) within the population? Within the body, cell hybridization might be a factor. However, it has been observed that cell fusion *in vitro* is less apt to occur at body temperature than when the cells are held at lower temperatures. Free viral nucleic acid has been demonstrated in the blood of animals, and there is no *a priori* reason to believe that viral nucleic acid would function differently in infections of man. Particularly in leukemias, emperipolesis is likely to play a role in the spread of disease. Emperipolesis was first observed in the cell cultures of frog's blood[86] but it has since been observed in the cells from a number of animal species.[26, 94, 114] Small motile lymphocytes have been shown to penetrate histocytes or monocytes, to move about within the cytoplasm or the nucleus, and then to escape. Some cells have been observed to contain more than one lymphocyte. This inexplicable behavior was observed in cell cultures of Burkitt African lymphoma by Pulvertaft.[101] The phenomenon has apparently not been studied in animals bearing tumors induced by an easily identifiable virus.

There are no answers to the question of the mode of spread of an oncogenic virus from one individual to another. Judging by the induction of tumors in lower animals, the development of tumors in humans may be the result of an infection acquired in childhood.

Insects are known vectors in the natural spread of some of the oncogenic viruses such as rabbit myxomatosis and rabbit fibroma,[77] while polyoma virus has been transmitted by insects under experimental conditions.[6] Since Burkitt lymphoma occurs in the areas of Africa infested by tsetse flies and mosquitoes, and is rare in high-altitude areas where the temperature drops below 60°F. and rainfall is below 20 inches annually, suspicion is strong that this condition is spread by an arthropod vector. To date, convincing evidence for such spread has not been obtained.

Some oncogenic viruses infect more than one animal species, and a virus oncogenic for man could conceivably be passed from animal to man. Many animals, such as dogs, cats, cattle, chickens, and horses, that are frequently in close contact with man develop tumors. A few cases of leukemia have been reported in persons who had been in contact with dogs suffering from leukemia, but such cases have been too few to be meaningful. Studies of cancer in many animals have proved to be almost as intricate as studies of cancer in man. There is need for development in the technology of cell cultures. Whether this can be accomplished by changes in nutrient media, by the use of cells from organs or animal species not yet investigated, or by changes in the temperature of incubation remains to be determined. It should be noted that SV-40 did not produce a recognizable cytopathic effect in rhesus monkey kidney cells and, as a result, undetected contamination of several poliovirus vaccine lots with this agent occurred. However, following inoculation of African green monkey kidney cells, SV-40 produces multiple small vacuoles in the cytoplasm and ultimately destroys the entire cell sheet.[28] An intermediate phenomenon was produced by the adenoviruses. When these viruses were grown in HeLa cells, titers based on cytopathic effect of $10^{2.0}$ to $10^{2.5}$ were observed. When these same virus preparations were titrated in primary human embryonic kidney cell cultures, titers of $10^{7.5}$ to $10^{8.0}$ were obtained.

Whether the spread of the elusive human oncogenic viruses can be reduced by the institution of simple precautionary measures remains speculative. Progress has been made in the chemotherapy of cancers, but the more desirable goal lies in prevention. Prevention of infection with oncogenic viruses in man could be approached in two ways: (1) by the use of vaccines to prevent tumors, a method dependent upon recovery and identification of human oncogenic viruses, which to date has not been accomplished, and (2) by extraordinary care in protecting babies from contact with people from whom they might acquire infections. In Africa, where Burkitt lymphoma is common, it has been proposed that children should be protected from mosquitoes. For most babies in Africa such protection would be impossible at present.

If viruses oncogenic for humans could be identified, it is probable that tumors induced by them could be prevented. However, there is little evidence that tumors, once they appear, can be eliminated by immunological means. Cases have been reported in which malignant tumors in humans have regressed without apparent reason and the patients have recovered. Whether recovery was due to the development of antibodies against the tumor is not known.

Experiments have been reported in which RNA from normal adult mouse liver or normal mouse fibroblasts inhibited the multiplication of polyoma virus inoculated into mouse cell cultures.[136] Heterologous yeast RNA exerted no influence on the multiplication of virus, and RNAase-treated RNA produced a growth-stimulating effect. These results were explained on the assumption that the excess of normal homologous RNA constituted an excess of normal genetic information which interfered with the faulty information produced in the cell as a result of the viral infection. The growth of a transplantable mouse tumor, L 1210, has also been shown to be inhibited by thymic DNA.[53]

Li et al.[87] and Schmeer[112] have each shown that clams produce an antitumor substance which is effective in destroying certain transplanted tumors and tumors induced in hamsters following inoculation of adenovirus type 12 or SV-40. Temperature is a factor in the clam's elaboration of the antitumor substance. Clams collected in cold weather lacked the substance but acquired it after being transferred to heated tanks of saline solution.[68]

Typhoid fever has been controlled principally through the institution of sanitary measures. Perhaps the incidence of tumors in man can be reduced in all age groups by the prevention of young children from acquiring infections which appear to be of minor clinical importance but in the future might be shown to be precursors of cancer. Cancer would not be the first disease to follow a mild beginning. The primary lesions of syphilis or the initial infection which precedes rheumatic fever are mild compared to the sequelae which can occur later.

## SUMMARY

If cancer in man is an infectious process, it is a more complex process than diseases such as measles or smallpox. It is probable that the oncogenic viruses are widespread in the population and that they may be common infectious agents for man, and possibly for animals, although not identifiable as causes of any serious diseases. Since both oncogenic and nononcogenic viruses are antigenic, tumors may develop only in individuals who receive an overwhelming dose of virus or who have lowered immunity to the virus. Judging by the induction of tumors in animals, tumors in human beings may be more likely to develop in those infected when very young, although the tumors may not appear until late in life.

The identification of the causative virus in many tumors is hampered because (1) infectious virus tends to disappear from malignant cells and (2) the methods of cell cultures in current use either are not suitable to sustain growth of the virus or, if growth occurs, no cytopathic changes are produced. The known oncogenic viruses do induce specific new cellular antigens, known as tumor, T, neo, or ICFA antigens, which are present in the cell nuclei, and others known as transplantation antigens which are confined to the cell surface.

Antibodies are produced in response to these new cellular antigens as well as to the infectious virus. Antibodies against the transplantation antigen or antigens tend to inhibit tumor development. The biological role of the tumor or T antigens is unknown. Antibodies against the infectious virus may prevent subsequent infection of an animal with the virus but have no deterring effect on the development of a tumor once it is initiated. Animals bearing virus-induced tumors may have high-titer humoral antibodies against the infectious virus or they may have none, and often no infectious virus can be recovered from the tumor.

The problems involved in cancer research are further complicated by the discovery that a defective oncogenic virus, one unable to elaborate a protein coat, may take on a protein coat of another virus which may be oncogenic or nononcogenic. The new hybrid virus is infectious and it takes on the antigenic characteristics of the virus which provided the protein coat, yet it remains oncogenic and induces tumor or T antigen characteristic of the defective virus following inoculation into a susceptible host.

It is reported that an oncogenic virus may be made up of different kinds of DNA. One kind of DNA is involved in cell lysis and will not hybridize with host genetic material; another type shows homology with the DNA of the host cell and will combine with host genetic material.

Two other nonspecific cellular substances, interferon and Forssman antigen, may be induced by oncogenic viruses.

Growth of oncogenic viruses, like that of nononcogenic viruses, may be either enhanced or interfered with by simultaneous infections with other microorganisms.

To date there is little evidence that a tumor, once it appears, can be successfully treated by immunological means. It is probable that tumors could be prevented if the etiological agent or agents were known.

With at least one oncogenic virus, SV-40, infectious virus has been recovered from virus-induced but "virus-free" tumor cells by fusion of the tumor cells with virus-susceptible indicator cells. Variations of this method offer some hope that the etiological entity can be recovered from human tumors.

It is possible that the incidence of cancer can be reduced by taking extraordinary care that individuals, especially the very young, are protected from infections, particularly those which cause but minor symptoms.

## ACKNOWLEDGMENT

I am grateful to Dr. Joseph P. O'Malley, Dr. P. Anthony Morris, and Dr. B. William Uhlendorf for reviewing this paper.

# *References*

1. Abercrombie, M., J. E. M. Heaysman, and H. M. Karthauser. 1957. Social behaviour of cells in tissue culture. III. Mutual influences of sarcoma cells and fibroblasts. Exp. Cell Res. *13:*276–291.
2. Allison, A. C. 1961. Interference with and interferon production by polyoma virus. Virology *15:*47–51.
3. Ambrus, J. L., and H. V. Strandström, 1967. Complement fixing antibodies against cultured neoplastic cells in sera from normal individuals. Proc. Amer. Assoc. Cancer Res. *8:*2.
4. Armstrong, D., G. Henle, and W. Henle. 1966. Complement-fixation tests with cell lines derived from Burkitt's lymphoma and acute leukemias. J. Bact. *91:*1257–1262.
5. Axelrod, D., E. T. Bolton, and K. Habel. 1967. Homology of polyoma DNA to DNA of polyoma-free tumors. Fed. Proc. *23*(Part 1):401.
6. Banfield, W. G., P. A. Woke, C. M. Mackay, and H. L. Cooper. 1965. Mosquito transmission of a reticulum cell sarcoma of hamsters. Science *148:*1239–1240.
7. Barski, G. 1961. Clones cellulaires "hybrids" isolés à partir de cultures cellulaires mixtes. C. R. Acad. Sci. (Paris), *253:*1186–1188.
8. Barski, G., S. Sorieul, and F. Cornefert. 1961. "Hybrid" type cells in combined cultures of two different mammalian cell strains. J. Nat. Cancer Inst. *26:*1269–1290.
9. Barski, G., S. Sorieul, and F. Cornefert. 1960. Production dans des cultures *in vitro* de deux souches cellulaires en association de cellules de caractère "hybride." C. R. Acad. Sci. (Paris), *251:*1825–1827.
10. Bendich, A., E. Borenfreund, A. D. Vizoso, and R. G. Harris. 1966. Malignant transformation and intercell communication involving DNA. *In:* Subviral Carcinogenesis. Aichi Cancer Center, Nagoya and Japanese Cancer Association, pp. 99–115.
11. Bendich, A., T. Wilczok, and E. Borenfreund. 1965. Circulating DNA as a possible factor in oncogenesis. Science *148:*374–376.
12. Benyesh-Melnick, M. 1966. Studies of acute leukemia and infectious mononucleosis in children. *In:* Viruses Inducing Cancer. University of Utah Press, Salt Lake City, pp. 305–319.
13. Bittner, J. J. 1936. Some possible effects of nursing on the mammary gland tumor incidence in mice. Science *84:*162.
14. Black, P. H., W. P. Rowe, H. C. Turner, and R. J. Huebner. 1963. A specific complement-fixing antigen present in SV40 tumor and transformed cells. Proc. Nat. Acad. Sci. *50:*1148–1156.

15. Haughton, G., and P. McGehee. 1967. Measurement of mouse transplantation antigens. Transplantation *6:*656–658.
16. Chany, C., and C. Brailovsky. 1967. Stimulating interaction between viruses (stimulons). Proc. Nat. Acad. Sci. *57:*87–94.
17. Crawford, L. V., E. M. Crawford, and D. H. Watson. 1962. The physical characteristics of polyoma virus. I. Two types of particles. Virology *18:*170–176.
18. Dalldorf, G., and H. Weigand. 1958. Poliomyelitis as a complex infection. J. Exp. Med. *108:*605–616.
19. Defendi, V. 1963. Effects of SV40 virus immunization on growth of transplantable SV40 and polyoma virus tumors in hamsters. Proc. Soc. Exp. Biol. Med. *113:*12–16.
20. Defendi, V. 1966. Transformation *in vitro* of mammalian cells by polyoma and simian 40 viruses. Progr. Exp. Tumor Res. *8:*125–188.
21. Defendi, V., and F. Jensen. 1967. Oncogenicity by DNA tumor viruses: Enhancement after ultraviolet and cobalt 60 radiation. Science *157:*703–705.
22. Defendi, V., and H. Koprowski. 1959. Influence of adult lymphoid tissues on polyoma-induced tumours. Nature *184:*1579–1580.
23. Diderholm, H. 1967. Transformation of bovine cells *in vitro* by polyoma virus, and the properties of the transformed cells. Proc. Soc. Exp. Biol. Med. *124:*1197–1201.
24. Diderholm, H., B. Stenkvist, J. Pontén and T. Wesslén. 1965. Transformation of bovine cells *in vitro* after inoculation of simian virus 40 or its nucleic acid. Exp. Cell. Res. *37:*152–159.
25. Di Mayorca, G. A., B. E. Eddy, S. E. Stewart, W. S. Hunter, C. Friend, and A. Bendich. 1959. Isolation of infectious deoxyribonucleic acid from SE polyoma-infected tissue cultures. Proc. Nat. Acad. Sci. *45:*1805–1808.
26. Dreyer, D. A., C. C. Shullenberger, and L. Dmochowski. 1964. A study on intracellular lymphocytes ("emperipolesis") in tissue culture of lymph nodes from patients with malignant lymphoma. Texas Rep. Biol. Med. *22:*61–69.
27. Eddy, B. E. Unpublished experiments.
28. Eddy, B. E. 1964. Simian virus 40 (SV40): an oncogenic virus. Progr. Exp. Tumor Res. *4:*1–26.
29. Eddy, B. E. 1966. Oncogenic Viruses. *In:* Basic Medical Virology. Williams & Wilkins Company, Baltimore, pp. 471–501.
30. Eddy, B. E. 1966. Factors which influence the induction of tumors in hamsters infected with adenovirus or simian virus 40 (SV40). Int. Cancer Confer. Tokyo *9:*235.
31. Eddy, B. E., G. S. Borman, W. H. Berkeley, and R. D. Young. 1961. Tumors induced in hamsters by injection of rhesus kidney cell extracts. Proc. Soc. Exp. Biol. Med. *107:*191–197.
32. Eddy, B. E., G. S. Borman, G. E. Grubbs, and R. D. Young. 1962. Identification of the oncogenic substance in rhesus kidney cell cultures as simian virus 40. Virology *17:*65–75.
33. Eddy, B. E., G. E. Grubbs, and R. D. Young. 1966. Immunity of hamsters to tumor development caused by oncogenic viruses. Proc. Int. Congress Microbiol. Moscow *9:*523.
34. Eddy, B. E., W. P. Rowe, J. W. Hartley, S. E. Stewart, and R. J. Huebner. 1958. Hemagglutination with the SE polyoma virus. Virology *6:*290–291.
35. Eddy, B. E., S. E. Stewart, and W. Berkeley. 1958. Cytopathogenicity in tissue cultures by a tumor virus from mice. Proc. Soc. Exp. Biol. Med. *98:*848–851.
36. Eddy, B. E., S. E. Stewart, and G. E. Grubbs. 1958. Influence of tissue culture passage, storage, temperature and drying on viability of SE polyoma virus. Proc. Soc. Exp. Biol. Med. *99:*289–292.
37. Eddy, B. E., R. D. Young, and G. E. Grubbs. 1965. Method for inhibiting oncogenesis in hamsters infected when newborn with SV40. *In:* Perspectives in Virology 4. Hoeber Medical Division, Harper & Row Publishers, Inc., New York, pp. 209–214.
38. Ellermann, V., and O. Bang. 1908. Experimentelle Leukämie bei Huhnern. Zbl. Bakt. [Orig.] *46:*595–609.
39. Enders, J. F., T. H. Weller, and F. C. Robbins. 1949. Cultivation of the Lansing strain of poliomyelitis virus in cultures of various human embryonic tissues. Science *109:*85–87.
40. Epstein, M. A., B. G. Achong, and Y. M. Barr. 1964. Virus particles in cultured human lymphoblasts from Burkitt's malignant lymphoma. Lancet *1:*702–703.
41. Evans, V. J., and W. F. Andresen. 1966. Effect of serum on spontaneous neoplastic transformations *in vitro*. J. Nat. Cancer Inst. *37:*247–249.
42. Fink, M. A., R. A. Malmgren, F. J. Rauscher, H. C. Orr, and M. Karon. 1964. Application of immunofluorescence to the study of human leukemia. J. Nat. Cancer Inst. *33:*581–588.

43. Fishbein, M., L. Hektoen, and E. M. Salmonsen (eds.). 1946. A Bibliography of Infantile Paralysis 1789–1944. J. B. Lippincott Company, Philadelphia.
44. Fogel, M., and L. Sachs. 1964. The induction of Forssman antigen synthesis in hamster and mouse cells in tissue culture as detected by the fluorescent-antibody technique. Exp. Cell. Res. *34:*448–462.
45. Freeman, A. E., P. H. Black, E. A. Vanderpool, P. H. Henry, J. B. Austin, and R. J. Huebner. 1967. Transformation of primary rat embryo cells by adenovirus type 2. Proc. Nat. Acad. Sci. *58:*1205–1212.
46. Fujinami, A., and K. Inamoto. 1914. Ueber Geschwülste bei Japinschen Haushühnern insbesondere über einen transplantablen Tumor. Z. Krebsforsch. *14:*94–119.
47. Gerber, P. 1966. Studies on the transfer of subviral infectivity from SV40-induced hamster tumor cells to indicator cells. Virology *28:*501–509.
48. Gerber, P., and S. M. Birch. 1967. Herpes-like virus particles in cultures of buffy coat from non-leukemic donors. Bact. Proc. *20:*153.
49. Gerber, P., and S. M. Birch. 1967. Complement-fixing antibodies in sera of human and nonhuman primates to viral antigens derived from Burkitt's lymphoma cells. Proc. Nat. Acad. Sci. *58:*478–484.
50. Gerber, P., and R. L. Kirschstein. 1962. SV40-induced ependymomas in newborn hamsters. I. Virus-tumor relationships. Virology *18:*582–588.
51. Girardi, A. J., M. R. Hilleman, and R. E. Zwickey. 1963. Search for virus in human malignancies. III. Sex segregation and neoplasia in ICR/Ha mice. Proc. Soc. Exp. Biol. Med. *114:*609–614.
52. Girardi, A. J., V. M. Larson, M. R. Hilleman, and R. E. Zwickey. 1966. Search for virus in human malignancies. IV. Tests of human neoplastic tissues in sex segregated mice. Proc. Soc. Exp. Biol. Med. *121:*428–432.
53. Glick, J. L., and A. R. Salim. 1967. Inhibition of tumour cell viability by DNA. Nature *213:*676–678.
54. Gotlieb-Stematsky, T., Z. Rotem, and S. Karby. 1966. Production and susceptibility to interferon by polyoma virus variants of high and low oncogenic properties. J. Nat. Cancer Inst. *37:*99–103.
55. Grace, J. T., Jr., E. A. Mirand, and D. T. Mount. 1960. Relationship of viruses to malignant disease. II. Oncogenic properties of cell-free filtrates of human tumors. Arch. Intern. Med. *105:*482–491.
56. Graffi, A., J. Gimmy, L. Baumbach, and F. Schneiders. 1962. Zür Histologie der durch den BB/T2—Polyoma—Virusstamm bei Kaninchen und Meerschweinchen induzierten Geschwülste. Acta Biol. Med. German. *9:*167–202.
57. Green, M. 1966. Comparative molecular structure of oncogenic and nononcogenic adenoviruses. *In:* Viruses Inducing Cancer. University of Utah Press, Salt Lake City, pp. 211–218.
58. Gross, L. 1951. "Spontaneous" leukemia developing in C₃H mice following inoculation in infancy with Ak-leukemic extracts, or Ak-embryos. Proc. Soc. Exp. Biol. Med. *76:* 27–32.
59. Gross, L. 1961. Oncogenic Viruses. Pergamon Press, New York, pp. 153–254, 281–345.
60. Habel, K. 1961. Resistance of polyoma virus immune animals to transplanted polyoma tumors. Proc. Soc. Exp. Biol. Med. *106:*722–725.
61. Habel, K. 1966. Virus tumor antigens: Specific fingerprints? Cancer Res. *26*(Part 1): 2018–2024.
62. Habel, K., and B. E. Eddy. 1963. Specificity of resistance to tumor challenge of polyoma and SV40 virus immune hamsters. Proc. Soc. Exp. Biol. Med. *113:*1–4.
63. Hanafusa, H., T. Hanafusa, and H. Rubin. 1963. The defectiveness of Rous sarcoma virus. Proc. Nat. Acad. Sci. *49:*572–580.
64. Hare, J. D. 1967. Transplant immunity to polyoma virus-induced tumor cells. IV. A polyoma strain defective in transplant antigen induction. Virology *31:*625-632.
65. Harris, H., and J. F. Watkins. 1965. Hybrid cells derived from mouse and man: artificial heterokaryons of mammalian cells from different species. Nature 205:640–646.
66. Hatano, M., R. Shimizu, O. Morita, and T. Yamagishi. 1967. Attempt for specificity determination of cell injuring reaction (CIR) by bacteria. Med. Biol. (Tokyo) *74:*293–298.
67. Heath, C. W., and R. J. Hasterlik. 1963. Leukemia among children in a suburban community. Amer. J. Med. *34:*796–812.
68. Hegyeli, A. 1964. Temperature dependence of the activity of the anti-tumor factor in the common clam. Science *146:*77–78.
69. Heidenhain, L. 1932. Ist Krebs durch Zerfallsprodukte übertragbar? Z. Krebsforsch. *36:* 360–364.
70. Hellström, I. 1967. A colony inhibition (CI) technique for demonstration of tumor cell destruction by lymphoid cells *in vitro.* Int. J. Cancer 2:65–68.

71. Henle, G., and W. Henle. 1966. Immunofluorescence in cells derived from Burkitt's lymphoma. J. Bact. *91:*1248–1256.
72. Henle, G., W. Henle, and V. Diehl. 1968. Relation of Burkitt's tumor-associated herpes-type virus to infectious mononucleosis. Proc. Nat. Acad. Sci. *59:*94–101.
73. Huang, C. H. 1943. Further studies on the titration and neutralization of the western strain of equine encephalomyelitis virus in tissue culture. J. Exp. Med. *78:*111–126.
74. Huebner, R. J., R. M. Chanock, B. A. Rubin, and M. J. Casey. 1964. Induction by adenovirus type 7 of tumors in hamsters having the antigenic characteristics of SV40 virus. Proc. Nat. Acad. Sci. *52:*1333–1340.
75. Huebner, R. J., W. P. Rowe, H. C. Turner, and W. T. Lane. 1963. Specific adenovirus complement-fixing antigens in virus-free hamster and rat tumors. Proc. Nat. Acad. Sci. *50:*379–389.
76. Ito, Y. 1960. A tumor-producing factor extracted by phenol from papillomatous tissue (Shope) of cottontail rabbits. Virology *12:*596–601.
77. Kilham, L., and P. A. Woke. 1953. Laboratory transmission of fibromas (Shope) in cottontail rabbits by means of fleas and mosquitoes. Proc. Soc. Exp. Biol. Med. *83:*296–301.
78. Kisch, A. L., and K. B. Fraser. 1964. Effect of pH on transformation of BHK21 cells by polyoma virus. I. Relationship between transformation rate and synthesis of viral antigen. Virology *24:*186–192.
79. Kisch, A. L., and J. H. Subak-Sharpe. 1966. Effect of pH on transformation of BHK21 cells by polyoma virus. II. Kinetic consideration. Virology *28:*188–201.
80. Klein, G., P. Clifford, E. Klein, and J. Stjernswärd. 1966. Search for tumor-specific immune reactions in Burkitt's lymphoma patients by the membrane immunofluorescence reaction. Proc. Nat. Acad. Sci. *55:*1628–1635.
81. Koch, M. A., and A. B. Sabin. 1963. Specificity of virus-induced resistance to transplantation of polyoma and SV40 tumors in adult hamsters. Proc. Soc. Exp. Biol. Med. *113:*4–12.
82. Kohn, A. 1965. Polykaryocytosis induced by Newcastle disease virus in monolayers of animal cells. Virology *26:*228–245.
83. Koprowski, H., F. C. Jensen, and Z. Steplewski. 1967. Activation of production of infectious tumor virus SV40 in heterokaryon cultures. Proc. Nat. Acad. Sci. *58:*127–133.
84. Larson, V. M., P. A. Gosnell, and M. R. Hilleman. 1967. Complement-fixation reaction of human neoplastic tissue with sera from hamsters bearing virus-induced tumors. Proc. Soc. Exp. Biol. Med. *125:*525–534.
85. Lemonde, P., and M. Clode-Hyde. 1966. Influence of bacille Calmette-Guérin infection on polyoma in hamsters and mice. Cancer Res. *26*(Part 1):585–589.
86. Lewis, W. H. 1925. The engulfment of living blood cells by others of the same type. Anat. Rev. *31:*43–49.
87. Li, C. P., B. Prescott, B. Eddy, G. Caldes, W. R. Green, E. C. Martino, and A. M. Young. 1965. Activity of paolins from clams. Ann. N. Y. Acad. Sci. *130:*374–382.
88. Macpherson, I., and L. Montagnier. 1964. Agar suspension culture for the selective assay of cells transformed by polyoma virus. Virology *23:*291–294.
89. Mattern, C. F. T., K. K. Takemato, and A. M. De Leva. 1967. Electron microscopic observations on multiple polyoma virus-related particles. Virology *32:*378–392.
90. Medina, D., and L. Sachs. 1961. Cell-virus interactions with the polyoma virus. The induction of cell transformation and malignancy *in vitro*. Brit. J. Cancer *15:*885–904.
91. Michel, M. R., B. Hirt, and R. Weil. 1967. Mouse cellular DNA enclosed in polyoma viral capsids (pseudovirions). Proc. Nat. Acad. Sci. *58:*1381–1388.
92. Minocha, H. C., and R. A. Consigli. 1967. Effect of FUDR on DNA and protein synthesis in polyoma-infected mouse embryo cells under selective cultural conditions. Bact. Proc. *67:*142.
93. Moore, A. E., and A. C. Caparó. 1964. Tumors occurring in newborn mice after inoculation of human cancer material. Cancer Res. *24:*765–769.
94. Moore, A. E., and J. Hlinka. 1964. Activities of lymphocytes inside fibroblasts. Proc. Amer. Assoc. Cancer. Res. *5:*46.
95. Morris, J. A., M. J. Casey, B. E. Eddy, W. J. Lane, and R. J. Huebner. 1966. Occurrence of SV40 neoplastic and antigenic information in vaccine strains of adenovirus type 3. Proc. Soc. Exp. Biol. Med. *122:*679–684.
96. Okado, Y. 1962. Analysis of giant polynuclear cell formation caused by HVJ virus from Ehrlich's ascites tumor cells. Exp. Cell Res. *26:*98–107.
97. Okado, Y. and J. Tadokoro. 1963. The distribution of cell fusion capacity among several cell strains or cells caused by HVJ. Exp. Cell Res. *32:*417–430.
98. Okamoto, H., M. Minami, S. Shoin, S. Koshimura, and R. Shimizu. 1966. Experimental anticancer studies. XXXI. On the streptococcal preparation having potent anticancer activity. Jap. J. Exp. Med. *36:*175–186.

99. Old, L. J., E. A. Boyse, H. F. Oettgen, E. De Harven, G. Geering, B. Williamson, and P. Clifford. 1966. Precipitating antibody in human serum to an antigen present in cultured Burkitt's lymphoma cells. Proc. Nat. Acad. Sci. 56:1699–1704.

100. Pope, J. H., and W. P. Rowe. 1964. Immunofluorescent studies of adenovirus 12 tumors and of cells transformed or infected by adenoviruses. J. Exp. Med. 120:577–588.

101. Pulvertaft, R. J. V. 1964. Cytology of Burkitt's tumour (African lymphoma). Lancet 1:238–239.

102. Rabson, A. S., G. T. O'Conner, I. K. Berezesky, and F. J. Paul. 1964. Enhancement of adenovirus growth in African green monkey kidney cell cultures by SV40. Proc. Soc. Exp. Biol. Med. 116:187–190.

103. Rapp, F., J. S. Butel, and J. L. Melnick. 1965. SV40-adenovirus "hybrid" populations. Transfer of SV40 determinants from one type of adenovirus to another. Proc. Nat. Acad. Sci. 54:717–724.

104. Rapp, F., J. L. Melnick, T. Kitahara, and R. Sheppard. 1965. Search for virus-induced antigens in human tumors using the SV40 hamster system as a model. Proc. Soc. Exp. Biol. Med. 118:573–576.

105. Rous, P. 1911. A sarcoma of the fowl transmissible by an agent separable from the tumor cells. J. Exp. Med. 13:397–411.

106. Rowe, W. P., and S. G. Baum. 1964. Evidence for a possible genetic hybrid between adenovirus type 7 and SV40 viruses. Proc. Nat. Acad. Sci. 52:1340–1347.

107. Rowe, W. P., J. W. Hartley, I. Brodsky, and R. J. Huebner. 1958. Complement-fixation with a mouse tumor virus (SE polyoma). Science 128:1339–1340.

108. Sabin, A. B. 1965. Manifestations of latent viral genetic material in experimentally-produced cancers and search for such manifestations in human cancers. Israel J. Med. Sci. 1:93–103.

109. Sachs, L., and D. Medina. 1961. In vitro transformation of normal cells by polyoma virus. Nature 189:457–458.

110. Sanarelli, G. 1898. Das myxomatogene Virus. Beitrag zum Studium der Krankheitserreger ausserhalb des Sichtbaren. Zlb. Bakt. [Orig.] 23:865–873.

111. Sanford, K. K. 1965. Malignant transformation of cells in vitro. Int. Rev. Cytol. 18:249–311.

112. Schmeer, M. R. 1966. Mercenene: Growth-inhibiting agent of Mercenaria extracts. Further chemical and biological characterization. Ann. N. Y. Acad. Sci. 136:211–218.

113. Schwartz, S. O., I. Greenspan, and E. R. Brown. 1963. Leukemia cluster in Niles, Illinois. Immunological data on families of leukemic patients and others. J.A.M.A. 186:106–108.

114. Sheldon, E., and A. J. Dalton. 1959. Electron microscopy of emperipolesis. J. Biophys. Biochem. Cytol. 6:513–514.

115. Shimizu, R., N. Nishida, I. Bando, S. Koshimura, M. Hayashi, and T. Kobayaski. 1963. [On the appearance of RNA in the medium as a result of cancer cell damage by hemolytic streptococci.] Japanese. Kanazawa Daigaku Kekken Nempo 22:27–34.

116. Shope, R. E. 1932. A filterable virus causing tumor-like condition in rabbits and its relationship to virus myxomatosum. J. Exp. Med. 56:803–822.

117. Shope, R. E. 1933. Infectious papillomatosis of rabbits. J. Exp. Med. 58:607–624.

118. Šimkovič, D., J. Svoboda, and N. Volentová. (1963) Clonal analysis of line XCtc rat tumour cells (derived from tumor XC) grown in vitro. Folia. Biol. (Praha) 9:82.

119. Sjögren, H. O. 1964. Studies on specific transplantation resistance to polyoma virus-induced tumors. II. Mechanism of resistance induced by polyoma virus infection. J. Nat. Cancer Inst. 32:375–393.

120. Sjögren, H. O. 1966. Tumor specific antigens in viral neoplasms and in unrelated virus-infected tumors. Ann. Med. Exp. Fenn. 44:227–231.

121. Sjögren, H. O. and Hellström, I. 1966. In vivo and in vitro demonstration of specific transplantation antigens in polyoma, Rous, and adeno 12 mouse sarcomas. In: Subviral Carcinogenesis. Aichi Cancer Center, Nagoya and Japanese Cancer Association, pp. 207–219.

122. Sjögren, H. O., and N. Ringertz. 1962. Histopathology and transplantability of polyoma-induced tumors in strain A/SN and three coisogenic resistant (IR) substrains. J. Nat. Cancer Inst. 28:859–895.

123. Sjögren, H. O., I. Sjögren, and G. Klein. 1961. Resistance of polyoma virus immunized mice to transplantation of established polyoma tumors. Exp. Cell Res. 23:204–208.

124. Stanners, C. P. 1963. Studies on the transformation of hamster embryo cells in culture by polyoma virus. II. Selective techniques for the detection of transformed cells. Virology 21:464–476.

125. Stanners, C. P., J. E. Till, and L. Siminovitch. 1963. Studies on the transformation of hamster embryo cells in culture by polyoma virus. I. Properties of transformed and normal cells. Virology 21:448–463.

126. Stewart, S. E., B. E. Eddy, and N. G. Borgese. 1958. Neoplasms in mice inoculated with tumor agent carried in tissue culture. J. Nat. Cancer Inst. *20:*1223–1243.

127. Stewart, S. E., B. E. Eddy, A. M. Gochenour, N. G. Borgese, and G. E. Grubbs. 1957. The induction of neoplasms with a substance released from mouse tumors by tissue culture. Virology *3:*380–400.

128. Stewart, S. E., J. Landon, E. Lovelace, and G. Parker. 1965. Burkitt tumor: Brain lesions in hamsters induced with an extract from the SL₁ cell line. Wistar Institute Symp. Monograph *4:*93–101.

129. Stoker, M. 1962. Studies on transformation by polyoma virus *in vitro. In:* Tumor Viruses of Murine Origin. Ciba Foundation, Little, Brown & Company, Boston pp. 365–376.

130. Stoker, M. 1963. The interaction of polyoma virus with hamster fibroblasts. *In:* Viruses, Nucleic Acids, and Cancer. Williams & Wilkins Company, Baltimore, pp. 487–497.

131. Stoker, M., and P. Abel. 1962. Conditions affecting transformation of polyoma virus. Cold Spring Harbor Symp. Quant. Biol. *27:*375–386.

132. Stoker, M., and I. Macpherson. 1961. Studies on transformation of hamster cells by polyoma virus *in vitro.* Virology *14:*359–370.

133. Stuck, B., L. J. Old, and E. A. Boyse. 1964. Antigenic conversion of established leukemias by an unrelated leukemogenic virus. Nature *202:*1016–1018.

134. Svoboda, J., P. Chýle, D. Šimkovič, and I. Hilgert. 1963. Demonstration of the absence of infectious Rous virus in rat tumor XC, whose structurally intact cells produce Rous sarcoma when transferred to chick. Folia Biol. (Praha) *9:*77–81.

135. Takemato, K. K., and K. Habel. 1966. Hamster tumor cells doubly transformed by SV40 and polyoma viruses. Virology *30:*20–28.

136. Tikhonenko, T. I., A. A. Shotkin, and I. S. Irlin. 1964. Inhibitory effect of normal cell RNA on virus multiplication. Fed. Proc. (Translation suppl.) *23:*998–1002.

137. Ting, R. C. 1964. A new approach for the demonstration of viral genes in virus-free polyoma tumor cells. Virology *24:*227–228.

138. Todaro, G. J., and H. Green. 1965. Successive transformations of an established cell line by polyoma virus and SV40. Science *147:*513–514.

139. Tournier, P., R. Cassingena, R. Wicker, J. Coppey, and H. Suarez. 1967. Étude du mécanisme de l'induction chez des cellules de hamster syrien transformées par le virus SV40. Int. J. Cancer *2:*117–132.

140. Trentin, J. J., Y. Yabe, and G. Taylor. 1962. The quest for human cancer viruses. Science *137:*835–841.

141. Trevethia, S. S., and F. Rapp. 1965. Demonstration of new surface antigens in cells transformed by papovavirus SV40 in cytotoxic tests. Proc. Soc. Exp. Biol. Med. *120:*455–458.

142. Vogt, M., and R. Dulbecco. 1960. Virus-cell interaction with a tumor-producing virus. Proc. Nat. Acad. Sci. *46:*365–370.

143. Vogt, M., and R. Dulbecco. 1963. Steps in the neoplastic transformation of hamster embryo cells by polyoma virus. Proc. Nat. Acad. Sci. *49:*171–179.

144. Watkins, J. F., and R. Dulbecco. 1967. Production of SV40 virus in heterokaryons of transformed and susceptible cells. Proc. Nat. Acad. Sci. *58:*1396–1403.

145. Weil, R. 1961. A quantitative assay for a subviral infective agent related to polyoma virus. Virology *14:*46–53.

146. Wigzell, H. 1965. Quantitative titrations of mouse H-2 antibodies using Cr 51 labelled target cells. Transplantation *3:*423–431.

147. Winocour, E. 1967. On the apparent homology between DNA from polyoma virus and normal mouse synthetic RNA. Virology *31:*15–28.

Reprinted from Journal of Cellular Physiology, *71*:43–60, Feb. 1, 1968.

*Chapter* 26

# INTERFERON INDUCTION AND UTILIZATION*

M. R. HILLEMAN

*Division of Virus and Cell Biology Research,*
*Merck Institute for Therapeutic Research,*
*West Point, Pennsylvania*

## ABSTRACT

The interferon mechanism offers the hope for moderate to high-level prophylactic immunity of broad antiviral spectrum but of relatively short duration. Economic and biological considerations offer little hope for utilization of exogenous interferon as a prophylactic or therapeutic substance, unless but a small part of the total molecule be found to carry the activity. The real promise for interferon application is in the administration of suitable inducers so as to cause the body to produce and distribute its own interferon. Certain ribonucleic acids (RNA's) offer hope for high-level potency as inducers without adverse effect. The condition for interferon induction by ribonucleic acids appears to be double- or multistrandedness and freedom from inhibitors. These can be of biological or synthetic origin. The mechanism of action of interferon is not fully understood but appears to fit into the Jacob-Monod model involving two phases: first, a derepression by the inducer to cause the cell to form interferon, and second, a derepression by interferon to cause recipient cells to form the active substance which acts by preventing translation from viral messenger RNA. Double- or multistranded RNA of viral or other origin appears to be unique to the cell and serves as the alert to it to produce interferon in phase 1. Greatest need for interferon is clearly for those diseases in which there is a multiplicity of immunological types in excess of the numbers which could be put into a vaccine as, e.g., the common cold and enteric viruses. There

* Presented in abbreviated form at the Gustav Stern Symposium on Perspectives in Virology, New York, New York, January 29-30, 1968.

might be some overall therapeutic benefit also if inducer were given early enough in infection. Special value for interferon induction might derive by administration in early life, before the development of immunological maturity, as a means for preventing infection with oncogenic or other viruses. Additionally, suitable inducers might be capable of interrupting the reinfection cycle in virus-dependent malignancies.

The favorable outlook for interferon utilization must always be tempered by the realization that under certain as yet undiscovered situations, adverse rather than beneficial effects might result from induction of interferon. It is not impossible that in certain special circumstances, as in ordinary immunological responses, it might be more beneficial to negate rather than to promote the effect.

# BACKGROUND

There are three approaches to specific control of viral diseases: immunological, chemical, and host resistance (see Table 1). Immunological control, spanning 17 decades, has been remarkably effective in affording protection of long-term or relatively long-term duration, but has the disadvantage of narrow spectrum. Chemoprophylaxis or chemotherapy, investigated extensively since World War II, has thus far given scant reward and suffers the disadvantage of both narrow spectrum and need for continuing administration to obtain a protective effect. Host resistance, as exemplified by the interferon mechanism, is still an object for exploratory research but offers the promise for broad-spectrum antiviral activity with the disadvantage of only short-term duration of effect.

The phenomenon of viral interference had its beginnings three decades past in the observation by Hoskins (1935) that the attenuated neurotropic variant of yellow fever virus protected monkeys against an otherwise fatal infection with virulent pantropic yellow fever virus given simultaneously. Findlay and MacCallum (1937) subsequently showed that the phenomenon was in no way related to a specific antibody immune reaction and gave support for this position by demonstrating interference between the antigenically unrelated Rift Valley fever and yellow fever viruses. Since that time, reports of interference between viral pairs have been legion.

TABLE 1. *Appraisal of Approaches to Specific Control of Viral Diseases*

| | CHARACTERISTIC | | |
| KIND | *Level of Effectiveness* | *Antiviral Spectrum* | *Duration* |
|---|---|---|---|
| 1. Immunological | Usually high | Very narrow | Relatively long to lifetime |
| 2. Chemical | Low to moderate | Narrow | Very short term |
| 3. Host resistance (interferon) | Moderate to high | Very broad* | Relatively short |

* But host species-specific.

Interference, in spite of its potential, lay dormant for 20 years until catapulted into sudden interest by the findings of Isaacs and Lindenmann (1957). These workers showed that resistance to viral infection could be imparted to cells by prior treatment with a virus-free protein, called interferon, which was excreted by cells that had been exposed to a virus. The importance of this discovery has become increasingly evident with the realization that the conventional antibody immune mechanisms may have little to do with the early stages of recovery from viral infections. Thus, interferon appears to provide a first line of defense, being produced early in infection and functioning at the intracellular locus to limit or prevent viral replication. Antibody is seen later and its importance seems to be mainly that of limiting late extracellular spread or of averting reinfection. Once the individual cell is infected, its fate, i.e., life or death, appears to depend on factors other than antibody.

Interferon and interference have received major attention in our laboratories during the past ten years, with orientation toward ultimate practicable utilization of the phenomenon in human and animal medicine. Our studies are carried out by a team which includes A. A. Tytell, A. K. Field, M. M. Nemes, G. P. Lampson, and the author. The present review seeks to highlight the present knowledge concerning interferon properties, function, and induction with assessment of the potential for clinical application. References are made to key papers and to reviews, wherever suitable, with no pretense toward completeness of bibliography. Many excellent reviews including a textbook are presently available (Baron and Levy, 1966; Burke and Skehel, 1967; Finter, 1966; Hilleman, 1963 and 1965; Ho, 1967; Ho and Postic, 1967; Isaacs, 1965; Merigan, 1967a and b; Paucker and Boxaca, 1967; Wagner, 1965; Wagner and Smith, 1967) and may be consulted for details.

# PROPERTIES OF INTERFERON

The initial demonstration of interferon as an active antiviral substance understandably stimulated a considerable interest in ascertaining its physical and chemical nature. Here was an essentially nontoxic antiviral substance and it was possible that characterization of the principle might provide clues for understanding nonspecific cellular resistance and recovery from viral infection. Furthermore, if its structure were simple, then similar substances with prophylactic and therapeutic efficacy might be synthesized in the laboratory. These hopes have not been realized to date.

The first and best studied of all the interferons are those elaborated by chick embryo cells in response to virus. The earliest characterization of interferon by Isaacs (Isaacs and Burke, 1959; Isaacs et al., 1957) and by others (Wagner, 1960; Zemla and Vilcek, 1961), employing mostly indirect methods, established the important properties of protein nature, low molecular weight, and stability over a wide pH range. First significant purification of interferon was achieved by our group (Lampson et al., 1963), employing interferon elaborated into allantoic fluid of hens' eggs which were infected with influenza A virus and which showed a very favorable activity: total protein ratio.

Purification, as carried out by us, consisted essentially of perchloric acid precipitation to remove virus and extraneous protein, concentration and purification by precipitation with $Zn^{++}$, column chromatography on CM-cellulose, and zone electrophoresis on pevikon. The interferon was purified 4500 times with respect to initial protein and one unit of interferon activity was about 0.0042 $\mu$g. of protein when assayed in the chick embryo cell culture-Eastern equine encephalomyelitis (EEE) virus system used. This activity is well in excess of the *in vitro* activity of antibiotic substances such as penicillin (0.05 $\mu$g. in 1 ml.) and tetracycline (0.2 $\mu$g. in 1 ml.) assayed with highly sensitive organisms. Analysis of the highly purified substance revealed a protein which displayed a characteristic ultraviolet absorption spectrum, which had a molecular weight of about 25,000, which contained a trace of carbohydrate, and which was stable at 76°C. for 1 hour and at pH 2 to 10. Since that time, a great many procedures for purification and for assay of interferon have been made and claims for purity up to five times that of the interferon described before have been made (Finter, 1966), based on comparisons of activity units per milligram of protein. Such may be difficult to substantiate because of differing sensitivities of assay procedures used for measuring activity. Whatever the degree of purity already achieved or attainable in the future, chick interferon appears to fall into the general molecular species described in Table 2.

The further work on interferons has shown that substances of similar quality and activity may be elaborated by cells or by intact animals of a wide range of avian or mammalian species including chicken, mouse, man, rabbit, calf, rat, monkey, and probably guinea pig, dog, pig, tortoise, and fish (Finter, 1966). Some evidence has also been presented (Finter, 1966) for presence of roughly comparable but nonidentical substances in plants and even bacteria, suggesting that the interferon mechanism might be of primordial origin. It is also established that a wide variety of nonviral substances may also induce interferons (see later), which are readily demonstrable in the tissues or blood of intact host animals. The careful studies which have been carried out have revealed that these substances have a remarkable diversity of molecular weights, ranging from 25,000 to 167,000, while still retaining the similar quality of broad-spectrum antiviral activity, host species specificity, and other properties permitting inclusion in the general class of substances regarded as interferons. Merigan (1967a, b) has emphasized that the pattern of production of these several molecular species of interferons depends upon

TABLE 2. *Principal Biochemical and Biophysical Properties of Chick Embryo Interferon*

---

1. Protein, containing a small amount of carbohydrate.
2. Contains all or nearly all amino acids, including glucosamine.
3. Groups:
    Essential—disulfide, $\gamma$-S-methyl (of methionine), amino.
    Nonessential—sulfhydryl, hydroxyl.
4. Molecular weight, 25–40,000.
5. Isoelectric point near neutral (pH 7.0 $\pm$ 0.5).
6. U.V. absorption max. 278 m$\mu$, min. 253 m$\mu$.
7. Stable pH 2–10, and at 65–70°C. for at least 1 hour.

---

the nature of the inducer, the animal species studied, the site of induction, and the time following induction. This same author has noted that interferon of the 110,000-molecular-weight species may appear in the blood of chickens three hours after injection of the polysaccharide statolon, to be followed by a 30,000 to 40,000-molecular-weight species after 16 hours. The exact relationship between the different size molecules is not known, although it is possible that they might represent varying multiples of a single molecular unit (Lampson et al., 1963; Merigan, 1967b). Alternatively, the proteins might be only carriers of a single active substance, viz., a prosthetic group. Interferons produced in certain mammalian species including man have to date appeared to be less stable to heat than chick interferon (Finter, 1966).

## POTENTIAL FOR UTILIZATION OF EXOGENOUS INTERFERON FOR PROPHYLAXIS AND THERAPY

The discovery of the soluble exogenous quality of interferon quite expectedly invited immediate exploration for its use as a therapeutic agent for treating viral disease, viz., an "antivirotic." To be clinically useful, however, any chemotherapeutic agent should be nontoxic at the dose levels used, should be nonantigenic so as to permit repeat administration, should be active therapeutically when given in a reasonable regimen, should be safe, and should be practical in terms of cost. Exogenous interferon meets so few of these requirements as to preclude practicable clinical utilization, at least for the present. Each of these may be considered in further detail (see Table 3).

Purified interferon applied *in vivo* and *in vitro* is clearly nontoxic and this is as might be expected for a naturally occurring substance which is concerned with normal host resistance processes. It shows no adverse effect when given in animals and has no measurable effect on host cell synthetic functions (Levy and Merigan, 1966) including synthesis of protein, DNA, or RNA or energy metabolism insofar as measured to date. Cell mitotic processes are unaffected by treatment with interferon and antibody synthesis is unimpaired, both *in vivo* and *in vitro* (Finter, 1966).

Even though of low molecular weight, interferon is antigenic and can induce neutralizing antibodies when given in multiple injections into animals for a long period of time. Chick and mouse interferons appear to be antigenically distinct and this might be generally true, considering that interferon is a product of the host genetic processes. For practicable utilization, interferon would necessarily need to be prepared in the same host species and even here, allogeneic species differences might be important from the antigenic standpoint.

Duration of antiviral effect resulting from interferon administration may vary widely, with longest duration in nondividing cells, in which resistance may persist for one to two weeks (Finter, 1966). Susceptibility to infection is regained in stepwise fashion in dividing cells with development of full sus-

TABLE 3. *Appraisal of Potential for Utilization of Exogenous Interferon*

1. Nontoxic *in vivo* and *in vitro*. No measurable effect on host synthetic function.
2. Weakly antigenic, likely precluding multiple repeat administration of interferon of heterologous source.
3. Limited duration of effect. 1–2 weeks *in vitro* with rapid loss on cell replication. Few days *in vivo*.
4. Broad spectrum against viruses but with varying efficacy including poor effect against herpes group viruses.
5. Host species specificity in utilization with very limited phylogenetic overlap.
6. Very limited effectiveness. Local best, systemic less.
7. Lack of practicable interferon source for use in man.
8. Costs for interferon preparation extremely prohibitive.
9. Outlook negative, in absence of other significant advance.

ceptibility after seven generations (Paucker and Cantell, 1963). Mice have been shown to be protected to slight extent against challenge three days following injection of largest possible doses of interferon (Finter, 1966). Except for certain cell systems such as bone marrow, hair follicles, or gastrointestinal tract epithelium, the cells of the intact host do not undergo rapid continuous replication. While reliable extrapolation cannot be made at this time from cell culture systems to the intact host, such findings do suggest that a single effective dose of interferon might show better than a fleeting effect in some organ systems in the whole animal.

All evidence to date indicates that while interferon is highly active as a prophylactic agent, it gives far less promise as a therapeutic substance. In cell cultures, interferon generally is beneficial only when given prior to or within a few hours following virus, at a time before the virus has taken over control of the synthetic activities of the cell. Interferon can scarcely be expected to reverse the process of viral replication in advanced cellular infection, and this has been confirmed in animal experiments. The basic problem in the clinical-therapeutic sense, therefore, is the relationship between the time of first appearance of symptoms in the patient and the ratio of the number of cells already infected to the number and kind of cells which ultimately would be committed to replicating the virus. This problem, of course, is one which would face any potentially useful viral chemotherapeutic agent. However, it is conceivable that interferon given during prodromata, at onset of symptoms, or on known exposure might be sufficiently early as to render a beneficial effect. Here, therapy denotes prophylaxis in cells which would otherwise be given over to the virus.

Although varying widely with respect to degree of efficacy and extending to relatively low-level resistance in the case of herpesvirus group agents (Finter, 1966), interferon does exhibit a remarkably broad-spectrum activity against heterologous virus species. This is in keeping with the mode of action of interferon in preventing translation of viral nucleic acid message which is a common event in all viral replication (see later). By contrast, however, there is very great host specificity with regard to utilization of interferon from heterologous species. Though phylogenetic overlap has been noted in some instances, e.g., monkey vs. man (Sutton and Tyrrell, 1961), such is insufficient and there appears to be no practical utility.

With present technology, interferon for human clinical use would necessarily have to be made in human cells. Primary cell culture is impractical. Present philosophy and United States Federal Regulations (1967) forbid the use of frank malignant or other "line" cell cultures for preparation of biologicals for human application. Human diploid cell strains, which have been reported to form interferon (Finter, 1966) and which retain certain qualities of "normalcy" on serial passage (Hayflick et al., 1963), as yet enjoy no consensus of safety in the scientific community. Further, human cells give low yields of interferon.

The least optimal aspect for interferon application as a prophylactic or therapeutic tool is its apparent lack of practicability from the aspect of dose and yield. In considering this problem some time past (Hilleman, 1965), we calculated what might be the dose requirement in man, extrapolating from the highly favorable chick embryo interferon-chick embryo cell culture-Eastern equine encephalomyelitis (EEE) virus system. General distribution to all body cells was assumed, disallowing destruction by proteinases, inequitable local binding to cells or to body fluid components, and renal excretion, which may be quite rapid (Ho and Postic, 1967) for certain interferons. Chick interferon, on a weight basis, is highly active, 0.004 $\mu$g. (1 unit) affording total protection to about $10^5$ cells against a lethal amount of EEE virus in a single static chick embryo cell culture. Assuming equal distribution and a cell population of $10^{13}$ in the average human being, the required dosage for man equivalent to the cell cultures would be 40 mg. Yields of egg interferon on purification have been poor, but even granting 100 per cent yield, the equivalent of fluids from 2000 embryonated hens' eggs (20,000 ml.) would be needed to prepare a single 40 mg. human dose. Under such circumstance, the cost for the treatment would be excessive.

This appraisal of interferon utility has been abundantly confirmed in animal experiments carried out to date and in trials in man (Ho and Postic, 1967; Finter, 1966). It has been evident in the animal tests that exogenous interferons can protect some animals against some viruses. Greatest effect was noted when interferon was given locally into sites such as eyes, skin, or peritoneum which were later challenged into the same site, though systemic protection has been noted also in some instances. Reports of trials in human subjects were generally consistent with the animal data. In one study, rhesus monkey kidney interferon infiltrated into the skin prevented "takes" of vaccinia virus given on the following day into the same site (Scientific Committee, 1962). In another study, topically applied monkey kidney interferon given in multiple doses suppressed epithelial changes in natural ocular keratitis caused by vaccinia virus (Jones et al., 1962). In studies by the Scientific Committee on Interferon (Great Britain) (1965), volunteers were given monkey interferon by nasal drops or by spray prior to, during, or following challenge into the respiratory tract with a rhinovirus, Coxsackie A2, or parainfluenza 1 virus. There was no evidence for protection in the treated groups compared with the controls. The Soviets, by contrast, using nasal administration of interferon prepared in human leukocytes and given prior to virus challenge, recorded a decrease in replication of influenza virus in the human respiratory tract (Soloviev, 1967). In the absence of a major development, however, utilization of exogenous interferon in medical practice is lacking in promise.

## QUEST FOR PRACTICABLE INTERFERON INDUCERS

In the absence of any real promise for prophylactic or therapeutic utility of exogenous interferon, attention has been diverted to the search for a practicable inducer whereby the body may be stimulated to produce and distribute its own interferon. For the purpose of this discussion, the term inducer shall be used in its broadest sense, that of eliciting an interferon response. The research of the past several years has uncovered a remarkable array of substances of wide chemical and biological diversity which are capable of eliciting an interferon or interferon-like response. The list now includes most viruses, many bacterial genera (including *Brucella, Salmonella, Escherichia, Bordetella,* pleuropneumonia-like organisms), bacterial endotoxins, rickettsiae, psittacosis group agents, fungal extracts (statolon, helenine, mannan), mitogenic agents (phytohemagglutinin, streptolysin O, poke weed mitogen), cycloheximide (an antibiotic), maleic divinyl ether copolymer (pyran), various synthetic polyanions, and nucleic acids (see later) (Finter, 1966; Friedman and Cooper, 1967; Merigan, 1967c). Even before the discovery of interferon, various extracts of bacteria, fungi, and plant cells were demonstrated to exhibit antiviral activity which, in retrospect, might be interpreted as likely involving the interferon mechanism (Finter, 1966). The extreme divergence of biological origin and chemical constitution of the active substances has presented an enigma concerning their mode of action. Kleinschmidt et al. (1964) noted the common presence of polyanionic macromolecules among the active inducers and was led to speculate that the common activity of such polyanions was to combine with or to remove histone repressor from cellular DNA responsible for coding the interferon molecule in the host cell. The validity of this hypothesis, while of great interest, remains to be established.

Certain minimal attributes seem requisite to consider interferon inducers as candidates for application to human and animal disease control. These include (1) freedom from significant toxicity, (2) nonantigenicity so as to permit repeat administration, (3) noninfectiousness, (4) elimination without incorporation into host cell genome, (5) significant efficacy both in height and duration, (6) acceptability for administration by a practicable route, (7) overall safety, (8) absence of carcinogenic and teratogenic potential, and (9) acceptable cost. Excluding nucleic acids now under investigation (see later), it is doubtful that any of the known inducers would qualify. The synthetic anionic polymers which are currently of special interest (Merigan, 1967c; Regelson, 1967) suffer the drawback of failure to be metabolized, with the resulting complication of their deposition in the reticuloendothelial system and the development of thrombocytopenia.

The studies in our laboratories during the past several years have been directed specifically to the discovery of a highly active interferon inducer which would be worthy of clinical evaluation. In these studies, we were guided by the belief that a likely source or lead for finding a nontoxic and acceptable interferon inducer would come from an examination of the cell response to viral infection. We consequently undertook fractionation of a number of viruses to ascertain which component or components of the virus was responsible for inducing interferon. We were surprised, at the time, to find that none of the fractions examined, not even nucleic acid, was active. This became understandable in the light of further work since all the viral nucleic acids we had tested were single-stranded. Around that time, we noted the reported activity (Braun and Nakano, 1965, 1967) of certain synthetic oligoribonucleotides in potentiating antibody responses and we wondered whether substances of such quality might also induce interferon. We therefore obtained a number of synthetic homopolymers of ribonucleic acid for testing and it was found that a complex of inosinic with cytidylic acid homopolymers (I:C) was active in gamma amount in inducing interferon and resistance to viral infection (Field et al., 1967a). Adenylic-uridylic homopolymer complex and inosinic acid homopolymer plus cytidylic acid dinucleotide were also active but usually to a lesser extent and less consistently in repeat tests. The individual single-stranded homopolymers were inactive. An apparent requirement of double- or polystrandedness of ribonucleic acid for interferon induction was thereby revealed and this led us to seek double-stranded ribonucleic acids from other sources to support the thesis and to be examined for possible utility as clinically useful inducers.

One such source was helenine, an extract of *Penicillium funiculosum* which had been found by Shope (1966) and Rytel et al. (1966) to evoke host resistance to virus and, more recently, to induce interferon. Our group had been doing purification work on this material at the time and it was soon found that helenine contained a very small amount of double-stranded RNA (HeI-RNA) (Lampson et al., 1967) which was a highly active inducer of interferon and host resistance once it had been freed of inhibitory protein. The RNA was purified by a process which involved initial concentration of mycelial extract by high-speed centrifugation, phenolic extraction to eliminate protein, and chromatography on ecteola-cellulose. We were puzzled as to why double-stranded RNA should be found in mold mycelium since double-stranded RNA is the replicative form of nucleic acid in RNA viruses and is not a component of normal cells. We postulated (Lampson et al., 1967) that the *Penicillium funiculosum* culture from which the helenine was derived might have carried a hypothetical viral infection. This theory found support in the recent demonstration by others (Ellis and Kleinschmidt, 1967) of virus-like particles in statolon, a polysaccharide derived from the closely related *Penicillium stoloniferum.*

In seeking further evidence for the requirement of double-strandedness of RNA for interferon induction, our group isolated a noninfectious nucleic acid from reovirus type 3 (Reo 3-RNA) virions (Tytell et al., 1967). This virus is unique in its having double-stranded rather than single-stranded RNA in the formed virus particle. Such nucleic acid also proved highly active in inducing interferon and cellular resistance to virus infection.

Finally, we sought to isolate double-stranded RNA in the viral replicative stage of MS2 bacteriophage infection of *Escherichia coli* (Field et al., 1967b). The virion of MS2 coliphage contains single-stranded RNA but artificial cell lysis about one hour following infection, prior to appearance of whole virus, permitted isolation of phage RNA (MS2-RF-RNA) which was extremely active in inducing interferon and resistance to viral infection.

Table 4 presents a summary of findings in tests of nucleic acids of diverse origin and type. The four double- or multistranded RNA's, viz., I:C, HeI-RNA, Reo 3-RNA, and MS2-RF-RNA, all induced interferon following intravenous injection into rabbits. Single-stranded RNA's of viral, microbial, or mammalian origin all were inactive, as was calf thymus DNA. It may be of some importance with regard to interferon-inducing capability that the x-ray diffraction pattern of I:C is quite similar to that of natural RNA and unlike that of A:U and A:I (Davies and Rich, 1958). The interferons which were elicited in rabbits by the double-stranded RNA's all exhibited the usual properties of interferon including trypsin sensitivity, host species specificity, and isoelectric point near neutral, pH $7.0 \pm 0.1$. The molecular weights, as determined by Sephadex gel filtration, ranged from 40,000 to 61,000. HeI-RNA and MS2-RF-RNA induced an additional interferon of a second species with molecular weights of 130,000 and 167,000, respectively.

The double-stranded RNA's were "early" inducers of interferon, as exemplified for I:C and shown in Figure 1. Maximal interferon titers were

TABLE 4. *Interferon Induction in Rabbits by Nucleic Acids*

| Source and kind of nucleic acid | Chemical nature | Intravenous dose per rabbit ($\mu$G.) | Interferon titers of sera from individual rabbits |
|---|---|---|---|
| Inosinic: cytidylic acid complex (I:C) | Double-stranded* RNA | 2 | >640, >640 |
| *Penicillium funiculosum* (HeI-RNA) | Double-stranded RNA | 8 | 80, 640 or > |
| Reovirus 3 virion (Reo 3-RNA) | Double-stranded RNA | 8 | 640, >640 |
| MS2 coliphage | | | |
|   Replicative RNA (MS2-RF-RNA) | Double-stranded RNA | 8 | 40, 160 |
|   Virion RNA | Single-stranded RNA | 8 | <10, <10 |
|   Whole virion | Contains single-stranded RNA | $1.1 \times 10^{11}$ PFU†/ml. | <10, <10 |
| *E. coli* RNA | Single-stranded RNA | 100 | <10, <10 |
| Newcastle disease virus virion | Single-stranded RNA | 10 | <5 |
| Influenza virus virion (WS) | Single-stranded RNA | 10 | <5 |
| Tobacco mosaic virus virion | Single-stranded RNA | 40 | <5 |
| Yeast ribosome | Single-stranded RNA | 1000 | <5 |
| Yeast sRNA | Single-stranded RNA | 200 | <5 |
| Yeast core RNA | Single-stranded RNA | 100 | <5 |
| Mouse liver (ribosomal) | Single-stranded RNA | 200 | <5 |
| Bovine liver sRNA | Single-stranded RNA | 200 | <5 |
| Calf thymus DNA | Double-stranded DNA | 200 | <5 |

\* Possible multistranding.
† Plaque-forming units.

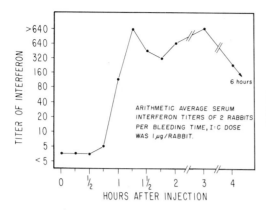

TITER OF INTERFERON

>640
640
320
160
80
40
20
10
5
<5

ARITHMETIC AVERAGE SERUM
INTERFERON TITERS OF 2 RABBITS
PER BLEEDING TIME, I:C DOSE
WAS 1 μg/RABBIT.

6 hours

0    ½    1    1½    2    3    4
HOURS AFTER INJECTION

*Figure 1.* Kinetics of serum interferon induction after single I:C intravenous injection.

usually achieved in the blood within two hours, followed by marked decline within six hours. In this respect, the RNA's resembled endotoxin in causing early appearance of interferon contrasted with viruses which usually cause maximal titers around five to six hours and later decline. This is discussed further later.

In addition to interferon, the double-stranded RNA's induced resistance to viral challenge which was measurable in cell culture *in vitro* and in the intact host animal. The amounts needed were extremely small. As shown in Table 5, the minimal required dosage for interferon induction in rabbits was less than 1 μg. per animal and direct interference in rabbit kidney cell culture against vesicular stomatitis virus required no more than 0.3 μg. Nasal administration of RNA to mice prior to and following nasal challenge protected mice against lethal infection with PVM and Sendai viruses and intraperitoneal injection of RNA protected against lethal subcutaneous challenge with Col. SK virus. Dosage was 7.9 to 131 μg. of RNA per animal; the minimal required amount has since been shown to be about one-fifth that amount. I:C was shown also to induce interferon *in vitro* within 7.5 hours in spinner flasks of trypsinized spleen cells of six-week-old rabbits.

All the double-stranded RNA's which were used were highly purified and displayed the usual ultraviolet absorption spectrum. Double-strandedness of the HeI, Reo 3, and MS2-RF RNA's was established on usual criteria including relative resistance to RNase, high thermal transition midpoint (Tm) (> 100°C. or 110°C.), depression of Tm by heating in the presence of formaldehyde, or low ionic strength. HeI-RNA was shown to contain ribose and phosphorus with the approximate theoretical values for RNA and the expected adenine, guanine, cytosine, and uracil base groups were found present. Protein, carbohydrate, and deoxyribose were absent and the molecular weight was about 1,600,000. The I:C complex appeared less firmly bound and less stable to RNase than the naturally occurring RNA's. The Tm was only 60.5°C. Effective complexing was prevented by reacting in distilled water rather than in saline solution, and by binding of amino groups of C with formaldehyde or by removal by deamination. Biological activity was destroyed and complex formation prevented by shortening the chain length of C by treatment with RNase prior to mixing. I:C was dissociated at pH 9.5 or greater with reduction in biological activity, and was vulnerable to degradation by RNase at 25°C., also with reduction in biological activity.

TABLE 5. *Summary of Biological Activities of Double-Stranded RNA's of Diverse Origin*

| RNA INJECTED | MINIMAL EFFECTIVE AMOUNT | | PROTECTIVE DOSE IN MICE AGAINST VIRUS* | | |
|---|---|---|---|---|---|
| | *Interferon Induction in Rabbits* | *Interference to VSV in Rabbit Kidney Cell Culture* | *PVM* | *Col. SK* | *Sendai* |
| *Synthetic* | | | | | |
| Polyinosinic-polycytidylic acid complex (I:C) | 0.5 µg. | 0.00125 µg. | 7.9 µg. | 131 µg. | 16 µg. |
| *Viral* | | | | | |
| Reovirus 3 (Reo 3-RNA) | 0.5 µg. | 0.04 µg. | 16 µg. | ND | ND |
| Coliphage (MS2-RF-RNA) | 0.5 µg. | 0.04 µg. | 18 µg. | ND | ND |
| *Fungal* | | | | | |
| Penicillium funiculosum (Hel-RNA) | 0.125 µg. | 0.3 µg. | 20 µg. | 50 µg. | ND |

* Minimal required dose not determined.

An established value of the studies of double-stranded RNA to date lies in the demonstration of double- or polystranding of RNA for induction of interferon. To what extent the minimal attributes of inducers worthy of clinical trial will be met by the double-stranded RNA's remains to be seen in the extensive studies now in progress.

The matter of induction of interferon by nucleic acids deserves special discussion to relate the present findings to those reported earlier by other workers. Isaacs et al. (1963) claimed to have induced interferon in cell culture by foreign RNA or by chemically altered homologous RNA. Characteristically, large amounts (100 µg. per cell culture) were required and the titer of inhibitor produced was very low, never more than 1:2. Recent studies in our laboratory have shown that double-stranded RNA added to cell cultures induced resistance to viral infection at a concentration of 0.002 µg./ml., whereas "foreign" single-stranded RNA did not induce resistance, even at a concentration of 100 µg./ml. It is open to question whether the very low titer inhibitor reported by Isaacs was induced by the added RNA. In a recent report (1965), Isaacs himself questioned the validity of his foreign nucleic acid hypothesis and stated that it "can no longer be maintained." This latest conclusion of Isaacs relating to his own use of RNA is probably valid since the ribonucleic acids he employed were all single-stranded and the inactivity of such single-stranded materials has been confirmed in the present report. The suggested induction of interferon by Jensen et al. (1963, 1964) and Takano et al. (1965) by many ribonucleic and deoxyribonucleic acids, and by nucleosides and nucleotides used at high concentration, can be dismissed because of lack of evidence for interferon induction, by failure to remove the inducer prior to virus challenge, by the inordinately long incubation period required, by the direct antiviral effect of certain breakdown products of nucleic acids, and by the failure of confirmation by others (Finter, 1966). Studies by others with nucleic acids and their derivatives can be similarly dismissed (Finter, 1966).

# THE INTERFERON MECHANISM

Much attention has been given in the contemporary period to studies of the mechanism whereby interferon is induced and whereby interferon exerts its antiviral action. Elucidation of such mechanism is of paramount importance because leads might be uncovered for stimulating any of the several stages of interferon action, with simple and chemically defined substances, it is hoped. Considerations of the mode of action of interferon must necessarily embrace two aspects: first, the interaction of the cell with the inducer with resultant synthesis of interferon; second, the action of the induced interferon upon new cells to prevent or limit viral replication. Although the mechanisms for interferon induction and utilization are incompletely understood, there is sufficient knowledge to permit a working hypothesis. The available data fit satisfactorily into the mechanics of the well known Jacob-Monod model (Jacob and Monod, 1961) for enzyme induction whereby, in simplest concept, a specific inducer effects a derepression of a corresponding host gene to cause formation of messenger RNA, with resultant translation of a corresponding protein. This concept will be used in further discussion of interferon mechanism, even though the data to establish all points are not available.

The early work on interferon induction by Heller (1963) and Wagner (1963) gave the first clue to interferon production in their demonstration that synthesis of interferon was inhibited by actinomycin D. A principal activity of this antibiotic is to bind the guanine residues of double-stranded DNA, thereby preventing the formation of messenger RNA by host cell DNA, and it became evident, therefore, that interferon was synthesized under the host genetic code in response to a viral stimulus. If introduced after messenger RNA was formed, actinomycin D had no effect on interferon synthesis. Further in the process, it was noted that inhibitors of protein synthesis, puromycin and p-fluorophenylalanine, prevented formation of interferon, presumably by acting at the messenger RNA level (Buchan and Burke, 1964, 1966). It thus appears that interferon is produced by the cell in response to viral infection by a mechanism involving derepression of host DNA to form a messenger RNA essential to production of interferon. There is some evidence that cells may also contain preformed interferon, since rapid appearance of interferon-like substance follows administration of endotoxin or of *Brucella* organisms and since the formation of such interferon is not prevented by actinomycin D or by puromycin or cycloheximide inhibitors of protein synthesis (Ke et al., 1966; Youngner et al., 1964). Further, evidence has been presented that interferon may be present in (Nagano et al., 1966) or synthesized in small amount by (Wagner and Smith, 1967) apparently normal macrophages. Clarification of the situation as applies to preformed versus newly synthesized interferon must await further investigation.

The action of the produced interferon to prevent or to limit viral replication appears not to be upon the virus directly. Thus, direct inactivation of virions or of infectious RNA is not involved. Further, virus attachment to cell, cell penetration, viral uncoating, viral assembly, and viral release are not prevented by interferon. Instead, as shown by Taylor (1964), interferon appears to act in some way to prevent synthesis of viral substance. As in interferon production, the activity displayed by interferon appears also to be indirect since it can be inhibited by actinomycin D and by inhibitors of protein synthesis (Friedman and Sonnabend, 1964; Levine, 1964; Taylor, 1964). The simple interpretation is that interferon itself may act only as a derepressor to cause the host DNA to produce the messenger RNA for yet another protein which is the true antiviral substance. Added credence is given to this by the fact that only brief exposure to a small amount of interferon is needed to permit development of resistance and such resistance may increase even after the interferon is removed, provided synthesis of RNA and protein is not impaired (Finter, 1966). Baron (Finter, 1966) has likened interferon to other message-carrying polypeptides and proteins in the body which are generally classified as hormones and which act apparently as derepressors of host DNA to form proteins required for cellular function.

The precise mechanism whereby the final antiviral protein prevents synthesis of new virus is likewise not known. Shortly after the discovery of interferon, Isaacs (1960, 1961; Isaacs et al., 1961) postulated that interferon altered carbohydrate metabolism and evolved a hypothesis that interferon acts in suppressing viral synthesis by uncoupling oxidative phosphorylation in the nucleus. This concept has been refuted on several bases (Finter, 1966; Hilleman, 1963) and need not be discussed further.

Sonnabend and Friedman (Finter, 1966) presented three possibilities for action of the interferon system based on the observation that formation of viral nucleic acid is clearly impeded, viz., (1) prevention of synthesis of viral RNA polymerase, (2) inhibition of viral RNA polymerase, or (3) degradation of newly synthesized viral RNA. Best available data support the concept of prevention of formation of virus-specific polymerase or other protein. Interferon-mediated interference shows a differential inhibition of viral messenger RNA and not of host messenger (m) RNA. Carter and Levy (1967) and Joklik and Merigan (1966), working with Mengo or vaccinia virus, have observed that the ribosomes derived from interferon-treated cells do not form or show reduced formation of the polysome complexes with viral messenger RNA; this precludes the synthesis of viral coded proteins at the translational level. Capacity of the ribosomes to associate with cell messenger RNA was preserved. Marcus and Salb (1966), working with Sindbis virus, noted that ribosomes derived from interferon-treated cells did react with either viral or host messenger RNA to form polysome complexes. The difference lay in the fact that there was suppression in the readout of the message from viral mRNA but not from host mRNA. This led Marcus and Salb to postulate the formation by interferon-treated cells of messenger RNA which then produced a substance which they called translation inhibitory protein (TIP). According to the theory, the TIP binds to ribosomes in the cytoplasmic pool. The polysomes composed of host mRNA and TIP-attached ribosomes translate normally, whereas those composed of viral mRNA and TIP-attached ribosomes do not translate, resulting in suppression of viral synthesis.

A current working thesis for interferon induction and interference is presented graphically in Figure 2. Phase 1 involves the production of interferon and phase 2 involves the action of interferon to prevent virus synthesis. Essentially, single-strand RNA virus penetrates the cell, is uncoated, releases

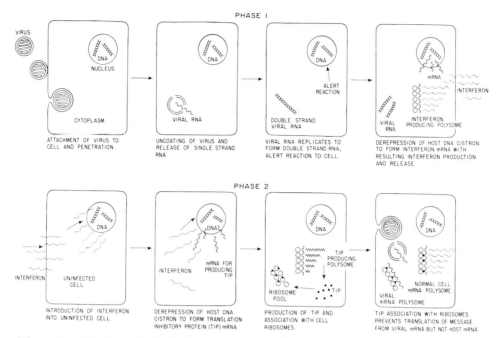

*Figure 2.* Working thesis for interferon induction and interference with viral synthesis. (Phase 2 after Marcus and Salb, in part.)

its RNA, and sets about to produce a complementary strand of RNA which is essential to its replication. Double-stranded RNA, formed in the process, or the annealing of only a very small portion of these strands should suffice to stimulate interferon formation. Double-stranded RNA is not normal to the cell and this is presumed to provide the alert, possibly by derepression, for cellular formation of interferon mRNA and interferon production. The interferon is transported via the blood or body fluids or by contact to uninfected cells, where it derepresses a second host cistron to form mRNA for translation inhibitory protein, TIP. The TIP associates with cell ribosomes which attach to viral mRNA following attack and to cell mRNA, forming polysomes. There is some alteration in the ribosome configuration by TIP such that translation of cell mRNA is not inhibited but viral mRNA is inhibited. In certain instances, polysome formation with viral mRNA may not occur; this also prevents readout of the viral messenger.

This working hypothesis does not attempt to explain the mode of action of all kinds of inducers of interferon and does not deal with the apparent release of preformed interferon by endotoxin without need for mRNA synthesis by the host cell. It does attempt, however, to show that the unique requirement for interferon induction by viral RNA or by synthetic RNA polymer is that it be double- or polystranded. Clearly, the single-stranded RNA's of viral, cellular, or synthetic origin have been inactive as interferon inducers, whereas the replicative-form double-stranded RNA of ordinary RNA viruses, the unique double-stranded RNA of reovirus 3 virion, double-stranded RNA of fungal origin, and certain complexed synthetic RNA's have shown activity. Insufficient work has been carried out to date to establish whether

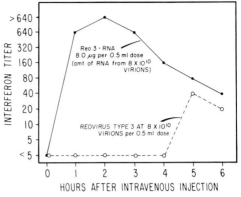

*Figure 3.* Comparison of kinetics for induction of interferon in rabbits by intravenous injection of Reo 3-RNA or reovirus type 3 virions.

induction of interferon by the double-stranded RNA's requires DNA-dependent RNA synthesis, and whether such activity is due to the relative resistance of multistranded RNA to ribonuclease, in contrast to single-stranded RNA, can only be speculated upon at this time. Isolated noninfectious reovirus 3 RNA induces interferon which is detectable within one hour following intravenous administration in rabbits (Tytell et al., 1967) (see Fig. 3). By contrast, whole virion requires about five hours and this is the expected time required for the intracellular removal of the protein overcoat from the virion. This suggests that the variable time lag in interferon appearance following certain of the interferon inducers may be more closely related to the time required to provide sufficient active inducing material within the cell than to any basic difference in the mode of action in inducing interferon. The mode of action of DNA viruses in stimulating interferon is not presently known, though it may well be by a mechanism similar to that for RNA viruses, possibly involving a special replicative form of double-stranded DNA (Korn, 1967), or a viral DNA-RNA complex. Presence of double-stranded DNA in the cytoplasm might also be important. Double-strandedness of DNA alone appears insufficient since double-stranded DNA is normal to the cell, and since double-stranded calf thymus DNA, as an example, does not stimulate interferon formation (Lampson et al., 1967).

Which cells in the body are ordinarily active in producing interferon in response to viral infection is not known, though it has been shown that many kinds of cells possess the capacity to do so. The fact that leukocytes commonly harbor viruses and are generally excellent interferon producers (Finter, 1966) makes it tempting to speculate that the leukocytes might be a first line of defense in resistance to virus infection, providing a ready supply of expendable sacrificial cells which can be given to this purpose.

Irrespective of whether the viral inhibitory factor (TIP) induced by interferon acts by preventing viral mRNA polysome formation or by preventing translation from the polysome, the end result is the same, viz., prevention of virus synthesis. The model explains the inhibition of both RNA and DNA viruses since the translation of viral mRNA nucleotide is an event which is common to the infectious cycle of both kinds of virus. Salb and Marcus (1965) have recently shown that inhibition of readout of mRNA may operate as a normal event during mitosis, thus bringing this mechanism into play in normal cells. The TIP of normal cells in mitosis has been found to be destroyed by trypsin, rendering the ribosomes capable of normal translation (Marcus and Salb, 1966; Salb and Marcus, 1965). Marcus and Salb (1966) have data to suggest that trypsin treatment converts TIP-ribosomes to ribosomes which will translate Sindbis virus mRNA.

## OUTLOOK AND APPRAISAL

The diversity in number and kind of viral disease agents is demanding of the broad perspective in seeking their control. Those viral diseases in which there is a paucity or unity of serotypes and which are naturally followed by long-term or lifelong immunity lend themselves best to the vaccine approach, especially live virus vaccines, as exemplified by measles, mumps, rubella, varicella, yellow fever, and poliomyelitis. A limited spectrum of the respiratory disease agents including the influenza, parainfluenza, respiratory syncytial, and Eaton's pleuropneumonia agents offers promise for medium to long-term immunity, by employment of killed vaccines, especially if the antibody response has been potentiated in height and duration through application of a suitable immunological adjuvant (Hilleman, 1965). The vaccine approach is clearly prophylactic. Chemical agents, which must surely evolve, are needed most for treating viral diseases once effective contact with the host has been made or when symptoms have already appeared. Already, iododeoxyuridine treatment may cure ocular herpes simplex, amantadine may afford some prophylactic benefit against influenza A2 virus, and isatin-$\beta$-thiosemicarbazone may give prophylactic or weak therapeutic effect in smallpox infections (Hilleman, 1965). The interferon mechanism, by its broad-spectrum antiviral activity, affords the greatest hope for eventual prophylactic control of those viral infections in which the plurality of serotypes is so great as to preclude successful application of vaccines, e.g., the common cold caused by rhinoviruses with probably hundreds of serotypes (Hilleman, 1965), and the enteric and systemic diseases caused by the diversity of enterovirus serotypes. Real hope for respiratory disease control is provided by the demonstration, to date, of high-level protective efficacy against respiratory infection afforded by the double-stranded RNA interferon inducers given nasally (Field et al., 1967a, b; Lampson et al., 1967; Tytell et al., 1967). Special situations might also apply, e.g., in the wake of pandemic influenza virus apprehended too late to permit significant vaccine production and administration prior to occurrence, or in the widespread dissemination of smallpox virus in areas where vaccine had been inadequately applied.

Clearly, the interferon mechanism is one which applies to man and is not unique to the experimental animal models in which it has been studied most extensively. Interferon appears in viral infections in man and is produced in human cells cultivated *in vitro*. Exogenous interferon placed in local sites in man can cause resistance to virus challenge, and human cells have been rendered resistant to viral infection *in vitro* by addition of the substance

(Finter, 1966). The greatest promise for benefit to be derived from the interferon system is in prophylaxis, though some degree of therapeutic activity might also be attained. Interferon resistance is a condition of the individual cell. The matter resolves itself simply into what proportion of the cells of the metazoan host which would otherwise have been committed to viral replication are actually infected at the time that the interferon mechanism is brought into effective play. Thus, limitation of clinical reaction might be attained even after first appearance of symptoms.

The situation as applies to cancer is worthy of special mention. The interferon system is broad-spectrum with respect to viruses and this includes oncogenic viruses as well as those which bring about lytic destruction of cells (Finter, 1966). Oncogenic viruses may stimulate interferon production and the replication and neoplastic transformation by such viruses may be inhibited by exogenous interferon. Further, interferon may prevent neoplastic transformation by oncogenic SV40 virus in cells in which it does not replicate the infectious agent. It is a quality of most oncogenic viruses of animals that infection must be accomplished early in life, during the period of immunological immaturity, if clinically apparent neoplasia is to occur. If this analogy extends to hypothetical cancer virus in man, continuing artificial stimulation of interferon during the early postnatal months in human subjects might provide the means for prophylaxis of cancer. Alternatively, it is well established that certain of the neoplasias of animals caused by RNA viruses are virus-dependent, requiring continued presence of virus and reinfection of new cells to perpetuate the disease. Conceivably, an effective interferon inducer might break an essential link in the chain of events in leukemia so as to bring about effective control of the process. Several workers have already recorded inhibition of Friend leukemia virus propagation and inhibition of splenomegaly in mice by administration of interferon inducers including divinyl ether maleic anhydride copolymer (pyran), the anionic polysaccharide statolon, and phytohemagglutinin (Merigan and Regelson, 1967 a, b; Regelson, 1967; Wheelock, 1967; Wheelock and Larke, 1967). Pyran is currently undergoing clinical trial in man in advanced cases of cancer (Merigan and Regelson, 1967a, b; Regelson, 1967).

The significant attempt to apply the interferon mechanism to human and veterinary medicine lies clearly in the future and there are many hurdles to be crossed. One important aspect of application of interferon inducers lies in the duration of protective effect. The early work (Kleinschmidt and Murphy, 1967) with statolon-induced resistance in mice has been promising in the demonstration of protection against fatal MM virus infection in mice for at least 29 days following a single injection of the inducer. The matter of maintaining an uninterrupted state of interferon protection is complicated by the fact that blood clearance of interferon is rapid and that once interferon is induced, cells *in vitro* and animals become refractory for a period of time before they can be restimulated. This phenomenon, referred to as tolerance, may last for a week or perhaps as long as resistance persists. Future research might well be directed toward breaking of such tolerance, even as breaking of immunological tolerance is being actively pursued in cancer therapy. A matter of further complication in maximal interferon utilization is the demonstration (Chany and Brailovsky, 1967; Isaacs et al., 1966; Kato et al., 1965; Truden et al., 1967) that virus-infected cells may contain substances called "stimulon," "enhancer," or "blocker" which may prevent the production of interferon or otherwise overcome its effect. Whether these substances actually prevent interferon formation, antagonize interferon action, or merely act to promote viral replication is not fully disclosed. The important lesson is that viruses may have their own defense against cellular defenses, an apt example in this age of antimissile missiles, and it may be important to pursue methods for negating such defensive action on the part of the virus. As noted earlier (Hilleman, 1965), the possibility must always be entertained that sustained or even temporary activity of interferon, naturally acquired or artificially induced, might not always be beneficial to the host and the development of means for nullifying rather than promoting interferon action might be advantageous in special circumstances.

# References

Baron, S., and H. B. Levy. 1966. Interferon. Ann. Rev. Microbiol., *20:*291–318.

Biological Products. 1967. Public Health Service Regulations, Title 42, Part 73. U. S. Department of Health, Education and Welfare, Publication 437.

Braun, W., and M. Nakano. 1965. Influence of oligodeoxyribonucleotides on early events in antibody formation. Proc. Soc. Exp. Biol. Med., *119:*701–707.

Braun, W., and M. Nakano. 1967. Antibody formation: Stimulation by polyadenylic and polycytidylic acids. Science, *157:*819–821.

Buchan, A., and D. C. Burke. 1964. Inhibition of interferon production by puromycin and p-fluorophenylalanine. Abstr. Sixth Internat. Congr. Biochem., New York, p. 46.

Buchan, A., and D. C. Burke. 1966. Interferon production in chick-embryo cells. The effect of puromycin and p-fluorophenylalanine. Biochem. J., *98:*530–536.

Burke, D. C., and J. J. Skehel. 1967. Interferons and other cell products influencing viral multiplication. Brit. Med. Bull., *23:*109–113.

Carter, W. A., and H. B. Levy. 1967. Ribosomes: Effect of interferon on their interaction with rapidly labeled cellular and viral RNA's. Science, *155:*1254–1257.

Chany, C., and C. Brailovsky. 1967. Stimulating interaction between viruses (stimulons). Proc. Nat. Acad. Sci., *57:*87–94.

Davies, D. R., and A. Rich. 1958. The formation of a helical complex between polyinosinic acid and polycytidylic acid. J. Am. Chem. Soc., *80:*1003–1004.

Ellis, L. F., and W. J. Kleinschmidt. 1967. Virus-like particles of a fraction of Statolon, a mould product. Nature, *215:*649–650.

Field, A. K., A. A. Tytell, G. P. Lampson, and M. R. Hilleman. 1967a. Inducers of interferon and host resistance. II. Multistranded synthetic polynucleotide complexes. Proc. Nat. Acad. Sci., *58:*1004–1010.

Field, A. K., G. P. Lampson, A. A. Tytell, M. M. Nemes, and M. R. Hilleman. 1967b. Inducers of interferon and host resistance. IV. Double-stranded replicative form RNA (MS2-RF-RNA) from *E. coli* infected with MS2 coliphage. Proc. Nat. Acad. Sci., *58:*2102–2108.

Findlay, G. M., and F. O. MacCallum. 1937. An interference phenomenon in relation to yellow fever and other viruses. J. Path. Bact., *44:*405–424.

Finter, N. B. (ed.). 1966. Interferons. W. B. Saunders Company, Philadelphia.

Friedman, R. M., and H. L. Cooper. 1967. Stimulation of interferon production in human lymphocytes by mitogens. Proc. Soc. Exp. Biol. Med., *125:*901–905.

Friedman, R. M., and J. A. Sonnabend. 1964. Inhibition of interferon action by p-fluorophenylalanine. Nature, *203:*366–367.

Hayflick, L., P. S. Moorhead, C. M. Pomerat, and T. C. Hsu. 1963. Choice of a cell system for vaccine production. Science, *140:*766–768.

Heller, E. 1963. Enhancement of Chikungunya virus replication and inhibition of interferon production by Actinomycin D. Virology, *21:*652–656.

Hilleman, M. R. 1963. Interferon in prospect and perspective. J. Cell. Comp. Physiol., *62:*337–353.

Hilleman, M. R. 1965. Immunologic, chemotherapeutic and interferon approaches to control of viral disease. Am. J. Med., *38:*751–766.

Ho, M. 1967. The induction of interferons and related problems. Japan. J. Exp. Med., *37:*169–182.

Ho, M., and B. Postic. 1967. Prospects for applying interferon to man. *In:* First International Conference on Vaccines Against Viral and Rickettsial Diseases of Man. Pan American Health Organization, Washington, D. C., pp. 632–649.

Hoskins, M. 1935. A protective action of neurotropic against viscerotropic yellow fever virus in Macacus rhesus. Am. J. Trop. Med., *15:*675–680.

Isaacs, A. 1960. Metabolic effects of interferon on chick fibroblasts. Virology, *10:*144–146.

Isaacs, A. 1961. Interferon. Sci. Am., *204:*51–57.

Isaacs, A. 1965. Studies on interferon. Aust. J. Exp. Biol. Med. Sci., *43:*405–412.

Isaacs, A., and D. C. Burke. 1959. Viral interference and interferon. Brit. Med. Bull., *15:*185–188.

Isaacs, A., R. A. Cox, and Z. Rotem. 1963. Foreign nucleic acids as the stimulus to make interferon. Lancet, *2:*113–116.

Isaacs, A., H. G. Klemperer, and G. Hitchcock. 1961. Studies on the mechanism of action of interferon. Virology, *13:*191–199.

Isaacs, A., and J. Lindenmann. 1957. Virus interference. I. The interferon. Proc. Royal Soc., B, *147:*258–267.

Isaacs, A., J. Lindenmann, and R. C. Valentine. 1957. Virus interference. II. Some properties of interferon. Proc. Royal Soc., B, *147:*268–273.

Isaacs, A., Z. Rotem, and K. H. Fantes. 1966. An inhibitor of the production of interferon ("blocker"). Virology, *29:*248–254.

Jacob, F., and J. Monod. 1961. Genetic regulatory mechanisms in the synthesis of proteins. J. Mol. Biol., *3:*318–356.

Jensen, K. E. 1964. Personal communication.

Jensen, K. E., A. L. Neal, R. E. Owens, and J. Warren. 1963. Interferon responses of chick embryo fibroblasts to nucleic acids and related compounds. Nature, *200:*433–434.

Joklik, W. K., and T. C. Merigan. 1966. Concerning the mechanism of action of interferon. Proc. Nat. Acad. Sci., *56:*558–565.

Jones, B. R., J. E. K. Galbraith, and M. K. Al-Hussaini. 1962. Vaccinial keratitis treated with interferon. Lancet, *1:*875–879.

Kato, N., A. Okada, and F. Ota. 1965. A factor capable of enhancing virus replication appearing in parainfluenza virus type 1 (HVJ[1])-infected allantoic fluid. Virology, *26:*630-637.

Ke, Y. H., S. H. Singer, B. Postic, and M. Ho. 1966. Effect of puromycin on virus and endotoxin-induced interferonlike inhibitors in rabbits. Proc. Soc. Exp. Biol. Med., *121:*181–183.

Kleinschmidt, W. J., J. C. Cline, and E. B. Murphy. 1964. Interferon production induced by statolon. Proc. Nat. Acad. Sci., *52:*741–744.

Kleinschmidt, W. J., and E. B. Murphy. 1967. Interferon induction with Statolon in the intact animal. Bact. Rev., *31:*132–137.

Korn, D. 1967. Inhibition of bacteriophage T4 deoxyribonucleic acid maturation by actinomycin D. J. Biol. Chem., *242:*160–162.

Lampson, G. P., A. A. Tytell, M. M. Nemes, and M. R. Hilleman. 1963. Purification and characterization of chick embryo interferon. Proc. Soc. Exp. Biol. Med., *112:*468–478.

Lampson, G. P., A. A. Tytell, A. K. Field, M. M. Nemes, and M. R. Hilleman. 1967. Inducers of interferon and host resistance. I. Double-stranded RNA from extracts of *Penicillium funiculosum.* Proc. Nat. Acad. Sci., *58:*782–789.

Levine, S. 1964. Effect of actinomycin D and puromycin dihydrochloride on action of interferon. Virology, *24:*586–588.

Levy, H. B., and T. C. Merigan. 1966. Interferon and uninfected cells. Proc. Soc. Exp. Biol. Med., *121:*53–55.

Marcus, P. I., and J. M. Salb, 1966. Molecular basis of interferon action: Inhibition of viral RNA translation. Virology, *30:*502–516.

Merigan, T. C. 1967a. Interferons of mice and men. New Eng. J. Med., *276:*913–920.

Merigan, T. C. 1967b. Various molecular species of interferon induced by viral and nonviral agents. Bact. Rev., *31:*138–144.

Merigan, T. C. 1967c. Induction of circulating interferon by synthetic anionic polymers of known composition. Nature, *214:*416–417.

Merigan, T. C., and W. Regelson. 1967a. Interferon induction in mouse and man by a synthetic polyanion of defined composition. Clin. Res., *40:*309. Abst.

Merigan, T. C., and W. Regelson. 1967b. Interferon induction in man by a synthetic polyanion of defined composition. New Eng. J. Med., *277:*1283–1287.

Nagano, Y., Y. Kojima, J. Arakawa, and R. S. Kanashiro. 1966. Production du facteur inhibiteur du virus par les phagocytes péritonéaux du lapin non inoculé. Japan. J. Exp. Med., *36:*481–487.

Paucker, K., and M. Boxaca. 1967. Cellular resistance to induction of interferon. Bact. Rev., *31:*145–156.

Paucker, K., and K. Cantell. 1963. Quantitative studies on viral interference in suspended L cells. V. Persistence of protection in growing cultures. Virology, *21:*22–29.

Regelson, W. 1967. Prevention and treatment of Friend leukemia virus (FLV) infection by interferon-inducing synthetic polyanions. *In:* The Reticuloendothelial System and Atherosclerosis (N. R. DiLuzio, and R. Paolctti, eds.). Plenum Press, New York, pp. 315–332.

Rytel, M. W., R. E. Shope, and E. D. Kilbourne. 1966. An antiviral substance from *Penicillium funiculosum.* V. Induction of interferon by helenine. J. Exp. Med., *123:*577–584.

Salb, J. M., and P. I. Marcus. 1965. Translational inhibition in mitotic HeLa cells. Proc. Nat. Acad. Sci., *54:*1353–1358.

Scientific Committee on Interferon. 1962. Effect of interferon on vaccination in volunteers. Lancet, *1:*873–875.

Scientific Committee on Interferon. 1965. Experiments with interferon in man. Lancet, *1:* 505–506.

Shope, R. E. 1966. An antiviral substance from *Penicillium funiculosum.* IV. Inquiry into the mechanism by which helenine exerts its antiviral effect. J. Exp. Med., *123:*213–227.

Soloviev, V. D. 1967. Interferon. Discussion. *In:* First International Conference on Vaccines Against Viral and Rickettsial Diseases of Man. Pan American Health Organization, Washington, D. C., pp. 658–659.

Sutton, R. N. P., and D. A. J. Tyrrell. 1961. Some observations on interferon prepared in tissue cultures. Brit. J. Exp. Path., *42:*99–105.

Takano, K., J. Warren, K. E. Jensen, and A. L. Neal. 1965. Nucleic acid-induced resistance to viral infection. J. Bact., *90:*1542–1547.

Taylor, J. 1964. Inhibition of interferon action by actinomycin. Biochem. Biophys. Res. Commun., *14:*447–451.

Truden, J. L., M. M. Sigel, and L. S. Dietrich. 1967. An interferon antagonist: Its effect on interferon action in mengo-infected Ehrlich ascites tumor cells. Virology, *33:*95–103.

Tytell, A. A., G. P. Lampson, A. K. Field, and M. R. Hilleman. 1967. Inducers of interferon and host resistance. III. Double-stranded RNA from reovirus type 3 virions (Reo 3-RNA). Proc. Nat. Acad. Sci., 58:1719–1722.

Wagner, R. R. 1960. Viral interference. Some considerations of basic mechanisms and their potential relationship to host resistance. Bact. Rev., *24:*151–166.

Wagner, R. R. 1963. Interferon control of viral infection. Trans. Assoc. Am. Phys., *76:*92–101.

Wagner, R. R. 1965. Interferon. A review and analysis of recent observations. Am. J. Med., *38:*726–737.

Wagner, R. R., and T. J. Smith. 1967. The interferons: Some unsolved problems of action and biosynthesis. *In:* First International Conference on Vaccines Against Viral and Rickettsial Diseases of Man. Pan American Health Organization, Washington, D. C., pp. 616–622.

Wheelock, E. F. 1967. Effect of statolon on Friend virus leukemia in mice. Proc. Soc. Exp. Biol. Med., *124:*855–858.

Wheelock, E. F., and R. P. B. Larke. 1967. Prolongation of life in mice with established Friend virus leukemia by inoculation with Sendai virus, interferon, or Statolon. Science, *158:* 537–538.

Youngner, J. S., W. R. Stinebring, and S. E. Taube. 1964. Influence of inhibitors of protein synthesis on interferon formation in mice. Virology, *1:*541–550.

Zemla, J., and J. Vilcek. 1961. Studies on an interferon from tick-borne encephalitis virus-infected cells (IF). II. Physical and chemical properties of IF. Acta Virol., *5:*367–372.

# Index

Page numbers in *italics* indicate illustrations.

Acidosis, in cholera, 293
Actinomycin D, and interferon induction, 604
Adaptive immunity, evolution of, 3
  in fish, 3
  limitation to vertebrates, 2
  origins of, 4
Adenovirus, capsid of, 467, *468*
    synthesis of "late" proteins of, 476, *479*
  cytopathology of, 456, *458, 459,* 466–486
  in autolyzing cell, *445*
  infection by, and host macromolecule bio-
    synthesis, 477–480
    process of, 469
  micrograph of, *453, 454, 455*
  multiplication of, 469, *469*
  type 5, cytopathic effects of, 471, *472*
  virion of, 467–470, *468*
    synthesis of, 473–477
Aedes mosquitoes, in yellow fever transmission, 432, 539, 544
African horse sickness virus, 543
  transmission of 548, *548*
Agammaglobulinemia, Bruton type, 94
    infections in, 96, 97
    lymph node in, *96*
    lymphatic leukemia in, 106
  Swiss type, 90
    lymphoid tissues in, *91*
    malignancy in, 106
Agglutinins, cold, in *Mycoplasma pneumoniae* infections, 417
Agglutinogen, of *Bordetella pertussis,* 249
Aging, and immunologic responses and malig-
  nancy, 107
Alastrim, 497
  complications of, 498
  transmission of, 511
Allergic reactions, IgE and, 99
Aluminum adjuvants, in pertussis vaccine,
  258

Amapari virus, 543
Anopheles A virus, transmission of, 548, *548*
Anopheles B virus, transmission of, 548, *548*
Antibiotics, and gonococci, 279
  and meningococci, 278
  in pertussis, 243
  resistance to, transduction of, in *Staphylo-
    coccus aureus,* 213
Antibody(ies), 120
  anti-M, 176
  cellular transportation of, 40
    functional significance of, 43
  complement fixing, in poliomyelitis, 529
  cytophilic, 33
  detection and measurement of, 506
  function of, 15
  immunosuppressive function of, 16
  in lower vertebrates, 13
  in smallpox, 507
  induction of, 13
  neutralizing, in poliomyelitis, 528
    in smallpox revaccination, *507*
  production of, 79
    evolution of, 12–16
    genetic approach to, 12
    neonatal thymectomy and, 82
  streptococcal, diagnostic value of studies of,
    178
  to oncogenic viruses, 574
  to Reiter antigen, 370, 374
  to treponemal carbohydrate fractions, 375
  treponemal immobilizing, 370, 372, 375,
    376
  Wassermann, 370, 371, 375, 376
Antigen(s), Brucella, delayed hypersensitiv-
    ity to, 330, 335
  C, of poliovirus, 522
  D, of poliovirus, 522
  Forssman, induction by oncogenic viruses,
    578

613